MW00987672

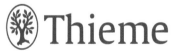

Differential Diagnosis in Neurology and Neurosurgery

A Clinician's Pocket Guide

2nd Edition

Sotirios A. Tsementzis, MD (B'ham), PhD (Edin)
Professor and Chairman Emeritus of Neurosurgery
Founder and Director
Neurosurgical Institute of Ioannina
University of Ioannina, Medical School
Ioannina, Greece;
Attending Neurosurgeon
Metropolitan General Hospital
Athens, Greece

417 illustrations

Thieme
Stuttgart • New York • Delhi • Rio de Janeiro

Library of Congress Cataloging-in-Publication Data

Names: Tsementzis, S. A., author.
Title: Differential diagnosis in neurology and neurosurgery : a clinician's pocket guide / Sotirios A. Tsementzis.
Description: 2nd edition. | Stuttgart ; New York : Thieme, [2019] | Includes bibliographical references and index.
Identifiers: LCCN 2018056410 (print) | LCCN 2018057120 (ebook) | ISBN | ISBN 9783132417182 (paperback) | ISBN 9783132417199 (e-book)
Subjects: | MESH: Nervous System Diseases–diagnosis | Diagnosis, Differential | Neurologic Examination | Signs and Symptoms | Handbook
Classification: LCC RC348 (ebook) | LCC RC348 (print) | NLM WL 39 | DDC 616.8/0475–dc23
LC record available at https://lccn.loc.gov/2018056410

© 2019 Georg Thieme Verlag

Rüdigerstrasse 14, D–70469 Stuttgart, Germany http://www.thieme.de

Thieme New York, 333 Seventh Avenue, New York, NY 10001, USA
http://www.thieme.com

Thieme Publishers Stuttgart
Rüdigerstrasse 14, 70469 Stuttgart, Germany
+49 [0]711 8931 421, customerservice@thieme.de

Thieme Publishers New York
333 Seventh Avenue, New York, NY 10001 USA
+1 800 782 3488, customerservice@thieme.com

Thieme Publishers Delhi
A-12, Second Floor, Sector-2, Noida-201301
Uttar Pradesh, India
+91 120 45 566 00, customerservice@thieme.in

Thieme Publishers Rio de Janeiro, Thieme Publicações Ltda.
Edifício Rodolpho de Paoli, 25º andar
Av. Nilo Peçanha, 50 - Sala 2508
Rio de Janeiro 20020-906 Brasil
+55 21 3172 2297 / +55 21 3172 1896

Cover design: Thieme Publishing Group
Typesetting by DiTech Process Solutions Pvt. Ltd., India

Printed in Germany by CPI Books   5 4 3 2 1

ISBN 978-3-13-241718-2

Also available as an e-book:
eISBN 978-3-13-241719-9

Important Note: Medicine is an ever-changing science undergoing continual development. Research and clinical experience are continually expanding our knowledge, in particular our knowledge of proper treatment and drug therapy. Insofar as this book mentions any dosage or application, readers may rest assured that the authors, editors, and publishers have made every effort to ensure that such references are in accordance with **the state of knowledge at the time of production of the book.**

Nevertheless, this does not involve, imply, or express any guarantee or responsibility on the part of the publishers with respect of any dosage instructions and forms of application stated in the book. **Every user is requested to examine carefully** the manufacturer's leaflets accompanying each drug and to check, if necessary in consultation with a physician or specialist, whether the dosage schedules mentioned therein or the contraindications stated by the manufacturer differ from the statements made in the present book. Such examination is particularly important with drugs that are either rarely used or have been newly released on the market. Every dosage schedule or every form of application used is entirely at the user's risk and responsibility. The authors and publishers request every user to report to the publishers any discrepancies or inaccuracies noticed.

Some of the product names, patents, and registered designs referred to in this book are in fact registered trademarks or proprietary names, even though specific reference to this fact is not always made in the text. Therefore, the appearance of a name without a designation as proprietary is not to be construed as a representation by the publisher that it is in the public domain.

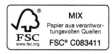

To Theoula Karouta in appreciation of her continuous support and the true love she has endlessly shown to me for more than 23 years of common life and companionship.

Contents

Contents

3 Developmental—Acquired Anomalies and Paediatric Disorders

Contents

Contents

Preface to the First Edition

A wealth of neurological textbooks, journals, and papers are available today. The student of clinical neuroscience is therefore faced with a large number of unrelated facts that can be very difficult to remember and apply. In neurology, one of the most difficult tasks is knowing how to reach the correct diagnosis by differentiating it from the other possibilities, so that the patient can receive the appropriate treatment for the disease concerned.

Physicians frequently encounter clinical symptoms and signs, as well as other data, that require interpretation. Establishing a differential diagnosis list is essential to allow correct interpretation of clinical and laboratory data, and it provides the basis for appropriate therapy. But it is difficult for physician, who is unable to remember everything on the spot, to compile a complete differential diagnosis list. Despite a firm intention to "check it," the physician does not always do so, because the information is located in multiple reference sources at the library or at home, but not at the bedside or prior to taking final examinations. Lists of differential diagnoses of neurological signs provide information that can be used logically when analyzing a neurological problem. But time-consuming searches in massive textbooks, trying to memorize lists, or—even worse—trying to construct them oneself, all involve time and effort that could be put to better use elsewhere. I felt that if this information could be brought together in a single source and made available in a paperback format, it would be a valuable aid to medical students, house staff, emergency room physicians, and specialist clinicians.

This book of differential diagnosis provides a guide to the differentiation of over 230 symptoms, physical and radiological signs, and other abnormal findings. The lists of differential diagnoses for the major disease categories are organized into a familiar pattern, so that completely different clinical problems can be approached using a common algorithm. The template is arranged under 15 major headings in neurology and neurosurgery, typically beginning with the most general and prevalent, to allow the physician to proceed in as much details as may be required, to the most rarely encountered disorders.

The aim of this book is to provide assistance with differential diagnosis in neurological and neurosurgical disease. It is not intended for use on its own, as it is not a complete textbook of neurology and neurosurgery.

I would like to express my thanks to the colleagues, trainees, and students who encouraged me to write this book. In particular, I am grateful to my patients who taught me how to look and how to differentiate. I am indebted to Dr. P. Toulas for providing several personal X-ray cases for the book. I am also grateful to Dr. Clifford Bergman, medical editor at Thieme, for excellent advice and collaboration in preparing this book.

Sotirios A. Tsementzis, MD (B'ham),
PhD (Edin)

Preface to the Second Edition

The past 15 years, since the first edition of this book was published, have witnessed tremendous progress in the fields of neurology and neurosurgery and a lot of new information has been acquired. In this new edition, I have maintained the general organization of the first edition but have expanded the information on several existing subjects and added new titles, especially those presenting problems of children with disorders of the nervous system. This edition also includes elaborate information on cerebrovascular diseases, cranial nerves pathology, intracranial tumors, infectious diseases as they are related to abnormalities of neuroimmunology, and peripheral nerve disorders. New diagrams and illustrations have also been added for a better understanding of clinical diagnosis of some of the complex problems that are difficult to describe in words.

Sotirios A. Tsementzis, MD (B'ham),
PhD (Edin)

1 Epidemiological Characteristics of Neurological Diseases

1.1 Prevalence of Neurological Diseases

Prevalence (per 1,000) of neurological disorders, by cause, WHO region and mortality stratum, projections for 2005, 2015, and 2030

	2005		2015		2030	
Population	6,441,919,466	Number per 1,000	7,105,297,899	Number per 1,000	7,917,115,397	Number per 1,000
Epilepsy	39,891,898	6.19	44,568,780	6.27	50,503,933	6.38
Alzheimer's disease	24,446,651	3.79	31,318,923	4.41	44,016,718	5.56
Parkinson's disease	5,223,897	0.81	5,967,673	0.84	7,236,712	0.91
Multiple sclerosis	2,492,385	0.39	2,823,092	0.40	3,279,190	0.41
Migraine	326,196,121	50.64	364,432,879	51.30	412,894,420	52.15
Cerebrovascular disease	61,537,499	9.55	67,212,050	0.46	76,826,240	9.70
Neuroinfection	18,169,479	2.82	15,714,399	2.21	13,290,180	1.68
Nutritional/ neuropathies	352,494,535	54.72	321,738,424	45.29	285,369,403	36.04
Neurological injuries	170,382,211	26.45	197,627,526	27.82	242,728,912	30.60

Source: Neurological disorders: public health challenges, WHO 2006.

1.2 Epidemiology of Worldwide Neurological Disorders

In order to improve the understanding of the global burden of neurologic conditions, the Public Health Agency of Canada launched the National Population Health Study of Neurological Conditions in 2009. One of its many aims was to examine the epidemiology, including the incidence and prevalence, of 15 common neurologic conditions. This effort involved the review of 65,529 abstracts and 4,650 full-text articles, with 1,242 research studies. In the following tables, the overall worldwide pooled prevalence or incidence data from the systemic reviews of neurologic conditions are presented. The table shows differences that exist. For example, in the Canadian systematic review of the epidemiology of epilepsy, the incidence was highest in Africa at 215.00 per 100,000 person-years, followed by South America at 162.45 per 100,000 person-years. The incidence of epilepsy in North America was 23.29 per 100,000 person-years and it was 42.63 per 100,000 person-years in Europe. These differences in incidence between continents are most likely attributable to the geographic differences in risk factors for epilepsy such as the high prevalence of central nervous system (CNS) infections (i.e., neurocysticercosis) in many developing countries compared to the developed countries. For many conditions, data on the prevalence or incidence of neurologic conditions in Africa and South America were scarce or unavailable, limiting the possibility of drawing firm conclusions in these areas.

Neurological condition	Overall pooled worldwide prevalence or incidence	Region-specific prevalence or incidence
Dementia	Prevalence (community-based, age 65+)	Prevalence (community-based, age 65+)
	4,628 per 100,000 persons	Asia 4,038 per 100,000 persons
	Incidence (community-based, 65+)	Europe 6,758 per 100,000 persons
	4,169 per 100,000 persons	North America 5,097 per 100,000 persons
		South America 3,668 per 100,000 persons
		Incidence (community-based, age 65+)
		Africa 1,350 per 100,000 persons
		Asia 870 per 100,000 persons
		Australia 1,289 per 100,000 persons
		Europe 2,317 per 100,000 persons
		North America 5,830 per 100,000 persons
Tourette syndrome	Prevalence (in children)	Region specific analysis not performed
	770 per 100,000 persons	
Epilepsy	Prevalence (active epilepsy)	Prevalence (community-based, age 65+)
	596 per 100,000 persons	Africa 863 per 100,000 persons
	Incidence (active epilepsy)	Asia 495 per 100,000 persons
	51.32 per 100,000 persons	Europe 457 per 100,000 persons
	Incidence	North America 5,097 per 100,000 persons
	49.06 per 100,000 persons	South America 934 per 100,000 persons
		Incidence (active epilepsy)
		Africa 78.39 per 100,000 person-years
		Asia 37.56 per 100,000 person-years

▲ *(Continued)*

Neurological condition	Overall pooled worldwide prevalence or incidence	Region-specific prevalence or incidence
		Europe 43.87 per 100,000 person-years
		North America 42.48 per 100,000 person-years
		South America 119.78 per 100,000 person-years
Parkinson disease	Prevalence	Prevalence
	315 per 100,000 persons	Asia 337 per 100,000 persons
	Incidence	Africa 77 per 100,000 persons
	Females 36.5 per 100,000 person-years	North America/Europe/Australia 1,398 per 100,000 persons
	Males 65.5 per 100,000 person-years	South America 1,046 per 100,000 persons
Cerebral palsy	Prevalence	Region specific analysis not performed
	221 per 100,000 live births	
Traumatic brain injury	Incidence (all age groups)	Incidence (all age groups)
	211.35 per 100,000 persons	Asia 380.35 per 100,000 persons
		Australia 414.56 per 100,000 persons
		Europe 227.74 per 100,000 persons
		North America 167.87 per 100,000 persons
Hydrocephalus	Prevalence (infants)	Region specific analysis not performed
	135 per 100,000 persons	
Spina bifida	Prevalence	Prevalence
	46.20 per 100,000 persons	Africa 78.81 per 100,000 persons
		Asia 66.36 per 100,000 persons
		Australia 48.11 per 100,000 persons
		Europe 66.23 per 100,000 persons

▲ (Continued)

Neurological condition	Overall pooled worldwide prevalence or incidence	Region-specific prevalence or incidence
		North America 35.72 per 100,000 persons
		South America 30.37 per 100,000 persons
Brain tumors	Incidence	Region-specific analysis not performed
	10.82 per 100,000 person-years	
Cervical dystonia	Prevalence	Prevalence
	4.98 per 100,000 persons	Japan 2.52 per 100,000 persons
		Europe 6.71 per 100,000 persons
Duchene muscular dystrophy	Prevalence (males)	Region specific analysis not performed
	4.78 per 100,000 persons	
Spinal cord injury	Incidence (excluding prehospital mortality)	Incidence (excluding prehospital mortality)
	2.88 per 100,000 persons	Europe/Asia/Australia 2.24 per 100,000 persons
	Incidence (including prehospital mortality)	North America 4.23 per 100,000 persons
	5.13 per 100,000 persons	
Huntington disease	Prevalence	Prevalence
	2.71 per 100,000 persons	Asia 0.40 per 100,000 persons
	Incidence	North America/Europe/Australia 5.7 per 100,000 persons
	0.38 per 100,000 persons	
Multiple sclerosis	Meta-analysis not performed	Meta-analysis not performed

Source: Jette N, Pringsheim T. Technical report for the Public Health Agency of Canada and the Neurological Health Charities of Canada: systemic reviews of the incidence and prevalence of neurological conditions. Ottawa, Canada: Public Health Agency of Canada; 2013 Neurology 2014;83(18):1661–1664.

Primary brain and other central nervous system tumors of children and adolescents diagnosed in the United States in 2009–2013

| | Age at diagnosis (Years) | | | | | | | | |
| | 0–14 Y | | | 0–19 Y | | | 0–4 Y | | |
	5-year total	Annual average	Rate	5-year total	Annual average	Rate	5-year total	Annual average	Rate
Neuroepithelial tumors	12,303	2,461	4.04	15,363	3,073	3.74	4,880	976	4.88
Astrocytoma									
Pilocytic	2,999	600	0.98	3,645	729	0.89	1,065	213	1.06
Diffuse	792	158	0.26	1,083	217	0.26	308	62	0.31
Anaplastic	275	55	0.09	375	75	0.09	69	14	0.07
Unique variant	343	69	0.11	461	92	0.11	89	18	0.09
Glioblastoma	467	93	0.15	692	138	0.17	113	23	0.11
Oligodendroglioma	110	22	0.04	203	41	0.05	19	4	0.02
Anaplastic	–	–	–	28	6	0.01	–	–	–
Astrocytic	70	14	0.02	127	25	0.03	19	4	0.02
Ependymal tumors	961	192	0.31	1,230	246	0.30	496	99	0.50
Malignant glioma, NOS	2,385	477	0.78	2,737	547	0.67	931	186	0.93
Choroid plexus	336	67	0.11	390	78	0.09	239	48	0.24
Other neuroepithelial tumor	30	6	0.01	34	7	0.01	–	–	–
Neuronal/mixed neuronal-glial tumors	1,091	218	0.36	1,631	326	0.40	276	55	0.28
Pineal tumors	139	28	0.05	183	37	0.04	57	11	0.06

▲ (Continued)

| | Age at diagnosis (Years) | | | | | | | | |
| | 0–14 Y | | | 0–19 Y | | | 0–4 Y | | |
	5-year total	Annual average	Rate	5-year total	Annual average	Rate	5-year total	Annual average	Rate
Embryonal tumors	2,295	459	0.75	2,544	509	0.62	1,188	238	1.19
Medulloblastoma	1,466	293	0.48	1,642	328	0.40	554	111	0.55
PNET	287	57	0.09	334	67	0.08	176	35	0.18
Atypical teratoid/rhabdoid tumor	353	71	0.11	359	72	0.09	316	36	0.32
Other embryonal histologies	189	38	0.06	209	42	0.05	142	28	0.14
Tumors of cranial and spinal nerves	809	162	0.27	1,218	244	0.29	277	55	0.28
Nerve sheath tumors	809	162	0.27	1,216	243	0.29	277	55	0.28
Tumors of meninges	500	100	0.16	1,012	202	0.24	151	30	0.15
Meningioma	273	55	0.09	615	123	0.15	59	12	0.06
Mesenchymal tumors	162	32	0.05	210	42	0.05	80	16	0.08
Primary melanocytic lesions	–	–	–	–	–	–	–	–	–
Other neoplasms related to the meninges	58	12	0.02	177	35	0.04	–	–	–
Lymphomas and hematopoietic neoplasms	79	16	0.03	120	24	0.03	17	3	0.02
Lymphoma	29	6	0.01	58	12	0.01	–	–	–

▲ (Continued)

	Age at diagnosis (Years)								
	0–14 Y			0–19 Y			0–4 Y		
	5-year total	Annual average	Rate	5-year total	Annual average	Rate	5-year total	Annual average	Rate
Other hematopoietic neoplasms	50	10	0.02	62	12	0.02	–	–	–
Germ cell tumors and cysts	635	127	0.21	918	184	0.22	156	31	0.16
Germ cell tumors, cysts, and heterotopias	635	127	0.21	918	184	0.22	156	31	0.16
Tumors of sellar region	1,415	283	0.47	3,472	694	0.83	169	34	0.17
Tumors of the pituitary	743	149	0.24	2,655	531	0.63	30	6	0.03
Craniopharyngioma	672	134	0.22	817	163	0.20	139	28	0.14
Unclassified tumors	912	182	0.30	1,419	284	0.34	318	64	0.32
Hemangioma	308	62	0.10	534	107	0.13	115	23	0.12
Neoplasm unspecified	585	117	0.17	862	172	0.21	194	39	0.19
All other	19	4	0.01	23	5	0.01	–	–	–
Total	16,653	3,331	5.47	23,522	4,704	5.70	5,968	1,194	5.98

Abbreviations: NOS, not otherwise specified.

Source: CBTRUS (Central Brain Tumor Registry of the United States); NPCR (National Programs of Cancers). 2016 Society for Neuro-Oncology Epidemiology and End Results program. Oxford Journals NEURO ONCOL, October 1, 2016;18(suppl 5).

Note: Annual average cases are calculated by dividing the five-year total by five.

Rates are per 100,000 and are age-adjusted to the 2000 US standard population.

Primary brain and other central nervous system tumors of children and adolescents diagnosed in the United States in 2009–2013

	5–9 Y			10–14 Y			15–19 Y		
	5-yr total	Annual average	Rate	5-yr total	Annual average	Rate	5-yr total	Annual average	Rate
Neuroepithelial tumors	**3,914**	**783**	**3.85**	**3,509**	**702**	**3.41**	**3,060**	**612**	**2.85**
Astrocytoma									
Pilocytic	1,017	203	1.00	917	183	0.89	646	129	0.60
Diffuse	227	45	0.22	257	51	0.25	291	58	0.27
Anaplastic	97	19	0.10	109	22	0.11	100	20	0.09
Unique variant	118	24	0.12	136	27	0.13	118	24	0.11
Glioblastoma	163	33	0.16	191	38	0.19	225	45	0.21
Oligodendroglioma	41	8	0.04	50	10	0.05	93	19	0.09
Anaplastic	–	–	–	–	–	–	18	4	0.02
Astrocytic	22	4	0.02	29	6	0.03	57	11	0.05
Ependymal tumors	229	46	0.23	236	47	0.23	264	54	0.25
Malignant glioma, NOS	893	179	0.88	561	112	0.55	352	70	0.33
Choroid plexus	48	10	0.05	49	10	0.05	54	11	0.05
Other neuroepithelial tumor	–	–	–	–	–	–	–	–	–
Neuronal/mixed neuronal-glial tumors	313	63	0.31	502	100	0.49	540	108	0.50
Pineal tumors	37	7	0.04	45	9	0.04	44	9	0.04
Embryonal tumors	699	140	0.69	408	82	0.40	249	50	0.23

▲ (Continued)

| | Age at diagnosis (Years) | | | | | | | | |
| | 5–9 Y | | | 10–14 Y | | | 15–19 Y | | |
	5-yr total	Annual average	Rate	5-yr total	Annual average	Rate	5-yr total	Annual average	Rate
Medulloblastoma	684	117	0.57	328	66	0.32	176	35	0.10
PNET	54	13	0.06	47	9	0.05	47	9	0.04
Atypical teratoid/rhabdoid tumor	25	5	0.02	–	–	–	–	–	–
Other embryonal histologies	25	5	0.03	21	4	0.02	20	4	0.02
Tumors of cranial and spinal nerves	259	52	0.26	273	55	0.27	409	82	0.38
Nerve sheath tumors	259	52	0.26	273	55	0.27	407	81	0.38
Tumors of meninges	112	22	0.11	237	47	0.23	512	102	0.47
Meningioma	61	12	0.06	153	31	0.15	342	68	0.32
Mesenchymal tumors	43	9	0.04	39	8	0.04	48	10	0.04
Primary melanocytic lesions	–	–	–	–	–	–	–	–	–
Other neoplasms related to the meninges	58	12	0.02	44	9	0.04	119	24	0.11
Lymphomas and hematopoietic neoplasms	34	7	0.03	28	6	0.03	41	8	0.04
Lymphoma	–	–	–	–	–	–	29	6	0.03
Other hematopoietic neoplasms	23	5	0.02	–	–	–	–	–	–

▲ *(Continued)*

	5–9 Y			10–14 Y			15–19 Y	
	5-yr total	Annual average	Rate	5-yr total	Annual average	Rate	5-yr total	Annual average	Rate
				Age at diagnosis (Years)					
Germ cell tumors and cysts	168	34	0.17	311	62	0.30	283	57	0.26
Germ cell tumors, cysts, and heterotopias	168	34	0.17	311	62	0.30	283	57	0.26
Tumors of sellar region	483	97	0.48	763	153	0.74	2,057	411	1.91
Tumors of the pituitary	175	35	0.17	538	108	0.52	1,912	382	1.77
Craniopharyngioma	308	62	0.30	225	45	0.22	145	29	0.13
Unclassified tumors	219	44	0.22	375	75	0.36	507	101	0.47
Hemangioma	66	13	0.07	127	25	0.12	226	45	0.21
Neoplasm unspecified	150	30	0.15	241	48	0.23	277	55	0.26
All other	–	–	–	–	–	–	–	–	–
Total	5,189	1,038	5.12	5,496	1,099	5.34	6,869	1,374	6.38

Abbreviations: NOS, not otherwise specified.

Source: CBTRUS (Central Brain Tumor Registry of the United States); NPCR (National Programs of Cancers). 2016 Society for Neuro-Oncology Epidemiology and End Results program. Oxford Journals NEURO ONCOL, October 1, 2016;18(suppl 5).

Note: Annual average cases are calculated by dividing the five-year total by five.

Rates are per 100,000 and are age-adjusted to the 2000 US standard population.

1.3 The Incidence and Lifetime Prevalence of Neurological Disorders in a Prospective Community-Based Study in the United Kingdom

A population of 100,230 patients registered with participating general practices was followed prospectively for the onset of neurological disorders. The lifetime prevalence of neurological disorders was surveyed in the 27,658 patients. The age- and sex-adjusted incidence rates per 100,000 persons per annum are presented in the following table with 95% confidence intervals (CI) in parentheses. Lifetime prevalence rates are expressed as rate per 1000 persons with 95% CI. Overall the onset of 625 neurological disorders was observed per 100,000 populations annually. Six percent (6%) of the population had at some time had a neurological disorder.

Neurological disorders		
Incidence	**Number**	**(CI)**
Cerebrovascular events	205	(183–230)
Shingles	140	(104–184)
Diabetic polyneuropathy	54	(33–83)
Compressive neuropathies	49	(39–61)
Epilepsy	46	(36–60)
Parkinson's disease	19	(12–27)
Peripheral neuropathies	15	(9–23)
CNS infections	12	(5–13)
Postherpetic neuralgia	11	(6–17)
Major neurological injuries	10	(4–11)
Prevalence		
Completed stroke	9	(8–11)
Transient ischemic attacks	5	(4–6)
Active epilepsy	4	(4–5)
Congenital neurological deficit	3	(3–4)
Parkinson's disease	2	(1–3)
Multiple sclerosis	2	(2–3)
Diabetic polyneuropathy	2	(1–3)
Compressive mononeuropathies	2	(2–3)
Subarachnoid hemorrhage	1	(0.8–2)

Source: MacDonald BK, Cockerell OC, Sander AS, and Sorinsen SD. The incidence and lifetime prevalence of neurological disorders in a prospective community-based study in the UK. Brain 2000;123(4):665–676.

1.4 Prevalence and Incidence of Neurological Disorders in the United States: A Meta-Analysis

Epidemiological figures were collected from the most recent, reliable data available in the research literature and population statistics were based on the most recent census from the US Census Bureau. The data of the leading studies for several neurological studies was compiled in order to obtain the most accurate extrapolations.

The **incidence** of the most common adult-onset brain disorders in the United States were obtained from sources that have been published during the past decade with the exception of amyotrophic lateral sclerosis (ALS), Huntington's disease, and traumatic brain injury. All efforts were made to locate the most accurate and recent data.

The **prevalence** figures were obtained from studies conducted within the past 10 years with the exception of Huntington's disease, the prevalence of which was obtained from sources published between 1955 and 1994.

Incidence[a] of the major causes of adult-onset brain disorders in the United States

Diagnosis/cause	People diagnosed annually
Alzheimer's disease	468,000
Amyotrophic lateral sclerosis	10,131
Brain tumor	50,656
Epilepsy	142,000
HIV dementia	20,789
Huntington's disease	1,053
Multiple sclerosis	12,000
Parkinson's disease	59,000
Stroke	825,848
Traumatic brain injury	1,500,000
Total estimated incidence	**3,089,477**

[a](Incidence rate/100,000 individuals) *Population estimates = Incidence

Prevalence[a] of the major causes of adult-onset brain disorders in the United States

Diagnosis/Cause	People currently living with disorder
Alzheimer's disease	2,459,000
Amyotrophic lateral sclerosis	36,480
Brain tumor	401,565
Epilepsy	2,008,000
HIV dementia	328,600
Huntington's disease	15,611
Multiple sclerosis	268,000
Parkinson's disease	921,020
Stroke	5,839,000
Traumatic brain injury	3,170,000
Total estimated prevalence	**15,535,276**

Source: Bortongan CV, Bums J, Naoki Tajirt, Stahl CE et al. htt://dx.dol.org/10.1371/journal.pone.0078490, Oct 24, 2013.
[a](Prevalence rate/100,000 individuals) *Population estimates = Prevalence

1.5 Primary Malignant Brain Tumors in Adults

1.5.1 Incidence

Brain, and other CNS and intracranial tumors are the ninth most common cancers in the United Kingdom, accounting for 3% of all new cancer cases (2015). There are around 11,500 new brain, and other CNS and intracranial tumor cases in the United Kingdom every year, i.e., 31 cases every day (2013–2015).

In UK males, brain and other CNS tumors are the 11th whereas in the females these are the 8th most common cancers. Incidence rates are highest in people aged 85–89 years. Over the past decade, incidence rates of brain and other CNS intracranial tumors have increased by 15% in the United Kingdom. The overall annual incidence rate of all brain tumors is 7 per 100,000 population.

Incidence rates for brain tumors are projected to rise by 6% in the UK between 2014 and 2035, i.e., 22 cases per 100,000 people by 2035. In Europe, around 57,100 new cases of brain and CNS cancer were estimated to have been diagnosed in 2012. The UK incidence rate is 20th lowest in Europe for males and 11th lowest for females. In 2012, more than 256,000 brain and other CNS tumors were estimated to have been diagnosed worldwide, with incidence rates varying across the world.

Brain and central nervous system tumors: The United Kingdom incidence

		England	Wales	Scotland	Northern Ireland	UK
Numbers	Males	2,092	159	196	81	2,528
	Females	1,529	136	165	37	1,867
	Persons	3,621	295	361	118	4,395
Age standardized rates[a]	Males	8.3	10.1	7.6	10.4	8.4
	Females	5.3	7.6	5.2	4.4	5.4
	Persons	6.8	8.8	6.3	7.2	6.8
95% confidence intervals	Males	(8.0–8.7)	(8.5–11.7)	(6.5–8.6)	(8.1–12.7)	(8.1–8.7)
	Females	(5.1–5.6)	(6.4–8.9)	(4.4–6.0)	(3.0–5.8)	(5.2–5.7)
	Persons	(6.5–7.0)	(7.8–9.8)	(5.6–6.9)	(5.9–8.5)	(6.6–7.0)

Source: www.concerresearchUK.org
[a]Directly age standardized (European) rate per 100,000 population at risk.

The largest proportion of adult tumors are supratentorial and the majority (86%) are gliomas which include astrocytomas, glioblastomas, oligodendrogliomas, and unspecific gliomas. Threefold differences in the incidence of brain tumors have been reported between countries worldwide and differences are also seen between ethnic groups within the same country. Brain cancer is more common in white people than in Asian or black.

1.5.2 Risk factors

Current thinking suggests that brain tumors develop as a consequence of accumulated genetic alterations that permit cells to evade normal regulatory mechanisms and destruction by the immune system. These alterations may be in part or wholly inherited but any agents (chemical, physical, or biological) that damage DNA are also possible neurocarcinogens. The following table lists the environmental factors which have received attention as possible causes of brain tumors.

Summary of environmental risk factors for brain tumors (epidemiological studies)

Factor	Specific aspects	Evaluation of risk
Ionizing radiation	Therapeutic, diagnostic	Therapeutic doses increase risk but diagnostic x-rays do not appear to be associated
Mobile phones	Radiofrequency exposure	Current epidemiological and biological evidence do not support any link between mobile use and the risk of brain tumors
Extremely low frequency electromagnetic fields	Residential and occupations exposure	Little consistent evidence but research is ongoing
Specific infections	Viruses, *Toxoplasma gondii*, in utero influenza and varicella	No candidate viruses consistently associated or found in tumor tissue. Few links to in utero exposure
Allergies	Atopy	The presence of atopy appears to be protective but further work needed to identify mechanisms
Diet	Nitrosamine/nitrosamide/nitrite/nitrite/aspartame consumption	No consistent evidence
Tobacco	Cigarettes, cigars, pipes	No associations
Alcohol		No associations
Chemical agents	Hair dyes, solvents, pesticides, traffic related air pollutants	No consistent evidence
Occupations	Rubber manufacture, vinyl chloride, petroleum refining	Small risks associated with working in the petroleum/oil industry but no mechanism or specific chemical known
Head trauma/injury		No consistent evidence

Source: McKinney PA. Brain tumors: incidence, survival, and etiology. J Neurol Neurosurg Psychiatry 2004;75(suppl II):ii12–ii17.

1.5.3 WHO's estimates for stroke incidence and prevalence

Reliable data on stroke incidence and prevalence are essential for calculating the burden of stroke and the planning of prevention and treatment of stroke patients. In the current study, we have reviewed the published data from EU countries,

Iceland, Norway, and Switzerland, and provide WHO estimates for stroke incidence and prevalence in these countries. Studies on stroke epidemiology published in peer reviewed journals during the past 10 years were identified using Medline/PubMed searches, and reviewed using the structure of WHO's stroke component of the WHO InfoBase. Forty-four incidence studies and 12 prevalence studies were identified. There were several methodological differences that hampered comparisons of data. WHO stroke estimates were in good agreement with results from ideal stroke population studies. According to the WHO estimates, the number of stroke events in these selected countries is likely to increase from 1.1 million per year in 2000 to more than 1.5 million per year in 2025 solely because of the demographic changes. Until better and more stroke studies are available, the WHO stroke estimates may provide the best data for understanding the stroke burden in countries where no stroke data currently exists.

1.5.4 WHO stroke incidence estimates, men and women per 100,000

The WHO's estimates for stroke incidence in men and women aged from 25 to 85+ years are presented in the following tables. In both men and women stroke rates increase exponentially with age, and in most countries, rates are higher for men than for women. In men, the lowest stroke incidence rates are estimated for France and Switzerland. Highest rates are estimated for Latvia where age-specific stroke incidence rates are more than twice that for France and Switzerland. In women, low incidence rates are estimated for France, Switzerland, and Slovakia, whereas high incidence rates are estimated for Greece and Latvia. Rates in the latter two are up to three times higher than in countries with the lowest estimated stroke incidence rates.

Age	Austria		Belgium		Cyprus		Czech Rep		Denmark		Finland	
	M	W	M	W	M	W	M	W	M	W	M	W
25–34	13	10	19	12	12	10	17	7	30	13	23	12
35–44	26	20	37	23	20	11	33	14	60	30	46	24
45–54	153	69	139	84	83	40	271	119	194	80	201	74
55–64	324	172	312	186	229	134	678	347	351	184	384	191
65–74	877	613	812	550	672	463	1,989	1,449	882	580	987	653
75–84	1,631	1,376	1,237	1,752	1,726	3,474	2,918	1,514	1,250	1,708	1,391	1,105
85+	2005	1,801	1,754	1,661	2,535	2,753	4,056	3,513	1,771	1,628	2,009	1,764

Epidemiological Characteristics of Neurological Diseases

Age	France M	France W	Germany M	Germany W	Greece M	Greece W	Iceland M	Iceland W	Ireland M	Ireland W	Italy M	Italy W
25–34	19	9	14	9	21	11	11	9	14	21	14	8
35–44	37	18	28	17	42	21	23	19	28	42	27	16
45–54	131	49	131	60	215	98	107	74	126	99	124	63
55–64	253	109	316	152	535	288	212	187	315	192	295	154
65–74	630	364	899	588	1,541	1,216	690	647	877	672	918	585
75–84	1,105	837	1,696	1,395	3,131	3,312	1,381	1,493	1,621	1,396	1,946	1,569
85+	1,325	1,113	2,096	1,857	4,032	4,671	1,697	1,990	1,992	1,732	2,521	2,214

Age	Luxembourg M	Luxembourg W	Malta M	Malta W	Netherlands M	Netherlands W	Norway M	Norway W	Portugal M	Portugal W	Spain M	Spain W
25–34	15	18	16	10	11	12	13	8	47	20	12	8
35–44	31	36	32	20	21	25	26	17	93	39	24	15
45–54	146	103	153	81	119	93	123	69	362	149	132	57
55–64	366	231	381	203	284	175	287	148	842	390	298	143
65–74	988	721	1,126	789	847	565	905	530	2,299	1,431	804	498
75–84	1,852	1,584	1,870	1,637	1,567	1,265	1,796	1,359	3,769	3,193	1,413	1,207
85+	2,314	2,087	2,098	2,021	1,889	1,657	2,234	1,887	4,262	4,153	1,682	1,647

Age	Sweden M	Sweden W	Switzerland M	Switzerland W	U.K. M	U.K. W	Estonia M	Estonia W	Latvia M	Latvia W	Hungary M	Hungary W
25–34	8	6	8	6	16	9	27	12	18	14	27	14
35–44	16	13	17	12	32	18	54	25	37	27	54	29
45–54	122	65	58	49	129	94	367	133	455	205	367	141
55–64	294	164	171	110	301	209	877	407	1,155	587	877	332
65–74	841	535	515	329	845	652	1,858	1,171	2,563	1,645	1,824	907
75–84	579	1,287	1,074	822	1,512	1,453	2,641	2,473	3,963	3,539	2,607	1,680
85+	943	1,767	1,401	1,158	1,809	1,925	2,953	3,284	4,656	4,757	2,953	2,070

Age	Lithuania M	Lithuania W	Poland M	Poland W	Slovakia M	Slovakia W	Slovenia M	Slovenia W
25–34	17	9	17	12	7	4	21	11
35–44	35	17	34	25	14	9	41	22
45–54	268	138	250	103	156	58	194	139
55–64	670	332	613	289	469	183	612	296
65–74	1,404	882	1,255	800	1,132	631	1,467	858
75–84	2,029	1,659	1,619	1,459	1,568	1,102	2,344	1,754
85+	2,320	2,081	1,706	1,792	1,654	1,251	1,784	2,344

Source: Truelsen T, Piechowski-Jozwiak B, Bonita R, et al. Stroke incidence and prevalence in Europe: a review of available data. Eur J Neurol 2006;13:581–598.

1.5.5 WHO stroke prevalence rate, estimates, men and women per 100,000

WHO estimates of stroke prevalence rates are presented in following table. Stroke prevalence rates increase exponentially with age and in most countries these are higher for men than for women. In men, the lowest stroke prevalence rates are estimated for Cyprus, Lithuania, Poland, and Slovakia, whilst the highest rates are estimated for Czech Republic, Greece, Portugal, and Slovenia. In women, low prevalence rates are estimated for Cyprus, France, Lithuania, Poland, and Slovakia, whilst high prevalence rates are estimated for Czech Republic, Greece, Hungary, and Portugal.

Age	Austria M	Austria W	Belgium M	Belgium W	Cyprus M	Cyprus W	Czech Rep M	Czech Rep W	Denmark M	Denmark W	Finland M	Finland W
25–34	77	56	114	65	59	25	99	39	196	87	150	67
35–44	147	106	218	124	113	48	189	74	374	165	285	127
45–54	1,163	634	1,072	804	380	171	2,037	1,103	1,607	775	1,652	695
55–64	2,246	1,304	2,185	1,476	929	553	4,604	2,637	2,658	1,484	2,887	1,490
65–74	5,359	3,791	5,052	3,568	2,354	1,507	11,959	8,965	5,869	3,820	6,529	4,168
75–84	8,656	6,807	7,830	6,260	4,215	3,112	18,711	15,171	8,974	6,554	10,032	7,148
85+	10,619	8,733	9,403	8,362	5,998	4,881	21,192	17,156	10,198	8,342	11,497	8,890

Epidemiological Characteristics of Neurological Diseases

Age	France M	France W	Germany M	Germany W	Greece M	Greece W	Iceland M	Iceland W	Ireland M	Ireland W	Italy M	Italy W
25–34	118	50	83	46	114	55	66	52	85	132	79	42
35–44	225	95	158	87	217	104	126	99	161	252	150	80
45–54	1048	465	992	535	1,481	838	788	702	950	1,044	868	548
55–64	1849	837	2,172	1,122	3,318	2,037	1,417	1,464	2,148	1,708	1,864	1,114
65–74	4064	2,324	5,472	3,524	8,497	6,996	3,998	4,140	5,318	4,777	5,095	3,416
75–84	6242	4,218	8,947	6,646	14,616	14,686	7,066	7,537	8,522	8,178	9,172	7,038
85+	7371	5,553	11,072	8,759	19,308	21,217	8,668	9,954	10,454	9,681	12,237	10,178

Age	Luxembourg M	Luxembourg W	Malta M	Malta W	Netherlands M	Netherlands W	Norway M	Norway W	Portugal M	Portugal W	Spain M	Spain W
25–34	95	107	99	58	62	73	72	42	282	109	68	40
35–44	180	203	188	111	119	139	138	80	538	208	130	76
45–54	1,129	1,022	1,180	787	893	919	851	589	2,770	1,400	965	509
55–64	2,552	1,914	2,666	1,639	1,924	1,464	1,798	1,060	5,841	3,020	1,973	1,061
65–74	6,149	4,854	6,968	5,167	5,059	3,780	4,962	3,049	14,151	9,038	4,714	3,017
75–84	9,872	8,441	10,582	8,878	8,260	6,752	8,583	6,060	21,026	16,185	7,306	5,698
85+	2,425	10,944	10,944	10,422	9,824	8,681	10,733	8,534	22,701	20,578	8,527	7,805

Age	Sweden M	Sweden W	Switzerland M	Switzerland W	U.K. M	U.K. W	Estonia M	Estonia W	Latvia M	Latvia W	Hungary M	Hungary W
25–34	47	32	48	33	93	50	106	52	72	57	95	55
35–44	81	63	91	55	177	94	222	108	150	119	198	104
45–54	827	554	415	455	952	857	1,363	647	1661	984	1,283	838
55–64	1,800	1,155	1,094	847	2,021	1,589	3,326	2,108	4,120	2,994	2,862	2,037
65–74	4,550	3,090	2,933	2,062	5,016	4,041	6,153	4,772	8,326	6,638	5,608	6,996
75–84	7,428	5,750	5,132	3,911	7,918	7,101	7,631	6,434	10,893	8,994	6,979	14,686
85+	9,127	7,953	6,926	5,639	9,315	9,288	7,391	6,669	11,456	9,548	5,942	21,217

Age	Lithuania		Poland		Slovakia		Slovenia	
	M	W	M	W	M	W	M	W
25–34	68	38	73	53	28	18	131	68
35–44	142	79	156	114	59	38	250	130
45–54	982	697	1,228	661	710	349	1566	1,418
55–64	2,517	1,769	2,877	1,523	2,032	902	4432	2,524
65–74	4,603	5,569	3,584	3,584	4,583	2,617	9714	5,966
75–84	5,710	4,741	6,492	4,920	5,816	3,726	13,444	9,760
85+	5,742	4,402	5,296	4,627	4,757	3,035	15,631	12,098

Source: Truelsen T, Piechowski-Jozwiak B, Bonita R, et al. Stroke incidence and prevalence in Europe: a review of available data. Eur J Neurol 2006;13:581–598.

1.6 Epidemiology of Epilepsy

1.6.1 Prevalence (per 1,000) of active epilepsy in Europe

Population-based European studies are not available from the majority of European countries. Studies including all ages have been reported from Italy, Poland, Denmark, and Iceland. The prevalence of active epilepsy in these countries varies from 3.3 to 7.8 per 1,000 inhabitants.

Studies where only adults with active epilepsy are included have been reported from three countries in northern Europe, Finland, Sweden, and Estonia. Prevalence rates in these countries range from 5.3 to 6.3 per 1,000 inhabitants.

Prevalence rates for children with active epilepsy are available from 8 countries in 11 studies. The ages of children included in these studies vary. Six studies included all or most childhood ages whilst the remaining five studies at preschool/school ages. Prevalence rates in these studies range from 3.2 to 5.1.

Author (year), country	Prevalence	Age	Number of cases
Zielinski (1974), Poland	7.8	All ages	33
Granieri et al (1983), Italy	6.2	All ages	278
Maremmani et al (1991), Italy	5.1	All ages	51
Beghi et al (1991), Italy	3.9	All ages	199
Giuliani et al (1992), Italy	5.2	All ages	235
Rocca et al (2001), Italy	3.3	All ages	81
Joensen (1986), Faeroes, Denmark	7.6	All ages	333
Olafsson and Hauser (1999), Iceland	4.8	All ages	428
Keranen et al (1989), Finland	6.3	Adults	1,233
Forsgren (1992), Sweden	5.5	Adults	713
Qun et al (2003a), Estonia	5.3	Adults	396
de la Court et al (1996), Netherlands	7.7	Adults 55–94 years	43
Luengo et al (2001), Spain	4.1	Children > 10 and adults	405
Brorson (1970), Sweden	3.5	Children 0–19 years	195
Sidenvall et al (1996), Sweden	4.2	Children)–16 years	155
Waaler et al (2000), Norway	5.1	Children 6–12 years	198
Sillanpaa (1973), Finland	3.2	Children 0–15 years	348
Eriksson and Koivikko (1997), Finland	3.9	Children 0–15 years	329
Endziniene et al (1997), Lithuania	4.3	Children 0–19 years	560
Cavazzuti (1980), Italy	4.5	Children 5–14 years	178
Sangrador and Luaces (1991), Spain	3.7	Children 6–14 years	62
Tidman et al (2001), England	4.3	Children 4–10 years	69

Source: Forsgren L, Beghi E, Qun A, Sillanpaa M. The epidemiology of epilepsy in Europe: a systematic review. Eur J Neurol 2005;12:245–253.
Note: Range and median, all ages: 3.3–7.8; 5.2.
　　　Range and median, adults: 5.3–6.3; 5.5.
　　　Range and median, children: 3.5–5.1; 4.1.

1.6.2 Annual incidence of epilepsy in Europe, men and women per 100,000

Incidence population-based studies of epilepsy in Europe and elsewhere are much more uncommon than prevalence studies due to the fact that the prospective incidence studies are often time consuming and costly.

Author (year), country	Incidence	Age	Number of cases
Joensen (1986), Faeroes, Denmark	43	All ages	118
Loiseau et al (1990), France	44	All ages	494[a]
Olafsson et al (1996), Iceland	47	All ages	42
Jallon et al (1997), Switzerland[b]	46	All ages	176[a]
MacDonald et al (2000), UK[c]	46	All ages	31
Keranen et al (1989), Finland	24	Adults > 15 years	230
Forsgren et al (1996), Sweden	56	Adults > 16 years	160[a]
Qun et al (2003b), Estonia	35	Adults > 19 years	81
Sillanpaa (1973), Finland	25	Children 0–15 years	397
Blom et al (1978), Sweden	82	Children 0–15 years	43
Brorson and Wranne (1987), Sweden	50	Children 0–19 years	68
Sidenvall et al (1993), Sweden	73	Children 0–15 years[d]	61[a]

Source: Forsgren L, Beghi E, Qun A, Sillanpaa M. The epidemiology of epilepsy in Europe: a systematic review. Eur J Neurol 2005;12:245–253.
[a]Single seizures.
[b]Rate calculated only on unprovoked seizures.
[c]Incidence 57 with single seizures included.
[d]Neonatal seizures excluded.

Studies including all ages have been identified mostly in northern and western parts of Europe. The annual incidence rates in these studies range from 43 to 47 per 100,000.

Studies in adults are reported from Estonia, Finland, and Sweden. The incidence rates varied from 24, 35–56 per 100,000 respectively.

The only European incidence studies limited to childhood populations are from Finland, Sweden, Faroes-Denmark, and Iceland. Incidence rates in the childhood population in these studies range from 25, 50–82, 71 and 67 respectively per 100,000.

1.6.3 Prospective studies of the incidence of epilepsy in Nordic countries per 100,000

Only five prospective incidence studies of epilepsy have been undertaken in the Nordic countries, in which only two include all age groups. The study with the largest population basis that included single, unprovoked seizures (Adelow 2009) found an annual incidence of 34 per 100,000. A prospective study from Iceland

(Olafsson 2005), in which single, unprovoked seizures had been included, found an incidence of 33 per 100,000.

A smaller prospective study among children (Braathen 1995) found an annual incidence of epilepsy of 53 per 100,000. A prospective study of adult patients (Forsgren 1995), in which single, unprovoked seizures had been included, found an incidence of 56 per 100,000.

First author	Year	Country	Age (years)	Incidence (per 100,000 person-years)
Olafsson et al	2005	Iceland	All	33
Adelow et al	2009	Sweden	All	34
Sidenval et al	1993	Sweden	Children (0–15)	73
Braathen et al	1995	Sweden	Children (0–16)	53
Forsgren et al	1996	Sweden	Children > 17	56

Source: Syvertsen M, Koht Jeanette, Nakken Karl O. Prevalence and incidence of epilepsy in the Nordic countries. Tidsskriften Den Norske Legeforening 2015;135:1641–1645.

1.7 Epidemiology of Spinal Cord Injuries and Risk Factors

Spinal cord injuries (SCIs) are highly disabling and deadly injuries, and etiologically can be divided into two different groups: traumatic spinal cord injuries (TSCIs) and nontraumatic spinal cord injuries (NTSCIs). At present, few studies focus on NTSCIs, and there is little information regarding the risk factors for complete injuries. This study aims to describe the demographics and the injury characteristics for both TSCI and NTSCIs and explore the risk factors for complete SCIs.

The incidence and prevalence of spinal injuries have been increasing with the estimated incidence rate of 15 to 40 cases per million worldwide. With the modernization of society, SCI incidence increases year after year. In addition to the substantial burden for the affected individuals and their families, society must bear the cost of healthcare treatments, rehabilitation, and lost productivity. The epidemiological characteristics of SCIs obviously vary in different countries, in regions with different economic levels, as well as in different economic periods.

The mean age of the SCI patient in developed countries is higher than in developing countries over the same time period; the reason may be related to the aging of the populations in developed countries and/or to the larger male-to-female ratio in developing countries in relation to developed countries. France reported an SCI incidence rate of 19.4 per million or an average of 934 new cases each year. Finland reported an annual SCI incidence of 28 per million in 2005. Canada reported that the incidence of TSCIs in people aged 15–64 years was 42.4 per million, and for people over the age of 65 years, the incidence was 51.4 per million between January 1997 and June 2001. Australia reported that the average estimated incidence rates of TSCI and NTSCIs were 3.8 and 6.5 per million, respectively in children younger than 15 years of age. The United States reported an annual average SCI incidence of 40 per million in 2012. Taiwan reported that the incidence rate of paediatric SCIs is 5.99 per million person-years. Young adults are the highest risk age group for SCIs: the 21–30-year age group has the highest number of patients and the number of SCIs is greater in males than in females. This finding is possibly related to the fact that more young men are engaged in dangerous outdoor activities, while most women work in the household or perform other relatively less dangerous work.

According to the international standards set forth by the American Spinal Injury Association (ASIA), an injury is categorized as either complete or incomplete on the basis of its severity. A complete injury is defined as the absence of sensory and motor function in the lowest sacral segments. In Beijing, complete injuries accounted for 67% of the total SCIS over the past 30 years; this value has decreased to 45% over the past decade. Canada reported that complete injuries accounted for 35% of the SCIs in 2006. The incidence of complete injury was higher in the thoracic segments than in the lumbar and cervical segments. Tianjin reported that 100% of thoracic SCIs resulted in complete injuries, whereas 46.7% of cervical and 60% lumbar SCIs presented as incomplete injuries. SCI is often associated with fractures at other locales and brain injuries.

The complications for SCI patients include fever, pulmonary complications, electrolyte disturbances, spasms, pain, urinary tract infections, autonomic dysreflexia, cardiovascular disease, osteoporosis and fractures, myositis ossificans, deep vein thromboses, bedsores, and pruritus. A group of Italian investigators reported that the most common complication among SCI patients was urinary tract infection, followed by pain and spasms. In addition, an Italian study reported that patients with multiple injuries, such as associated brain injuries, are affected by more severe neurological lesions.

The level of injury at admission for the patients with SCIs (Yang et al) was a cervical injury (1,720 cases), followed by thoracic and lumbar injuries (1,264 and 941 cases, respectively). The sum of the injuries at all three levels was higher than 3,832 cases because an SCI patient might have more than one level of injury. Regarding the severity of the injury, there were more cases of incomplete injuries than complete injuries, and the percentages of complete and incomplete injuries were 17.70 and 82.30%, respectively. This result revealed that the proportion of complete injuries was as follows: 21.8% in the cervical spine, 14.6% in the thoracic spinal region, and 15.0% in the lumbar spine. The distributions of injury severity at the different spinal levels were all statistically significant at $P < 0.05$.

Distribution of spine level injuries for SCI patients by the severity of injury

Level of injury	Severity of injury, n (%)			P-value
	Complete	Incomplete	Total	
Cervical				< 0.001
Yes	375 (21.8)	1345 (78.2)	1720 (44.9)	
No	303 (14.3)	1809 (85.7)	2112 (55.1)	
Thoracic				< 0.001
Yes	185 (14.6)	1079 (85.4)	1264 (33.0)	
No	493 (19.2)	2075 (80.8)	2568 (67.0)	
Lumbar				0.016
Yes	141 (15.0)	800 (85.0)	941 (24.6)	
No	537 (18.6)	2354 (81.4)	2891 (75.4)	
Total	678 (17.7)	3154 (82.3)	3832 (100.0)	

Another worldwide literature review (Wyndaele and Wyndaele 2006) revealed that 2 studies gave prevalence of SCI, whereas 17 studies gave incidence of SCI. The published data on prevalence of SCI was insufficient to consider the range of 223–755 per million inhabitants to be representative for a worldwide estimate. Reported incidence of SCI lies between 10.4 and 83 per million inhabitants per year. One-third of patients with SCI are reported to be tetraplegic and 50% of patients with SCI have a complete lesion. The mean age of patients sustaining their injury is reported as 33 years, and the sex distribution (men/women) as 3.8/1.

Epidemiology of spinal cord injury, literature data

	Paraplegia (%)	Tetraplegia (%)	Complete (%)	Incomplete (%)	Age (years)	Men/Women
Kurtzke	86.40	13.60	40.00	60.00	15–34	5.0/1
Tricot	42.68–91.3	8.7–57.32			38.2	4.6/1
van Asbeck et al	43.00	57.00	48.70	51.30		3.0/1
Maharaj	69.00	31.00	52.10	47.90	16–30	4.0/1
Dahlberg et al	54.00	46.00	43.00	57.00	31.00	3.0/1
Karacan et al	67.80	32.18			35.5 ± 15.1	2.5/1
Karamehmetoglu et al	67.00	33.00			33.00	3.0/1
Karamehmetoglu et al	57.80	41.30			31.30	5.8/1
Chen et al					46.10	3.0/1
Martins et al					50.00	3.0/1
Surkin et al						4.4/1

Source: Springer Nature © 2018 MacMillan Publishers Ltd.

1.7.1 Prevalence of spinal cord injuries

Only two manuscripts of SCI prevalence were found. One study is based on information on SCI in Australia, and the other one relates to SCI in Helsinki, Finland. Both studies used different methods to measure prevalence.

In the Australian study, based on the Australian Spinal Cord Injury Register (ASCIR), prevalence was estimated based on the relationship of prevalence (*P*) to the multiplicative product of disease incidence (*I*) and disease duration (*D*): $P = I \times D$. In the Finnish study, cases were identified using SCI registers.

Wyndaele (2006) also found three other reports dealing with the same subject: the Stockholm Spinal Cord Injury Study (SSCIS, 1996) used SCI registers to estimate SCI prevalence and estimated it to be 223 per million inhabitants. The National Center for Injury Prevention and Control (NCIPC) estimated 200,000 inhabitants of the United States to have SCI in 2001, which converts to a prevalence of about 700 per million population. The National Spinal Cord Injury Statistical Centre (NSCISC) database, which has recently been positively evaluated, estimated the number of people in the United States, who are alive and have an SCI, to be approximately 250,000 persons in July 2005, with a range of 225,000–288,000 persons. This converts to a prevalence of about 755 per million population, with a range of 679–870 per million population.

Prevalence rates of Stockholm (223 per million) and of Helsinki (280 per million) are comparable. The same goes for the prevalence rates of Australia (681 per million) and of the United States (700–755 per million). Unfortunately, we found only these five studies on prevalence of SCI, and all of them are from developed countries. We have not found data on Asia, Africa, South America, and the rest of Europe and therefore we cannot produce a worldwide SCI prevalence estimate.

1.7.2 Incidence of spinal cord injuries

In all, 17 studies of SCI incidence were found. To be able to make a comparison with prevalence estimates, we included only incidence studies based on a post-injury acute care and on a rehabilitation population. Most studies (15 out of 17) were retrospective.

Seven of these studies were related to SCI in Europe (Turkey, Russia, Portugal, The Netherlands, and France) with an incidence variation from 10.4 per million per year to 29.7 per million per year. Five studies were based on information from Northern America (Alaska, Mississippi, Kentucky, Indiana, Ontario, and Alberta), showing an incidence between 27.1 per million per year and 83 per million per year. A report from the NSCISC estimated the annual incidence of SCI, not including those who die at the scene of the accident, to be approximately 40 cases per million population or approximately 11,000 new cases each year. Four studies were from in Asia (Jordan, Japan, Taiwan, and Fiji Islands) with an incidence between 18.0 per million per year and 40.2 per million per year. From Australia, there was one study, estimating the age-standardized SCI incidence at 14.5 per million per year. The crude SCI incidence is 16.8 per million per year.

Again, most studies are from developed countries. No studies from South America or from Africa were found. The global estimate of SCI incidence from literature lies between 10.4 per million per year and 83 per million per year when only patients that survived before hospital admission were included.

Three studies also contained data including the prehospital mortalities. Martins et al estimated this total incidence to be 57.8 per million per year in Portugal, Surkin et al estimated it to be 77 per million per year in Mississippi (USA) and Dryden et al estimated it to be 52.5 per million per year in Alberta (Canada). This results in a prehospital mortality rate ranging from 15 to 56%.

1.7.3 Evolution of SCI incidence and prevalence over 30 years

Older studies produced an average of the available data (sum divided by the number), whereas recent studies produce a range of data. Which method is preferable will be discussed further in the section. In order to compare older and recent rates, we calculated the average of the latter (within brackets).

Evolution of incidence and prevalence of spinal cord injury over 30 years

Year of review	Authors	Incidence per million inhabitants per year	Prevalence per million inhabitants
1977	Kurtzke	30	520
1981	Tricot	21.7	Not mentioned
1975–1995	Blumer and Quine	13–71 (34.4)	110–1120 (554)
1995–2005	Wyndaele M	10.4–83 (29.5)	223–755 (485)

Note: Average of incidence and prevalence is given in brackets.

Important is from which regions, the reviews give the data. Tricot reviewed four studies from Europe (Russia, Switzerland, Norway, and France), two studies from Australia (Victoria and Brisbane), two studies from Northern America (Northern California) and one study from Asia (Japan). Blumer and Quine reviewed 10 studies from Northern America (Northern California, Minnesota, Canada and Greenland, USA global), two studies from Europe (France and Iceland), one study from Asia (Kashmir) and one study from Australia. The following table summarizes the averages of the data found.

Evolution of incidence and prevalence of spinal cord injury in literature over 30 years per continent

Review	North America		Europe		Australia		Asia
	Incidence	Prevalence	Incidence	Prevalence	Incidence	Prevalence	Incidence
Tricot	43.3	13.9	15.8		27.1		
Blumer and Quine	46	681	15.5	250	19	370	
Wyndaele[a]	51	755	19.4	252	16.8	681	23.9

Note: Incidence: average number per million inhabitants per year. The Australian incidence number used is the crude rate as opposed to the age-standardized rate.
Prevalence: Average number per million inhabitants.
[a]Wyndaele M, Wyndaele JJ. Incidence, prevalence and epidemiology of spinal cord injury: what learns a worldwide literature survey? Spinal Cord. 2006;44(9):523–529.

1.7.4 Associated injuries

Of total SCI patients, 73.7% had associated injuries. Spinal fractures were found in 48.6% of the SCI patients, other fractures were reported in 16.0% of the patients, and brain injuries were observed in 9.1% of the patients. Spinal fractures were observed in 23.7% of the patients with complete injuries; 26.3 and 25.4% of the patients with other fractures and brain injuries, respectively, had complete SCIs. Statistically significant differences were noted among all the associated injury groups with regard to the severity of injury ($P < 0.001$).

Characteristics of associated injuries in the 3,832 patients by the severity of injury

Associated injury	Severity of injury, n (%)			P-value
	Complete	Incomplete	Total	
Spinal fracture				< 0.001
Yes	442 (23.7)	1422 (76.3)	1864 (48.6)	
No	236 (12.0)	1732 (88.0)	1968 (51.4)	
Fracture of other parts				< 0.001
Yes	161 (26.3)	452 (73.7)	613 (16.0)	
No	517 (16.1)	2702 (83.9)	3219 (84.0)	
Brain injury				< 0.001
Yes	89 (25.4)	261 (74.6)	350 (9.1)	
No	589 (16.9)	2893 (83.1)	3482 (90.9)	
Total	678 (17.7)	3154 (82.3)	3832 (100.0)	

1.7.5 Clinical complications of SCI

In a large retrospective study from China (Rui Yang et al 2014), 12.8% of the SCI patients experienced clinical complications. The number of complication cases increased from 13 to 491 cases during the study period. The four main complications were pulmonary infections (37.6%), urinary tract infections (26.3%), bedsores (13.6%), and electrolyte disturbances (10.3%). As shown in the following table, the percentages of patients with complete SCIs who experienced pulmonary infections, urinary tract infections, bedsores, and electrolyte disturbances were 51.4, 38.0, 32.8, and 25.5%, respectively.

Complication	Severity of injury, n (%)		Total
	Complete	Incomplete	
Pulmonary infection	95 (51.4)	90 (48.6)	185 (37.6)
Urinary tract infection	49 (38.0)	80 (62.0)	129 (26.3)
Bedsores	22 (32.8)	45 (67.2)	67 (13.6)
Electrolyte disturbance	13 (25.5)	38 (74.5)	51 (10.3)
Deep venous thrombosis	4 (28.6)	10 (71.4)	14 (2.8)
Digestive system disease	4 (28.6)	10 (71.4)	14 (2.8)
Urinary calculus	4 (40.0)	6 (60.0)	10 (2.0)
Spasms	0 (0)	4 (100.0)	4 (0.8)
Autonomic dysreflexia	2 (66.7)	1 (33.3)	3 (0.6)
Cardiovascular diseases	1 (33.3)	2 (66.7)	3 (0.6)
Osteoporosis	0 (0)	1 (100.0)	1 (0.2)
Other	6 (60.0)	4 (40.0)	10 (2.0)
Total	200 (40.7)	291 (59.3)	491 (100.0)

Note: The total number in this table was 491, which referred to the number of patients with complications; the total number (n) of patients in this study was 3,832.

Moreover, the multivariate logistic regression model was used to screen the related risk factors for a complete injury. The results revealed that male gender (OR=1.25, 95% CI: 1.07–1.89), having a spinal fracture (OR=1.56, 95% CI: 1.35–2.60), having a thoracic injury (OR=1.23, 95% CI: 1.10–2.00), and having complications (OR=2.47, 95% CI:1.96–3.13) were the major risk factors for a complete SCI. High falls, traffic accidents, low falls, and nontraumatic injuries, compared with being struck by falling objects, had ORs < 1, so they were the protective factors against complete SCIs.

Epidemiological Characteristics of Neurological Diseases

Epidemiology of spinal cord injuries and risk factors for complete injuries

Variables	Odds ratio (95% confidence interval)	P-value
Age (years)		
</= 20	0.83 (0.53–1.29)	0.410
21–40	1.08 (0.80–1.47)	0.630
41–60	1.04 (0.77–1.41)	0.780
>/= 60	1.00 (reference)	
Gender		
Male	1.33 (1.06–1.67)	0.013
Female	1.00 (reference)	
Spinal fracture		
Yes	2.34 (1.97–2.79)	< 0.001
No	1.00 (reference)	
Complication(s)		
Yes	3.42 (2.76–4.23)	< 0.001
No	1.00 (reference)	
Cervical injury		
Yes	1.69 (1.43–2.00)	< 0.001
No	1.00 (reference)	
Thoracic injury		
Yes	2.25 (1.85–2.73)	< 0.001
No	1.00 (reference)	
Lumbar injury		
Yes	0.78 (0.64–0.96)	0.021
No	1.00 (reference)	

Source: Wyndaele M, Wyndaelee JJ. Incidence, prevalence epidemiology of spinal cord injury: what learns a worldwide literature survey? Spinal Cord 2006;44:523–529.
Singh A, Tetreault JJ, Kalsi-Ryan E et al. Global prevalence and incidence of traumatic spinal cord injury. Clin. Epidemiol 2014;6:309–331.
Yang R, Guo L, Wang Peng et al. Epidemiology of spinal cord injuries and risk factors for complete injuries in Guangdong, China: a retrospective Study. J Neurorestoratol 2014;9(1): e84733.

2 Neuroradiology

2.1 Imaging Findings of Various Calvarial Bone Lesions

CT and MRI have been incorporated into the basic imaging tools for evaluating calvarial lesions with their increasing frequency. Therefore, it is useful to categorize diagnostic features of images taken by CT and MRI and not the conventional radiography. It is possible to categorize different types of calvarial lesions based on four key features: thickening or thinning of calvarial bone, sclerosis or lysis of bone, focal or generalized lesions, and singularity or multiplicity of lesions. On CT and MRI, **sclerotic** lesions appear as thickening of calvarial bone (either the inner/outer tables, or bone marrow, or both). They can be further subdivided into *focal (solitary)* or *diffuse* lesions. The **lytic** category can be subdivided into either *single (solitary)* or *multiple* lesions. Furthermore, we can expect to get additional information about matrix characteristics with contrast enhancement and diverse advanced MR sequences such as diffusion-weighted imaging, perfusion-weighted imaging, and MR spectroscopy.

CT scan is considered to be the best examination to characterize bone alterations whereas MRI depicts bone marrow abnormalities and invasion of adjacent tissues.

2.1.1 Clinical features for evaluation of a calvarial lesion

Patient age, symptoms, clinical history, and laboratory findings are important clinical factors in making radiological diagnosis. The imaging appearance of calvarial lesions can indicate the lesion growth rate and sometimes suggest a specific diagnosis or limit the differential diagnosis. Systematic analysis of certain radiological features can be used for imaging evaluation of a calvarial lesion.

2.1.2 Radiological features for evaluation of a calvarial lesion

Size and number of lesions

The number of lesions, either single or multiple, can suggest a specific diagnosis. For example, in patients over 50 years of age, multiple osteolytic lesions with variable size are highly suggestive of multiple metastases.

Pattern of bone destruction and margins (transitional zone)

Benign tumors usually exhibit geographic/sharp bone destruction and a clear narrow transitional zone between normal and abnormal bone. Sclerotic margin may be present. Aggressive tumors often have poorly defined, moth-eaten, or permeated bone destruction and a wide zone of transition.

Periosteal reaction

A unilamellate uninterrupted pattern is usually associated with slow-growing lesions, and an interrupted periosteal reaction signifies an aggressive lesion.

Soft-tissue component and local extension

Malignant tumors often have a soft-tissue component that can extend to the scalp or to extra-axial spaces and/or the cerebral cortex.

Type of matrix and internal characteristics

The type of tumor matrix or other internal characteristics can suggest a specific diagnosis. Chondroid- and osteoid-producing tumors are usually easily detected by CT. Bone-forming tumors most often display amorphous or cloud-like mineralization, but the amount and degree of matrix mineralization are widely variable. Cartilage-forming tumors typically exhibit punctuate, comma-like, ring, or popcorn-like mineralization. Nonmineralized chondroid matrix, vascular tissue, fibrous matrix, and fatty, cystic, hemorrhagic contents within the lesions are more easily detected by MRI.

2.2 Solitary Radiolucent Skull Lesion without Sclerotic Margins in Adults

1. Normal
   a) Foramina, canals, and unfused sutures
   b) Vascular markings and emissary channels
   c) Arachnoidal granulations (near midline or superior sagittal sinus)
2. Variants
   a) Parietal thinning: Involves only the outer table of elderly individuals.
   b) Sinus pericrania: Anomalous venous diploic channel between the extracranial and intracranial venous system most commonly seen in the frontal bones; clinically it appears as a soft mass under the scalp that changes in size with alteration in the intracranial blood volume.

3. Congenital and developmental defects
   a) Encephaloceles: Extracranial protrusions of brain and/or meninges through skull defects; occipital in 70% and frontal in 15%. Congenital midline masses include encephaloceles, nasal gliomas, and dermoid and epidermoid cysts. These lesions occur in the nasofrontal region, the occiput, or the cranial vertex. Transsphenoidal encephaloceles occur at the skull base and are not visible at clinical examination but may be seen as nasopharyngeal masses and are part of the spectrum of encephaloceles seen in children. (▶ Fig. 2.1)

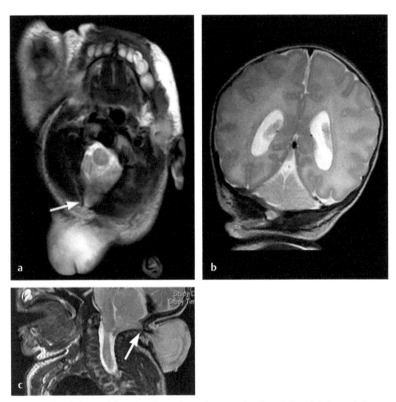

Fig. 2.1 (a–c) Chiari III (Chiari II malformation with an associated cervical-occipital encephalocele). Multiplanar T2W images demonstrate an intracranial Chiari II hindbrain malformation with a high cervical/occipital encephalocele. The *arrows* **(a, c)** indicate the site of the occipital calvarial defect resulting in herniation of disorganized cerebellar tissue. (Reproduced from Case 116. In: Tsiouris A, Sanelli P, Comunale J, ed. Case-Based Brain Imaging. 2nd edition. Thieme; 2013.)

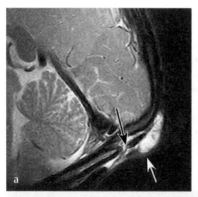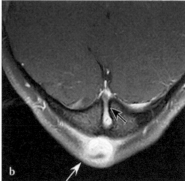

Fig. 2.2 (a, b) Occipital dermoid cyst. Sagittal T2-weighted **(a)** and axial contrast-enhanced T1-weighted **(b)** surface coil MR images show a midline suboccipital cystic lesion (*white arrow*), with a sinus tract in the occipital bone (*black arrow*), and an infratorcular intracranial connection. The enhancement is due to infection of the cyst.

- b) Dermoid cyst: Midline orbital in 80% lesion originating from ectodermal inclusions. (▶ Fig. 2.2)
- c) Neurofibroma: May cause a lucent defect in the occipital bone usually adjacent to the left lambdoidal suture.
- d) Intradiploic arachnoid cyst: Expansion of diploic space and thinning of the outer table.
4. Traumatic and iatrogenic defects
    - a) Linear skull fracture
    - b) Suture diastasis
    - c) Burr hole, craniectomy (very well defined)
    - d) Leptomeningeal cyst or "growing fracture"

2.3 Solitary Radiolucent Skull Lesion without Sclerotic Margins in Children

1. Normal
    - a) Parietal foramina
    - b) Fontanelle
    - c) Venous lakes and emissary channels
    - d) Arachnoidal granulations (near midline or superior sagittal sinus)

2. Trauma
   a) Burr hole, craniotomy
   b) Leptomeningeal cyst or "growing fracture": Under a skull fracture if the dura is torn, the arachnoid membrane can prolapse, and the cerebrospinal fluid (CSF) pulsations can cause over several weeks' time a progressive widening and scalloping of the fracture line.
   c) Intraosseous hematoma
3. Congenital and developmental defects
   a) Cranium bifidum, meningocele, encephalocele, dermal sinus
   b) Epidermoid or dermoid cyst (▶ Fig. 2.3): Midline orbital in 80% lesion originating from ectodermal inclusions.
   c) Intradiploic arachnoid cyst: Expansion of diploic space and thinning of the outer table
   d) Neurofibromatosis (▶ Fig. 2.4)
4. Infection
   a) Osteomyelitis: bacterial or fungal
   b) Hydatid cyst
   c) Tuberculosis
   d) Syphilis
5. Neoplasia
   a) Metastasis: commonly from a neuroblastoma and leukemia
   b) Langerhans cell histiocytosis (▶ Fig. 2.5)
      i. Eosinophilic granuloma: A solitary lesion which causes only local pain. Only has sclerotic margins if it is in the healing process.

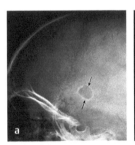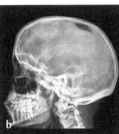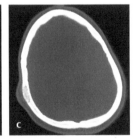

Fig. 2.3 (a–c) An epidermoid in 1-year-old infant. **(a)** Arrows point to a small oval defect in the parietal bone with a sharply defined sclerotic border. **(b)** An epidermoid in another child shows that these lesions may not be as well demarcated by sclerotic edges. **(c)** A computed tomography scan reveals the lesion and soft-tissue swelling.

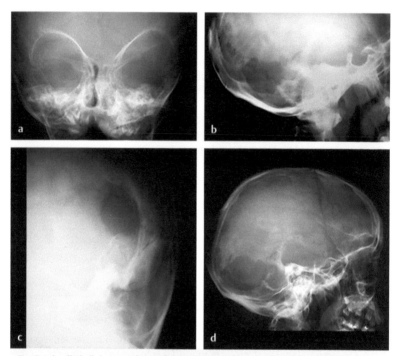

Fig. 2.4 (a–d) Skull changes of neurofibromatosis (NF) type 1. A frontal view of the orbits reveals an elevated sphenoid wing (bilateral) and hypoplasia of the left sphenoid bone **(a)**. A 5-year-old boy with NF has a defect in the left lambdoid suture seen on lateral **(b)** and oblique **(c)** views. A lateral view of another child with NF who has a large skull defect seen in the left lambdoid suture **(d)**. (These images are provided courtesy of Peter Strouse, MD, Ann Arbor, MI.)

ii. Hand–Schüller–Christian disease: "Geographic" as well as multiple lytic lesions are common, associated with systemic symptoms such as exophthalmos, diabetes insipidus, chronic otitis media, "honeycomb lung." There are solitary or multiple areas of bone destruction. The edges of the individual lesions are sharp, having a slightly cupped shape or irregular, but do not have a transitional zone sclerosis. Typically, the lesion originates in the diploe and involves one or both of the bone plates, causing a well-defined

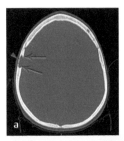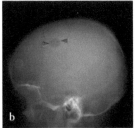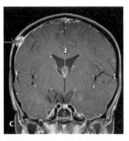

Fig. 2.5 Langerhans cell histiocytosis. **(a)** Axial bone algorithm computed tomographic image shows a lytic lesion within the right parietal bone, that has extended through the inner table of the skull, with a sharp "beveled" margin (*red arrows*) and with early extension through the outer table (*red arrowhead*). **(b)** Sagittal thick-section reformatted image from a computed tomographic scan, simulating a lateral radiograph of the skull, shows a lytic lesion with circumscribed margins within the right parietal bone (*red arrowheads*). **(c)** Coronal T1 W plus contrast image shows an enhancing soft tissue component causing the lytic lesion (*red arrow*), and reactive dural thickening in the region (*red arrowhead*). (Reproduced from Calvarial Defects. In: Choudhri A, ed. Pediatric Neuroradiology. Clinical Practice Essentials. 1st edition. Thieme; 2016.)

radiolucent defect and slightly irregular "punched-out" lesion with beveled edge, which is caused by asymptomatic destruction of the inner and outer cortices of the skull bone.

In the Hand–Schuller–Christian disease, the lesions can coalesce, become similar to a very large map, a finding referred to as a "geographic skull," whereas eosinophilic granuloma lesions tend to be smaller, of the order of 1–2 cm.

Skull lesions can be asymptomatic but may manifest with focal pain and soft-tissue swelling in the scalp. At MRI, the soft-tissue component is hyperintense on T2-weighted images (T2WI) and isointense on T1-weighted images (T1WI), with enhancement after gadolinium-based contrast agent administration.

c) Sarcoma (i.e., Ewing's brown tumor, osteosarcoma)
d) Solitary plasmacytoma
6. Miscellaneous
   a) Aneurysmal bone cyst (▸ Fig. 2.6)
   b) Arteriovenous malformation
   c) Osseous hemangioma (▸ Fig. 2.7)

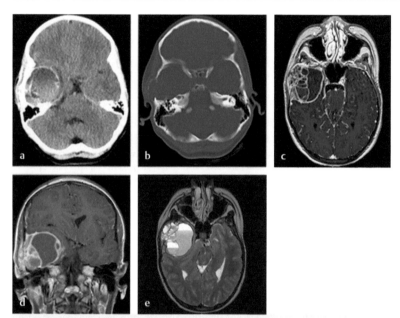

Fig. 2.6 Aneurysmal bone cyst. This 12-year-old girl presented with a nontender firm mass in the right temple. **(a, b)** Computed tomography shows calcification surrounding the lesion; bone windows show a thin shell of intact bone externally. **(c, d)** Axial and coronal T1-weighted images with contrast reveal an enhancing soft tissue portion of the tumor. **(e)** Axial T2-weighted image shows typical fluid–fluid levels of nonclotted blood. (Reproduced from Surgical Concepts. In: Albright A, Pollack I, Adelson P, ed. Principles and Practice of Pediatric Neurosurgery. 3rd edition. Thieme; 2014.)

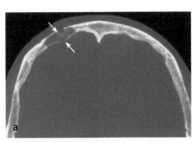
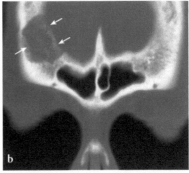

Fig. 2.7 Intraosseous hemangioma. **(a)** Serial reformatted sagittal CT scans, showing a frontal bone hemangioma encroaching on the superior orbit. This may be mistaken for a benign fibro-osseous lesion such as fibrous dysplasia. **(b)** Coronal CT scan in another patient, showing a histologically proven hemangioma of the right frontal bone (*arrows*). (Reproduced from Mafee M. Pathology. In: Valvassori G, Mafee M, Becker M, ed. Imaging of the Head and Neck. 2nd edition. Stuttgart: Thieme; 2004.)

2.4 Solitary Radiolucent Skull Lesion with Sclerotic Margins

1. Congenital and developmental
   a) Epidermoid (▶ Fig. 2.8): Arises from the diploic region and so it can expand both the inner and the outer tables. Most common location is the squamous portion of the occipital bone, less common are the frontal and temporal portions. It is the most common erosive lesion of the cranial vault.
   b) Meningocele: Midline skull defect with a smooth sclerotic margin and an overlying soft-tissue mass. In 70% of the cases, it appears in the occipital bone; in 15%, occurs in the frontal and less commonly in the basal or parietal bones.
2. Neoplastic
   a) Langerhans cell histiocytosis (▶ Fig. 2.9): Only has a sclerotic margin if it is in the healing process.
   b) Hemangioma: Originates in the diploic area and rarely has a sclerotic margin.
3. Infective
   a) Frontal sinus mucocele (secondary to chronic sinusitis)
   b) Chronic osteomyelitis: Most commonly pyogenic but may be fungal, syphilitic, or tubercular. Reactive sclerosis dominates particularly with fungal infections, i.e., actinomycosis, with only a few lytic areas.

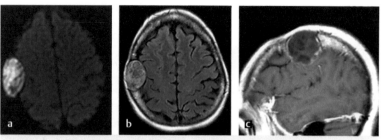

Fig. 2.8 (a) Axial DWI and (b) T2W FLAIR images reveal restricted diffusion in a heterogeneously hyperintense intradiploic calvarial lesion. (c) Sagittal postcontrast T1W image shows both inner and outer skull table involvement of this intradiploic epidermoid cyst. (Reproduced from Case 37. In: Tsiouris A, Sanelli P, Comunale J, ed. Case-Based Brain Imaging. 2nd edition. Thieme; 2013.)

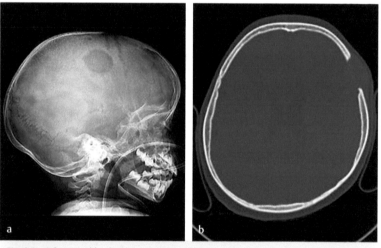

Fig. 2.9 Eight-year-old girl with Langerhans cell histiocytosis. (a) Radiograph shows lesion without sclerotic solitary osteolytic border. (b) Axial CT image with bone window reveals small lesion with well-defined contours; inner and outer tables are unequally affected, giving lesion its characteristic beveled edges on CT.

4. Miscellaneous
   a) Fibrous dysplasia: The normal medullary space is replaced by fibroosseous tissue. It involves the craniofacial bones in 20% of the cases. It appears as solitary or multiple lytic lesions with or without sclerotic regions on MRI.

2.5 Multiple Radiolucent Skull Lesions

1. Normal
   a) Fissures, parietal foramina, and channels
   b) Pacchionian depressions from arachnoidal granulations (near midline or superior sagittal sinus)
   c) Venous lakes and diploic channels
2. Metabolic
   a) Hyperparathyroidism: The multiple punctate lytic changes in the cranium cause the so-called pepperpot appearance. The focal lucencies are made of fibrous tissue and giant cells known as brown tumors, indicated by the old term *osteitis fibrosa cystica*.
   b) Renal osteodystrophy: Excessive excretion or loss of calcium due to kidney disease results in calcium mobilization and in a skull appearance identical to primary hyperthyroidism.
   c) Osteoporosis: Loss of protein matrix results in lytic areas in the diploic and inner table of the skull in elderly and in patients with endocrine diseases such as Cushing's disease.
3. Neoplasm
   a) Metastatic tumors: The most frequent neoplastic involvement of the skull is by hematogenous metastases from breast, lung, prostate, kidney, and thyroid or by invasion from adjacent primary neoplasms with osteolytic metastases such as the medulloblastoma.
   b) Multiple myeloma: Produces small, discrete round holes of variable size, also referred as punched-out lesions. (▶ Fig. 2.10)

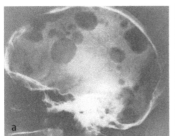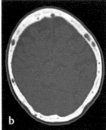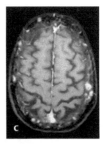

Fig. 2.10 (a) Multiple myeloma. Lateral x-ray demonstrates multiple lytic lesions. (Reproduced from XI. Differential Diagnosis by Location. In: Citow J, Macdonald R, Refai D, ed. Comprehensive Neurosurgery Board Review. 2nd edition. Thieme; 2009.) (b) Multiple osteolytic lesions from multiple myeloma are seen in the skull on axial CT. (c) The lesions show gadolinium contrast enhancement on axial fat-suppressed T1-weighted imaging. (Reproduced from Table 1.3 Multiple lesions involving the skull. In: Meyers S, ed. Differential Diagnosis in Neuroimaging: Head and Neck. 1st edition. Thieme; 2016.)

c) Leukemia and lymphoma: Produce small, not well-defined, or separated multiple lesions which tend to coalesce.

d) Neuroblastoma: In infants, it is the most common metastatic tumor of the skull.

e) Ewing's sarcoma (may rarely metastasize to the skull)

4. Miscellaneous

a) Radiation necrosis: Focal irradiation results in multiple small areas of bone destruction localized in the area treated.

b) Avascular necrosis: A few months following local ischemia from trauma destructive changes occur in the outer and diploic region of the cranium.

c) Hand–Schüller–Christian disease: Multiple large areas of bone destruction with irregular edges and without marginal sclerosis; the latter feature differentiates this form of histiocytosis X from eosinophilic granuloma which is believed to be the more benign form of the two.

d) Osteoporosis circumscripta: Represents the first stage of an idiopathic decalcification/ossification condition which results in areas of lucency sharply separated from normal bone. The second stage is characterized by an abnormal recalcification and ossification, suggesting an initial insult followed by disordered repair. The coexistence of these two stages of bone destruction and sclerosis characterize the pathological changes seen in Paget's disease.

2.6 Localized Increased Density or Hyperostosis of the Skull Vault

1. Traumatic

a) Depressed skull fracture: Occurs due to overlapping bone fragments.

b) Cephalohematoma: Old calcified hematoma under elevated periosteum. It is commonly found in the parietal area; may be bilateral.

2. Miscellaneous

a) Calcified sebaceous cyst

b) Paget's disease: It involves all skull layers and is characterized with the appearance of both lytic, osteogenesis circuscripta, and sclerotic phases. (▶ Fig. 2.11)

c) Fibrous dysplasia: Affects the craniofacial bones in approximately 20% cases and it may be monostotic or polyostotic and diffuse. It consists of abundant myofibromatous tissue woven with dysplastic, nonmaturing, or atypical bone. CT imaging shows thickened, sclerotic bone with a "ground glass" appearance (70–130 HU), with cystic components found in the early stages of the disease. On MRI, the expanded, thickened bone is typically of low to intermediate signal intensity on both T1WI and

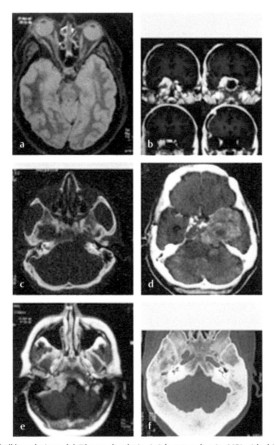

Fig. 2.11 Skull base lesions. **(a)** Fibrous dysplasia. Axial proton density MRI with thickening of the right sphenoid bone and reduction of the size of the orbit and associated exophthalmos. **(b)** Meningioma of the right cavernous sinus. Coronal T1 WI shows expansion of the right cavernous sinus and a very high signal intensity following contrast enhancement. **(c)** Metastasis. Axial CT demonstrating an osteolytic lesion of the sphenoid tip of the petrous bone. **(d)** Chordoma. Axial CT with a high-density space-occupying lesion of the left temporal fossa and the parasellar region. The mass is eroding the apex of the petrous bone and is extending to the cerebellopontine angle of the same side. **(e)** Paraganglioma or glomus jugulare. Axial CT shows a space-occupying lesion of the right CP angle that occupies the right jugular foramen and demonstrates intense, heterogeneous postcontrast enhancement. **(f)** Paget's disease. Axial CT shows a marked thickening of all bones of the skull base with reduction of the size of the posterior fossa.

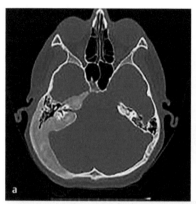 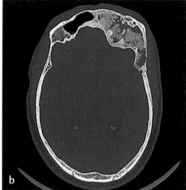

Fig. 2.12 Fibrous dysplasia. **(a)** Axial CT images with bone windows show expanded masses localized in right occipito-temporal, **(b)** and left frontal bone and containing characteristic ground-glass matrix. It displaces outer table more than the inner one.

T2WI, although scattered hyperintensity areas may be present. Following gadolinium injection, a variable enhancement occurs. (▶ Fig. 2.12)

  d) Hyperostosis frontalis interna: This idiopathic condition refers to the thickening of the inner table. It is commonly found in the frontal bone of sexually active females indicating a true endocrine relationship.
3. Neoplasia
   a) Osteoblastic metastases: Metastatic prostatic carcinoma is most frequently osteoblastic and is the most common cause of osteoblastic metastasis in the males. Medulloblastoma is a rare example of blastic metastasis.
   b) Neuroblastoma
   c) Primary skull tumors
      i. Benign skull tumors
         – Osteoid osteoma: When arising from the dura, it stimulates a calvarial lesion. In order to be disclosed, the neurosurgeon needs to open the dura.
         – Osteoblastoma
      ii. Malignant skull tumors: Chondrosarcoma, osteosarcoma, fibrosarcoma, and angiosarcoma.
         The distinct radiological aspects of conventional osteosarcoma are bone marrow lesions, cortical bone destruction, an aggressive periosteal reaction, a soft-tissue mass, and a tumor matrix in the

destructive lesion, as well as within the soft-tissue mass. Although the tumors can present as purely sclerotic or purely osteolytic, most are a combination of the two. The borders are generally indistinct, with a broad zone of transition. The bone destruction is infiltrative, with a "moth-eaten" appearance, and only rarely geographic. The most common forms of periosteal reaction seen in osteosarcomas are the speculated (sunburst) type and Codman's triangle with the laminated (onion-skin) type being less common.

d) Meningioma: Focal hyperostosis and enlargement of meningeal arterial grooves are the classic findings in a plain skull x-ray.

2.7 Diseases Affecting the Temporal Bone

2.7.1 Destructive (lucencies with irregular margins)

1. Petrous ridge or apex
   a) Inflammatory: Acute petrositis is a nondestructive inflammatory condition (rare complication of otomastoiditis) affecting only 30–50% of the cases with the aerated petrous apex and is characterized by irregular spotty opacifications scattered through the petrous pyramid. Spread of the inflammation may lead to osteomyelitis and abscess formation in the petrous pyramid. The involvement of the surrounding tissues causes the irritation of cranial nerve Vth with periorbital pain, VIth nerve palsy causing diplopia and ipsilateral ottorhea which is referred to as *Gradenigo's syndrome*, although it may not be present in every patient. The facial pain is due to focal meningitis over the petrous apex with irritation of the Gasserian ganglion in the Meckel cavity. Abducens nerve involvement occurs at its course through the Dorello canal. Imaging studies demonstrate erosive changes of the petrous apex with abnormal enhancement of the adjacent meninges. Differential diagnosis should be performed with neoplastic disease (rhabdomyosarcoma, metastasis) and epidermoid tumors. On MRI, it presents typically of low signal intensity on T1WI and high intensity on T2WI. In chronic petrositis, the high content of protein and viscosity causes high signal on T1WI and/or lower signal intensity on T2WI. (▶ Fig. 2.13)
   b) Malignant neoplasm
      i. Nasopharyngeal carcinoma: Usually large area of destruction in the floor of the middle cranial fossa are also seen.
      ii. Metastatic tumors: Any site of the petrous pyramid, particularly lung, breast, and kidney carcinoma (▶ Fig. 2.14)
      iii. Parotid gland neoplasia

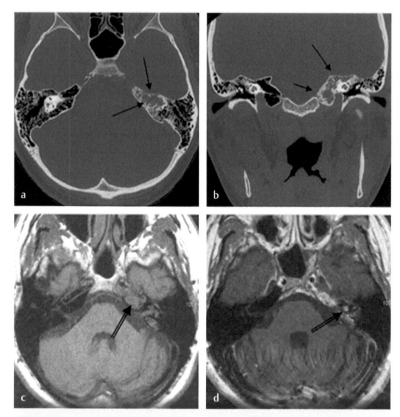

Fig. 2.13 Petrous apicitis. **(a)** Axial and **(b)** coronal computed tomography images demonstrate diffuse opacification localized to the petrous apex with loss of septations (*arrows*), indicating coalescent disease. **(c)** Axial precontrast T1-weighted magnetic resonance image (T1WI) reveals petrous apex disease (*arrow*). **(d)** Axial post-contrast T1WI reveals intensely enhancing debris. Leptomeningeal disease is manifest most notably by enhancement of the facial and superior vestibular nerves within the internal auditory canal (*arrow*). (Reproduced from Pathology and Treatment. In: Swartz J, Loevner L, ed. Imaging of the Temporal Bone. 4th edition. Thieme; 2008.)

    iv. Chordoma: Arises from a notochordal remnant, usually in the midline at the spheno-occipital synchondrosis. The origin is 35% from the clivus, 50% sacrococcygeal, and 15% spinal. The presence of dense retrosellar calcification with bone destruction of the

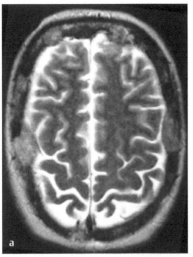 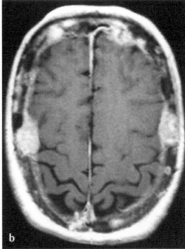

Fig. 2.14 A 68-year-old woman with metastatic breast carcinoma who has multiple lesions in skull marrow associated with bone destruction and extraosseous tumor extension.
(a) The tumors have intermediate to slightly high signal on axial T2-weighted imaging and
(b) show gadolinium contrast enhancement on axial T1-weighted imaging. Thickened contrast enhancing dura is also seen from neoplastic invasion. (Reproduced from Table 1.3 Multiple lesions involving the skull. In: Meyers S, ed. Differential Diagnosis in Neuroimaging: Head and Neck. 1st edition. Thieme; 2016.)

clivus, dorsum sellae, and petrous bones is characteristic of clivus chordoma. Frequent tumor calcification shows lytic destruction of bone, and has mild enhancement. On T1WI, the lesions are usually isointense (75%) or hypointense (25%) but nearly all are hyperintense on T2WI.

The classic appearance of intracranial chordoma at high-resolution CT is that of a centrally located, well-circumscribed, expansile soft-tissue mass that arises from the clivus with associated extensive lytic bone destruction. The bulk of the tumor is usually hyperattenuating relative to the adjacent neural axis. Intratumoral calcifications appear irregular at CT and are usually thought to represent sequestra from bone destruction rather than dystrophic calcifications in the tumor itself. (Fig. 2.15)

MRI is the single best modality for radiologic evaluation of intracranial chordomas. It is similar to CT in detecting intracranial

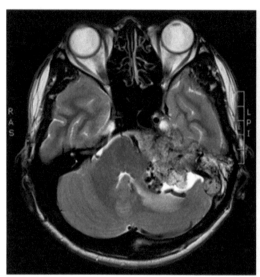

Fig. 2.15 T2 axial MRI of a C3 Di3 jugular paraganglioma that has caused significant compression of the brainstem with associated edema. The patient required a ventriculoperitoneal shunt. (Reproduced from 39.1 Introduction. In: Sekhar L, Fessler R, ed. Atlas of Neurosurgical Techniques: Brain, Volume 2. 2nd edition. Thieme; 2015.)

chordomas. However, it is considerably superior to CT in the delineation of lesion extent because it provides excellent tissue contrast and exquisite anatomic detail. The multiplanar capability of MRI is also helpful in this regard. Sagittal images are generally most valuable in defining the posterior margin of the tumor, showing the relation between the tumor and brainstem, and depicting nasopharyngeal extension of the tumor. Sagittal imaging is also useful in disclosing transdural transgression by a tumor, an important factor in surgical planning. Coronal images, on the other hand, are helpful in detecting tumor extension into the cavernous sinus and depicting the position of the optic chiasm and tract.

Angiographic evaluation of intracranial chordomas is nonspecific. Abnormal tumor vascularity or staining is rare. Angiographic evaluation is reserved for cases in which there is significant displacement, encasement, or narrowing of the internal carotid or vertebral artery at MR angiography. Cerebral angiography can better demonstrate the degree of luminal narrowing or occlusion and the extent of collateral circulation.

c) Benign tumors
   i. Glomus jugulare or ganglioglioma or chemodectoma: Arise from chemoreceptor organs on the promontory in the jugular fossa in the superior portion of the jugular bulb. Usually, these tumors spread

superiorly and laterally through the inferior surface of the petrous pyramids. At this stage, they show an irregular enlargement of the jugular foramen and an irregular destruction of the inferior aspect of the petrous pyramid. As the tumor grows, it causes further destruction involving the ossicular system, the internal jugular vein, the posterior margin of the carotid canal, and the posterior fossa. On CT scan, it seems this mass erodes the jugular foramen of the temporal bone. The mass may grow inferiorly into the jugular vein or may grow from the jugular bulb region into the sigmoid and transverse sinuses or the vein. Mass within the vessel plexus may be distinguished from thrombosis by the presence of enhancement in the former. On MRI, the glomus jugulare has a typical "salt and pepper" appearance. Characteristically, they reveal undulating channel-like voids, especially on T2WI. Following gadolinium injection, there is moderate enhancement. Angiography was needed in the definitive diagnosis of these lesions previously but now the location of the lesion at or extending into the jugular bulb plus the vascularity and the "salt and pepper" appearance of MR images makes this an easy diagnosis.

   d) Miscellaneous
      i. Langerhans granulomatosis
2. Middle ear and mastoid
   a) Infection
      i. Acute or chronic bacterial: There are four main mechanisms of extension of the infection in acute mastoiditis: preformed pathways, osseous erosion, thrombophlebitis, and hematogenous seeding. When mastoid region inflammation cannot be arrested, the suppuration under pressure causes local acidosis and osseous decalcification, ischemia, and osteoclastic dissolution of the pneumatic cell walls. The pneumatic cells can coalesce into larger cavities filled with purulent exudates and granulations, resulting in empyema and the stage of coalescent mastoiditis. This osteoclastic osseous resorption proceeds in all directions, and intratemporal or intracranial complications threaten to occur before spontaneous resolution. Spread of the inflammatory debris anteriorly to the middle ear via the aditus ad antrum can result in spontaneous resolution if the tympanic membrane was previously perforated. The infection may also spread laterally and produce a subperiosteal abscess or spread medially to the petrous air cells, causing petrositis. Coalescent mastoiditis is diagnosed when temporal bone CT scan demonstrates erosion of the mastoid septa or mastoid walls. This complication

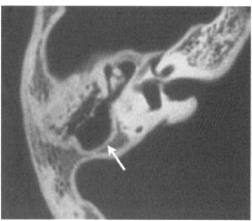

Fig. 2.16 Chronic otitis media in a 12-year-old female. Axial CT shows opacification of the right middle ear and mastoid air cells. The mastoid is small, with zones of lysis of mastoid bone septa related to an intra-mastoid empyema (referred to as coalescent mastoiditis) (*arrow*). (Reproduced from Table 1.8 Lesions involving the middle ear. In: Meyers S, ed. Differential Diagnosis in Neuroimaging: Head and Neck. 1st edition. Thieme; 2016.)

can follow a more acute and aggressive course (coalescent acute mastoiditis) or a more subclinical progression (latent or "masked" mastoiditis). (▶Fig. 2.16) Chronic mastoiditis was commonly associated with benign intracranial hypertension due to the contiguous extension of the inflammation to the neighboring sigmoid and lateral sinuses.

    ii. Tuberculosis: Very rare; causes bone destruction without sclerosis.

b) Malignant neoplasm

    i. Squamous-cell carcinoma: The most common malignant tumor of the middle ear. Irregularly marginated lucent defects, without any evidence of sclerosis.

    ii. Adenocarcinoma: Less common than squamous-cell carcinomas.

    iii. Sarcoma (rare)

c) Benign neoplasm

    i. Glomus hypotympanicum tumor—Chemodectoma: Most common benign tumor of the middle ear. Arises from the receptor organs on the promontory in the hypotympanum. These are locally invasive and extremely vascular tumors.

d) Miscellaneous

    i. Langerhans granulomatosis: This disease has a propensity for the mastoid portion of the temporal bone of children and young adults. It presents as a lytic process clinically resulting in loss of hearing without pain or tenderness. The patients are afebrile and otherwise healthy children. The lesion is intense on T1WI and hyperintense and enhanced on T2WI.

2.7.2 Erosive (lucencies with well-defined margins, with or without sclerosis)

1. Petrous pyramid or apex (▶ Fig. 2.17)
   a) Acoustic neurinoma
   b) Bone neoplasm, benign, or malignant: Such as hemangioma, osteoblastoma, chordoma, chondroma, metastasis.

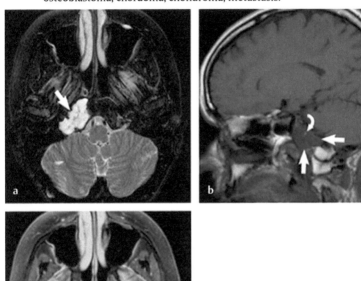

Fig. 2.17 Chondrosarcoma. **(a)** Axial T2-weighted magnetic resonance image (MRI) shows an irregular mass (*arrow*) that is hyperintense but located laterally at the petroclival synchondrosis and invading the right petrous apex. **(b)** The mass is minimally hypointense compared with brain on sagittal T1-weighted MRI, with a focal area of T1 hyperintensity (*curved arrow*) that may represent hemorrhage or calcification. **(c)** Axial gadolinium-enhanced T1-weighted image shows uniform intense contrast enhancement. (Reproduced from Pathology. In: Swartz J, Loevner L, ed. Imaging of the Temporal Bone. 4th edition. Thieme; 2008.)

    c) Epidermoid: In the cerebellopontine angle (CPA) cistern.

    d) Aneurysm of the intracavernous or intrapetrous internal carotid artery

    e) Meningioma of Meckel's cave

    f) Subarachnoid cyst

    g) Neurinoma of V, IX, or X nerve

    h) Langerhans granulomatosis

2. Internal auditory canal

    a) Acoustic neurinoma: It represents 8% of all intracranial tumors. It arises from the Schwann cells which invest the eighth nerve as it enters the internal auditory canal (IAC). Ninety-five percent (95%) of these tumors originate within the auditory canal and the other 5% arise from the nerve at its CPA course, proximal to the canal. Often bilateral in neurofibromatosis. Most acoustic neuromas arise from the superior vestibular branch of the eighth cranial nerve. As vestibular schwannomas enlarge, they may expand medially into the CPA and laterally toward the fundus and/or into the cochlear aperture. The most noticeable X-ray change caused by these tumors is erosion of the superior and posterior lips of the porus acusticus. On CT images, most vestibular schwannomas are isoattenuating with the cerebellum and are difficult to delineate without contrast material enhancement. However, if the tumor is large and causes expansion of the porus acusticus, this may be readily seen on CT bone window images, with the porus acusticus asymmetrically wider on the affected side. Calcification and hemorrhage are rare unless the tumor has not been treated. (▶ Fig. 2.18)

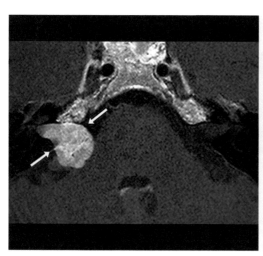

Fig. 2.18 Axial contrast-enhanced T1-weighted MR image of vestibular schwannoma. This middle-aged man presented with sudden asymmetric sensorineural hearing loss on the right. Image demonstrates an avidly enhancing tumor in the internal auditory canal extending through an expanded porus acusticus (*between arrows*) into the cerebellopontine angle, where it forms an acute angle with the posterior petrous ridge.

On MR images, schwannomas are usually isointense to mildly hypointense to brain parenchyma and hyperintense to CSF on T1WI, whereas on T2WI, these are mildly hyperintense to brain parenchyma and isointense to hypointense to CSF and enhance avidly. Large tumors may be heterogeneous, with intra- or extramural cystic components, and may deform and displace the brainstem, causing parenchymal edema, and compress the fourth ventricle. Heavily T2-weighted sequences are helpful for outlining the tumor, as most structures except CSF appear quite dark. CSF, thus, provides natural contrast around the dark tumor mass. Heavily T2-weighted sequences may also reveal decreased signal intensity of the labyrinthine fluid ipsilateral to the tumor, thought to be related to higher protein content in the fluid; this may also be seen as increased signal intensity on fluid-attenuated inversion recovery images. Enhancement is always evident and homogeneous in approximately 70% of patients. Peritumoral edema may be seen in 30–35% of cases with larger lesions and less frequent calcification, cystic change, and hemorrhage. (▶ Fig. 2.19 and ▶ Fig. 2.20)

b) Facial nerve neuroma: Very rare tumors but may cause similar roentgenographic changes to that of an acoustic neuroma.

c) Meningioma of the Gasserian cavity: Meningiomas of the auditory canal may cause erosion of the canal and usually extend to involve the posterior surface of the petrous apex. In contrast to vestibular schwannomas,

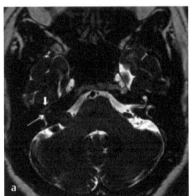
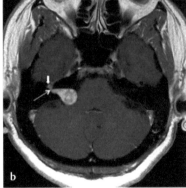

Fig. 2.19 Facial schwannoma on a heavily T2-weighted sequence (T2 DRIVE) **(a)** and corresponding postgadolinium T1 section **(b)**. The enhancing "ice-cream cone"–like cisternal and IAC component of the mass is similar to a vestibular schwannoma. The distinguishing feature is the involvement of the labyrinthine segment of the facial nerve (*thin arrow*) and the geniculate ganglion (*thick arrow*). (Reproduced from Role of Neuroimaging in Skull Base Surgery. In: Di Ieva A, Lee J, Cusimano M, ed. Handbook of Skull Base Surgery. 1st edition. Thieme; 2016.)

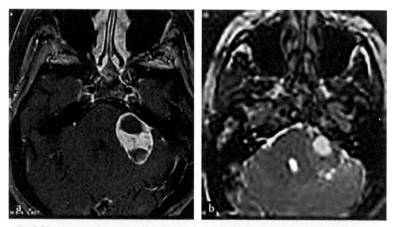

Fig. 2.20 Acoustic schwannoma (large with cystic change). **(a)** Axial T1 C+ fat sat. Left cerebellopontine angle extra-axial mass with cystic component. It shows typical extension through the internal auditory meatus and displays avid enhancement in post contrast study. **(b)** Axial T2 of facial nerve neuroma. Very rare tumors but may cause similar roentgenographic changes to that of an acoustic neuroma.

meningiomas are often eccentric to the porus acousticus, centered at the CPA; when they do extend into the IAC, they seldom expand the porus or the IAC. Meningiomas may extend into the middle cranial fossa by means of herniation, growth through the tentorium, or growth through the temporal bone. They may also extend into the middle ear and cavernous sinus. As mentioned above, meningiomas tend to be broad-based along the tposterior petrous wall, forming an obtuse angle at the bone–tumor interface, appearing either hemispherical or plaquelike. Dural enhancement extending outward from the margins of the tumor is often seen. (▶ Fig. 2.21)

d) Chordomas
e) Vascular lesions
   i. Aneurysm of the intracavernous or intrapetrous carotid artery
   ii. Arteriovenous malformation or occlusive disease of the anterior inferior cerebellar artery may cause erosion of the IAC causing it to have a funnel-shaped appearance.
   iii. Aneurysm at the origin of the internal auditory artery may cause erosion of the canal.
f) Miscellaneous
   i. Epidermoid adjacent to the apex
   ii. Leptomeningeal cyst

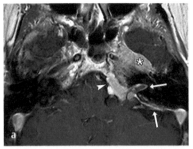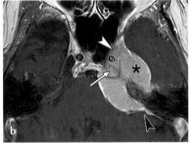

Fig. 2.21 Axial contrast-enhanced T1-weighted MR images of meningioma. **(a)** Lesion having a broad-based component against the posterior petrous surface (*arrowhead*) and an en plaque component extending into the internal auditory canal (IAC) and along the posterior surface of the mastoid (*arrows*). The IAC is not expanded. There is extension to the middle cranial fossa (*). **(b)** Extension into the middle cranial fossa is well seen in this image from the same sequence at a more cranial level (*), along with invasion of the Meckel cave (*arrow*) and cavernous sinus (*white arrowhead*). Tumor surrounds the internal carotid artery, causing mild narrowing. Note the obtuse angles between the tumor and the bone surfaces (*black arrowhead*).

      iii. Langerhans granulomatosis
      iv. Metastasis
      v. Glioma of the brain stem
      vi. Neurofibromatosis
3. Middle ear or mastoid
  a) Infection
      i. Acute or chronic bacterial: Chronic mastoiditis was commonly associated with benign intracranial hypertension due to the contiguous extension of the inflammation to the neighboring sigmoid and lateral sinuses.
      ii. Tuberculosis: Very rare; causes bone destruction without sclerosis.
  b) Trauma (postoperative changes)
  c) Cholesteatoma: Primary cholesteatomas are developmental in origin and less common than the secondary ones that result from inflammatory ear disease; although their x-ray findings are identical. The earliest x-ray sign is partial to complete destruction of the bony ridge or drum spur of the innermost portion of the roof of the external auditory canal in 80% of the cases. More than 95% of cholesteatomas are visible on otoscopic examination. The mastoid antrum is enlarged and may often be sclerotic due to the associated chronic infection. A soft-tissue mass within the tympanic cavity with destruction or demineralization of the ossicular chain may also be seen. These latter x-ray changes may also be seen after involvement of

the tympanic cavity by granulation tissue due to chronic inflammation, in which case are indistinguishable roentgenographically. On CT, cholesteatomas appear as noninvasive, erosive, and well-circumscribed lesions in the temporal bone with scalloped margins. On MR imaging, they usually hypointense on T1WI and hyperintense on T2WI. (▶ Fig. 2.22)

d) Neoplasm
   i. Metastases: Hematogenous from breast, lung, prostate, kidney, other primary neoplasms with osteolytic metastases
   ii. Carcinoma of the middle ear: It is associated with chronic otitis media in 30% of the cases; pain and bleeding appear late. Bone destruction is seen in 12% cases, particularly in the temporal fossa of the temporomandibular joint.
   iii. Glomus jugulare tumor: The jugular foramen is enlarged and destroyed. It is a very vascular lesion.
   iv. Nasopharyngeal tumor invasion.
   v. Rhabdomyosarcoma: This is a tumor of children and young adults with a predilection for the nasopharynx. It may be very vascular and may displace the posterior antral wall forward, thus stimulating angiofibroma. Imaging studies show a bulky soft-tissue mass with areas of bone destruction. Signal intensity is similar to muscle on T1WI but becomes hyperintense on T2WI. Some contrast enhancement is usual.

e) Dermoid cyst

f) Cholesterol granuloma: In the setting of eustachian tube dysfunction, there may be build-up of negative pressure or vacuum phenomenon in the middle ear cavity, leading to mucosal edema and rupture of blood vessels. The breakdown of erythrocytes and tissue elements release cholesterol, which incites a foreign body giant cell reaction leading to formation of a chronic granuloma termed cholesterol granuloma. This lesion is also referred to as a cholesterol cyst, chocolate cyst, or blue-domed cyst. Common locations for this entity include the middle ear and the petrous apex; it can also rarely occur in a mastoidectomy cavity. In the middle ear, patients will present with a blue tympanic membrane, hemotympanum, or conductive hearing loss.

In the petrous apex, an expansile lesion with imperceptible bone margins may be seen on CT scans. On MR images, the characteristic finding is the presence of intrinsic T1 shortening (hyperintensity) due to the presence of blood products. On T2WI, signal intensity is usually heterogeneously hyperintense. A hypointense rim on T2WI may be present, which is believed to represent hemosiderin or a preserved rim of bone. Cholesterol granulomas do not enhance. An important differential diagnosis for this entity is entrapped simple fluid or a petrous apex

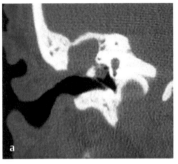
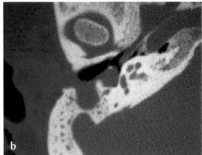
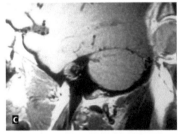

Fig. 2.22 A 76-year-old woman with an epidermoid/cholesteatoma originating in the middle ear and extending into bone at the upper medial external auditory canal (EAC), resulting in an automastoidectomy, which caused extrusion of eroded ossicles out of the external auditory canal. (a) Coronal and (b) axial CT images show absence of the ossicular chain in the middle ear, residual cholesteatoma deep to the tympanic membrane, and bony erosion at the epitympanum and upper medial wall of the right EAC. (Reproduced from Table 1.7 Acquired lesions involving the external auditory canal (EAC). In: Meyers S, ed. Differential Diagnosis in Neuroimaging: Head and Neck. 1st edition. Thieme; 2016.) (c) Cholesteatoma, congenital, petrous pyramid. The cholesteatoma appears in the T2W image as a high signal intensity mass involving the anterior aspect of the petrous pyramid and middle ear cavity. In the sagittal spin-density-weighted sections, the signal intensity is less than in T2W. (Reproduced from Valvassori G. Cholesteatoma of the Middle Ear. In: Valvassori G, Mafee M, Becker M, ed. Imaging of the Head and Neck. 2nd edition. Stuttgart: Thieme; 2004.)

effusion. However, although an effusion may mimic a cholesterol granuloma by way of MR signal characteristics, it does not cause expansion or destruction of the petrous apex air cells, a distinction that is best evaluated with CT.

g) Langerhans granulomatosis

h) Tuberculosis: Rare and may be present without evidence of TB elsewhere. Lytic lesions with no sclerotic margins.

4. Sphenoid wing
   a) Meningioma (CT, MRI)
   b) Benign bone neoplasm (e.g., Chondroma, giant cell tumor)
   c) Chordoma
   d) Craniopharyngioma
   e) Glioma (e.g., optic)
   f) Metastasis
   g) Parasellar aneurysm
   h) Pituitary tumor (e.g., chromophobe adenoma)
   i) Langerhans granulomatosis
   j) Plexiform neurofibroma

2.8 Abnormalities of the Craniovertebral Junction

These abnormalities may involve either the bones and joints, or the meninges and the nervous system, or all of the above.

2.8.1 Congenital anomalies and malformations

1. Malformations of the occipital bone
   a) Manifestations of occipital vertebrae: These are ridges and outgrowths around the bony margins of the foramen magnum. Even though the bony anomaly occurs extracranially at the anterior margin, it is often associated with an abnormal angulation of the craniovertebral junction resulting in a ventral compression of the cervicomedullary junction. This particular anomaly is frequently associated with primary syringomyelia and Chiari malformation.
   b) Basilar invagination: The term *basilar invagination* applies to the primary form of invagination of the margins of the foramen magnum upward into the skull. The roentgenographic diagnosis is based on pathologic features seen on plain x-rays, CT, and MRI. Basilar invagination is often associated with anomalies of the notochord of the cervical spine, i.e., atlanto-occipital fusion, stenosis of foramen magnum, Klippel–Feil syndrome, and maldevelopments of the syringomyelia. The term *basilar impression* applies to the secondary acquired form of basilar invagination that is due to softening of the bone secondary to diseases such as Paget's disease, osteomalacia, hyperparathyroidism, osteogenesis imperfecta, renal rickets, and achondroplasia.

   The term *platybasia* applies to a condition in which the basal angle formed by joining the planes of the clivus and of the anterior cranial fossa is greater than 140°. By itself it causes no symptoms or sings but if associated with basilar invagination then obstructive hydrocephalus may occur. (▶ Fig. 2.23)

c) Condylar hypoplasia: The elevated position of the atlas and axis may lead to vertebral artery compression, compensatory scoliotic changes, and lateral medullary compression.

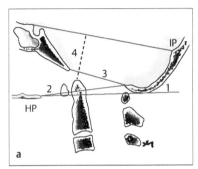
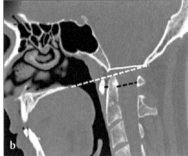
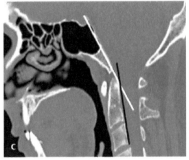

Fig. 2.23 (a) Radiographic criteria for basilar impression. 1: McGregor's line between hard palate (HP) and the lowest point of occiput. Basilar impression is present if the dens protrudes more than 5 mm above this line. 2: Chamberlain's line between hard palate and opisthion. Positive diagnosis if dens protrudes more than 2.5 mm above line. 3: McRae's line between basion and opisthion should be above the dens. 4: Klaus index, distance between tip of dens and the tuberculum-cruciate line between tuberculum (T) and internal occipital protuberance (IP). This measures depth of the posterior fossa. (This image is provided courtesy of Dept of Neurological Surgery, University of California, Davis Sacramento CA, USA. [PangTV@aol.com] **(b, c)** Craniometric measures. (b) *Solid black*: ADI normal is more than 3 mm adults and more than 5 mm children, dotted black: PADI normal is more than 13 mm. *Dotted white*: Chamberlain's line and *solid white*: McRae's line. (c) *White*: Wacken-Heim Clivus line: It should fall tangent to the posterior aspect of the tip of the odontoid. It forms clivus canal angle along the posterior surface of the axis body. (*Continued*)

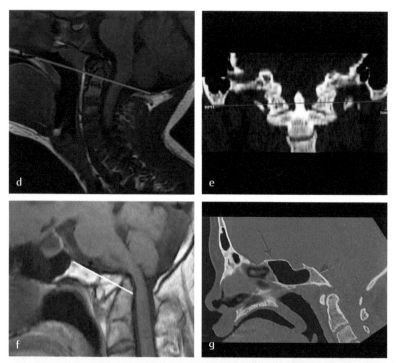

Fig. 2.23 (*Continued*) Basilar invagination. Sagittal T1 W image of the craniocervical junction of a 6-year-old boy shows the primary ossification center of the odontoid process projecting several millimeters above the line between the posterior hard palate and the opisthion (*red line*), with the unossified secondary ossification center of the odontoid apex projecting even further above this line, representing basilar invagination. There is a somewhat sharp angle between the posterior clivus and the posterior cortex of the odontoid process, and there is borderline platybasia as well. Coronal CT showing basilar invagination (**e**). The tip of the dens lies above the bimastoid line. Sagittal CT shows the Wackenheim clivus baseline intersecting the anterior one third of the dens (abnormal) (**f**). Associated platybasia is evident. The Welcher basal angle is >140°. (Reproduced from Anomalies of the Occiput. In: Goel A, Cacciola F, ed. The Craniovertebral Junction. Diagnosis – Pathology – Surgical Techniques. 1st edition. Thieme; 2011.) (**g**) Platybasia. Sagittal bone algorithm computed tomographic image of the skull base and craniocervical junction of a 15-year-old girl demonstrates a wide angle between the planum sphenoidale (*red arrow*) and the dorsal clivus (*red arrowhead*), known as platybasia ("flat base"). (Images d and g are reproduced from Anatomy and Pathology of the Craniocervical Junction. In: Choudhri A, ed. Pediatric Neuroradiology. Clinical Practice Essentials. 1st edition. Thieme; 2016.)

2. Malformations of atlas
   a) Assimilation or occipitalization of atlas: Occurs in 0.25% of the popu-lation and in only 1/4 or 1/3 of the affected population does it cause neurologic symptoms and signs.
   b) Atlanto-axial fusion: Very rare except when associated with Klippel–Feil syndrome.
   c) Aplasia of atlas arches
3. Malformations of the axis
   a) Irregular atlanto-axial segmentation
   b) Dens dysplasias
      i. Ossiculum terminale: Results from the persistence of the summit ossification center; seldom appears before the age of 5 years.
      ii. Os odontoideum: Results from the nonfusion of the epiphyseal plate and separation of the deformed odontoid process from the axial centrum. Increased incidence in patients with Down's syndrome, spondyloepiphyseal dysplasia, and Morquio syndrome. (▶ Fig. 2.24)
      iii. Hypoplasia-aplasia
   c) Segmentation failure of C2–C3

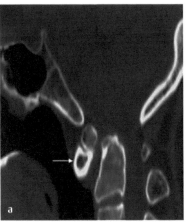 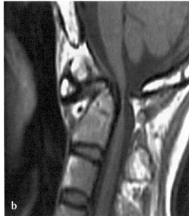

Fig. 2.24 Os Odontoideum. **(a)** Sagittal CT image, **(b)** T1W MRI in a young patient with tetraparesis showing rounded bony fragment lying above and anterior to the base of dens. Dens is hypoplastic, smooth, and well corticated, and anterior arch is hypertrophied (*arrow*) and rounded differentiating the condition from fracture. MRI also showing marked ligament thickening, spinal canal narrowing with cord compression, and myelomalacia.

2.8.2 Developmental and acquired abnormalities

These lesions may be misdiagnosed as: multiple sclerosis (MS) (31%), syringomyelia or syringobulbia (18%), tumor of brain stem or posterior fossa (16%), lesions of the foramen magnum or Arnold–Chiari malformation (13%), cervical fracture or dislocation or cervical disc prolapse (9%), degenerate disease of the spinal cord (6%), cerebellar degeneration (4%), hysteria (3%), or chronic lead poisoning (1%).

Chief complaints of patients with symptom-producing bony anomalies at the craniovertebral junction are: weakness of one or both legs (32%), occipital or suboccipital pain (26%), neck pain or paresthesias (13%), numbness or tingling of fingers (12%), and ataxic gait (9%). The average age of onset of symptoms in such patients is 28 years.

1. Abnormalities at the foramen magnum
   a) Secondary basilar invagination: Such as Paget's disease, osteomalacia, rheumatoid cranial setting.
   b) Foraminal stenosis: Such as achondroplasia, occipital dysplasia, rickets
2. Atlantoaxial instability
   a) Down's syndrome: High incidence of craniovertebral anomalies and increased incidence of general ligamentus laxity may lead to instability in 30–40% of such patients. The usual onset of neurological symptoms is between 7 and 12 years.
   b) Inflammatory
      i. Rheumatoid arthritis (96%): The cervical spine is variably affected in 44–88% of patients from minor symptomatic atlantoaxial subluxation to total incapacity from severe and progressive myelopathy. Autopsies showed that severe atlantoaxial dislocation and high spinal cord compression was the most common cause of sudden death in patients with rheumatoid arthritis. (▶ Fig. 2.25)
      ii. Postinfections (2.5%): Upper respiratory tract infections, mastoiditis, parotitis, tuberculosis.
      iii. Gout (1.5%)
   c) Traumatic lesions of the craniovertebral junction
      i. Occipito-atlantal dislocation: Excessive hyperflexion of the skull with distraction which is usually fatal.
      ii. Atlantoaxial luxations: The anterior predental space is greater than 5 mm indicating that the transverse and alar ligaments are incompetent.
   d) Tumors: Meningiomas, neurinomas, chordomas, dermoids, epidermoids, lipomas, primary bone tumors, metastases, and multiple myelomas.

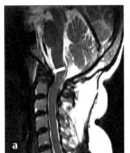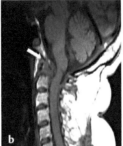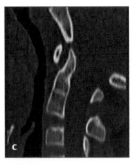

Fig. 2.25 Rheumatoid arthritis (RA). **(a)** Sagittal T2W and **(b)** T1W MRI images showing T2 hypodense and T1 isointense pannus formation (*arrows*) and thickened TAL. There is destruction of odontoid and compression of cervicomedullary junction. **(c)** Reformatted sagittal CT image showing hook shaped odontoid in another patient with RA.

e) Inborn errors of metabolism: Odontoid dysplasia or absence is characteristic in the various types of dwarfism, such as Morquio syndrome, pseudoachondroplastic dysplasia, Scott's syndrome, spondyloepimetaphyseal dysplasia

f) Miscellaneous syndromes: Marfan's syndrome, Hurler's syndrome, neurofibromatosis, and the fetal warfarin syndrome.

2.9 Craniosynostosis

2.9.1 Types (▶Fig. 2.26)

1. Scaphocephaly or dolichocephaly (40–55% of synostosis): Elongated skull from front to back with the biparietal diameter the narrowest part of the skull; e.g., boat or keel-shaped head due to premature closure of the sagittal suture.

2. Trigonocephaly (5–15% of craniosynostosis): Triangular head; angular and pointed forehead with a prominent midline bony ridge due to the premature closure of the metopic suture.

3. Frontal plagiocephaly: Ipsilateral flattened frontal region with a contralateral outward bulging and marked facial asymmetry, "harlequin eye," due to the unilateral coronal suture synostosis. (Plagiocephaly in general constitutes 20–25% of craniosynostosis).

4. Occipital plagiocephaly: Flattening of the involved occipital region with prominence in the ipsilateral frontal region due to the unilateral lambdoid suture synostosis.

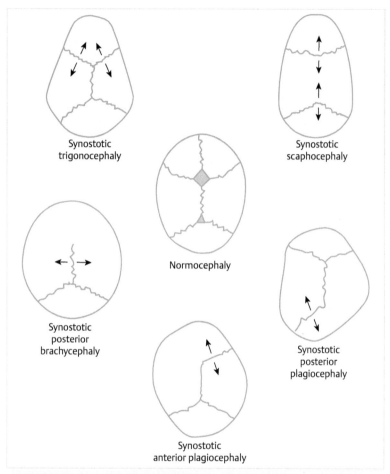

Fig. 2.26 Craniosynostosis. There are numerous types of craniosynostosis each of which involves a different suture or combination of sutures and results in a distinctive head shape

5. Oxycephaly or turricephaly or acrocephaly: Tall and pointed head with overgrowth of bregma and flat, underdeveloped posterior fossa due to the premature closure of the coronal and lambdoid sutures.
6. Brachycephaly: Short, wide, slightly high head due to bilateral coronal suture synostosis.

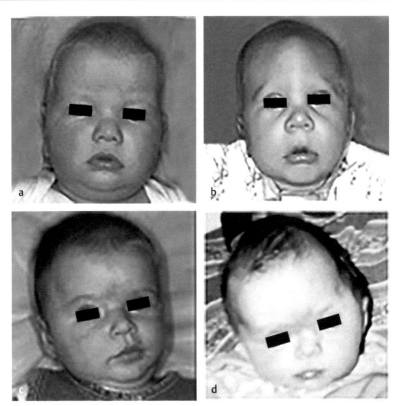

Fig. 2.27 (a) Sagittal suture synostosis, **(b)** metopic suture synostosis, **(c)** coronal suture synostosis, and **(d)** lambdoidal suture synostosis.

7. Triphyllocephaly or cloverleaf head or Kleeblattschädel: Trilobular skull with temporal and frontal bulges due to intrauterine closure of the sagittal, coronal, and lambdoid sutures. (▶ Fig. 2.27)

2.9.2 Associated craniofacial syndromes

1. Crouzon's syndrome: Coronal synostosis, maxillary hypoplasia, shallow orbits with exophthalmos, hypertelorism and often strabismus. Hydrocephalus, mental retardation, seizures, conductive deafness, and optic atrophy may be present. (▶ Fig. 2.28 and ▶ Fig. 2.29)

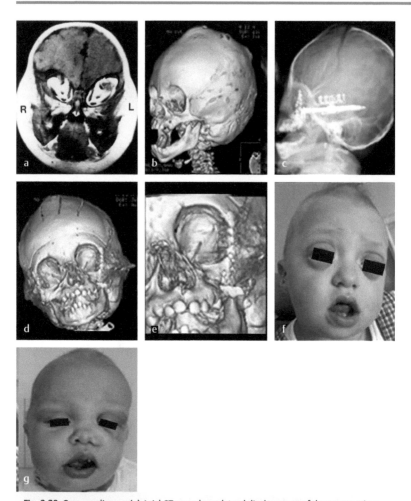

Fig. 2.28 Crouzon disease. **(a)** Axial CT scan shows lateral displacement of the greater wings of the sphenoid, ballooning of the ethmoid complex, and recession of the lateral wall of the orbits. Note increased convolutional markings along the lateral aspect of both temporal fossae. Frontofacial advancement in a baby boy with Crouzon syndrome. (Reproduced from Mafee M. Pathology. In: Valvassori G, Mafee M, Becker M, ed. Imaging of the Head and Neck. 2nd edition. Stuttgart: Thieme; 2004.) **(b)** Preoperative 3D CT. **(c)** Postoperative x-ray image. **(d, e)** Left maxillary fracture. Pictures of the patient **(f)** before and **(g)** after osteodistraction. (Reproduced from 17.3 Outcomes and Postoperative Course. In: Cohen A, ed. Pediatric Neurosurgery: Tricks of the Trade. 1st edition. Thieme; 2015.)

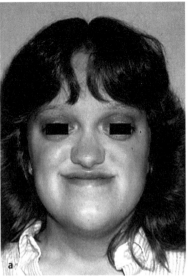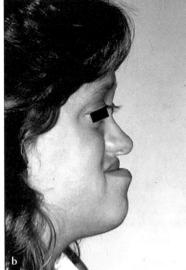

Fig. 2.29 (a, b) Typical appearance of a patient with Crouzon's syndrome, with maxillary retrusion, exorbitism, and pseudoprognathism. (These images are provided courtesy of Chaiyasate K. Craniofacial syndromes. Medscape 1280034.)

2. Apert syndrome or acrocephalosyndactyly: Craniosynostosis most commonly coronal, midfacial hypoplasia, hypertelorism, downslanting of the palpebral features, and strabismus. Associated anomalies include osseous or cutaneous syndactyly, pyloric stenosis, ectopic anus, and pyloric aplasia. (▶ Fig. 2.30 and ▶ Fig. 2.31)

3. Carpenter's syndrome: Brachycephaly, lateral displacement of the inner canthi, brachydactyly of the hands, syndactyly of the feet, and hypogenitalism. (▶ Fig. 2.32)

4. Kleeblattschädel syndrome: Trilobe skull, low set ears, and facial deformities. Dwarfism and aqueductal stenosis and hydrocephalus may be seen.

5. Pfeiffer's syndrome: Brachycephaly, hypertelorism, upslanting palpebral fissures, a narrow maxilla, and broad thumbs and toes (▶ Fig. 2.33 and ▶ Fig. 2.34). Mental retardation, Chiari malformation, and hydrocephalus are often present.

6. Saethre–Chotzen syndrome: Brachycephaly, maxillary hypoplasia, prominent ear crus, syndactyly, and often mental retardation. (▶ Fig. 2.35)

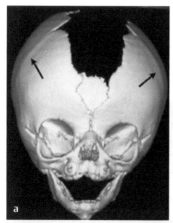
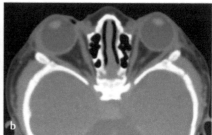

Fig. 2.30 A 5-month-old child with Apert syndrome. **(a)** Coronal volume-rendered CT shows craniosynostosis consisting of premature closure of the coronal suture (*arrows*), resulting in a widened sagittal suture. Also seen is midface hypoplasia/underdevelopment. **(b)** Axial CT shows hypertelorism. (Reproduced from Table 2.1 Congenital and developmental abnormalities. In: Meyers S, ed. Differential Diagnosis in Neuroimaging: Head and Neck. 1st edition. Thieme; 2016.)

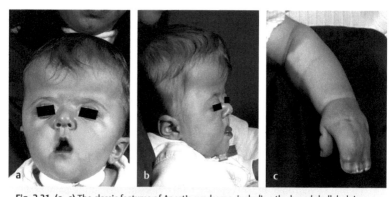

Fig. 2.31 (a–c) The classic features of Apert's syndrome, including the broad skull, bulging the temporal area, and retrusion and vertical shortening of the maxilla. Note hand syndactyly of all fingers. (These images are provided courtesy of Chaiyasate K. Craniofacial syndromes. Medscape 1280034.)

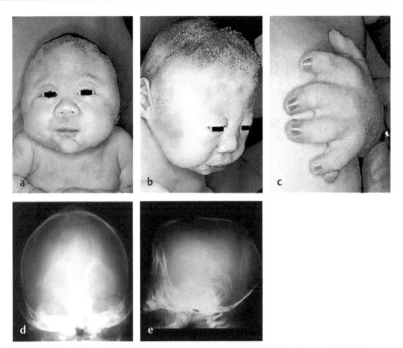

Fig. 2.32 Carpenter's syndrome. **(a, b, c)** In infants with Carpenter's syndrome the facial appearance is similar to that of infants with Apert's syndrome; in addition, there is polysyndactyly. Oblique view shows high steep forehead and turribrachycephaly. **(d, e)** Radiographs show the premature fusion of the coronal sutures and the turribrachycephaly. (These images are provided courtesy of RR school of nursing—Newborns 2016.)

7. Baller–Gerold syndrome: Craniosynostosis, dysplastic ears, and radial aplasia-hypoplasia. Optic atrophy, conductive deafness, and spina bifida occulta may be present.
8. Summitt's syndrome: Craniosynostosis, syndactyly, and gynecomastia.
9. Herrmann–Opitz syndrome: Craniosynostosis, brachysyndactyly, syndactyly of the hands, and absent toes.
10. Herrmann–Pallister–Opitz syndrome: Craniosynostosis, microcrania, cleft lip and palate, symmetrically malformed limbs, and radial aplasia.
11. Moebius syndrome (Congenital facial diplegia): 6th and 7th CN palsy, bilateral facial paralysis, convergent strabismus, micrognathia, high broad nasal bridge, atrophy of tongue, droopy angles of the mouth, mental retardation. MRI demonstrates brainstem hypoplasia and absence of facial colliculus.

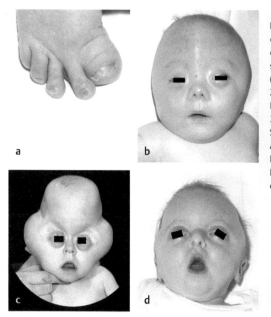

Fig. 2.33 Pfeiffer's syndrome. (a) Typical hallux deformity. (b) Pfeiffer syndrome type 1. (c) Pfeiffer syndrome type 2; cloverleaf pattern. (d) Pfeiffer syndrome type 3. (Reproduced from The Syndromes. In: Albright A, Pollack I, Adelson P, ed. Principles and Practice of Pediatric Neurosurgery. 3rd edition. Thieme; 2014.)

2.9.3 Associated congenital syndromes

1. Achondroplasia (base of skull)
2. Asphyxiating thoracic dysplasia
3. Hypophosphatasia (late)
4. Mucopolysaccharidoses (Hurler's syndrome); mucolipidosis III; fucosidosis
5. Rubella syndrome
6. Trisomy 21 or Down's syndrome
7. Trisomy 18 syndrome
8. Chromosomal syndromes (5p-, 7q+, 13)
9. Adrenogenital syndrome
10. Fetal hydantoin syndrome
11. Idiopathic hypercalcemia or Williams syndrome
12. Meckel syndrome
13. Metaphyseal chondrodysplasia or Jansen syndrome
14. Oculo-mandibulo-facial or Hellermann–Streiff syndrome

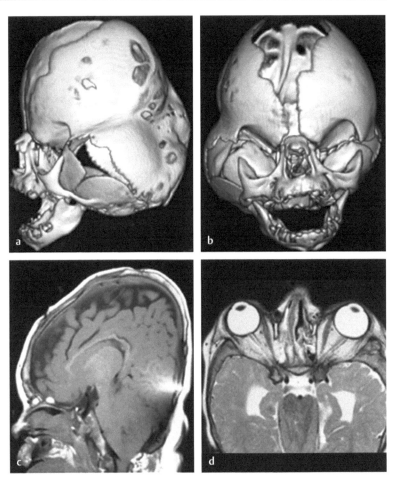

Fig. 2.34 A 1-year-old male with Pfeiffer syndrome 1. **(a)** Lateral and **(b)** coronal volume-rendered CT shows a cloverleaf-shaped skull from premature closure of the coronal and lambdoid sutures, resulting in turri-brachycephaly. Expansion of calvarial bone is seen between sutures. **(c)** Chiari I malformation on sagittal CT and **(d)** hypertelorism on axial CT are also present. (Reproduced from Table 1.1 Congenital and developmental abnormalities involving the skull. In: Meyers S, ed. Differential Diagnosis in Neuroimaging: Head and Neck. 1st edition. Thieme; 2016.)

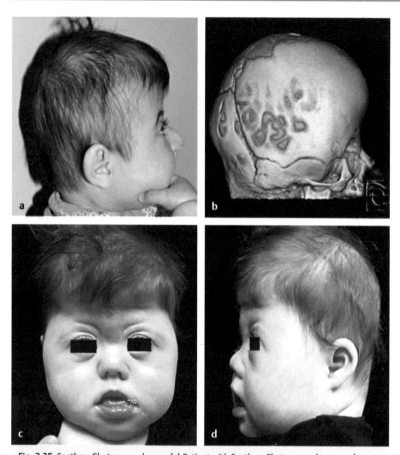

Fig. 2.35 Saethre–Chotzen syndrome. **(a)** Patient with Saethre–Chotzen syndrome and bicoronal synostosis resulting in significant turribrachycephaly. The sagittal, lambdoid, and squamosal sutures were patent with a large fontanelle, characteristic of Saethre–Chotzen syndrome. **(b)** Initial 3D CT volume rendering show bicoronal craniosynostosis. **(c, d)** Six month old with Saethre–Chotzen syndrome. Note the high forehead, low hairline, shallow eye orbits, and beak-shaped nose. The craniosynostosis had resulted in retrusion above the eyes and a tall short head shape. (These images are provided courtesy of Bartlett-Taylor 2014-Children's Hospital, Philadelphia.)

2.9.4 Associated disorders

1. Rickets
2. Hyperthyroidism
3. Hypocalcemia
4. Polycythemia
5. Thalassemia

2.10 Macrocephaly/Macrocrania

Macrocephaly refers to large cranial vault.

1. Thickened skull
   a) Thalassemia or anemias with increased marrow activity
   b) Rickets
   c) Osteopetrosis
   d) Osteogenesis imperfecta
   e) Epiphyseal dysplasia
2. Hydrocephalus
   a) Noncommunicating/congenital: Aqueduct stenosis, stenosis of the foramen of Monro causing asymmetrical enlargement, Dandy–Walker cyst, Chiari malformation.
   b) Communicating/acquired
      i. Meningeal fibrosis (postinflammatory, posthemorrhagic, posttraumatic)
      ii. Malformation, destructive lesions (hydranencephaly, holoprosencephaly, porencephaly).
      iii. Choroid plexus papilloma.
3. Extra-axial fluid collection
   a) Subdural effusion/hygroma
   b) Subdural hematoma
4. Brain edema
   a) Toxic: e.g., lead encephalopathy
   b) Endocrine: e.g., hypoparathyroidism, galactosemia
5. Megalencephaly (refers to a large brain)
6. Familial macrocephaly
7. Congenital syndromes
   a) Chondrodystrophies: e.g., achondroplasia, achondrogenesis, thanatophoric dwarfism and metaphoric dwarfism, cleidocranial dysplasia, Soto's syndrome.

b) Mucopolysaccharidoses: e.g., Hurler, Hunter, Morquio, GM gangliosidosis.

c) Neurocutaneous syndrome: e.g., neurofibromatosis, tuberous sclerosis.

2.11 Microcephaly/Microcrania

1. Perinatal damage: e.g., cortical atrophy from hypoxia or ischemia.
2. Craniosynostosis
3. Encephalocele
4. Genetic abnormalities
   a) Familial microcephaly: Autosomal, recessive, and X-linked.
   b) Hereditary nonchromosomal syndromes: e.g., Fanconi syndrome, Prader–Willi syndrome, Seckel syndrome, Rubinstein–Taybi syndrome.
5. Metabolic abnormalities
   a) Neonatal hypoglycemia
   b) Phenylketonuria
   c) Aminoaciduria
   d) Homocystinuria
6. Chromosomal abnormalities
   a) Trisomy 21 (Down's syndrome)
   b) Trisomy 18
   c) Trisomy 13–15
   d) Cat cry syndrome (5p-)
7. Intrauterine injury or infection
   a) Radiation
   b) Infection: e.g., toxoplasmosis, rubella, cytomegalic inclusion disease, herpes simplex (TORCH)
   c) Diabetes
   d) Uremia
   e) Malnutrition
   f) Fetal alcohol syndrome
   g) Maternal phenytoin use
8. Miscellaneous
   a) Chronic cardiopulmonary disease
   b) Chronic renal disease
   c) Xeroderma pigmentosa

2.12 Pneumocephalus

1. Trauma: e.g., penetrating injury or fracture of the ethmoid, frontal, or of the mastoid sinuses is most common.

2. Iatrogenic: e.g., postoperative, pneumoencephalography, ventriculography.
3. Brain abscess (infection with gas-forming organisms).
4. Neoplasm of base of skull
    a) Osteoma (if it erodes cribriform plate)
    b) Nasopharyngeal/ethmoid carcinoma

2.13 Small Pituitary Fossa

1. Normal variant
2. Hypopituitarism; growth hormone deficiency
3. Decreased intracranial pressure: e.g., brain atrophy, shunted hydrocephalus
4. Fibrous dysplasia
5. Radiotherapy during childhood
6. Dystrophia myotonica: Hereditary, affecting early adult life and being associated with cataracts, testicular atrophy, frontal baldness, thick skull, and large frontal sinus
7. Deprivational dwarfism
8. Trisomy 21 (Down's syndrome)

2.14 Enlarged Pituitary Fossa

2.14.1 Intrasellar, parasellar, or juxtasellar masses

1. Neoplastic disorders
    a) Pituitary adenoma: e.g., chromophobe, eosinophilic; the basophilic virtually never expands.
    b) Craniopharyngioma
    c) Meningioma
    d) Hypothalamic/chiasmatic gliomas
    e) Clival lesions: e.g., metastases, chordomas
    f) Teratomas including dysgerminoma
    g) Epidermoid and dermoid cysts
2. Nonneoplastic disorders
    a) Nonneoplastic cysts: e.g., Rathke's cleft cyst, mucocele, arachnoid cyst.
    b) Vascular lesions: e.g., aneurysm or ectasia of the cavernous or suprasellar segment of the internal carotid artery (ICA) and caroticocavernous fistula.
    c) Inflammatory disorders: e.g., abscesses, sarcoidosis, histiocytosis, lymphoid adenohypophysitis.

2.14.2 Empty sella

1. Primary syndrome: Due to a deficiency in the diaphragma sella and associated herniation of the subarachnoid space into the sella turcica which allows pulsating CSF to expand the sella. Associated with benign intracranial hypertension.
2. Secondary: The result of prior operation or radiation therapy of usually a pituitary tumor.

2.14.3 Raised intracranial pressure, chronic

Obstructive hydrocephalus, dilated third ventricle, neoplasm, craniosynostosis are some examples.

2.15 Suprasellar and Parasellar Lesions

Most frequent suprasellar masses are: suprasellar extension of pituitary adenoma, meningioma, craniopharyngioma, hypothalamic/chiasmatic glioma, and aneurysm. These five entities account for more than three-fourth of all sellar/juxtasellar masses. Metastases, meningitis, and granulomatous diseases account for another 10%. Other suprasellar masses are uncommon, each is seen in less than 1–2% of all cases.

2.15.1 Neoplastic lesions

The two most common suprasellar tumor masses in adults are suprasellar extension of pituitary adenoma and meningioma; whereas in children, craniopharyngiomas and hypothalamic/chiasmatic glioma are common. (▶ Fig. 2.36)

1. Pituitary tumor
   a) Pituitary adenoma: Autopsy series indicate that asymptomatic microadenomas account for 14–27% of cases, pars intermedia cysts for 13–22%, and occult metastatic lesions for 5% of patients with known malignancy. The primary source of pituitary metastases in descending order of frequency is:
      i. Women: Breast cancer is by far the most common, accounting for over half of all secondary pituitary tumors followed by lung, stomach, and uterus cancers.
      ii. Men: Most frequent primary tumors are neoplasms of the lung, followed by prostate, bladder, stomach, and pancreas. Suprasellar extension accounts for 30–50% of all suprasellar masses, e.g., chromophobe or eosinophilic; the basophilic virtually never expands. On CT, the microadenoma (< 10 mm) is of low density compared with the normal gland, with or without enhancement. On MRI,

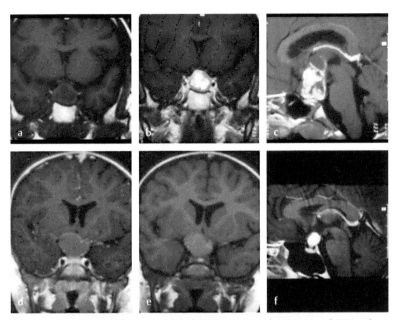

Fig. 2.36 Suprasellar lesions (neoplastic). **(a, b)** Pituitary macroadenoma, coronal T1WI with a pituitary macroadenoma in close relationship with the optic chiasm presenting a heterogeneous, postcontrast high-intensity signal. **(c)** Pituitary macroadenoma, sagittal T1WI shows a pituitary tumor with a heterogeneous postcontrast high-intensity signal with cystic and/or necrotic features in its posterior section filling the suprasellar cisterns and exerting compression on the optic chiasm. **(d, e)** Craniopharyngioma., a suprasellar space-occupying mass with no postcontrast enhancement on coronal T1WI. **(f)** Meningioma, sagittal T1WI shows a suprasellar space-occupying neoplastic lesion with a postcontrast high-intensity signal showing an unusual development alongside the pituitary stalk. (*Continued*)

the microadenomas are generally hypointense compared with the normal gland on T1WI and display a variable intensity on T2WI. Macroadenomas have roughly the same signal characteristics as microadenomas, although these have a propensity for hemorrhage and infarction because of their poor blood supply. Cystic areas produce low intensity on T1WI and high intensity on T2WI. Nowadays MRI has assumed a major role in the evaluation of adenomas of the pituitary. It locates deformation of the optic tracks, chiasm, and optic nerves, and also demonstrates invasion of the cavernous sinuses or the surrounding structures by neoplasms. MRI is particularly helpful in outlining blood vessels and ruling out aneurysms.

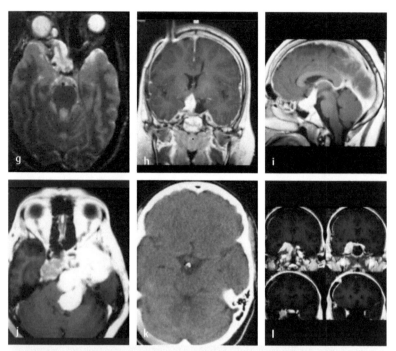

Fig. 2.36 (*Continued*) **(g)** Optic nerve glioma, axial T2WI shows a right optic nerve glioma with widening of the optic foramen in a patient with neurofibromatosis type I. **(h, i)** Pilocytic astrocytoma, a highly enhanced mass, occupying part of the sella and the suprasellar cisterns and extending behind the optic chiasm, is seen on coronal and sagittal T1WI respectively. **(j)** Chordoma, axial T1WI demonstrates a multilobular space-occupying neoplastic lesion which is heterogeneously and highly enhanced, developing into the left parasellar region and ipsilateral temporal and posterior fossae along the ridge of the petrous bone. **(k)** Dermoid tumor, calcification with elements of fat in the retrochiasmatic suprasellar cisterns. **(l)** Meningioma, coronal T1WI shows a postcontrast highly enhancing neoplastic lesion of the right cavernous sinus.

    b) Pituitary carcinoma or carcinosarcoma
    c) Granular cell tumor of the pituitary or choristoma
2. Craniopharyngiomas: These account for 20% of tumors in the adult and 54% in children. Three neuroimaging hallmarks have been identified which may be present from none to all of these in an individual lesion: (1) Calcification in 80% of cases, (2) cyst formation observed in 85% of cases, and (3) solid or nodular enhancement. MRI is relatively insensitive to calcification and can

have a variable intensity to cystic fluid, and it is not as specific as CT for the diagnosis of calcification and the low-density appearance of cyst formation.

3. Meningiomas: They represent 15–20% of all primary intracranial tumors and are the second most frequent suprasellar neoplasm in adults. Rarely, meningiomas may arise from the parasellar lateral wall of the cavernous sinus and extend posteriorly along the tentorial margin with a dovetail appearance. Extra-axial mass is non-cystic and heterogenous in texture which on CT imaging reveals hyperostosis, blistering of the tuberculum and erosion of the dorsum sellae. On T1W1 these are isointense and on T2W1 isointense to slightly hyperintense to brain, enhancing dramatically.

4. Hypothalamic and optic nerve/chiasm gliomas: These are the second most common paediatric suprasellar tumors and account for 25–30% of such cases. Bilateral optic nerve gliomas are associated with neurofibromatosis type I in 20–50% of these patients. On CT, these are isointense to hypointense and frequently enhance following contrast injection. On MRI, these lesions are hypointense on T1WI and hyperintense on T2WI. The MRI may show no contrast enhancement, variable enhancement, or intense uniform enhancement. The contrast pattern does not correlate with the pathological grade of the tumors.

5. Dermoid tumors: They are midline tumors found most commonly in the posterior fossa and only rarely in the suprasellar region. Imaging reflects the high fat content of these lesions. Calcification is relatively common. CT shows a hypodense lesion. The signals on MRI reflect a higher fat content than that of the brain. These tumors with the lipomas are two uncommon causes of suprasellar "bright spots."

6. Epidermoid tumors or "pearly tumors": These are located along the cisterns in the CPA or in the parasellar area and elsewhere as in the fourth ventricle, lateral ventricles, cerebrum, cerebellum, and brain stem. The CT appearance of epidermoids is that of low-density lesions that do not enhance with contrast. The MRI appearance is hypointense compared to brain on T1WI and hyperintense on the T2WI.

7. Teratomas and teratoid tumors including dysgerminomas: These are found in the pineal, intra- or suprasellar, and the sacrococcygeal region. Teratomas include tissues from all three germ cell layers. MRI demonstrates an infiltrating mass isointense to brain on T1WI, moderately hyperintense on protein density WI and T2WI. Homogeneous enhancement is common in both CT and MR studies.

8. Lipomas: Most intracranial lipomas are considered as congenital abnormalities rather than neoplasms. The most common sites are the interhemispheric fissure (50%), the quadrigeminal cistern and pineal region, the suprasellar cistern, and CPA cistern. CT imaging shows attenuation values

that are in the negative range, usually 30 to 100 HU, and are isodense to subcutaneous fat. MRI demonstrates lipomas high in intensity on T1WI and intermediate to low on T2WI.

9. Metastases: Represent approximately 1% of sellar and parasellar masses.
   a) Hematogenous spread: The most frequent metastatic lesions in this region from systemic primary cancer come from lung, breast, and prostate.
   b) Perineural spread
      i. Head and neck tumors may demonstrate perineural spread through the foramen at the skull base into the brain; e.g., basal cell carcinoma, melanoma, adenoid cystic carcinoma, schwannoma, lymphoma.
      ii. Infections; e.g., actinomycosis, Lyme disease, herpes zoster. Metastases are typically isointense on T1WI and moderately hyperintense on T2WI. Moderate enhancement occurs after gadolinium injection.

10. Chondrosarcoma: Rare tumor arising from embryonal rests, endochondral bone, or cartilage and located at the skull base, parasellar region, in the meninges, or in the brain. CT demonstrates the calcified (in 60% of cases) mass and enhancing neoplastic tissue. MRI shows the enhanced mas. The CT is probably more specific for this tumor because of its sensitivity to calcium.

11. Lymphoproliferative disorders
    a) Lymphoma: Intra- and suprasellar component. May involve the pituitary gland, hypothalamus, infundibular stalk in older adults.
    b) Granulocytic sarcoma or chloroma: Primitive myeloid cell tumor; rarely involving the CNS.

12. Olfactory neuroblastoma

13. Trigeminal schwannoma: Rare tumors (0.4% of brain tumors) arising most commonly from the parasellar region of the Gasserian ganglion or the posterior fossa. On CT imaging, particularly with bone windows, erosion can be demonstrated at the petrous apex. On MRI, they are smooth masses, isointense on T1WI and high intensity on T2WI with avid enhancement and intratumoral "cystic" changes observed within the enhancing mass.

2.15.2 Nonneoplastic lesions

1. Nonneoplastic cysts (▶ Fig. 2.37)
   a) Rathke's cleft cyst: These are benign cysts containing mucous protein, arising from Rathke's pouch and located in the anterior sellar and/or anterior suprasellar region. Resemble craniopharyngiomas, which calcify. CT is useful here because of its sensitivity to calcification as compared to MRI. The MRI of these lesions demonstrates a variable intensity depending on the cyst contents and these lesions enhance much less than craniopharyngiomas.

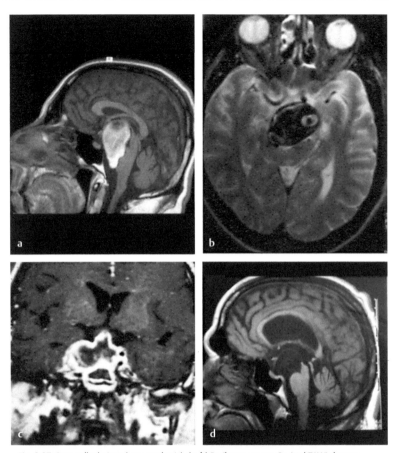

Fig. 2.37 Suprasellar lesions (nonneoplastic). **(a, b)** Basilar aneurysm. Sagittal T1WI shows a partially thrombosed (flow void appearance) giant aneurysm of the tip of the basilar artery extending retrochiasmatically into the suprasellar cisterns compressing the brain stem. **(c)** Pituitary bacterial abscess: Coronal T1WI demonstrates a sellar/suprasellar ring enhancing lesion containing necrotic fluid. **(d)** Arachnoid cyst: Sagittal T1WI with a retrochiasmatic cyst extending into the suprasellar cisterns with an intensity signal identical to that of cerebrospinal fluid.

b) Sphenoid sinus mucoceles: Mucoceles are most common in the frontal and ethmoidal sinuses, with sphenoid sinus mucoceles the least common. CT demonstrates an isodense smooth mass (with an enhancing ring). MRI manifests variable intensities depending on the protein concentration and viscosity but mostly are hyperintense on T1WI and T2WI with peripheral (not solid as in neoplasms) enhancement.

c) Arachnoid or leptomeningeal cysts: Approximately 15% of all arachnoid cysts occur in the suprasellar region. They enlarge and produce mass effects on adjacent structures. CT density and MR intensities of these cysts are those of CSF; they are not associated with enhancement or calcification. Cisternography can be helpful in differentiating these cysts from an ependymal cyst of the third ventricle or an enlarged third ventricle due to aqueduct stenosis.

2. Vascular lesions
   a) Aneurysms of the cavernous or suprasellar portion of the ICA or anterior communicating artery (ACoA): MRI is variable, depending on the presence and age of thrombus.
      i. The typical patent aneurysm lumen with rapid flow is seen as a well-delineated suprasellar mass that shows high-velocity signal loss (flow void) on T1WI and T2WI.
      ii. The completely thrombosed aneurysms may show variable MR findings. Subacute thrombus is predominately hyperintense on T1WI and T2WI images. Multilayer clots can be seen in thrombosed aneurysms that have undergone repeated episodes of intramural hemorrhage. Acutely thrombosed aneurysms may be isointense with brain parenchyma and difficult to differentiate from other intracranial masses.
   b) Vascular ectasias
   c) Cavernous hemangiomas: Located in Meckel's cave and in the cavernous sinus. Due to lack of a hemosiderin rim, central large hemorrhage and calcification is extremely difficult to diagnose with MRI.
   d) Caroticocavernous fistula or dural malformation
   e) Cavernous sinus thrombosis: May occur following a septic process, after an interventional procedure or postsurgery. CT manifests an irregular filling defect in an irregularly enhancing sinus. MRI without enhancement demonstrates a high intensity in the occluded sinus; enhancement is not helpful because nonthrombosed regions of the sinus enhance, and blood clot is also high in intensity.

3. Infectious/inflammatory lesions
   a) Parasitic infections: Cysticercosis and echinococcus parasitic cysts in this region are usually inhomogeneous and may be calcified.
   b) Abscesses: This can occur after surgery but also in situations that predispose to bacterial infection, including sinusitis. Exudative bacterial meningitis and tuberculous meningitis have a predilection for the basal subarachnoid spaces.

c) Granulomatous disease: Giant cell granuloma, sarcoidosis, and syphilis can affect the pituitary and suprasellar region often causing hypopituitarism and rarely diabetes insipidus.

d) Langerhans granulomatosis: e.g., Hand–Schüller–Christian and Letterer–Siwe diseases. Cranial involvement occurs in more than 90% of patients, who present with diabetes insipidus, and thickened and enhancing infundibular stalk with or without hypothalamic mass.

e) Lymphoid adenohypophysitis or lymphocytic hypophysitis: A rare inflammatory process affecting the anterior pituitary gland causing hypopituitarism and an expanding suprasellar mass. Affects women during late pregnancy or postpartum period. Imaging findings are nonspecific and resemble macroadenoma.

2.16 Intracranial Calcifications (ICC)

Refer to ▶ Fig. 2.38 and ▶ Fig. 2.39.

2.16.1 Physiological

Physiologic calcification is extremely rare below the age of 9 years old. For example, physiologic calcification in the pineal gland and choroid plexuses happens in only 2% of children below 9 years of age but increases fivefold by 15 years and is common in adults.

1. Pineal gland: In about 60% of all persons over 20 years of age.
2. Habenula: About 30% of all persons
3. Choroid plexus: Usually seen in the glomus and is bilateral.
4. Dura: e.g., falx, superior sagittal sinus, tentorium, petroclinoid ligaments, and diaphragma sellae.

2.16.2 Familial, congenital, or metabolic

1. Sturge–Weber syndrome: "Railroad track" type of calcification. (See ▶ Fig. 2.40)
2. Tuberous sclerosis: Calcification is seen most commonly centrally or near the lateral ventricles in nearly 50% of the patients.
3. Basal ganglion and dentate nucleus calcification
4. Lissencephaly: Calcification in a small nodule in the roof of the cavum septi pellucidi just behind the foramen of Monro.
5. Pseudoxanthoma elasticum: calcification of the dura, thickening of the cranial vault and platybasia.
6. Congenital cerebral granuloma

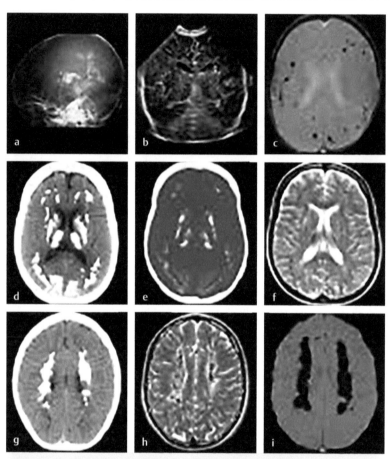

Fig. 2.38 The identification of intracranial calcification (ICC) using different imaging modalities. (Read from top left to right) **(a)** Dense calcification is readily apparent on a plain-film skull radiograph. **(b)** Ultrasound image of a child with congenital cytomegalovirus infection. ICC is readily seen as highly echogenic areas in the left periventricular region. **(c)** Gradient echo axial MRI of an infant with congenital toxoplasmosis showing multiple low-signal spots within the cortex and white matter. The spatial resolution is poor in gradient echo images. Different imaging modalities provide complementary information. **(d)** CT image at normal brain window settings, **(e)** CT image at bony window settings, and **(f)** T2-weighted axial MRI of the same patient. The location of ICC may be difficult to determine on normal brain window settings **(d)**, whereas on the bone window settings **(e)** the cortical location is apparent. This is confirmed on the T2-weighted MR **(f)** by the low-signal ribbon seen at the depths of the gyri. **(g)** CT, **(h)** T2-weighted axial MRI, and **(i)** susceptibility-weighted axial MRI from the same patient illustrating the differing appearances of ICC depending on the modality used.

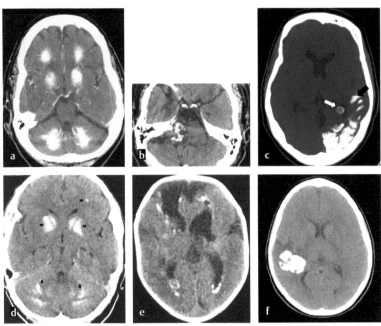

Fig. 2.39 **(a)** Hypoparathyroidism and ocular calcification. Axial CT scan shows marked calcification of the cerebellar dentate nuclei and supratentorial basal ganglia. **(b)** Epidermoid cyst. CT scan shows an intradural CPA epidermoid cyst. On rare occasions epidermoid like this may show calcification. (Reproduced from Mafee M. Pathology. In: Valvassori G, Mafee M, Becker M, ed. Imaging of the Head and Neck. 2nd edition. Stuttgart: Thieme; 2004.) **(c)** Computed tomography (CT) of the head without contrast shows multiple calcifications in the left parietal and occipital lobes (*black arrow*). There is calcification of an enlarged choroid plexus in the left atrium (*white arrow*). (Reproduced from Case 213. A 29-year-old man with a history of progressive seizures and right-sided hemiparesis since childhood. The visual acuity on the left is severely decreased. In: Riascos R, Bonfante E, ed. RadCases Plus Q&A: Neuro Imaging. 2nd edition. Thieme; 2018.) **(d)** Axial computed tomography image shows dense bilateral calcification of the basal ganglia, cerebellum, and left cerebral subcortical white matter (*black arrows*). (Reproduced from Endocrine Dysfunction. In: Kanekar S, ed. Imaging of Neurodegenerative Disorders. 1st edition. Thieme; 2015.) **(e)** An 8-day-old male with prenatal cytomegalovirus infection resulting in diffuse and focal zones of brain encephalomalacia, with dilated lateral ventricles, porencephaly involving the right frontal lobe, schizencephaly involving the left cerebral hemisphere, and multiple intra-axial calcifications as seen on axial CT. (Reproduced from Introduction. In: Meyers S, ed. Differential Diagnosis in Neuroimaging: Brain and Meninges. 1st edition. Thieme; 2016.) **(f)** Noncontrast head computed tomography (CT) scan of a paediatric patient with a right temporoparietal oligodendroglioma. Note the significant hyperdensity consistent with calcification and some underlying hypodensity that likely represents tumor. There is also mild peritumoral edema anterior to the lesion with essentially no mass effect on the surrounding parenchyma. (Reproduced from Radiographic Presentation. In: Keating R, Goodrich J, Packer R, ed. Tumors of the Pediatric Central Nervous System. 2nd edition. Thieme; 2013.)

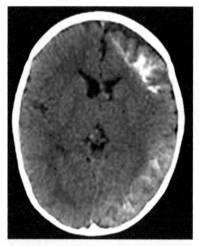

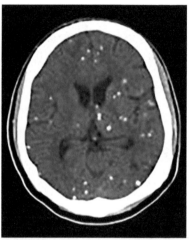

Fig. 2.40 Sturge–Weber syndrome. Characteristic gyral calcifications in Sturge–Weber syndrome.

Fig. 2.41 Neurocysticercosis.

2.16.3 Inflammatory disorders

1. Bacterial infections
   a) Tuberculosis: Tuberculous granuloma, healed meningitis.
   b) Pyogenic infections: Calcification occurs late following a healed brain abscess, purulent meningitis, or other pyogenic intracranial infection.
   c) Syphilitic granuloma or gumma
2. Parasitic infestations
   a) Cysticercosis: Cysts of the *Taenia solium* form in the basal cisterns or brain in 5% of infections. Only the dead cysts calcify.
   b) Hydatid cysts: Only 2% of infections produce cysts in the brain and these rarely calcify. (See ▸ Fig. 2.41)
   c) Paragonimiasis: Cysts of the oriental lung fluke occur commonly in the posterior parts of the cerebral hemispheres. Massive regions of calcification may be seen.
3. Fungal disease: Cryptococcosis, coccidioidomycosis.

2.16.4 Vascular

1. Arterial aneurysms
   a) Giant aneurysms: show curvilinear calcification outlining part of the aneurysmal sac in 50% of cases.

b) Dilatation of the vein of Galen: In older children or adults, a ring-like calcification may be seen in the region of the pineal gland.
2. Arteriovenous malformation: Curvilinear, amorphous and patchy, or nodular calcifications are seen in 6–29% of cases.
3. Intracranial hemorrhage
   a) Chronic subdural hematoma: 1–5% cases calcify.
   b) Extradural hematoma: Calcification rarely occurs.
4. Arteriosclerotic vascular disease: Especially at the carotid siphon

2.16.5 Neoplasm

1. Glioma: Overall 9–10% calcify; 6% of astrocytomas and 47% of oligodendro-gliomas. Grade I gliomas show 25% incidence of calcification and grade IV show 2% incidence. Ependymomas showed calcification in 15% of cases. Calcification is seen only in 1% in medulloblastomas.
2. Craniopharyngioma: The incidence of calcification in most series varies between 55 – 94%. Calcification is less likely in older patients.
3. Chordoma: About 15% show some amorphous or nodular calcification.
4. Chondroma and osteochondroma: Dense and nodular calcification in the ethmoid or sphenoid air cells or the CPA.
5. Meningioma: In most series, a variable appearance calcification has been reported in 6–9% of cases.
6. Pituitary adenoma: Approximately 6% show calcification commonly in the posteroinferior surface of the tumor.
7. Brain metastasis: Calcification is found in about 2% of all patients with brain metastasis.
   a) Mucinous adenocarcinoma
      i. Colon
      ii. Stomach
      iii. Ovary
      iv. Breast
   b) Osteocarcinoma
   c) Chondrosarcoma
8. Pinealoma: About 50% of pinealomas show a dense and homogeneous or scattered calcification.
9. Choroid plexus papilloma: About 20% show calcification; most common site is the fourth ventricle in children and the temporal horn in adults.
10. Dermoid and epidermoid tumors and teratoma: Calcification is rare in the dermoid and epidermoid tumors, but common in teratomas.
11. Lipoma of the corpus callosum: Characteristically two curvilinear bands of calcification, one on each side of the corpus callosum.
12. Hamartoma: Usually in the temporal lobe.
13. Neoplasms post radiotherapy.

2.17 Calcifications of the Basal Ganglia

Basal ganglia calcifications are seen in 0.6% of CT scans (▶ Fig. 2.42). They affect usually the globus pallidus, and are bilateral and symmetric, but can be unilateral. These lesions are mainly idiopathic and are often associated with *Dentate nuclei calcification*.

1. Idiopathic: These account for more than 50% of cases and can be familial.
2. Disorders of calcium metabolism: hyperparathyroidism, hypoparathyroidism, and pseudohypoparathyroidism.
3. Fahr's disease: It is also known as familial cerebrovascular ferrocalcinosis and characterized by microcephaly, spasticity, epilepsy, progressive deterioration of nervous system, and fine iron and calcium deposits in the basal ganglia, dentate nuclei, and periventricular areas.
4. Parasitic disease: Toxoplasmosis, cysticercosis. About half the cases of congenital toxoplasmosis result in intracranial calcification, such as in caudate nucleus, choroid plexus, ependyma.
5. Radiation therapy (mineralization microangiography).
6. Tuberous sclerosis.
7. Trisomy 21 (Down's syndrome).
8. Encephalitis (i.e. rubella, measles, chickenpox).
9. Birth anoxia.
10. Carbon monoxide intoxication.
11. Methotrexate therapy.
12. Lead toxicity.
13. Addison's disease.
14. Leigh's disease.
15. Neurofibromatosis.
16. Cockayne syndrome.

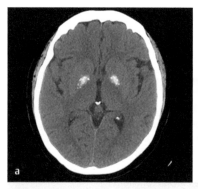 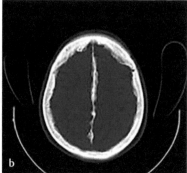

Fig. 2.42 (a) Calcification of basal ganglia. (b) Calcification of falx cerebri.

2.18 Parasellar Calcification

1. Neoplastic
   a) Craniopharyngioma
   b) Meningioma
   c) Pituitary adenoma (chromophobe)
   d) Chordoma
   e) Optic chiasm glioma
   f) Cholesteatoma
2. Vascular
   a) Aneurysm (circle of Willis or basilar artery)
   b) Atheroma (carotid siphon)
3. Infective
   a) Tuberculous meningitis (calcification in the basal meninges)

2.19 Posterior Fossa Tumors

Following table shows differentiation among medulloblastoma, ependymoma, and astrocytoma based on radiological characteristics. (▶ Fig. 2.43)

Radiological characteristic	Astrocytoma	Ependymoma	Medulloblastoma
CT scan (enhancement)	Hypodense (nodule enhances; cyst does not)	Isodense (minimal)	Hyperdense (moderate)
T1W1	Hypointense	Hypointense	Hypointense
T2WI	Hyperintense	Isointense	Isointense
Location	Eccentric	Midline	Midline
Origin	Cerebral hemisphere	Fourth ventricle, ependymoma	Fourth ventricle, superior medullary velum
Calcification	Uncommon (< 10%)	Common (40–50%)	Uncommon (< 10–15%)
Cystic degeneration	Typical	Common	Rare
Hemorrhage	Uncommon	Common	Uncommon (> 10%)
Subarachnoid seeding	Very rare	Common	Very common (25–50%)
Hydrocephalus	Unusual	Common	Very common
Fourth ventricle appearance	Unaffected	Enlargement (shape unaffected)	Distortion (posteroinferiorly)
Age (years)	10–12	2–10 & 40	5–12

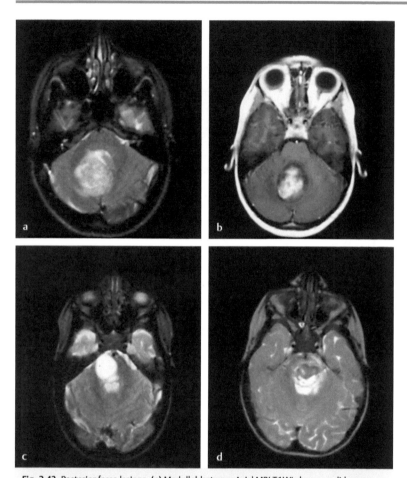

Fig. 2.43 Posterior fossa lesions. **(a)** Medulloblastoma: Axial MRI T1WI shows a solid space-occupying lesion with a moderate signal intensity on T2WI which occupies the area behind the fourth ventricle exerting pressure on it. **(b)** Ependymoma: Axial MRI T1WI shows a multi-lobular space-occupying lesion with solid features which are enhanced without homogeneity and cystic features in the periphery and focal calcifications. **(c)** Pilocytic astrocytoma of the brain stem on axial MRI T1WI with well-delineated margins and a highly pathological signal; mild compression on the fourth ventricle. **(d)** Chronic hematoma within a ruptured cavernous hemangioma of the pons in a child. Axial T2WI with a heterogeneous signal of a parenchymal lesion within the pons. This lesion displaces the fourth ventricle and is characterized by low and high intensity and surrounding edema.

2.20 Postoperative Brain Scar versus Residual Brain Tumor

There is nothing more infuriating to a neurosurgeon than a postoperative CT scan or MRI showing residual tumor after its supposedly "complete resection." Granulation tissue, which enhances on CT and MR scanning because of its fibrovascular nature, develops 72 hours after surgery. Therefore, it becomes difficult to differentiate between an enhancing surgical bed tissue and marginal residual tumor, provided that there was a preoperative tumor enhancement. The scan enhancement may persist for several months postoperatively, therefore, neurosurgeons scan their patients within 48 hours of operation. Scan enhancement in the surgical site within 48 hours should be compatible with a residual tumor.

Radiological characteristic	Postoperative scar	Residual tumor
Contrast enhancement		
Within 48–72 hours	No	Yes
After 48–72 hours	Yes	Yes
Type of enhancement	Linear (at the periphery of the preoperative tumor bed area)	Solid and nodular (within the tumor bed area)
Peritumoral edema (with time)	Decreases	Increases
Change in size (with time)	Stays the same or decreases	Increases
Blood (in the tumor bed area)	Resolves while the granulation tissue stays the same or decreases	May be present while the residual tumor mass increases

2.21 Differential Diagnosis of Infarction versus Mass (Tumor, Abscess)

Even though their pathophysiologies are completely different, it can sometimes be difficult to differentiate an ischemic infarct from a mass lesion, such as neoplasm or abscess on imaging studies. Many nontumorous lesions can mimic a brain tumor. Abscesses can mimic metastases. MS can present with a mass-like lesion with enhancement, also known as tumefactive MS. In the parasellar region, one should always consider the possibility of an aneurysm.

Some of these features are shown in the following table.

Imaging features	Infarction	Mass lesion
Vascular distribution	Single arterial distribution	May cross arterial territories
Shape	Wedge shaped (cortical infarcts)	Round or infiltrating shape
Mass effect	Mild mass effect related to the size of lesion; may not be present immediately or after one week	Marked mass effect relative to size of lesion
Edema	Cytotoxic type; involves white and gray matter (wedge shaped)	Vasogenic type; edema pattern follows white matter (finger-like shape)
Progression of mass effect and edema	Decreases with time, eventually volume loss	Increases with time
Enhancement	Gyral enhancement (cortical infarct)	Absent, ring, patchy, or homogeneous
Progression of enhancement	Decreases with time, eventually volume loss	Persists or increases with time
Gray matter involvement	Yes	Infrequently
Clinical course	Sudden onset of symptoms, improves after presentation	Gradual onset of symptoms, deterioration after presentation

2.22 Stages and Estimation of Age of Hemorrhage on MRI

Recognition of cerebral hemorrhage is critically important, and therefore, knowledge of the complex parameters that influence the MRI appearance of an evolving hematoma is essential. The MRI of a hematoma depends on whether T1-shortening proton electron dipole–dipole interactions or T2-shortening preferential T2 proton relaxation enhancement occur. The interaction that predominates thereafter depends on the particular heme moiety present (e.g., oxyhemoglobin, deoxyhemoglobin, methemoglobin, or hemosiderin), and on the fact whether it is in free solution or compartmentalized into red blood cells or macrophages. (▶ Fig. 2.44)

Stage	Time	Compartment	Hemoglobin	T1 signal intensity	T2 signal intensity
Hyperacute	<24 hours	Intracellular	Oxyhemoglobin	Medium (isointense)	Medium (hyperintense)
Acute	1–3 days	Intracellular	Deoxyhemoglobin	Long (= ↓) (isointense to low intensity)	Short (↓ ↓) (low intensity)
Subacute					
Early	3+ days	Intracellular	Methemoglobin	Short (↑) (high intensity)	Short (↓ ↓) (low intensity)
Late	7+ days	Extracellular	Methemoglobin	Short (↑) (high intensity)	Long (↑) (high intensity with rim of Low intensity)
Chronic					
Center	14+ days	Extracellular	Hemichromes	Medium (isointense to low intensity)	Medium (isointense to low intensity)
Rim		Intracellular	Hemosiderin	Medium (↓) (isointense)	Short (↓ ↓) (very hypointense)

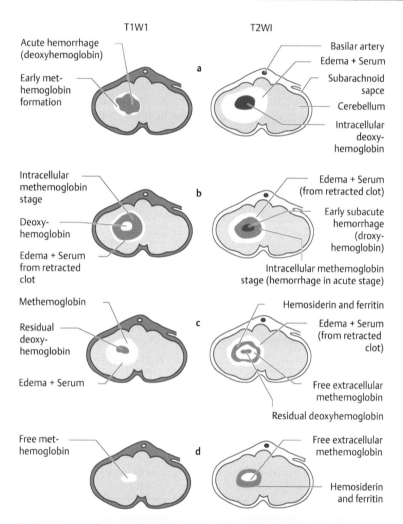

T1W1   T2WI

a

Acute hemorrhage (deoxyhemoglobin)

Early met- hemoglobin formation

Basilar artery

Edema + Serum

Subarachnoid sapce

Cerebellum

Intracellular deoxy- hemoglobin

b

Intracellular methemoglobin stage

Deoxy- hemoglobin

Edema + Serum from retracted clot

Edema + Serum (from retracted clot)

Early subacute hemorrhage (droxy- hemoglobin)

Intracellular methemoglobin stage (hemorrhage in acute stage)

c

Methemoglobin

Residual deoxy- hemoglobin

Edema + Serum

Hemosiderin and ferritin

Edema + Serum (from retracted clot)

Free extracellular methemoglobin

Residual deoxyhemoglobin

d

Free met- hemoglobin

Free extracellular methemoglobin

Hemosiderin and ferritin

Fig. 2.44 Stages and estimation of age of hemorrhage on MRI. **(a)** MRI scenarios of posterior fossa (right cerebellar) hemorrhage during: the acute stage, i.e., within 48 hours of ictus. On the T1WI, hemorrhage appears slightly hypodense to cerebellar parenchyma, due to the T2 effect of deoxyhemoglobin. There is a small amount of peripheral high density due to early intracellular methemoglobin formation. The T2WI demonstrates marked hypointensity caused by intracellular deoxyhemoglobin in intact red blood cells.

Fig. 2.44 (*Continued*) **(b)** Early subacute stage, i.e., within 3–7 days from ictus, during the time in which there is oxidation of the deoxyhemoglobin to methemoglobin inside the red blood cells at the periphery of the clot. On the T1WI, the central hemorrhage shows a high signal due to intracellular deoxyhemoglobin, whereas on the T2WI there is a marked hypointensity. The peripheral area of the hemorrhage, which represents the intracellular methemoglobin stage is isointense on the T1WI, and on the T2WI appears hypointense. Furthermore, surrounding this hemorrhage is a high-intensity area composed of edema and serum from the retracted blood clot. **(c)** Late subacute stage, i.e., within 7 to 10 days, during which time the heme-free molecule of the methemoglobin and/or other exogenous compounds including peroxide and superoxide can produce red blood cells lysis and accumulation of extracellular methemoglobin within the hematoma cavity. Methemoglobin in free solution is very hyperintense on T1- and T2WI. Inside this high signal rim of metHb a hypointense area appears, representing residual deoxyhemoglobin. Around the hematoma, on the T2WI, there is a hypointense rim (hemosiderin and ferritin) and peripherally, surrounding this rim there is a high signal intensity, representing vasogenic edema. **(d)** Chronic stage, i.e., more than 14 days, during which there is a pool of dilutefree metHb surrounded by the ferritin and hemosiderin, containing vascularized wall. These iron cores produce a thin hypo- or isointense rim on the T1WI and a very hypointense rim on the T2WI.

2.23 Normal Pressure Hydrocephalus versus Brain Atrophy

Although brain atrophy and normal pressure hydrocephalus (NPH) often share the finding of dilatation of the ventricular system, the prognostic and therapeutic implications of the two entities are markedly different. Atrophy reflects the loss of brain tissue, be it cortical cell bodies, axonal subcortical degeneration, or demyelination. Generally, there is no treatment for atrophy, whereas hydrocephalus can often be treated with ventricular or subarachnoid space shunts and/or removal of the obstructing or overproducing lesion.

The diagnosis of NPH requires very close correlation between clinical findings and imaging results. The best diagnostic test for the NPH still remains clinical improvement following ventricular shunting. It is difficult to distinguish NPH from atrophic ventriculomegaly on a single examination. Follow-up with serial CT or MRI, therefore, is necessary and it may show that the dilated ventricles have returned to normal size, remain enlarged, or, most importantly, that there has been no further interval enlargement.

Current radiologic diagnosis of NPH requires a subjective judgment of whether or not lateral ventricular enlargement is disproportionate to cerebral atrophy based on visual inspection of brain images. It has been investigated whether quantitative measurements of lateral ventricular volume and total cortical thickness (a correlate of cerebral atrophy) could be used to more objectively distinguish NPH from normal controls (NC), Alzheimer's disease (AD). Volumetric MRIs were obtained prospectively from these types of patients. Although mean ventricular volume was significantly greater in the NPH group than all others, the range of values overlapped those of the AD group. Individuals with NPH could be better distinguished when ventricular volume and total cortical thickness were considered in combination. This pilot study suggests that volumetric MRI measurements hold promise for improving NPH differential diagnosis. (▶ Fig. 2.45)

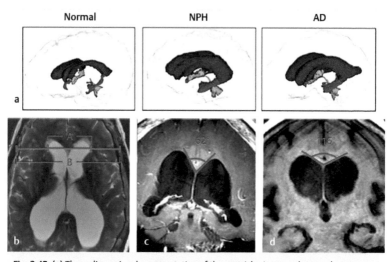

Fig. 2.45 (a) Three-dimensional representation of the ventricles in normal, normal pressure hydrocephalus (NPH), and Alzheimer's disease (AD) participant (left to right). The ventricles of the NPH and the AD participants are enlarged relative to the normal participant. The cortex of the AD participant is notably thinner, particularly in posterior regions, than that of the normal and NPH participant. (Reproduced from Moore DW et al. A pilot study of quantitative MRI measurements of ventricular volume and cortical atrophy for the differential diagnosis of normal pressure hydrocephalus. Neurol Res Int 2012;2012, Article ID 718150, 6 pages.)
(b) Radiographic indices used in the diagnosis of normal pressure hydrocephalus (NPH). Measurement of Evan's index on an axial T2-weighted magnetic resonance image (MRI) of the brain in a patient with NPH. A = 4.49 cm, B = 10.5 cm, Evan's index = A/B = 0.43 (≥ 0.3 is consistent with NPH). (c, d) Measurement of the callosal angle on T1-weighted MRI of the brain in (c) a patient with NPH and (d) a patient with Alzheimer's disease. A callosal angle of < 90° is consistent with NPH, while values > 90° are seen in ventriculomegaly related to Alzheimer's disease or other dementias. (Reproduced from 10.4 Diagnosis and Neuroimaging. In: Torres-Corzo J, Rangel-Castilla L, Nakaji P, ed. Neuroendoscopic Surgery. 1st edition. Thieme; 2016.)

The following table shows differentiation based on radiological features.

Radiological characteristic	Hydrocephalus	Brain atrophy
Ventricular system		
Temporal horns	Enlarged	Normal (except in Alzheimer's disease)
Frontal horns (ventricular angle)	More acute	More obtuse
Third ventricle	Convex	Concave
Fourth ventricle	Normal or enlarged	Normal (except in cerebellar atrophy)
Periventricular edema	Present (transependymal migration of CSF, especially to the frontal and occipital horns. Edema resolves quickly after ventricular decompression by shunting, within 24 hours)	Absent (rule out ischemia)
Aqueduct flow void	Accentuated (in normotensive hydrocephalus)	Normal
Corpus callosum	Thin, distended, rounded elevation. Increased fornico-callosal distance	Normal or atrophied. Normal fornico-callosal distance
Sulci	Flattened	Enlarged disproportionately to age
Fissures		
(Choroidal hippocampal)	Normal to mildly enlarged	Markedly enlarged (in Alzheimer's disease)

Abbreviation: CSF, cerebrospinal fluid.

2.24 Meningeal Enhancement

1. Postcraniotomy meningeal enhancement: In 80% of patients indicating inflammatory or chemical arachnoiditis from blood.
2. Meningitis: Bacterial, viral, syphilitic, and granulomatous.
3. Meningioma en plaque
4. Meningeal carcinomatosis
5. Meningeal fibrosis from:
   a) Aneurysmal subarachnoid hemorrhage
   b) CSF leaks, CSF shunting, and intracranial hypotension
   c) Dural sinus thrombosis
6. Nonneoplastic meningeal disorders
   a) Histiocytosis
   b) Sarcoidosis
   c) Rheumatoid disease
   d) Idiopathic pachymeningitis (▶ Fig. 2.46)
7. Lymphoma, leukemia
8. Extraskeletal mesenchymal osteocartilaginous tumors
   a) Osteochondroma
   b) Chondrosarcoma
9. Miscellaneous and rare causes of dural enhancement
   a) Amyloid
   b) Mucopolysaccharidoses (e.g., Gaucher disease)
   c) Glioblastoma multiforme
   d) Wegener's granulomatosis

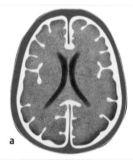 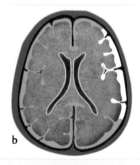

Fig. 2.46 (a) Diagram illustrates the enhancement pattern, which follows the pial surface of the brain and fills the subarachnoid spaces of the sulci and cisterns (i.e. carcinomatous meningitis). (b) Diagram illustrates gyral enhancement that is localized to the superficial gray matter of the cerebral cortex (i.e. herpes encephalitis). There is no enhancement of the arachnoid, and none in the subarachnoid space or sulci.

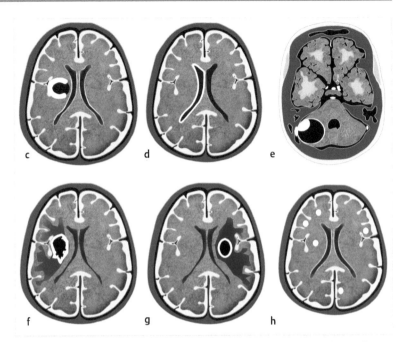

Fig. 2.46 (*Continued*) **(c)** Diagram illustrates a lesion with an incomplete rim (only part of the rim enhances). This appearance may be seen in multiple sclerosis (without mass effect as in this drawing), tumefactive demyelination (with mass effect), and fluid-secreting neoplasms (with associated mass effect and occasionally with surrounding vasogenic edema). **(d)** Axial nonenhanced CT scan shows a thick rim of periventricular hyperattenuation, with surrounding vasogenic edema (i.e. primary CNS lymphoma). **(e)** Diagram illustrates a "cystic" mass with a "mural nodule" which is the classic description for a pilocytic astrocytoma. This pattern is seen in a variety of fluid-secreting neoplasms, including hemangioblastoma, ganglioglioma, and pleomorphic xanthoastrocytoma. **(f)** Diagram illustrates a lesion with an enhanced rim that is very thick medially; the ring is thicker and more irregular than that seen in a typical abscess (i.e. necrotic ring pattern of high-grade neoplasm). The lesion is surrounded by a crown of vasogenic edema spreading into the white matter. **(g)** Diagram illustrates a thin (< 10 mm) rim of enhancement which is usually very smooth along the inner margin; this pattern is characteristic of an abscess. The lesion is surrounded by a crown of vasogenic edema spreading into the white matter. Smooth ring enhancing pattern in late cerebritis and subsequent cerebral abscess. **(h)** Diagram illustrates nodular lesions near the gray matter–white matter junction and one near the deep gray matter. This pattern is typical for metastatic cancer and clot emboli. Due to their typical subcortical location, metastases often manifest with cortical symptoms or seizures while the lesions are small (often < 1 cm in diameter). Subcortical nodular enhancement in metastatic melanoma.

2.25 Gyriform Enhancement

1. Cerebral infarction
2. Encephalitis
3. Infiltrating primary or subpial metastatic neoplasm
4. Cortical contusion
5. Postepilepsy (e.g., transient blood–brain barrier disruption)
6. Cortical hamartomas in tuberous sclerosis

2.26 Corpus Callosum Lesions

1. Neoplasmas: Near the top of the list of lesions involving the corpus callosum are:
   a) Glioblastoma multiforme
   b) Lymphoma
   c) Metastases
   d) Lipoma
2. Trauma: There is a propensity for shearing injuries in this location because of its relative fixed location spanning the interhemispheric fissure.
3. White matter lesions
   a) Multiple sclerosis: The frequent localization of acute and chronic MS lesions in the corpus callosum is thought to be due to tracking of these lesions along the ependymal veins from the ventricular surface into the adjacent white matter. T2 lesions of the corpus callosum have recently become important in diagnosing MS because they improve the sensitivity and specificity of MRI for that disease.
   b) Leukodystrophies: The hallmark of the leukodystrophies is demyelination of the cerebral white matter; they are due to disorders of the peroxisomes as in adrenal leukodystrophy (ADL), or of the lysosomal enzymes as in Krabbe's disease.
      i. Adrenal leukodystrophy (ADL)
      ii. Krabbe's disease (globoid cell leukodystrophy)
   c) Marchiafava–Bignami syndrome: It is a rare disorder of demyelination or necrosis of the corpus callosum and adjacent subcortical white matter, which occurs in the malnourished alcoholics.
   d) In severe hydrocephalus and after ventricular shunting.
4. Infection
   a) Lyme disease (Neuroborreliosis)
   b) Progressive multifocal leukoencephalopathy
5. Radiation damage
6. Infarction: Rare, because the blood supply is bilateral through the anterior cerebral arteries.

2.27 Ring-Enhancing Lesions

The triad tumor, pus, or blood account for most cases in adults. (▶ Fig. 2.47)

1. Tumor
    a) Primary brain tumors: Such as anaplastic astrocytoma, glioblastoma multiforme.
    b) Metastatic brain tumors (especially lung)
2. Abscess
    a) Pyogenic brain abscess: Common organisms causing pyogenic cerebral abscess are:
        i. Aerobic bacteria
            – *Staphylococcus aureus*
            – *Streptococcus*
            – Gram negative bacteria (*Escherichia coli, Klebsiella, Proteus, Pseudomonas, H. Influenzae*)
        ii. Anaerobic bacteria
            – *Streptococcus*
            – *Bacteroides*
            – *Peptostreptococcus*
    b) Fungal abscess
        i. Cryptococcosis: *Cryptococcus* ranks third after HIV and toxoplasmosis as a cause of CNS infection in AIDS.
        ii. Coccidioidomycosis
        iii. Mucormycosis
        iv. Nocardiosis: Nocardia lesions show a well-formed enhancing capsule containing multiple loculations.
        v. Aspergillosis: Contrary to *Nocardia*, intracranial aspergillosis rarely presents with ring enhancement.
        vi. Candidiasis: *Candida* is the most common cause of autopsy-proved non-AIDS cerebral mycosis.
    c) Parasitic abscess
        i. Toxoplasmosis: *Toxoplasma Gondii* infects the CNS in 10% of patients with AIDS and also immunocompromised adults.
        ii. Cysticercosis
3. Subacute resolving hematoma with capsule
4. Infarct
5. Miscellaneous
    a) Tuberculosis
    b) Granuloma
    c) Demyelinating disease (e.g., MS)
    d) Radiation necrosis

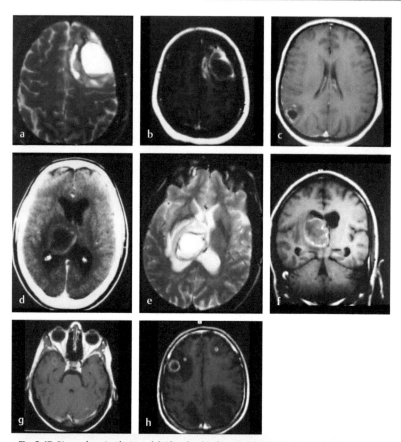

Fig. 2.47 Ring enhancing lesions. **(a)** Oligodendroglioma. Axial T2 WI shows a space-occupying lesion with a high intensity heterogeneous signal with solid and cystic features. **(b)** Oligodendroglioma. Axial T1 WI of the same case demonstrates an irregular postcontrast ring enhancement. **(c)** Astrocytoma grade III. Axial T1 WI shows a space-occupying lesion with a postcontrast ring enhancement, central necrosis, and peritumoral edema. **(d)** Bacterial abscess. A postcontrast axial CT with a space-occupying lesion in the right basal ganglia with an irregular ring enhancement and marked surrounding edema. **(e)** Bacterial abscess. Axial T2 WI of the same case with a space-occupying lesion in the right basal ganglia with a thick capsule and marked perifocal edema. **(f)** Bacterial abscess. Coronal T1 WI of the same case. **(g)** Toxoplasmosis. Axial T1 WI shows a small subcortical postcontrast ring enhancing toxoplasmosis brain abscess within the right temporal lobe. **(h)** Cerebral metastases. Axial T1 WI with multiple secondary focal lesions demonstrating postcontrast ring enhancement and an extensive infiltrating edema disproportionate to the size of the lesions.

e) Lymphoma (e.g., primary CNS lymphoma in AIDS or secondary systemic lymphoma)
f) Trauma
g) Thrombosed vascular malformation or aneurysm

2.28 Multifocal White Matter Lesions

1. Multiple sclerosis (▶ Fig. 2.48)
2. Hypertension and ischemic white matter lesions—Leukoaraiosis (e.g., increases as one ages and has also been chronic hypertensive). Ischemic white matter lesions are of two variants:
   a) Lesions involve the watershed distribution of the major brain arteries
   b) Lesions are caused by intrinsic disease of the small penetrating medullary arteries (arteriolar sclerosis)
3. Perivascular (Virchow–Robin) spaces: Enlargement of these perivascular spaces with age and hypertension is called État criblé. It is associated with thinning, pallor, and atrophy of the adjacent myelin.
4. Metastases
5. Trauma (Nonvascular white matter injury): Diffuse axonal shearing caused by acceleration–deceleration–rotation forces on the brain
6. Inflammatory (e.g., Lyme disease, cysticercosis)
7. Vasculitides
   a) Systemic lupus erythematosus
   b) Sjogren syndrome
   c) Behcet disease
   d) "Moya moya" disease
   e) Amyloid angiopathy
   f) Polyarteritis nodosa
8. Primary CNS lymphoma
9. Migraine: Mystery lesions of the frontal lobe, centrum semiovale, basal ganglia possibly due to microemboli from increased platelet aggregation during migrainous attacks
10. Inherited leukoencephalopathy
11. Secondary leukoencephalopathy
    a) Acute disseminated encephalomyelitis (ADEM)
    b) Progressive multifocal encephalopathy (PML)
    c) Binswanger's disease (Subcortical arteriosclerotic encephalopathy)
    d) Postanoxic encephalopathy
    e) Osmotic demyelination or central pontine myelolysis
    f) Alcoholism (Marchiafava–Bignami syndrome)

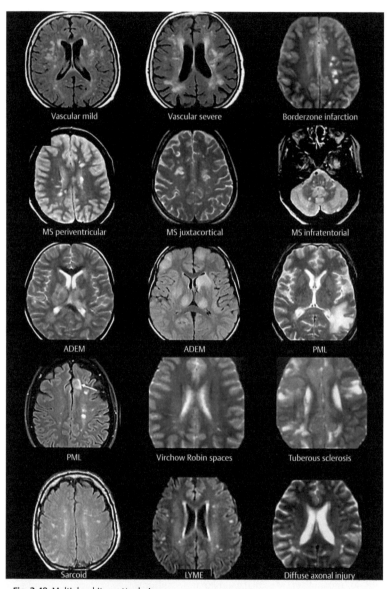

Fig. 2.48 Multiple white matter lesions.

g) Drugs and toxins
  i. Drugs: Methamphetamine, cocaine, heroin.
  ii. Toxins: Hexachlorophene, lead, isoniazid, chemotherapeutic agents, eclampsia
h) Radiation changes
12. Dysmyelinating diseases
  a) Metachromatic leukodystrophy (MLD): The most common type resulting from a deficiency in the enzyme arylsulfatase A
  b) Adrenoleukodystrophy: Associated with adrenal cortical insufficiency and accumulation of very-long-chain fatty acids in the white matter, adrenal cortex, and plasma from impairment in peroxisomes of the, oxidation
  c) Alexander's disease
  d) Canavan's disease: deficiency in the enzyme aspartoacylase
  e) Krabbe's disease: deficiency of the enzyme galactocerebrosidase (GALC), which is necessary for the metabolism of the spingolipids galactosylceremide and psychosine, resulting in degeneration of the myelin sheath surrounding nerves in the brain (demyelination)

2.29 Multiple Enhancing Lesions in White Matter

2.29.1 Vasculitis

Most diseases with vasculitis are characterized by punctiform enhancement. Vasculitis in the brain is seen in SLE, PAN, Behcet's disease, syphilis, Wagener, Sjogren, and primary angiitis of CNS.

2.29.2 Behcet's disease

It is more commonly seen in Turkish patients. Typical findings are brain stem lesions with nodular enhancement in the acute phase.

2.29.3 Metastases

Metastases mostly surrounded by a lot of edema.

2.29.4 Border zone infarction

Peripheral border zone infarction may enhance in the early phase. (▶ Fig. 2.49)

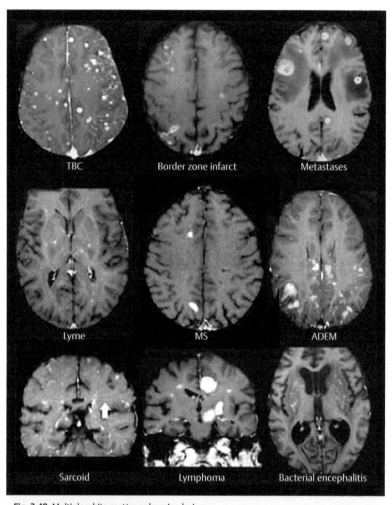

Fig. 2.49 Multiple white matter enhancing lesions.

3 Developmental—Acquired Anomalies and Paediatric Disorders

3.1 Movements Resembling Neonatal Seizures

In the newborn infant, there are several nonepileptic motor phenomena. They may be difficult to differentiate from seizures. *Tremor, jitteriness, and myoclonus* may be benign signs in an otherwise healthy infant, but may also signal a pathological condition. Examples include metabolic disturbance, infection, stroke, drug withdrawal, etc. These conditions show similarities to reflex behaviors of the neonate; however, they are not associated with ictal electroencephalogram (EEG) changes. They are often seen in hypoxic-ischemic encephalopathy. These types of seizures are considered exaggerated reflex behaviors due to release of brainstem facilitatory centers (for generating reflex behaviors) without cortical inhibition. They are also called brainstem release phenomena.

1. **Benign nocturnal myoclonus/Benign neonatal sleep myoclonus:** Sudden jerking movements of the limbs during sleep occur in normal people and requires no treatment. May occur focally during nonrapid eye movement (non-REM) sleep. Video EEG monitoring shows no electrographic seizures.
2. **Jitteriness or tremulousness:** Low-frequency, high-amplitude shaking of the limbs and jaw in response to stimulation. Occurs in newborns with perinatal asphyxia some of whom have seizures and require an EEG monitoring for differential diagnosis. Jitteriness is not associated with ocular deviation. It is stimulus sensitive (e.g., easily stopped with passive movement of the limb). The movement resembles a tremor, and no autonomic changes are associated with it. *Seizures often are associated with ocular deviation and are not stimulus sensitive. Autonomic changes frequently accompany them. The movements are clonic, unlike the tremor like movements or jitteriness.*
3. **Nonconvulsive apnea:** Irregular respiratory patterns of 3–6 seconds, followed by 10–15 seconds of hyperpnea without significant changes in heart rate, blood pressure, temperature, or skin color. It affects premature infants and is caused by immaturity of the respiratory centers in brain stem and not by a pathologic condition.
4. **Opisthotonos:** A prolonged arching of the back probably caused by meningeal irritation. It is observed in the infantile Gaucher's disease and kernicterus, and must be differentiated from tonic seizures and decerebrate posturing.
5. **Benign myoclonus:** Spasms in clusters increasing in frequency and intensity over weeks, then usually stop after 3 months with the exception of a few episodes, but no spasms occur after 2 years of age. The infants are neurologically normal, their EEG and CT scan of head are normal.

6. **Neonatal hyperekplexia or motor automatisms (startle disease):** Clinically hyperekplexia is characterized by pathological and excessive startle responses to unexpected auditory and tactile stimuli (sudden noise, movement, or touch) and severe generalized stiffness (hypertonia in flexion which disappears in sleep). It is usually a familial condition which is inconsistently associated with EEG seizures and are considered as nonepileptic.

Reuber M, Elger CE. Psychogenic nonepileptic seizures: review and update. Epilepsy Behav 2003;4(3):205–216

3.2 Pallid Breath-Holding Spells

These episodes are precipitated by a sudden, unexpected unpleasant stimulus such as a mild head injury (without associated crying) followed by collapse with pallor, diaphoresis, bradycardia and loss of consciousness. The patient may be limp, and have posturing and clonic movements, and may progress into a generalized tonic–clonic seizure presumably due to cerebral ischemia.

Breath-holding spells are often mistaken for epileptic seizures and it is important to differentiate the two to avoid unnecessary treatment with anticonvulsants.

Characteristics	Breath-holding spells	Epileptic seizures
Trigger	Crying, injury	Spontaneous, fever, sleep deprivation
Occurrence during sleep	No	May occur during sleep
Event	Sequence: provocation, apnea, cyanosis/pallor, limpness	Associated with stiffening and jerking of extremities
Postictal state	Usually brief	Maybe prolonged
Epileptiform abnormalities on EEG	Absent	Usually present
Treatment	Parental reassurance	Anticonvulsant therapy

Swaiman KF, Ashwal S, Ferrieto DM, eds. Pediatric Neurology: Principles and Practice. Nonepileptiform paroxysmal disorders and disorders of sleep. 4th ed. St Louis: Mosby Elsevier; 2006

3.3 Pseudoseizures

Pseudoseizures are episodic, behavioral spells that mimic true epileptic seizures. They are common, accounting for 5–20% of the outpatient epilepsy population. Of patients with pseudoseizures, 10–40% also have epileptic seizures. Majority of patients are female between 15–35 years of age, however these are also seen in young children.

The clinical features that differentiate nonepileptic seizures (pseudoseizures) from epileptic form seizures are presented in the following table.

Characteristics	Nonepileptic seizures	Epileptic seizures
Duration	Prolonged (several minutes)	Usually less than 2–3 minutes
Clinical features	Fluctuating features	Stereotyped features
	Usually during wakefulness	May occur in sleep
	Preserved consciousness	Altered consciousness
	Side-to-side head movements	Head unilaterally turned
	Out of phase extremity movements	In phase extremity movements
	Forward pelvic trusting	Retropelvic thrusting
	Emotional vocalization	Monotonous vocalization
	Pupillary reflex retained	Pupillary reflex absent
Incontinence	Rare	Present
Tongue bite	Occasional	Common
Postictal changes	None	Usually present
Effect	Indifferent	Concerned

Cragar DE, Berry DT, Fakhoury TA, Cibula JE, Schmitt FA. A review of diagnostic techniques in the differential diagnosis of epileptic and nonepileptic seizures. Neuropsychol Rev 2002;12(1):31–64

Reuber M, Elger CE. Psychogenic nonepileptic seizures: review and update. Epilepsy Behav 2003;4(3): 205–216

William TH. Pseudoseizures: differential diagnosis. J Neuropsychiatr Clin Neurosci 1981;1(1):67–69

3.4 Neonatal Seizures by the Time of Onset

Neonatal seizures are seizures occurring within the first 28 days in a full-term infant and extending to the 44 completed weeks gestational age in the preterm infant. The prevalence is approximately 1.5% and overall incidence approximately 3 per 1,000 live births. The neonatal period is the most vulnerable of all periods of life for developing seizures, particularly in the first 1–2 days to the first week from birth. They may be short-lived events lasting for a few days only. However, they often signify serious malfunction of or damage to the immature brain and constitute a neurological emergency.

3.4.1 Differential diagnosis

Differential diagnosis of neonatal seizures depends on the time of onset of the seizures.

1. **Seizures during the first 24 hours:** In order of frequency especially the first 12 hours.
   a) Hypoxic–ischemic encephalopathy
   b) Sepsis and bacterial meningitis
   c) Subarachnoid hemorrhage
   d) Intrauterine infection
   e) Trauma (Laceration of tentorium or falx)
   f) Direct drug affects
   g) Intraventricular hemorrhage at term
   h) Pyridoxine dependency
2. **Seizures during the period from 24 to 72 hours:** In order of frequency and importance.
   a) Intraventricular hemorrhage in premature infants
   b) Subarachnoid hemorrhage
   c) Cerebral contusion with subdural hemorrhage
   d) Sepsis and bacterial meningitis
   e) Cerebral infarction or intracerebral hemorrhage
   f) Cerebral dysgenesis
   g) Drug withdrawal
   h) Metabolic disorders
      i. Glycine encephalopathy
      ii. Glycogen synthetase deficiency
      iii. Hypoparathyroidism-hypocalcemia
      iv. Pyridoxine encephalopathy
      v. Urea cycle disturbances
   i) Tuberous sclerosis
3. **Seizures during the period from 72 hours to 1 week:** In order of frequency and importance.
   a) Inborn errors of metabolism especially organic acid disorders
      i. Hypoglycemia (fructose dysmetabolism, maple syrup disease)
      ii. Hypocalcemia (hypoparathyroidism)
      iii. Hyperammonemia (propionic acidemia, methylmalonic acidemia, etc.)
      iv. Hyperlactatemia (glycogen storage disease, mitochondrial disease, etc.)
      v. Metabolic acidosis (maple syrup disease, fructose dysmetabolism, multiple carboxylase deficiency)
      vi. No rapid screening test (neonatal adrenoleukodystrophy, glycine encephalopathy, infantile Gm, gangliosidosis, Gaucher's disease type 2)
   b) Cerebral dysgenesis
   c) Cerebral infarction
   d) Intracerebral hemorrhage
   e) Familial neonatal seizures

f) Kernicterus
g) Tuberous sclerosis
4. **Seizures during the period from 1 to 4 weeks**
   a) Inborn errors of metabolism especially organic acid disorders
      i. Hypoglycemia (fructose dysmetabolism, maple syrup disease)
      ii. Hypocalcemia (hypoparathyroidism)
      iii. Hyperammonemia (propionic acidemia, methylmalonic acidemia, etc.)
      iv. Hyperlactatemia (glycogen storage disease, mitochondrial disease, etc.)
      v. Metabolic acidosis (maple syrup disease, fructose dysmetabolism, multiple carboxylase deficiency)
      vi. No rapid screening test (neonatal adrenoleukodystrophy, glycine encephalopathy, infantile Gm gangliosidosis, Gaucher's disease type 2)
   b) Herpes simplex encephalitis
   c) Cerebral dysgenesis
   d) Familial neonatal seizures
   e) Tuberous sclerosis

3.5 Neonatal Seizures

Neonatal epileptic syndromes present with different seizure types. Understanding the conceptual difference between seizure and epileptic syndrome is important.

An *epileptic seizure* is defined as a transient neurologic dysfunction resulting from an excessive abnormal electrical discharge of cerebral neurons. The clinical manifestations are numerous, including disturbances of consciousness, changes in emotions, changes in sensation, abnormal movements, and changes in visceral functions or behavior.

Epilepsy syndromes is a group of disorders characterized by chronic, recurrent paroxysmal changes in neurologic function caused by abnormalities in electrical activity of the brain. The 2001 International League Against Epilepsy proposed a new diagnostic scheme for epilepsy syndromes and related conditions which is described below.

1. **Benign familial neonatal seizure**
   Autosomal dominant channelopathy with brief seizures within the first days of life (80% on the 2nd and 3rd day) typically in premature infants. The diagnosis is suspected when seizures occur without obvious precipitants in an otherwise normal newborn with a family history of similar seizures in the neonatal period. Prognosis is good.
2. **Early myoclonic encephalopathy**
   Clinically characterized by erratic or massive myoclonus, partial seizures, tonic spasms, and a suppression-burst pattern on EEG. It is believed to have various prenatal etiologies that often remain unknown; inborn errors of metabolism and genetic disorders are sometimes found. Prognosis is poor.

3. **Ohtahara syndrome**

It is one of the earliest developing forms of epileptic encephalopathy. The main characteristics of the syndrome are tonic seizures and a suppression-burst pattern on EEG. The etiology is symptomatic, with the majority of cases associated with structural brain damage, but recent cases due to genetic mutation and metabolic abnormalities have been described. Prognosis very poor.

4. **Benign neonatal seizures (nonfamilial)**

These are characterized by a single episode of repetitive clonic seizures, mainly unilateral, often of alternating sides in a full-term, previously healthy neonate; all investigations, except EEG, are normal. Due to the tendency of the seizures to occur on the 4th–5th day of life, the term "fifth day fits" has been commonly been used.

Panayiotopoulos CP. Neonatal seizures and neonatal syndromes. Chapter 5. In: Panayiotopoulos CP ed. The Epilepsies: Seizures and Management. Oxfordshire (UK): Bladon Medical Publishing; 2005

Plounin P. Benign familial neonatal convulsions and benign idiopathic neonatal convulsions. In: Engel J jr, Pedley TA, eds. Epilepsy. A Comprehensive Textbook. Lippincott-Raven; 1997:2247–2255

Heron SE, Crossland KM, Andermann E, et al. Sodium-channel defects in benign familial neonatal-infantile seizures. Lancet 2002;360(9336):851–852

Silverstein FS, Jensen FE. Neonatal seizures. Ann Neurol 2007;62(2):112–120

Pisani F, Sisti L, Seri S. A scoring system for early prognostic assessment after neonatal seizures. Pediatrics 2009;124(4):e580–e587

3.6 First Nonfebrile Tonic–Clonic Seizure after 2 Years of Age

1. Viral encephalitis
   a) Herpes simplex encephalitis
   b) Arboviral encephalitis
      i. St. Louis encephalitis
      ii. Western and Eastern equine encephalitis
      iii. Japanese B encephalitis
      iv. California-La Crosse encephalitis
   c) Retrovirus encephalitis (e.g., AIDS encephalitis)
   d) Rhabdovirus encephalitis (e.g., Rabies encephalitis)
2. Idiopathic isolated seizure
3. Partial complex seizures with secondary generalization (any seizure originating in the cortex may discharge into the brain stem)
   a) Benign rolandic epilepsy of childhood
   b) Benign occipital epilepsy of childhood
   c) Epilepsia partialis continua

4. Progressive encephalopathy
   a) Infectious diseases (e.g., subacute sclerosing panencephalitis)
   b) Lysosomal enzymes disorders
      i. Glycoprotein disorders
      ii. Mucopolysaccharidoses types II and VII
      iii. Sphingolipidoses
   c) Genetic disorders of gray matter
      i. Huntington disease
      ii. Mitochondrial disorders
      iii. Xeroderma pigmentosum
   d) Genetic disorders of white matter
      i. Alexander disease
      ii. Adrenoleukodystrophy

Pohlmann-Eden B, Beghi E, Camfield C, Camfield P. The first seizure and its management in adults and children. BMJ 2006;332(7537):339–342

3.7 Posttraumatic Epilepsy

If a case of posttraumatic epilepsy (PTE) demonstrates atypical features and the seizures continue despite treatment, the possibility of pseudoseizures should be considered. In patients with refractory PTE following moderate traumatic brain injury, about 20–30% proved to have been misdiagnosed and were actually having psychogenic attacks. This percentage is similar to that in patients with seizures after nontraumatic brain injury.

Therefore, the diagnosis should be verified by video-EEG monitoring which shows that the nature of the seizures is psychogenic rather than epileptic.

3.7.1 Differential diagnoses

- Benign childhood epilepsy
- Complex partial seizures
- Confusional states and acute memory disorders
- Dizziness, vertigo, and imbalance
- Frontal lobe epilepsy
- Head injury
- Neonatal seizures
- Psychogenic nonepileptic seizures
- Temporal lobe epilepsy
- Tonic–clonic seizures

Garga N, Lowenstein DH. Posttraumatic epilepsy: a major problem in desperate need of major advances. Epilepsy Curr 2006;6(1):1–5

3.8 Causes of Confusion and Restlessness

1. Epileptic (e.g., partial complex seizures, absence type seizures)
2. Metabolic and systemic disorders
   a) Osmolality disorders (e.g., hyponatremia, hypoglycemia)
   b) Endocrine disorders (e.g., adrenal insufficiency, parathyroid and thyroid disorders)
   c) Hepatic encephalopathy
   d) Metabolic disorders (e.g., carnitine deficiency, urea cycle and pyruvate disorders)
   e) Renal disease (e.g., hypertensive and uremic encephalopathy)
3. Infectious disorders
   a) Bacterial infections (e.g., meningitis, cat scratch disease)
   b) Rickettsial infections (e.g., Lyme disease)
   c) Viral infections (e.g., Herpes simplex, arboviruses, measles and postinfectious encephalitis, Reye syndrome)
4. Vascular
   a) Congestive heart failure
   b) Subarachnoid hemorrhage
   c) Embolic infarction
   d) Vasculitis and connective tissue disorders
   e) Migraine
5. Toxic
   a) Substance abuse
   b) Prescription drugs
   c) Toxins
6. Psychogenic (e.g., panic disorder, schizophrenia)
7. Postoperative (most common)
   a) Cerebrovascular disease
   b) Drugs, delirium tremens
   c) Chest infection or atelectasis
   d) Renal infection
   e) Abdominal sepsis, superficial or deep
   f) Over-full bladder or rectum

3.9 Hypotonic Infant or "Floppy Baby or Infant"

The term "floppy baby or infant" is used to denote an infant with poor muscle tone affecting the limbs, trunk, and the craniofacial musculature (▶ Fig. 3.1). The condition is usually evident at birth or is identified during early life as poor musculature results in an inability to maintain normal posture during movement and rest.

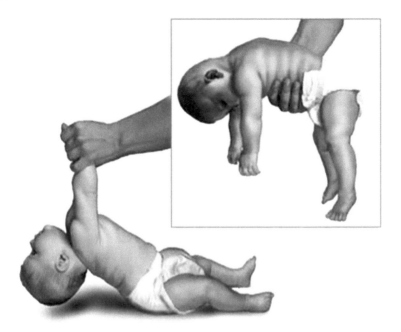

Fig. 3.1 Floppy baby. (These images are provided courtesy of Case Western Reserve University School of Medicine.)

Lesions at any level of the nervous system, including upper and lower motor units, can cause hypotonia. Hypotonia combined with severe muscle weakness usually is associated with lower motor neuron disease, including diseases affecting anterior horn cells of the spinal cord, peripheral nerves, neuromuscular junctions, and muscles. Hypotonia without obvious weakness often points to diseases of the central nervous system (CNS) as a result of a perinatal insult or may manifest later in infants with mental retardation or cerebral palsy. It may be a manifestation of a connective tissue disorder, chromosomal disease, or those involving metabolic, endocrine, or nutritional problems. It may also be an incidental and nonspecific feature of an acutely ill child and it is completely physiologic in the premature infant.

Irrespective of the cause, the floppy infant is likely to present a somewhat similar *clinical picture*, which one usually recognizes on the basis of three clinical signs: (a) bizarre or unusual posture, (b) diminished resistance of the joints to passive movements, and (c) increased range of joint movement. In the newborn period, the infant usually presents with the above features, together with a paucity of active movement; the older infant usually presents with delay in motor milestones. Central causes account for 60–80% of cases and that the diagnosis can usually be made by a careful history and examination. However, there may be a mixed picture. Infants with a peripheral cause for their hypotonia may be at increased risk for problems during labor, delivery, and resuscitation and develop hypoxic ischemic encephalopathy.

3.10 Causes of "Floppy" Infant

1. Systemic disease
   The most important and by far the most frequent cause of hypotonia in the newborn infant is systemic disease that influences the entire CNS (brain/brain stem) diffusely to cause hypotonia. The most frequent examples include:
   a) Congestive heart failure (significant congenital heart disease)
   b) Sepsis
   c) Hypoxic-ischemic insult (after they regain consciousness hypotonia persists for months, sometimes until they begin to get increased tone and reflexes and become spastic after the first 2–3 months.
2. Cerebral hypotonia
   Clues of diagnosis are:
   a) Other brain dysfunction,
   b) dysmorphic features,
   c) fisting of the hands,
   d) malformations of other organs,
   e) movement through postural reflexes,
   f) normal or brisk tendon reflexes, scissoring on vertical suspension.
      i. Benign congenital hypotonia: Hypotonic at birth, but later on have normal tone and increased incidence of cerebral abnormalities, e.g., retardation, learning difficulties, and other disabilities.
      ii. Chromosomal disorders
         - Trisomy
         - Prader–Willi syndrome: Deletion of the long arm of chromosome 15 causing hypotonia, mental retardation, obesity, short stature, and hypogonadism
      iii. Cerebral dysgenesis: It is suspected when hypotonia is associated with malformations in other organs or abnormalities in the size and shape of the head
      iv. Peroxisomal dysfunctions
         - Cerebrohepatorenal syndrome (Zellweger syndrome): Severe hypotonia, arthrogryposis, dysmorphic features, seizures. Death from aspiration, gastrointestinal bleeding, or liver failure within 1 year.

- Neonatal adrenoleukodystrophy: X-linked characterized by hypotonia, dysmorphia, failure to thrive, seizures, retardation, and spasticity. Death in early childhood.
- Infantile Refsum disease
  - v. Genetic disorders
    - Familial dysautonomia (Riley–Day syndrome): Autosomal recessive hypotonia from disturbances in the brain, dorsal root ganglia, and the peripheral nerves.
    - Oculocerebrorenal syndrome (Lowe syndrome): X-linked recessive hypotonia, hyporeflexia, cataracts, and glaucoma. Normal life span.

3. Spinal cord disorders
   a) Hypoxic-ischemic myelopathy: In severe perinatal asphyxia causing hypotonia and areflexia
   b) Spinal cord injury: Cervical spinal cord injury occurs exclusively during vaginal delivery; approximately 75% with breech presentation and 25% with cephalic presentation. Sphincter dysfunction and a sensory level at mid chest suggest myelopathy.

4. Motor unit disorders
   Clues to diagnosis are:
   a) Absent or depressed tendon reflexes,
   b) Failure of movement on postural reflexes,
   c) Fasciculations,
   d) Muscle atrophy,
   e) No abnormalities of other organs.
      i. Spinal muscular atrophies
         Genetic degeneration of anterior horn cells in the spinal cord and motor nuclei of the brain stem.
         - Acute infantile spinal muscular dystrophy (Werdnig–Hoffmann disease)
         - Chronic infantile spinal muscular dystrophy
         - Infantile neuronal degeneration
         - Neurogenic arthrogryposis
      ii. Polyneuropathies
         - Axonal
           ○ Familial dysautonomia
           ○ Hereditary motor-sensory neuropathy type II
           ○ Idiopathic with encephalopathy
           ○ Infantile neuronal degeneration
         - Demyelinating
           ○ Acute inflammatory (Guillain-Barre syndrome)

- o Congenital hypomyelinating neuropathy
- o Hereditary motor-sensory neuropathies, type I and type III
- o Metachromatic leukodystrophy
- iii. Disorders of neuromuscular transmission
  - – Infantile botulism
  - – Familial infantile myasthenia
  - – Transitory neonatal myasthenia
- iv. Congenital myopathies (fiber-type disproportion)
  - – Central core disease: Tightly packed myofibrils in the center of all type I fibers are undergoing degeneration.
  - – Fiber-type disproportion myopathy: Predominance of type I fiber and hypotrophy
  - – Myotubular myopathy: Predominance of type I fiber and hypotrophy, many internal nuclei, and a central core of increased oxidative enzyme and decreased myosin ATPase activity
  - – Nemaline myopathy: Multiple rodlike particles are present within most or all muscle fibers.
- v. Muscular dystrophies
  - – Congenital muscular dystrophy: Various size fibers present nucleation, extensive fibrosis, and proliferation of adipose tissue, regeneration and degeneration, and thickening of the muscle spindle capsule.
    - o Fukuyama type
    - o Leukodystrophy
    - o Cerebro-ocular dysplasia
  - – Neonatal myopathic dystrophy: Maturational arrest in muscles surrounding a fixed joint, and predominance of type II fibers.
- vi. Metabolic myopathies
  - – Acid maltase deficiency (Pompe's disease)
  - – Carnitine deficiency
  - – Cytochrome-c-oxidase deficiency
  - – Phosphofructokinase deficiency
  - – Phosphorylase deficiency
- vii. Infantile myositis: Diffuse inflammation and proliferation of connective tissue, and muscle fiber degeneration.
- viii. Endocrine myopathies
  - – Hyper/hypothyroidism
  - – Hyper/hypoparathyroidism
  - – Hyper/hypoadrenalism

3.10.1 Differential diagnosis

1. **Hypotonia with prominent weakness (lower motor unit disorders)**
   Spinal muscular atrophy, congenital myotonic dystrophy, congenital muscular dystrophy, neonatal myasthenia gravis, congenital myasthenic syndrome, congenital myopathies, metabolic myopathies (Pompe's disease, mitochondrial myopathy), hereditary motor and sensory neuropathies, Guillain–Bare syndrome, tick paralysis, infantile botulism.

2. **Hypotonia without prominent weakness**
   a) Cerebral hypotonia: perinatal hypoxia, birth trauma, Down's syndrome, Prader–Willi syndrome, Zellweger syndrome, Riley–Day syndrome, neonatal adrenoleukodystrophy, infantile Gm1 gangliosidosis
   b) Intrauterine infections: Toxoplasmosis, rubella, herpes, cytomegalovirus
   c) Metabolic, endocrine, nutritional problems: amino acidosis, biotinidase deficiency, organic acidosis, renal tubular acidosis, calcium abnormalities, hypothyroidism, celiac disease, malnutrition
   d) Connective tissue disorders: Ehlers–Danlos syndrome, Marfan's syndrome
   e) Benign congenital hypotonia
   f) Acute illness

Bodensteiner JB. The evaluation of the hypotonic infant. Semin Pediatr Neurol 2008;15(1):10–20

Peredo DE, Hannibal MC. The floppy infant: evaluation of hypotonia. Pediatr Rev 2009;30(9):e66–e76

Prasad AN, Prasad C. The floppy infant: contribution of genetic and metabolic disorders. Review article. Brain Dev 2003;2; 5(7):457–476

3.11 Precocious Puberty or Accelerated Sexual Maturity

Precocious puberty is the appearance of signs of pubertal development at an abnormally early age (▶ Fig. 3.2). In girls, this age has traditionally been considered to be 8 years, although guidelines from the United States have recommended that puberty be considered precocious only with appearance of breast development or pubic hair before 7 years of age in white girls and before 6 years of age in black girls. In boys, the onset of puberty before 9 years of age is considered to be precocious. The female-to-male ratio is 10:1. Precocious puberty is often a benign central process in girls but precocious puberty is rarely idiopathic in boys and early signs of puberty in boys are a particular cause for concern.

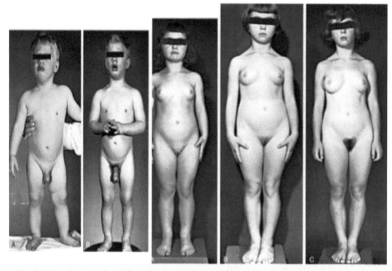

Fig. 3.2 Precocious puberty based upon attainment of secondary sex characteristics that include genital development in males, breast development in females, and pubic hair development in both genders. (These images are provided courtesy of Dr Santosh, MAGALI.)

Precocious puberty can be divided into two distinct categories.

1. **Gonadotrophin-dependent precocious puberty (central precocious puberty, (CPP) "true"):** This involves the premature activation of the hypothalamic–pituitary–gonadal (HPG) axis. Most children (especially girls) suspected of having CPP do not have any specific abnormality but lie at one end of the normal distribution curve.
   The causes may be:
   a) Idiopathic (sporadic or familial)
   b) CNS abnormalities or lesions
      i. Hypothalamic hamartomas
      ii. Tumors: astrocytoma, craniopharyngioma, ependymoma, glioma Germinoma, pineal tumors, human chorionic gonadotrophin (HCG)-secreting tumors, hypothalamic teratomas
      iii. Congenital malformations: arachnoid cyst, suprasellar cyst, phakomatosis, hydrocephalus (+ spina bifida), septo-optic dysplasia
      iv. Acquired disease: Inflammatory CNS disease, abscess, radiation, chemotherapy, trauma, ischemia, surgery

     v. Dysmorphic syndromes: Williams–Beuren syndrome, Klinefelter syndrome (rare)

    vi. Prolonged exposure to sex steroids: Congenital adrenal hyperplasia, sex steroid-producing tumors

c) Absence of CNS abnormalities, the causes of early normal puberty include:

     i. Genetic: Early puberty is familial and autosomal dominant

    ii. Russell–Silver syndrome

   iii. McCune–Albright syndrome

   iv. Hypothyroidism

    v. Obesity: in girls, but not in boys, early puberty is associated with increase in body mass index (BMI).

2. **Gonadotrophin-independent precocious puberty (or precocious pseudopuberty):** In this, the presence of sex steroids is independent of pituitary gonadotrophin release. This accounts for about 20% of cases of precocious puberty. The gonad matures independently of gonadotrophin-releasing hormone (GnRH) stimulation and levels of testosterone and estradiol, luteinizing hormone (LH) and follicle-stimulating hormone are usually at pubertal levels (in the absence of gonadotrophin pulsatility). There is a flat GnRH response and no response to treatment with GnRH analogues.

The causes may be:

a) Adrenal disorders

     i. Adrenal adenoma

    ii. Adrenal carcinoma

   iii. Congenital adrenal hyperplasia

b) Ovarian disorders: can cause masculinization or feminization

     i. Granulosa cell tumor

    ii. Theca cell tumors

   iii. Other estrogen-secreting tumors: teratoma, teratocarcinoma, dysgerminoma, luteoma, mixed cell tumor, lipoid tumor

   iv. Sex-cord or Sertoli-cell tumor of the ovary, and aromatase activity in Peutz–Jeghers syndrome

    v. McCune–Albright syndrome (ovarian cysts)

   vi. Autonomous isolated ovarian cysts

c) Testicular disorders

     i. Leydig cell adenoma

    ii. Constitutively activating LH receptor mutations (male-limited precocious puberty, i.e., *testotoxicosis*)

d) Human chorionic gonadotrophin (HCG)-secreting tumors
   i. Dysgerminoma
   ii. Teratoma
   iii. Chorioepithelioma
   iv. Choriocarcinoma
   v. Hepatoblastoma
   vi. Pinealoma
e) Exogenous
   i. Sex steroid exposure: pills (estrogens, anabolics), food additives, cosmetics, creams, etc.

Muir A. Precocious puberty. Pediatr Rev 2006;27(10):373–381

Kaplowitz P. Precocious puberty: update on secular trends, definitions, diagnosis, and treatment. Adv Pediatr 2004;51:37–62

3.12 Arthrogryposis

Arthrogryposis multiplex congenita is a collective term applied to a very large number of different syndromes characterized by nonprogressive, multiple joint contractures present at birth. (▶ Fig. 3.3) The joints usually develop normally in early embryonic life but as gestation progresses, movements are required to facilitate normal development. Abnormalities, such as neurological or connective-tissue disorders or physical restriction, lead to this condition. The basic cause is fetal akinesia. The underlying cause can be environmental (lack of ability to

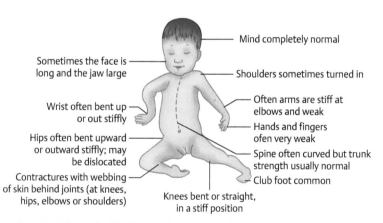

Sometimes the face is long and the jaw large

Mind completely normal

Shoulders sometimes turned in

Wrist often bent up or out stiffly

Often arms are stiff at elbows and weak

Hands and fingers ofen very weak

Hips often bent upward or outward stiffly; may be dislocated

Spine often curved but trunk strength usually normal

Contractures with webbing of skin behind joints (at knees, hips, elbows or shoulders)

Club foot common

Knees bent or straight, in a stiff position

Fig. 3.3 Typical baby with arthrogryposis.

move) or genetic (single gene conditions). The muscles involved are partially or completely replaced by fat and fibrous tissue. The most common form, accounting for 40% of cases, is amyoplasia (**A** = no, **myo** = muscle, **plasia** = growth).

3.12.1 Differential diagnosis

There is a wide and varied range of rare conditions to be considered in the diagnosis. Conditions causing arthrogryposis include:

1. **Fetal abnormalities**
   a) Neurogenic disorders
      i. Myelomeningocele
      ii. Sacral agenesis
      iii. Spinal muscular atrophy (anterior horn cell disease of prenatal origin (SMA 0), not Werding–Hoffman (SMA 1)
      iv. Congenital contracture syndrome (lethal)
      v. Cerebro-oculo-facial syndrome
      vi. Marden–Walker syndrome
      vii. Pena–Shokeir syndrome
   b) Myopathic disorders
      i. Congenital myopathies
      ii. Congenital muscular dystrophy
      iii. Myasthenic syndromes
      iv. Intrauterine viral myositis
      v. Mitochondrial disorders
   c) Connective tissue disorders
      i. Diastrophic dysplasia
      ii. Osteochondrodysplasia
      iii. Metatropic dwarfism
   d) Mechanical limitations to movement
      i. Oligohydramnios as in Potter's syndrome and multiple births
2. **Maternal disorders**
   a) Maternal infection (including rubella, Coxsackie, and enterovirus infections)
   b) Drugs (including alcohol, phenytoin, and methocarbamol)
   c) Trauma
   d) Intrauterine vascular abnormalities/compromise
   e) Other maternal illnesses (including myotonic dystrophy, myasthenia gravis, and multiple sclerosis)

Barnshad M, Van Heest A, Pleasure D. Arthrogryposis: a review and update. J Bone Joint Surg 2009;91 (Suppl 4):40–46

3.13 Progressive Proximal Weakness

It occurs commonly due to myopathy, usually a muscular dystrophy.

1. Myopathies
   a) Muscular dystrophies
      i. Duchene and Becker muscular dystrophy
      ii. Facioscapulohumeral syndrome
      iii. Limb-Girdle dystrophy
   b) Inflammatory myopathies
      i. Dermatomyositis
      ii. Polymyositis
   c) Metabolic myopathies
      i. Acid maltase deficiency
      ii. Carbohydrate myopathies (McArdle disease)
      iii. Muscle carnitine deficiency
      iv. Lipid myopathies
   d) Endocrine myopathies
      i. Hyper/hypothyroidism
      ii. Hyper/hypoparathyroidism
      iii. Hyper/hypoadrenalism
2. Juvenile spinal muscular atrophies: Wohlfart–Kugelberg–Welander disease
   a) Autosomal recessive form
   b) Autosomal dominant form
   c) GM2 Gangliosidosis (Tay–Sachs disease)
3. Myasthenic syndromes
   a) Familial limb-girdle myasthenia
   b) Slow channel syndrome
4. Spinal cord disorders
   a) Congenital malformations
      i. Arteriovenous malformations
      ii. Myelomeningocele
      iii. Chiari malformation (Type I and II)
      iv. Tethered spinal cord
      v. Atlantoaxial dislocation: Aplasia of odontoid process, Morquio syndrome, Klippel–Feil syndrome
   b) Familial spastic paraplegia
   c) Trauma
      i. Spinal cord concussion
      ii. Compressed vertebral body fractures

  iii. Fracture dislocation and spinal cord transection
  iv. Spinal epidural hematoma
 d) Tumors of the spinal cord
  i. Astrocytoma
  ii. Ependymoma
  iii. Neuroblastoma
  iv. Other tumors (sarcoma, neurofibroma, dermoid/epidermoid, meningioma, teratoma)
 e) Transverse myelitis
 f) Neonatal cord infarction
 g) Infections
  i. Diskitis
  ii. Epidural abscess
  iii. Tuberculous osteomyelitis

Chawla J. Stepwise approach to myopathy in systemic disease. Front Neurol 2011;2:49

McDonald CM. Clinical approach to the diagnostic evaluation of hereditary and acquired neuromuscular diseases. Phys Med Rehabil Clin N Am 2012;23(3):495–563

3.14 Progressive Distal Weakness

This condition mostly occurs due to myopathies, followed by neuropathies.

1. Myopathies

The myopathies are primary disease of muscle, and all produce weakness with variable pain and wasting of skeletal muscles.

 a) Muscular dystrophies
  i. Duchene muscular dystrophy
  ii. Becker muscular dystrophy
  iii. Facioscapulohumeral dystrophy
  iv. Limb girdle dystrophy
  v. Myotonic dystrophy
 b) Metabolic myopathies
  i. Glycogenoses: Myophosphorylase deficiency, acid maltase deficiency, phosphofructokinase deficiency
  ii. Lipidoses: Carnitine deficiency, carnitine palmityl transferase deficiency
  iii. Endocrine myopathies: Hyperthyroidism, hypothyroidism, hyperparathyroidism, corticosteroid myopathy
  iv. Periodic paralysis: Hyperkalemic, hypokalemic
  v. Mitochondrial myopathies

- Kearns-Sayre syndrome (external ophthalmoplegia, retinitis pigmentosa, heart block elevated CSF protein)
- Myoclonic epilepsy with ragged red fibres (MERRF)
- Mitochondrial encephalopathy with lactic acidosis and stroke-like episodes (MELAS)
- Pure skeletal myopathy

c) Inflammatory myopathies
Acquired muscle diseases in which muscle inflammation produces variable amounts of weakness and pain.
  i. Dermatomyositis
  ii. Polymyositis
  iii. Inclusion body myositis

2. Peripheral neuropathies
This type of neuropathy produces signs and symptoms in a distal-to-proximal gradient, the so-called stocking-glove pattern.
  a) Idiopathic chronic neuropathy
    i. Axonal form
    ii. Demyelinating form
  b) Hereditary motor and sensory neuropathy
    i. Type I: Charcot–Marie–Tooth disease
    ii. Type II: Charcot–Marie–Tooth disease, neuronal type
    iii. Type III: Dejerine–Sottas disease
    iv. Type IV: Refsum disease
  c) Other genetic neuropathies
    i. Giant axonal neuropathy
    ii. Metachromatic leukodystrophy
  d) Toxic/metabolic neuropathies
    i. Toxins: Mercury, lead, zinc, arsenic, thallium, alcohol, organophosphates
    ii. Drugs: Amiodarone, Cis-platinum, dapsone, INH, phenytoin, pyridoxine, vincristine, Nitrofurantoin, ddi, ddc
  e) Neuropathies associated with systemic disease
    i. Systemic diseases: Diabetes mellitus, uremia, porphyria, vitamin B12 deficiency, amyloidosis, hypothyroidism, benign monoclonal gammopathy
    ii. Systemic infections: Leprosy, syphilis, diphtheria, HIV
    iii. Vasculitis due to ischemic infarction of vasa vasorum: Systemic lupus erythematosus, rheumatoid arthritis, polyarteritis nodosa, cryoglobulinemia
    iv. Cancer: Hodgkin's disease, multiple myeloma, oat cell carcinoma

  f) Immune-mediated neuropathies
    i. Guillain–Barre syndrome
    ii. Chronic inflammatory demyelinating polyneuropathy
3. Motor neuron disease (anterior horn cell diseases)
  a) Lower motor neuron signs present
    i. Spinal muscular atrophy
    ii. Infantile (Werding–Hoffman disease)
    iii. Juvenile (Kugelberg–Welander disease)
    iv. Adult (Aran–Duchene)
  b) Lower and upper motor signs present
    i. Amyotrophic lateral sclerosis (motor neuron disease)
    ii. Progressive bulbar palsy
  c) Upper motor signs present
    i. Lateral sclerosis
4. Spinal cord disorders
  a) Congenital malformations
    i. Arteriovenous malformations
    ii. Myelomeningocele
    iii. Chiari malformation (type I and II)
    iv. Tethered spinal cord
    v. Atlantoaxial dislocation: Aplasia of odontoid process, Morquio syndrome, Klippel–Feil syndrome
  b) Familial spastic paraplegia
  c) Trauma
    i. Spinal cord concussion
    ii. Compressed vertebral body fractures
    iii. Fracture dislocation and spinal cord transection
    iv. Spinal epidural hematoma
  d) Tumors of the spinal cord
    i. Astrocytoma
    ii. Ependymoma
    iii. Neuroblastoma
    iv. Other tumors: sarcoma, neurofibroma, dermoid/epidermoid, meningioma, teratoma
  e) Transverse myelitis
  f) Neonatal cord infarction
  g) Infections
    i. Diskitis
    ii. Epidural abscess
    iii. Tuberculous osteomyelitis

Differential diagnosis of various types of weaknesses

| | | Clinical characteristics | | | | |
Weakness	Distribution	Muscle tone	Reflexes	Sensation/Pain	Atrophy	Coordination
Upper motor neuron	Lower face Arm extensors Leg flexors	Spasticity Increased resistance overcoming arm flexion, leg extension (clasp knife)	DTR increased Clonus at patella and ankle Babinski+		None Mild from disuse	Slowness or incoordination of fine movements (tapping fingers/ wiggling toes)
Lower motor neuron	Peripheral neuropathy, Symmetrical, distal, or follows root Plexus, nerve	Decreased in the affected muscles	Decreased or absent		Present in the affected muscles	Motor ataxia related to degree of weakness
Spinal cord lesion	UMN below level of cord lesion		Brisk below level of lesion	All modalities affected fairly equal (Brown-Sequard) Root pain at compression level		
Myasthenia gravis	Cranial n., diplopia, dysphagia, dysarthria, proximal/ distal symmetric	Normal	Normal or increased			Affected in proportion to degree of weakness

▶ (Continued)

		Clinical characteristics				
Weakness	Distribution	Muscle tone	Reflexes	Sensation/Pain	Atrophy	Coordination
Nerve root lesion	Upper/lower extremity, chest or abdominal wall Weakness in distribution of involved nerve root	Decreased in the affected muscles	Decreased or absent in affected dermatomes or myotomes	Pain in a radicular fashion Paresthesia in sensory distribution on the affected nerve root Worsening by activities such as straight leg raising	Present in affected muscles Fasciculations may be noted	Usually unaffected
Myopathic weakness	Proximal (neck flexors, shoulder, and hip girdle muscles) Problems climbing stairs, getting out of deep chairs, holding arms over head for long	Normal or decreased severe weakness and contractures may occur	Normal or diminished proportional to weakness	Pain, tenderness, and sometimes swelling on involved muscles	Present with moderate to severe involvement	

Abbreviations: DTR, deep tendon reflexes; UMN, upper motor neuron

van den Berg-Vos RM, Visser J, Franssen H, et al. Sporadic lower motor neuron disease with adult onset: classification of subtypes. Brain 2003;126(Pt 5);1036–1047

Pina-Garza JE. In: Fenichel's Clinica; Pediatrics Neurology: A sign and symptom approach. 7th ed. Elsevier Saunders; 2013

Swash M, Schwartz MS. Neuromuscular Diseases. 3rd ed. Springer-Verlag; 2013

3.15 Acute Generalized Weakness or Acute Flaccid Paralysis

Acute flaccid paralysis (AFP) is a clinical syndrome with a broad array of potential etiologies, characterized by rapid onset of weakness, including (less frequently) weakness of the muscles of respiration and swallowing, progressing to maximum severity within several days to weeks.

The list of underlying causes of AFP is broad and may vary by age and geographic region. The etiologies of AFP are often associated with specific pathophysiologic mechanisms or anatomic-morphologic changes, which may help in establishing the correct clinical diagnosis.

The sudden onset of flaccid weakness in the absence of encephalopathy is always due to motor unit disorders. From all listed disorders, Guillain–Barre syndrome is the most common cause.

3.15.1 Differential diagnosis

1. Lesions of the anterior horn cells of the spinal cord
   a) Viruses targeting motor neurons
      i. Polioviruses
      ii. Poliomyelitis
      iii. Vaccine-associated paralytic poliomyelitis
      iv. Nonpolio enteroviruses
   b) Other neurotropic viruses
      i. Rabies virus and rabies vaccines
      ii. Herpesviridae (cytomegalovirus, Epstein–Barr virus, varicella-zoster virus)
      iii. Viral encephalomyelitis (paramyxovirus [parainfluenza virus, mumps virus], togo virus, arbo virus, herpesviridae), parasites (*Trichinella spiralis*), or stroke of the spinal cord.
      iv. Japanese encephalomyelitis virus
2. Polyradiculoneuropathies
   a) Guillain–Barre syndrome: The diagnostic criteria based on the pathophysiologic and morphologic understanding of Guillain–Barre syndrome correspond to those of acute inflammatory demyelinating polyradiculoneuropathy. In the absence of wild virus-induced poliomyelitis, Guillain–Barre syndrome is the most common cause of AFP worldwide, and it accounts for over 50% of AFP cases. The incidence is 1–2 per 100,000 increasing with age and it is most common in the elderly.

b) Subacute and chronic inflammatory demyelinating polyradiculoneuropathy

c) Acute motor axonal neuropathy

d) Neurologic disorders associated with HIV infection, AIDS, or opportunistic infections

3. Acute myelopathies

a) Acute transverse myelitis: The initial spinal shock phase presents with weakness of the lower extremities, AFP, urinary distention (neurogenic bladder), constipation, hyporeflexia, sensory level, severe pain, and paresthesia. After 2–3 weeks, hyperreflexia and spasticity appear. Acute transverse myelitis has been associated with *Mycoplasma pneumoniae*, Herpesviridae, rabies virus, hepatitis A virus, enteric fever, parasitic infections, following administration of oral poliovirus vaccine, tetanus toxoid and cholera, typhoid fever.

b) Acute myelopathy due to spinal cord compression (paraspinal or epidural abscess, tumor or hematoma) or anterior spinal artery syndrome

4. Trauma

a) Acute traumatic sciatic neuritis associated with intramuscular gluteal injection

b) Spinal cord injury

c) Cardiovascular disorders, surgical complications
Postoperative spinal cord damage due to ischemia may result in total paraplegia or paraparesis. High aortic clamping and hypotension may also cause ischemic cord damage. Clinically there is AFP, areflexia, sensory loss, patulous sphincter, and reflex neurogenic bladder.

5. Peripheral neuropathies
Polyradiculopathies (spinal roots and peripheral nerve trunks) and *polyneuropathies* which result in bilaterally symmetrical disturbance of function, tend to be associated with agents that act diffusely on the peripheral nervous system, such as toxic substances, deficiency states, systemic metabolic disorders, and autoimmune reactions.

a) Toxic neuropathies: Distal axonal degeneration is the neuronal dysfunction in most toxic neuropathies. Neuropathies may occur in the course of infectious diseases such as diphtheria, borreliosis, and rabies. Acute peripheral neuropathy with features similar to those of Guillain–Barre syndrome can occur in acute beriberi, acute intermittent porphyria, AIDS, paralytic rabies, cytomegalovirus infection, Epstein–Bar virus infection, and hepatitis B virus infection and following the administration of Semple-type rabies vaccine. A variety of chemicals, metals, and drugs have been associated with motor-sensory neuropathies. Many antimicrobial, antirheumatic drugs (gold, colchicine), or chemotharapeutic

(Vinca alkaloids and platinum-containing compounds) agents may cause mainly sensory and distal weakness.

6. Diseases of the neuromuscular junction

A variety of naturally occurring toxins of animal, plant, and bacterial origin are capable of causing disorders of neuromuscular transmission leading to symmetrical weakness or paralysis of the extremities and trunk. Botulism, tetanus exotoxin, animal toxins (venom of various snakes, arthropods, and marine creatures, frogs, poisonous fish, shellfish, and crabs), plant toxins (curare, decamethonium), may cause neuroparalytic syndromes (baby, absent eye movements, bulbar symptoms, normal DRTs, hypoventilation). Organophosphorus esters (used as insecticides, pesticides, helminthicides, or war gases), petroleum additives and modifiers of plastics produce acute weakness of the hands, calf pain preceding paresthesia and weakness of the limbs, absent in ankle jerks, foot-drop, and claw-hand leading to muscle paralysis by delayed neuropathy.

7. Weakness associated with critical illness

Neuromuscular dysfunction in patients with sepsis is increasingly being reported. The common underlying pathogenic process appears to be systemic inflammatory response syndrome accentuated by the administration of steroids or neuromuscular blocking agents. Flaccid quadriplegia with inability to wean from ventilatory support despite full cardiopulmonary recovery is the typical presentation.

8. Neuropathies occurring in systemic or metabolic disorders

Acute hypokalemic periodic paralysis, usually familial (affects male Caucasian children), is a rare cause of AFP. *Thyrotoxic periodic paralysis* characterized by acute symmetrical weakness leading to AFP induced by excess level of thyroid hormones (Grave's disease), heavy exertion and high carbohydrate ingestion. *Acute intermittent propfyria* may cause a rapidly progressing peripheral neuropathy with motor-sensory signs and symptoms and consequent AFP. Sporadic cases of *hypokalemic paralysis* are associated with various disorders, such as renal tubular acidosis, Cron's disease and secondary hyperaldosteronism from licorice ingestion.

9. Other clinical syndromes causing AFP

Such entities include osteoarticular trauma, acute cerebellitis, retroperitoneal tumors, infection in an intervertebral disc, scurvy, Geoffrey's disease, postictal hemiparesis (Todd's paralysis), and "floppy infant" syndrome.

10. Paralytic syndromes or periodic paralysis
    a) Familial hyperkalemic periodic paralysis
    b) Familial hypokalemic periodic paralysis
    c) Familial normokalemic periodic paralysis

Antoniuk SA. Acute muscle weakness: differential diagnoses Rev Neurol 2013;57(Suppl 1):S149–S154

Hughes RA, Cornblath DR. Guillain–Barré syndrome. Lancet 2005;366(9497):1653–1666

Marx A, Glass JD, Sutter RW. Differential diagnosis of acute flaccid paralysis and its role in poliomyelitis surveillance. Epidemiol Rev 2000;22(2):298–316

3.16 Periodic Paralysis

Periodic paralysis (PP) is a group of disorders of different etiologies, with epi-sodic, short-lived, and hyporeflexic skeletal muscle weakness, with or without myotonia but without sensory deficit and without loss of consciousness. PP is divided into primary or familial periodic paralysis, and secondary periodic paralysis.

The serum potassium levels in both primary and secondary PP are usually abnormal during the attacks. If the level is below normal, the PP is known as hypokalemic type and if the level is higher than normal as hyperkalemic type.

Primary or familial PP is a group of disorders that occur due to single gene mutation resulting in abnormalities of calcium (hypokalemic PP), sodium (hyper-kalemic PP, paramyotonia congenita, potassium-aggravated myotonia), potas-sium (Andersen's syndrome, some cases of hyper- and hypokalemic PP), and chloride (myotonia congenita) channels on muscle cell membranes (aka channel-opathies or membranopathies).

Secondary PP may occur due to known causes:

1. Hypokalemic PP
   a) Thyrotoxicosis
   b) Thiazide or loop diuretics
   c) Potassium loosing nephropathy
   d) Drug induced (gentamycin, carbenicillin, amphotericin-B, tetracyclines, vitamin B12, alcohol)
   e) Primary or secondary hyperaldosteronism
   f) Acute human toxicity from ingestion of carbonate or rodenticide
   g) Gastrointestinal potassium loss
2. Hyperkalemic PP
   a) Chronic renal failure
   b) High dose of angiotensin-converting enzyme (ACE) inhibitor therapy, chronic renal failure, or advanced diabetic nephropathy.
   c) Potassium supplements if used with potassium-sparing diuretics and/or ACE inhibitors.
   d) Andersen's cardiodysrythmic syndrome
   e) Paramyotonia congenita PP
   f) Potassium-aggravated myotonia

Differential diagnosis of various types of primary periodic paralysis

Clinical features	Hypokalemic periodic paralysis	Hyperkalemic periodic paralysis	Paramyotonia congenita
Age of onset	Second decade	First decade	Early childhood
Inheritance	Autosomal dominant	Autosomal dominant	Autosomal dominant
Male:female ratio	3:1	1:1	No sex predilection
Timing of attack	Early morning or night	Day	Anytime
Duration of attack	Hours to days (2–12 hours)	Minutes to hours (1–2 hours)	2–24 hours
Precipitating factors	Rich carbohydrate meal, alcohol, rest after exercise	Rest after exercise, cold exposure	Spontaneously or after exposure to cold
Severity of attacks	Moderate to severe weakness	Mild to moderate weakness, may be local	Very mild
Myotonia	No	Yes	No
Effect of muscle cooling	No change	Increased myotonia	Increased myotonia, then weakness
Serum potassium during attack	Low	Usually high, may be normal	Usually normal
Ionic channel disorder	Calcium channel	Sodium channel	Sodium channel
EMG: during attack	Electrical silence	Electrical silence	
EMG: interictal	Fibrillation and complex repetitive discharge increased by cold and decreased by exercise	Myotonic discharges in some	Myotonic discharges hyper-irritability and after discharge. Weakened muscles show a dropping out of some motor unit potentials and reduced voltage and duration of others
Muscle biopsy	Presence of single or centrally placed vacuoles	Vacuoles and tubular aggregate	No change or at most a few vacuoles

Streib EW. AAEE minimonograph #27: differential diagnosis of myotonic syndromes. Muscle Nerve 1987; 10(7):603–615

Lin SH. Thyrotoxic periodic paralysis. Mayo Clin Proc 2005;80(1):99–105

3.17 Sensory and Autonomic Disturbances

These include pain, dysesthesias, and loss of sensibility.

1. Brachial neuritis
   a) Acute idiopathic brachial neuritis
   b) Familial recurrent brachial neuritis
   c) Reflex sympathetic dystrophy
2. Congenital insensitivity to pain: There is no sensory neuropathy; pain indifference is due to severe mental retardation, e.g, Lesch–Nyham syndrome.
3. Hereditary sensory and autonomic neuropathy
4. Hereditary metabolic neuropathy
5. Foramen magnum tumors (e.g., neurofibroma)
6. Syringomyelia
7. Multiple sclerosis
8. Thalamic syndromes of Dejerine and Roussy (e.g., ischemia of thalamus or of the primary sensory cortex and in thalamic gliomas)
9. Lumbar disc herniation

Reichgetti MJ. Clinical evidence of dysautonomia. In: Walker K, et al., eds. Clinical Methods. 3nd ed. Butterworths; 1990

Vnik Al, Maser RE, Mitchel BD. Diabetic autonomic neuropathy: evaluation of paraesthesia BMJ 2003; 26(5):1553–1579

3.18 Ataxia

1. Acute ataxia
   The most common causes in otherwise healthy children are drug ingestion, postinfectious cerebellitis, and migraine.
   a) Drug ingestion: E.g., overdose of hypnotics, tranquilizers, psychoactive, anticonvulsants (phenytoin, carbamazepine), antihistamines
   b) Postinfectious neuroimmune
      i. Acute postinfectious cerebellitis [preceded by an exanthema (varicella), infectious mononucleosis, or other viral infections (polio, mumps, coxsackie, herpes simplex, or echo viruses)]
      ii. Multiple sclerosis
      iii. Miller-Fisher syndrome (e.g., ataxia, ophthalmoplegia, areflexia)
      iv. Myoclonic encephalopathy and neuroblastoma (Dancing eye syndrome)
   c) Migraine (e.g., basilar migraine, benign paroxysmal vertigo)
   d) Brainstem encephalitis (e.g., echoviruses, coxsackieviruses, adenoviruses are the implicated etiologic agents)

e) Brain tumor (acute complication from existing neuroblastoma, e.g., bleeding, sudden foraminal shift, or hydrocephalus)
f) Conversion reaction (especially in girls aged 10–15 years)
g) Trauma (e.g., postconcussion syndrome, vertebrobasilar occlusion)
h) Vascular disorders
   i. Cerebellar hemorrhage (commonly due to an AVM)
   ii. Vasculitis (e.g., lupus erythematosus, Kawasaki disease)
i) Genetic disorders causing metabolic deficiencies
   i. Hartnup disease
   ii. Maple syrup urine disease
   iii. Carnitine acetyltransferase deficiency
   iv. Pyruvate decarboxylase deficiency
   v. Dominant recurrent ataxia

2. Chronic ataxia
It is progressive ataxia with/without headache in a previously healthy child that occurs most commonly due to a posterior fossa brain tumor.
a) Brain tumors
   i. Medulloblastoma
   ii. Cerebellar astrocytoma
   iii. Ependymoma
   iv. Cerebellar hemangioblastoma (Von Hippel-Lindau disease)
   v. Brainstem glioma
   vi. Supratentorial tumors
b) Congenital malformations
   i. Basilar impression
   ii. Cerebellar malformations (e.g., Hemispheric-vermian aplasia, Dandy–Walker cyst)
c) Hereditary disorders
   i. Autosomal recessive inheritance
      – Ramsay-Hunt syndrome
      – Ataxia-telangiectasia
      – Friedreich ataxia
      – Hartnup disease
      – Abetalipoproteinemia, hypolipoproteinemia
      – Maple syrup urine disease
      – Pyruvate dysmetabolism
   ii. Autosomal dominant inheritance
      – Olivopontocerebellar degeneration
   iii. X-linked inheritance
      – Adrenoleukodystrophy

3.18.1 Common causes of ataxia in different age groups

1. Children before 1 year of age
   a) Congenital malformations
   b) Mild arrested hydrocephalus
   c) Cerebral palsy
   d) Marinesco–Sjogren syndrome
2. Children between 1–5 years of age
   a) Drug ingestion
   b) Acute cerebellar ataxia
   c) Myoclonic encephalopathy and neuroblastomas
   d) Inborn errors of metabolism
   e) Brain tumors
   f) Ataxia telangiectasia
   g) Refsum's disease
3. Children between 5–10 years of age
   a) Drug ingestion
   b) Acute cerebellar ataxia
   c) Brain tumors
   d) Wilson's disease
   e) Adrenoleukodystrophy
   f) Hereditary ataxias
4. Children above 10 years of age
   a) Friedreich's Ataxia
   b) Miller-Fisher syndrome
   c) Cerebellar hemorrhage
   d) Multiple sclerosis
   e) Olivopontocerebellar degeneration
   f) Hereditary ataxias

Schulz JB, Boesch S, Bürk K, et al. Diagnosis and treatment of Friedreich ataxia: a European perspective. Nat Rev Neurol 2009;5(4):222–234

Gomez MR. Neurocutaneous Diseases: A Practical Approach. Boston: Butterworths; 1987

Fogel BL. Childhood cerebellar ataxia. J Child Neurol 2012;27(9):1138–1145

3.19 Acute Hemiplegia

The acute onset suggests either a vascular or an epileptic etiology.
1. Stroke
   a) Arteriovenous malformation
   b) Brain tumors and systemic cancer

    c) Carotid disorders (e.g., fibromuscular dysplasia, cervical infection, trauma)

    d) Drug abuse (e.g., cocaine, amphetamine)

    e) Heart disease (e.g., congenital, rheumatic)

    f) Moyamoya disease

    g) Vasculopathies (e.g., lupus, Kawasaki disease, Takayasu arteritis)

    h) Sickle cell anemia

2. Migraine

    a) Complicated migraine (causing hemiplegia or ophthalmoplegia)

    b) Familial hemiplegic migraine

3. Epilepsy

    a) Absence status

    b) Hemiparetic seizures (Todd's paralysis)

4. Diabetes mellitus: Insulin-dependent diabetes causing a complicated migraine as a pathophysiological mechanism

5. Infections: Bacterial or viral infections causing hemiplegia preceded by prolonged and persistent focal seizures, resulting from vasculitis or venous thrombosis

6. Trauma

    a) Hematomas (e.g., epidural, subdural, intracerebral)

    b) Brain edema

7. Tumors (following complications such as hemorrhage, epilepsy)

Uldry PA, Regli F. [Hemiplegia: diagnosis and differential diagnosis] Schweiz Rundsch Med Prax 1990; 79(43):1285–1290

Bhate S, Ganesan V. A practical approach to acute hemiparesis in children. Dev Med Child Neurol 2015; 57(8):689–697

Yew KS, Cheng E. Acute stroke diagnosis. Am Fam Physician 2009;80(1):33–40

Gondolo T. Neurology Study Guide: Oral Board Examination Review. Springer; 2005

3.20 Progressive Hemiplegia

1. Brain tumor
2. Brain abscess
3. Arteriovenous malformation
4. Demyelinating disease
5. Phakomatosis (e.g., Sturge–Weber disease)

3.21 Acute Monoplegia

When a child does not use a limb it signifies there is pain, weakness, or both in the limb. Pain is usually caused by injury, infection, or tumor. Complicated migraine may cause weakness. Pain and weakness together are signs of plexopathy, syringomyelia, and tumors of the cervical cord or brachial plexus.

The leading causes of monoplegia are plexopathies and mononeuropathies.
1. Plexopathies
    a) Acute idiopathic plexitis: A demyelinating disorder of the brachial and lumbar plexi
    b) Osteomyelitis-neuritis: Ischemic nerve damage due to vasculitis
    c) Hopkins syndrome: Postasthmatic viral spinal paralysis from infection of the anterior horn cells
    d) Injuries
        i. Neonatal brachial neuropathy (e.g. upper and lower plexus injuries)
        ii. Motor vehicle and sports related postnatal plexopathies
    e) Tumors of the brachial plexus
        i. Malignant schwannoma
        ii. Neuroblastoma
2. Mononeuropathies (e.g., lacerations, pressure and traction injuries of the radial, ulnal, and peroneal nerves)
3. Spinal muscular atrophy (e.g., hereditary degeneration of the anterior horn cells)
4. Stroke
5. Syringomyelia
6. Congenital malformations of the spinal cord
7. Tumor of the spinal cord

Misulis KE. Hemiplegia and Monoplegia. In: Bradley's Neurology in Clinical Practice. 6th ed. Chapter 23 Elsevier/Saunders; 2012

Dhammi IK, Singh S, Jain AK. Hemiplegic/monoplegic presentation of cervical spine (C1-C2) tuberculosis. Eur Spine J 2001;10(6):540–544

Fenichel GM. Monoplegia. In: Clinical Paediatric Neurology. A Sign and Symptom Approach. 6th ed.; 2009: 285 and 249

3.22 Agenesis of the Corpus Callosum

Agenesis of the corpus callosum (ACC) is a rare disorder that is present at birth (congenital). It is characterized by a partial or complete absence (agenesis) of the transverse fibers that connect the two cerebral hemispheres. The cause of ACC is usually not known, but it can be inherited as either an autosomal recessive trait or an x-linked dominant trait. It can also be caused by an infection or injury during the 12th to the 22nd week of pregnancy (intrauterine) leading to developmental disturbance of the fetal brain. Intrauterine exposure to alcohol (fetal alcohol syndrome) can also result in ACC. (▶ Fig. 3.4)

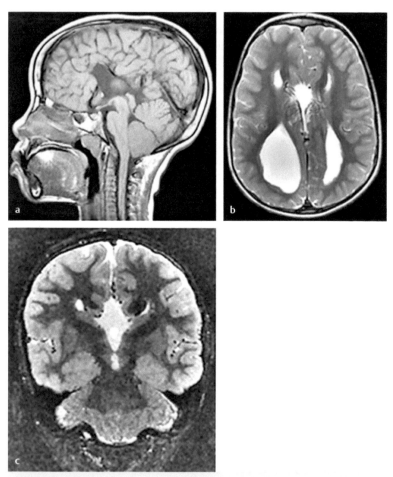

Fig. 3.4 Sagittal T1 magnetic resonance image (a) demonstrates absence of the corpus callosum with a high-riding third ventricle and extension of the medial cerebral hemisphere gyri to the ventricular margin in a radial configuration. Axial T2 image (b) shows a parallel configuration of the lateral ventricles with colpocephaly. Nodular foci of gray matter are visualized along the subependymal surfaces of the ventricles, consistent with heterotopia. Coronal T2 image (c) reveals a "longhorn" configuration of the frontal horns of the lateral ventricles secondary to medial indentation by white matter fibers (Probst bundles). The third ventricle is elevated in the midline. (Reproduced from Case 13. In: O'Brien W, ed. Top 3 Differentials in Neuroradiology. 1st edition. Thieme; 2015.)

ACC is frequently diagnosed during the first two years of life. An epileptic seizure can be the first symptom indicating that a child should be tested for a brain dysfunction. Other symptoms that may begin early in life are feeding problems and delays in holding the head erect, sitting, standing and walking, impairment of mental and physical development, and/or hydrocephalus. Nonprogressive mental retardation, impaired hand–eye coordination, and visual or auditory memory impairment can be diagnosed through neuro examination. Some patients may have deep-seated eyes, prominent forehead, microcephaly, macrocephaly, one or more bent fingers (camptodactyly), wide-set eyes (telecanthus), small nose, short hands, hypotonia and abnormalities of the larynx, and heart defects.

3.22.1 Differential diagnosis

1. Isolated ACC may be confused with *moderate hydrocephaly*. One of the clues that differentiate hydrocephaly from ACC is the presence of the cavum septum pellucidum.
2. Empiric evidence suggests that over 5% of patients with ACC will have an affected family member, due to complex genetic interactions and sporadic genetic disorders (chromosomal deletions and duplications.
3. Severe early-onset autosomal recessive hereditary neuropathies (i.e., those classified as *Charcot–Marie–Tooth hereditary neuropathy type 4, CMT4)*, may be considered as a differential diagnosis.
4. *Infantile neuroaxonal dystrophy (INAD) or Seitelberger disease*, comprises a classic form and an atypical form. PLA2G6 is the only gene known to be associated with NAD.
5. *Arylsulfatase A deficiency (metachromatic leukodystrophy, MLD)*: late infantile MLD (50–60%), juvenile MLD (20–30%), and adult MLD (15–20%) present with CNS and/or peripheral nervous system symptoms with death most commonly resulting from pneumonia or other infection.
6. *Giant axonal neuropathy (GAN)* characterized by severe early-onset peripheral motor and sensory neuropathy, intellectual disability, seizures, cerebellar signs, and pyramidal tract signs; death occurs within the third decade. The pathologic hallmark is so-called giant axons caused by the accumulation of neurofilaments.
7. *Aicardi syndrome*, thought to be inherited as an x-linked dominant disorder, involves ACC, infantile spasms, and abnormal eye structure, frequent seizures, striking abnormalities of the eyes (choroid, retinal layers), severe mental retardation. Only females are affected.
8. *Andermann syndrome*, a genetic disorder characterized by ACC, mental retardation, and progressive sensory–motor disturbances (neuropathy). Identified in an area of Quebec, Canada.

9. *X-linked lissencephaly with ambiguous genitalia (XLAG)* in which males have small and smooth brains (lissencephaly), small penis, severe mental retardation, and intractable epilepsy.
10. *Communicating and noncommunicating (fluid filled) cyst of the septum*
11. *Pellucidum*
12. *Lipoma of the septum pellucidum*
13. *Symmetrical tumors of the septum pellucidum*

Associated midline abnormalities include:
1. Interhemispheric arachnoid cyst
2. Interhemispheric lipoma
3. Agyria or lissencephaly
4. Pachygyria
5. Schizencephaly
6. Heterotopias
7. Dandy–Walker syndrome
8. Holoprosencephaly
9. Olivopontocerebellar degeneration
10. Encephalocele
11. Septo-optic dysplasia
12. Chiari I and II malformations
13. Trisomy 13–15 and 18
14. Spina bifida, meningocele or meningomyelocele

Dávila-Gutiérrez G. Agenesis and dysgenesis of the corpus callosum. Semin Pediatr Neurol 2002;9(4): 292–301

Barkovich AJ. Anomalies of the corpus callosum and cortical malformations. In: Barth PG, ed. Disorders of Neuronal Migration (International Review of Child Neurology). London, UK: Mac Keith Press; 2003:83–103

Hetts SW, Sherr EH, Chao S, Gobuty S, Barkovich AJ. Anomalies of the corpus callosum: an MR analysis of the phenotypic spectrum of associated malformations. AJR Am J Roentgenol 2006;187(5):1343–1348

3.23 Megalencephaly

It refers to brain with excessive weight or large brain.

A large head—*macrocephaly*—may be due to hydrocephalus, megalencephaly, a space-occupying lesion, or a thick skull. Megalencephaly (also called *macrencephaly*) describes an enlarged brain whose weight exceeds the mean (the average weight for that age and sex) of the general population by at least 2.5 standard deviations. It is associated with some cerebral degenerative disorders, as well as with other conditions (i.e., neurofibromatosis and achondroplasia) which are usually recognized by associated physical stigmata. The incidence of megalencephaly is estimated between 2 and 6%. Males predominate females (4:1), and at least one-half of the patients appear to have a familial basis of their megalencephaly.

Isolated megalencephaly, while described in some gifted individuals (i.e., Byron, Turgenev, Bismarck), is generally considered to be associated with convulsive disorders, delayed development, and corticospinal (brain cortex and spinal cord) dysfunction. It is thought that the condition results from an increased number of cells, an increased size of cells, or accumulation of a metabolic byproduct or abnormal substance due to an inborn error of metabolism.

3.23.1 Causes of megalencephaly

1. Metabolic/toxic
   a) Cerebral edema
      i. Benign intracranial hypertension
      ii. Intoxication (e.g., lead, vitamin A, tetracycline, cyclosporine)
      iii. Galactosemia
      iv. Endocrine (e.g., hypoparathyroidism, hypoadrenocorticism, steroid use/withdrawal)
      v. Iron deficiency anemia
   b) Leukodystrophy
      i. Canavan's disease (▶ Fig. 3.5)
      ii. Alexander's disease (▶ Fig. 3.6)
   c) Lysosomal diseases
      i. Tay–Sachs disease (▶ Fig. 3.7)
      ii. Metachromatic leukodystrophy

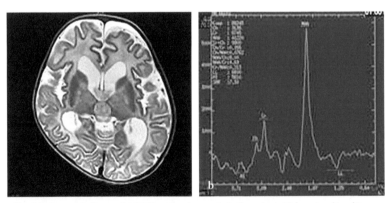

Fig. 3.5 Canavan's disease. **(a)** MRI imaging demonstrates large brain T1 low signal in white matter, T2 high signal in white matter. **(b)** MR spectroscopy: markedly elevated NAA and NAA:creatine ratio. (NAA, N-acetylaspartoacylase: key enzyme in myelin synthesis. In Alexander's disease: No NAA peak)

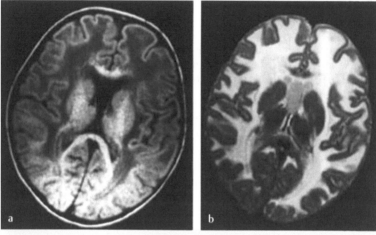

Fig. 3.6 Alexander's disease. A characteristic imaging feature is the predominantly frontal reversal of white-matter signal intensity due to demyelination. **(a)** T1-weighted axial MRI. **(b)** T2-weighted axial MRI. (Reproduced from Congenital White-Matter Diseases (Leukodystrophies). In: Sartor K, ed. Diagnostic and Interventional Neuroradiology. 1st edition. Thieme; 2002.)

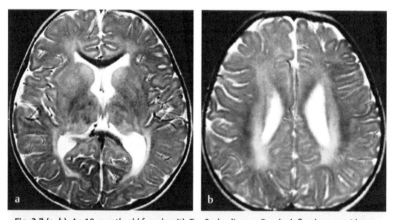

Fig. 3.7 (a, b) An 18-month-old female with Tay-Sachs disease. Poorly defined zones with abnormal high signal on axial T2-weighted imaging are seen in the periventricular white matter. Abnormal high signal is also seen in the caudate nuclei, putamina, and posterior thalami. (Reproduced from Fetal Brain MRI. In: Meyers S, ed. Differential Diagnosis in Neuroimaging: Brain and Meninges. 1st edition. Thieme; 2016.)

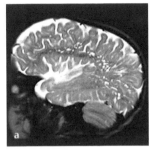
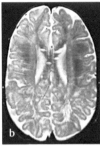
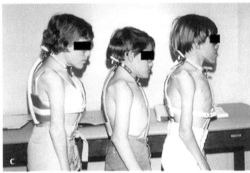

Fig. 3.8 A 2.5-year-old child with Hurler syndrome (MPS IH) shows foci of high signal on **(a)** sagittal and **(b)** axial T2-weighted imaging in the periventricular white matter and corpus callosum. Diffuse brain atrophy is seen. (Reproduced from Fetal Brain MRI. In: Meyers S, ed. Differential Diagnosis in Neuroimaging: Brain and Meninges. 1st edition. Thieme; 2016.) **(c)** Clinical photo of three Morquio siblings in extension braces. (Reproduced from Heritable Disorders of Connective Tissue. In: Dickson R, Harms J, ed. Modern Management of Spinal Deformities: A Theoretical, Practical, and Evidence-based Text. 1st edition. Thieme; 2018.)

   d) Mucopolysaccharidoses (▶ Fig. 3.8)
      i. Hurler's disease
      ii. Hunter's disease
      iii. Morquio syndrome
      iv. Maroteaux–Lamy syndrome
2. Structural
   a) Cerebral gigantism (Soto's syndrome)
   b) Familial megalencephaly (dominant and recessive)
   c) Neurocutaneous syndromes
      i. Neurofibromatosis
      ii. Tuberous sclerosis
      iii. Multiple hemangiomatosis
   d) Fragile X syndrome
   e) Congenital neuronal migrational anomaly
   f) Genetic disorders
      i. Bannayan-Riley-Ruvalcaba syndrome: Macrocephaly, multiple cutaneous tumors and tumor-like growths called hamartomas, dark freckles on the penis.

ii. Proteus syndrome: Mosaic mutation in the AKT1 gene, which helps regulate cell growth and division and cell death

iii. Cranio-cerebello-cardiac syndrome or Ritscher–Schinzel syndrome: Autosomal recessive disease, mutation of gene 8 at 8q24.13, heart defects, cerebellar hypoplasia, cranial dysmorphism

g) Tumors

h) Obstructive, noncommunicating, internal hydrocephalus

i. Posthemorrhagic

ii. Chiari II

iii. Aqueductal stenosis

iv. Dandy–Walker malformation

v. Congenital infection (especially toxoplasmosis)

i) Noncommunicating, communicating, external hydrocephalus

i. Subdural hematoma/hygroma

ii. Nonaccident trauma

iii. Cerebral malformations

iv. Cavernous vein/sinus thrombosis

v. Postmeningitis

vi. Cerebral malformations

Differential diagnosis of megalencephaly

Achondroplasia	Most are new mutations. True megalencephaly, normal cognitive development
Soto's syndrome	Variable inheritance, megalencephaly with gigantism
Hemimegalencephaly	Unilateral cerebral enlargement, associated with poor development and intractable seizures/infantile spasms
Neurocutaneous disorders	Hypomelanosis of Ito, incontinentia pigmenti, neurofibromatosis, tuberous sclerosis, epidermal nevus syndrome
Metabolic megalencephaly	Alexander's disease Cavanan's disease Glutaric aciduria type I: Normal development with macrocephaly until experiencing an encephalopathic event around age 2–3 years. After this, spasticity and movement disorders may be prominent, with variable cognition

McCaffery P, Deutsch CK. Macrocephaly and the control of brain growth in autistic disorders. Prog Neurobiol 2005;77(1–2):38–56

DeMeyer WE. Microcephaly, micrencephaly, megalencephaly. In: Swaiman K, Ashwal S, Ferriero DM, eds. Pediatric Neurology Principles and Practice. 4th ed. Philadelphia: Mosby-Elsevier, Inc; 2006:362–490

3.24 Unilateral Cranial Enlargement or Hemimegaloencephaly

Hemimegaloencephaly (or unilateral megalencephaly) is a related condition in which brain enlargement occurs in one hemisphere of the brain. It is a congenital malformation in which defective cellular organization and neuronal migration results in hamartomatous overgrowth of a hemisphere. In addition to overgrowth, abnormal cortical development is present in areas of *lissencephaly, agyria, pachygyria,* and *polymicrogyria* in varying proportions, with other areas appearing normal. (▶ Fig. 3.9)

3.24.1 Classification

1. Isolated form
2. Syndromic form: associated with a variety of syndromes typically including hemicorporal hypertrophy of the ipsilateral part of the body. Such associated syndromes include:
   a) Epidermal nevus syndrome
   b) Klippel–Trenaunay syndrome
   c) McCune–Albright syndrome
   d) Proteus syndrome

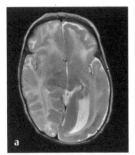 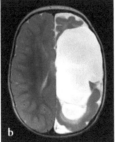 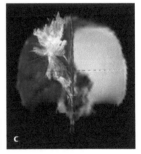

Fig. 3.9 Hemimegalencephaly/hemispherectomy. (**a**) Axial T2 W image in a 1-month-old female with intractable seizures shows hamartomatous overgrowth of the left cerebral hemisphere, with dysplastic cortex and ipsilateral ventricular enlargement. (**b**) Axial T2 W image at 20 months of age after the patient underwent a functional hemispherectomy, in which the temporal lobe, insula, and a majority of the frontal and parietal lobes were resected, with the remnant parenchyma of the frontal and occipital poles disconnected through a corpus callosotomy. (**c**) Fiber tracking on diffusion tensor imaging shows no fibers traversing the midline through the corpus callosum to the remnant left-hemispheric parenchyma, confirming disconnection of the two cerebral hemispheres. (Reproduced from Congenital Malformations. In: Choudhri A, ed. Pediatric Neuroradiology. Clinical Practice Essentials. 1st edition. Thieme; 2016.)

    e) Unilateral hypomelanosis of Ito

    f) Hemimegalencephaly (neuronal migrational anomaly)

    g) Neurofibromatosis type 1 (NF1): rare (▶ Fig. 3.10)

    h) Tuberous sclerosis: rare (▶ Fig. 3.11)

3. Total hemimegalencephaly: hemihypertrophy also involves the *brain stem* and *cerebellum*.

3.24.2 Differential diagnosis

1. Enlarged hemisphere
   a) Gliomatosis cerebri
2. Small hemisphere (making normal hemisphere appear large)
   a) Rasmussen encephalitis
   b) Dyke–Davidoff–Masson syndrome
   c) Sturge–Weber syndrome

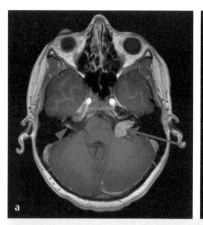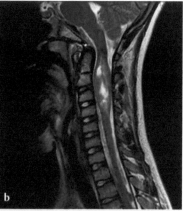

Fig. 3.10 Neurofibromatosis type 2 (NF2) vestibular schwannoma/spinal ependymoma.
(a) Axial T1 plus contrast image of the internal auditory canals (IACs) in an 11-year-old boy shows a mass filling and expanding the left IAC (*arrow*), extending through the porus acusticus and effacing the cerebellopontine angle cistern. A smaller enhancing lesion is seen in the right IAC (*arrowhead*), representing bilateral vestibular scwannomas in the setting of NF2.
(b) Sagittal T2 W image of the cervical spine shows an expansile intramedullary lesion extending from C1 through C4, which in the setting of NF2 probably represents an ependymoma. (Reproduced from Neurofibromatosis Type II. In: Choudhri A, ed. Pediatric Neuroradiology. Clinical Practice Essentials. 1st edition. Thieme; 2016.)

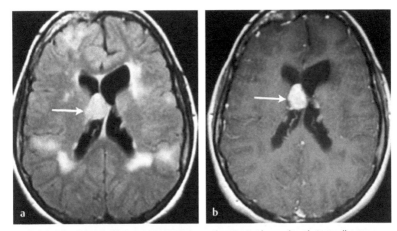

Fig. 3.11 An 18-year-old woman with tuberous sclerosis. A subependymal giant cell astrocytoma is seen at the right foramen of Monro that **(a)** has high signal on axial FLAIR (*arrow*) and **(b)** shows gadolinium contrast enhancement on axial T1-weighted imaging (*arrow*). Also seen are cortical tubers, peri-atrial white matter signal abnormalities, and ependymal hamartomas on axial FLAIR. The ependymal hamartomas also show gadolinium contrast enhancement on axial T1-weighted imaging. (Reproduced from Introduction. In: Meyers S, ed. Differential Diagnosis in Neuroimaging: Brain and Meninges. 1st edition. Thieme; 2016.)

3. Other neuronal migration anomalies without overgrowth
   a) Polymicrogyria, lissencephaly, agyria, pachygyria

Griffiths PD, Gardner SA, Smith M, Rittey C, Powell T. Hemimegalencephaly and focal megalencephaly in tuberous sclerosis complex. AJNR Am J Neuroradiol 1998;19(10):1935–1938

3.25 Microcephaly

In most cases, microcephaly results from failure of the brain to grow at an appropriate rate at some point during development. As the degree of microcephaly increases, so does the probability of mental retardation. A young child with an occipito-frontal circumference (OFC) more than 3 standard deviation below the mean for age has an approximate 50% chance of being mentally retarded. However, this risk may be modified by OFC growth velocity and family history. If possible, the parent's OFCs should always be measured. Among individuals with microcephaly and cognitive disability, acquired causes are more common than the inherited disorders. (▶ Fig. 3.12)

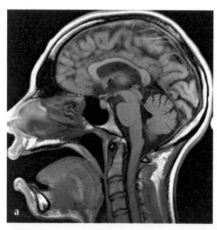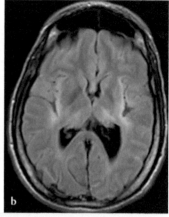

Fig. 3.12 Sagittal T1 magnetic resonance image **(a)** demonstrates microcephaly with a decreased craniofacial ratio. Axial fluid-attenuated inversion recovery image **(b)** reveals abnormal signal intensity involving the thalami, as well as abnormal signal intensity and encephalomalacia within the bilateral insular cortex and subcortical white matter. (Reproduced from Case 12. In: O'Brien W, ed. Top 3 Differentials in Neuroradiology. 1st edition. Thieme; 2015.)

3.25.1 Conditions associated with microcephaly

1. Acquired causes
   a) Fetal alcohol exposure
   b) Hypoxic–ischemic injury (pre- and postnatal events)
   c) Congenital infections (TORCHS, HIV)
   d) Untreated maternal phenylketonuria
   e) Postnatal meningoencephalitis (bacterial and viral)
   f) Early nonaccident trauma
   g) Severe malnutrition
2. Genetic forms
   a) Familial and nonfamilial microcephaly
   b) Chromosomal abnormalities
   c) Aminoaccidopathies (e.g., PKU)
   d) Metabolic disease
      i. Neuronal ceroid lipofuscins
      ii. Mitochondrial disorders
      iii. Carbohydrate-deficient-glycoprotein syndrome
   e) Angelman syndrome
   f) Fanconi anemia

g) Miller–Dieker syndrome
h) Rubinstein–Taybi syndrome
i) Rett syndrome
j) Seckel syndrome
k) Smith–Lemil–Opitz syndrome
l) Williams syndrome

Woods CG. Human microcephaly. Curr Opin Neurobiol 2004;14(1):112–117

3.26 Tethered Spinal Cord Syndrome

Tethered spinal cord syndrome (TCS) is a neurological disorder associated with the fixation (tethering) effect of inelastic tissue on the caudal spinal cord, thus limiting its movement within the spinal column. As a child ages, these attachments cause an abnormal progressive stretching of the spinal cord potentially resulting in a variety of neurological and other symptoms. Due to the variation of the growth rate of the spinal cord and the spinal canal, the progression of neurological signs and symptoms is highly variable. Some individuals present with tethered cord syndrome at birth (so-called congenital), while others develop the symptomatology in infancy, early childhood, or in adulthood (so-called acquired). The majority of cases are developmental, corresponding to the progressive development of excess fibrous connective tissue (fibrosis) in *the filum terminale*. The latter is a strand of tissue that bridges the spinal cord tip and the sacrum. (▶ Fig. 3.13)

Pathophysiologically, neuronal dysfunction in TCS results partly from inability for the spinal cord neurons to utilize oxygen (impaired oxidative metabolism), partly due to lack of oxygen supply (ischemic effect), and partly to ion channel dysfunction directly related neuronal membrane stretching.

3.26.1 Causes

Congenital (primary)

The inelastic structures in children originate from defective closure of the neural tube during embryonic development, eventually forming a condition known as *spina bifida* (incomplete closure of the posterior spinal cord and bony vertebrae-laminae). (▶ Fig. 3.14)

Many cases of this anomaly leave a portion of the spinal cord protruded through the spinal canal, typically forming a *myelomeningocele.* In this anomaly, the spinal cord fails to separate from the skin of the back during development, preventing it from ascending normally, so the spinal cord is low-lying or tethered. In patients with a *lipomyelomeningocele*, the spinal cord will have fat at the tip and this may connect to the fat which overlies the thecal sac.

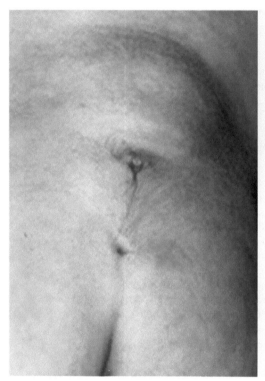

Fig. 3.13 Clinical photo of the back of a neonate with three cutaneous signatures of occult spinal dysraphism (focal hirsutism, subcutaneous mass [neurenteric cyst], and dermal sinus). (Reproduced from 35.1 Introduction and Background. In: Cohen A, ed. Pediatric Neurosurgery: Tricks of the Trade. 1st edition. Thieme; 2015.)

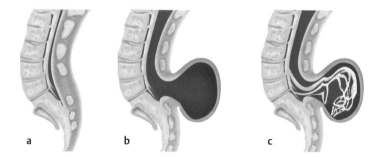

Fig. 3.14 (a) Spina bifida occulta, (b) meningocele, and (c) myelomeningocele.

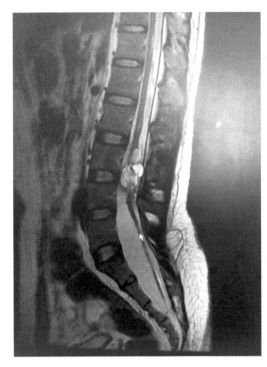

Fig. 3.15 Spinal lipoma with tethered spinal cord syndrome—spinal cord is pulled till sacrum due to lipoma.

Other types of spina bifida associated with TCS include an *abnormal connection of inelastic tissue to the spinal cord,* dermal sinus tract, which extends from the intraspinal tissue to the skin *(dermal sinus tract),* a split spinal cord *(diastematomy-elia),* and a benign fatty mass or tumor *(lipoma)* continuous to the cord. (▶ Fig. 3.15)

Acquired (secondary or developmental)

Secondary causes of tethered cord syndrome include *tumors, infection* or the development of scar tissue *(fibrosis)* connected to the spinal cord. TCS may develop as a complication of *spinal surgery,* and *trauma to the spine* resulting in a band of scar formation attached to the spinal cord.

3.26.2 Symptoms

Children with TSC show cutaneous tufts or hair, skin tags, dimples, benign fatty tumors, skin discoloration, or hemangiomas. Additional symptoms include lower back pain that worsens with activity and improves with rest, leg pain or numbness, difficult walking (gait disturbance), foot and spinal deformities (scoliosis, hyperlordosis), high-arched feet and hammertoes, and less commonly, difference in leg strength. TCS may also cause incontinence (involuntary urination or defecation) and repeated urinary tract infections.

This condition presents differently, and sometimes less obviously, *in adults* than in children. For example, children experience difficult walking, and adults usually have pain and weakness in the legs, back, and foot. Adults' symptoms also include limb muscle atrophy, sensory deficit (numbness), and urinary frequency and urgency accompanied by a sense of incomplete emptying and even incontinence. In adults, symptoms are aggravated by trauma, manoeuvres associated with stretching of the spine (flexion), disc herniation, and spinal stenosis.

3.26.3 Diagnosis

A diagnosis of TCS is made based upon a detailed patient history and a thorough clinical evaluation and detailed MRI studies.

In *children* typical imaging features such as a low-lying spinal cord and a thickened filum terminale is confirmed by MRI or CT scan and ultrasound studies.

Adult TCS is determined by MRI which shows a low level of the conus medullaris (below L2) and a thickened filum terminale.

3.26.4 Differential diagnosis

The diagnosis of TCS is confirmed on the basis of clinical signs and symptoms, which include pain, sensory changes, spasticity, and progressive scoliosis. However, *uncontrolled hydrocephalus* and *Chiari II malformation* must be excluded as causes of these symptoms. Moreover, symptoms similar to those of TCS can also be caused by other intraspinal pathologies, such as the following:

- Mass lesions of the cord
- Diastematmyelia
- Cord cavitation and narrowing
- Adhesions
- Dural bands

Düz B, Gocmen S, Secer HI, Basal S, Gönül E. Tethered cord syndrome in adulthood. J Spinal Cord Med 2008; 31(3):272–278

Bui CJ, Tubbs RS, Oakes WJ. Tethered cord syndrome in children: a review. Neurosurg Focus 2007;23(2):E2

Agarwalla PK, Dunn IF, Scott RM, Smith ER. Tethered cord syndrome. Neurosurg Clin N Am 2007;18(3): 531–547

Gupta SK, Khosla VK, Sharma BS, Mathuriya SN, Pathak A, Tewari MK. Tethered cord syndrome in adults. Surg Neurol 1999;52(4):362–369, discussion 370

Lew SM, Kothbauer KF. Tethered cord syndrome: an updated review. Pediatr Neurosurg 2007;43(3):236–248

3.27 Diastematomyelia

It refers to a type of spinal dysraphism when there is a longitudinal split in the spinal cord. It has been distinguished from *diplomyelia* in which the cord is duplicated rather than split (▶ Fig. 3.16). The term *split cord malformation (SCM)* is advocated to encompass both conditions.

Patients with diastematomyelia frequently are associated with other anomalies such as meningocele, neurenteric cyst, dermoid, club foot, spinal cord lipoma, and hemangioma overlying spine.

Split cord malformations are classified into two types according to presence of a dividing septum and a single vs dual dural sac:

- **Type I:** duplicate dural sac, with common midline spur (osseous or fibrous), and usually symptomatic; hydromyelia common, and usually presenting with scoliosis, spina bifida and tethered cord syndrome. Skin pigmentation, hemangioma and hair patch common.

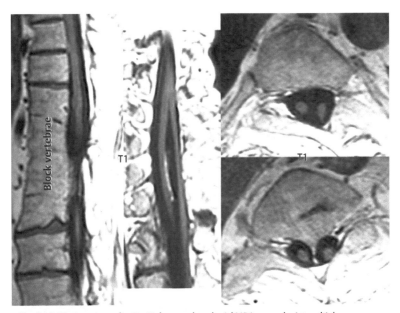

Fig. 3.16 Diastematomyelia: Sagittal, coronal, and axial MR images depict multiple nonsegmental midthoracic vertebral bodies, two hemicords, and on the final axial image a bony spur separating the two cords. Vertebral segmentation anomalies are common with diastematomyelia, in particular block vertebrae, and thus the presence of the latter finding (on plain film or CT) should raise the question of diastematomyelia.

- **Type II:** single dural sac containing both hemicords; hydromyelia and spina bifida may be present but no other anomalies; patients are less symptomatic or even be asymptomatic.

3.27.1 Clinical presentation

The majority of patients with diastematomyelia are symptomatic, presenting with signs and symptoms of tethered cord. Presenting symptoms include:

- Stigmata or having cutaneous lesions (hemangioma, dimples, hair patches, teratoma, or lipoma)
- Spinal deformities
- Weakness of the lower part of the body
- Low back pain
- Scoliosis
- Urinary incontinence or even bowel control
- Motor as well as sensory problems

3.27.2 Diagnosis

The problem is usually detected during prenatal (third semester) ultrasound. This is why adult detection rarely happens, but there are cases where it still happens. Split cord malformations are more common in the lower cord but sometimes occur at multiple levels.

- 50% occur between L1 and L3
- 25% occur between T7 and T12

There are also other problems seen such as spina bifida, hemivertebrae, or the butterfly vertebrae.

MRI is the modality of choice for assessing children with split cord malformations. MRI demonstrates the cord and presence of hydromyelia (if present), and the presence or not of other anomalies. CT scan is able to better image many of the features seen on plain films (i.e., widening of interpeduncular distance, scoliosis, multilevel spina bifida) and in addition may demonstrate the bony septum.

3.27.3 Differential diagnosis

Usually there is little in the way of a differential diagnosis when the cord has been adequately imaged and features are typical.

- Diastematomyelia
- Myelomeningocele

- Syringomyelia
- Diplomyelia
- Tethered cord syndrome
- Closed spina bifida

Pang D, Dias MS, Ahab-Barmada M. Split cord malformation: part I: a unified theory of embryogenesis for double spinal cord malformations. Neurosurgery 1992;31(3):451–480

Pang D. Split cord malformation: Part II: Clinical syndrome. Neurosurgery 1992;31(3):481–500

Schijman E. Split spinal cord malformations: report of 22 cases and review of the literature. Childs Nerv Syst 2003;19(2):96–103

Goldbloom RB. Pediatric Clinical Skills. 4th ed. Saunders/Elsevier; 2010

4 Cranial Nerve Disorders

4.1 Anosmia

Anosmia denotes the complete inability to detect odors on both sides of the nose, whereas decreased ability to detect odors is known as hyposmia. There are several other types of disorders related to ability to detect odors, such as dysosmia that is the distorted identification of smell. Parosmia is altered perception of smell in the presence of an odor, usually unpleasant. Phantosmia refers to the perception of smell without an odor present. Agnosiais the inability to classify or contrast odors, although in this case people are able to detect odors.

The common causes of primary olfactory deficits are aging, nasal and/or sinus disease, prior viral upper respiratory tract infections, and head trauma. These four causes comprise more than two-thirds of all patients with olfactory dysfunction.

Disturbances of olfaction can be classified as *conductive (i.e., transport) defects* where transmission of an odorant stimulus to the olfactory neuroepithelium is disrupted; and *sensorineural defects* that involve more central neural structures.

4.1.1 Conductive defects

1. Inflammatory processes cause a large proportion of olfactory defects.
   a) Bacterial rhinosinusitis
   b) Allergic rhinitis
   c) Vasomotor rhinitis
   d) Fungal rhinosinusitis
   e) Chronic inflammatory rhinitis (syphilis, tuberculosis, sarcoidosis, leprosy, Wegener's granulomatosis)
   f) Nasal polyposis
   g) Sjogren's syndrome
   h) Osteomyelitis of frontal and ethmoidal sinuses
2. Trauma—fracture causing airway obstruction
   a) Mucosal edema
   b) Foreign body
   c) Nasal surgery
3. Patients with laryngectomies or tracheostomies experience hyposmia due to decreased or absent nasal airflow. Children with tracheostomies are cannulated for a long time.
   a) Fixed nasal obstruction
   b) Paradoxical turbinates

    c) Nasal septal deformity
    d) Turbinate hypertrophy
    e) Rhinoplasty
    f) Sinus surgery
    g) Atrophic rhinitis
4. Neoplasia—masses may block the nasal cavity
    a) Benign (papilloma (most common), angiofibroma, osteoma, schwannoma)
    b) Malignant (squamous cell carcinoma, adenocarcinoma, esthesioneuroblastoma, lymphoma, salivary carcinoma, metastasis)
    c) Tumors of the nasopharynx with extension
5. Developmental anomalies may cause obstruction
    a) Encephaloceles
    b) Dermoid cysts

4.1.2 Central/sensorineural defects

1. Aging
Sense of smell decreases with age. The number of fibers in the olfactory bulb decrease throughout one's lifetime.
2. Head trauma, brain surgery, or subarachnoid hemorrhage may stretch, damage, or transect the delicate fila olfactoria or damage brain parenchyma resulting in anosmia.
3. Infectious and inflammatory processes
    a) Viral infections (damage of neuroepithelium)
    b) Sarcoidosis (affecting neural structures)
    c) Wegener's granulomatosis
    d) Multiple sclerosis (MS)
    e) Chronic rhinosinusitis (irreversible loss of olfactory receptors through upregulated apoptosis)
4. Intracranial neoplasm
    a) Benign (papilloma, meningioma, craniopharyngioma, glioma)
    b) Malignant (leukemia, esthesioneuroblastoma, metastasis)
    c) Temporal lobe tumors
5. Endocrine disturbances may affect olfactory function
    a) Hypothyroidism
    b) Hypoadrenalism
    c) Diabetes mellitus
    d) Cushing's syndrome

  e) Vitamin deficiency (vitamin A, B complex)
  f) Renal failure
  g) Cirrhosis of the liver
6. Congenital syndromes—aplasia of the olfactory bulbs
   a) Absence of neuroepithelium (agenesis/intrauterine infection)
   b) Turner's syndrome
   c) Kallmann syndrome (hypogonadism with eunuchoid gigantism, absence of puberty, and occasional color blindness)
7. Toxicity of systemic or inhaled drugs
   a) Aminoglycosides
   b) Formaldehyde
   c) Methotrexate
   d) Ethyl alcohol
   e) Organic solvents
   f) Zinc nasal sprays
   g) Nasal steroid sprays
   h) Cocaine
   i) Lead
8. Degenerative processes of the central nervous system (CNS)
   a) Parkinson's disease
   b) Alzheimer's disease
   c) Huntington's disease
   d) Motor neuron disease
   e) MS
   f) Temporal lobe seizures
   g) Amyotrophic lateral sclerosis
   h) Essential tremor
   i) Multiple system atrophy
9. Psychiatric disorders
   a) Depression
   b) Schizophrenia
   c) Seasonal affective disorder
10. Local radiation therapy: radiotherapy of head and neck
11. Heavy smoking
12. Albinism

Patten J. Neurological Differential Diagnosis. 2nd ed. Springer; 1995

Freda PU, Post KD. Differential diagnosis of sellar masses. Endocrinol Metab Clin North Am 1999; 28(1):81–117, vi

Katzenschlager R, Lees AJ. Olfaction and Parkinson's syndromes: its role in differential diagnosis. Curr Opin Neurol 2004;17(4):417–423

4.2 Oculomotor Nerve Palsy

Third cranial nerve (CN III) dysfunction can present with diplopia, ptosis, eye pain, headache, pupillary dilatation, monocular blurry near vision, or any combination thereof. The primary symptom is mixed horizontal and vertical binocular diplopia from deviation of the two visual axes. The clinical presentation is remarkably varied, as the CN III supplies seven different muscles, and almost any combination of these can be affected to varying degrees.

With the extremely rare unilateral CN III palsy, the involved eye usually is deviated down and out (infraducted, abducted), and there is ptosis which may be severe enough to cover the pupil. In addition, pupillary dilatation can cause symptomatic glare in bright light (if the ptotic lid does not cover the pupil), and paralysis of accommodation causes blurred vision for near objects. CN III is most often affected in combination with other cranial nerves, particularly II, IV, V, and VI (▶ Fig. 4.1).

With a complete CN III palsy, the eye in primary position is depressed and abducted, i.e., "down and out." It cannot elevate or adduct but has full abduction and some residual depression. Depression is accompanied by intorsion, maximally when the eye is abducted, and is due to the action of the superior oblique. This evidence of *superior oblique function* should be sought, as the differential diagnosis of CN III nerve palsy differs considerably from that of combined III and IV nerve palsies. Ptosis is severe, accommodation is impaired, and the pupil is large and does not constrict to light or vergence efforts.

Incomplete CN III palsies are more common than complete ones. If so, the examination should seek to determine whether the partial involvement conforms to a superior or inferior *divisional palsy*.

The most frequently identified causes of III nerve palsies are ischemia and aneurysms. Tumors and trauma account for another 10% each, and a cause is not

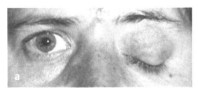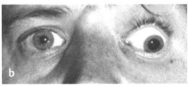

Fig. 4.1 Complete left oculomotor nerve palsy. **(a)** Complete ptosis of the left eye. **(b)** The examiner lifts the ptotic eyelid to reveal the mydriatic, fixed (i.e., unreactive) pupil. The eye is also mildly abducted through the predominant effect of the lateral rectus and superior oblique muscles, which are innervated by the abducens and trochlear nerves. (Reproduced from 12.3 Disturbances of Ocular and Pupillary Motility. In: Mattle H, Mumenthaler M, Taub E, ed. Fundamentals of Neurology: An Illustrated Guide. 2nd edition. Thieme; 2017.)

found in 20%. Two clinical signs that help differentiate aneurysmal and neoplastic palsies from the more benign ischemic palsy are: pupillary involvement and oculomotor synkinesis.

1. **Pupillary involvement**

   The pupil is spared in 75% of ischemic III nerve palsies, but involved in over 90% of aneurysmal palsies. Furthermore, pupil-sparing in aneurysmal palsies almost never occurs with complete dysfunction of all other III nerve muscles. Hence the correct "pupil rule" is that *complete pupil-sparing with otherwise complete and isolated palsy of the III nerve is never due to an aneurysm.* A small degree anisocoria (< 1 mm) occurs in 30% of microvascular CN III palsies. Relative pupil-sparing in an otherwise complete III nerve palsy, and complete pupil-sparing with incomplete palsy of extraocular muscles and the levator do not reliably exclude an aneurysm or other mass lesion. Also, the presence of pain and the degree of associated external ophthalmoplegia do not distinguish microvascular from compression causes of relative pupil-sparing III nerve palsies. The presence of other cranial nerve palsies or neurologic signs should prompt investigation for a mass lesion. Caution is required to ensure that a coexistent Horner's syndrome or aberrant regeneration of the pupil are not mimicking pupil-sparing, as these may indicate a mass.

2. **Oculomotor synkinesis(anomalous cocontraction of muscles)**

   The most common sign is *lid elevation on adduction. Pupillary constriction* on attempted adduction or depression also occurs often with light reaction. Synkinesis between extraocular muscles causes adduction or globe retraction with attempted vertical gaze. Any of these signs in an adult implies CN III nerve compression by an aneurysm or tumor until proven otherwise, since microvascular or idiopathic lesions are rare if ever responsible. Oculomotor synkinesis also occurs after trauma, including neurosurgical procedures and migraine.

4.2.1 Topographic diagnosis of oculomotor nerve paralysis

1. Intra-axial (midbrain)
   a) Ischemia—paramedian/basal midbrain infarction produces:
      i. Benedikt's syndrome: Ipsilateral CN III palsy, ipsilateral hand tremor (rubral tremor), and ataxia
      ii. Weber's syndrome: Ipsilateral CN III palsy and contralateral hemiplegia or hemiparesis
      iii. Millard–Gubler syndrome: Characterized by cross paralysis, contralateral limbs, ipsilateral face due to the involvement of CN VI and VII, and the corticospinal tract.

    b) Tumor (e.g., glioma, metastasis)

    c) Inflammation/demyelination (e.g., herpes zoster encephalitis, poliomyelitis, MS)

    d) Hemorrhage (e.g., intracranial hematoma, subarachnoid hemorrhage)

    e) Tuberculoma

    f) Congenital hypoplasia of CNIII nucleus

2. Basilar subarachnoid space

    a) Aneurysm: It is the most common lesion to affect the CN III in this location following a subarachnoid hemorrhage, therefore, sudden severe headache, stiff neck and loss of consciousness may be present. For example, posterior communicating, less commonly, posterior cerebral, basilar tip or superior cerebellar).

    b) Temporal lobe herniation

    c) Basal infectious meningitis (e.g., bacterial, fungal/parasitic, viral)

    d) Basal meningeal neoplastic infiltration and miscellaneous inflammatory lesions may involve the third and all the other cranial nerves with the primary symptoms of meningitis, such as headache, stiff neck, fever, and altered level of consciousness. The examples are carcinomatous/lymphomatous/leukemic infiltration, granulomatous inflammation (sarcoidosis, lymphomatoid granulomatosis, Wegener's granulomatosis), and meningovascular syphilis.

3. Cavernous sinus and superior orbital fissure

    a) Aneurysm (internal carotid)

    b) Tumor—Isolated CN III palsy may result from lateral extension of pituitary adenoma or other primary intrasellar mass (e.g., sphenoid wing meningioma, pituitary adenoma, nasopharyngeal, and other metastases).

    c) Inflammatory—Tolosa–Hunt syndrome (idiopathic or granulomatous inflammation). Inflammatory diffused lesions within the cavernous sinus typically give rise to simultaneous involvement of the CNs III, IV, VI, and first divisions of the V in various combinations that serve to define a cavernous sinus syndrome (CSS).

    d) Cavernous sinus thrombosis

    e) Pituitary apoplexy (infarction within existing pituitary adenoma)

    f) Carotid artery–cavernous sinus fistula

    g) Carotid dural branch–cavernous sinus fistula: Typically present with CN III palsy plus other cranial nerve involvement in the cavernous sinus and proptosis with arterialized conjunctival veins, due to a large volume of arterial blood into the anterior draining veins of the cavernous sinus. Isolated CN III palsy without the orbital congestion can occur when the primary drainage is posterior from the cavernous sinus, the so-called white eye fistulas.

h) Diabetic infarction of the nerve trunk—microvascular disease in vasa vasorum (pupil spared in 80% of cases; classically described as painful although it can be painless; reversible within 3 months).

i) Fungal infection (e.g., mucormycosis, usually found in diabetics)

j) Ophthalmic herpes zoster

4. Orbit

a) Inflammatory: Nonspecific or granulomatous inflammation in the orbit is referred to as orbital inflammatory pseudotumor.

b) Orbital blowout fracture: Lesions in the orbit tend to produce associated proptosis, lid swelling, conjunctival injection, and chemosis. There also may be involvement of the other cranial nerves that innervate extraocular muscles (IV and VI) or involvement of the muscles themselves.

c) Orbital tumors (e.g., meningioma 40%, hemangioma 10%, carcinoma of the lacrimal duct, neurofibroma, lipoma, epidermoid, fibrous dysplasia, sarcoma, and melanoma 35%).

d) Endocrine (thyroid orbitopathy)

5. Miscellaneous

a) Ophthalmoplegic migraine: Presents mainly in children under the age of 10 years with recurring bouts of unilateral headache and ipsilateral CN III palsy that may last for several weeks.

b) Arteritis, giant-cell arteritis

c) Guillain–Barre syndrome (GBS) (Fisher syndrome of isolated polyradiculitis)

d) Sarcoidosis (Schaumann's syndrome)

e) Infectious mononucleosis and other viral infections

f) After immunization

g) Mucormycosis

h) Albers-Schonberg syndrome (marble bone disease, osteopetrosis)

i) Associated with aspirin poisoning

j) Lupus erythematosus (Kaposi–Libman–Sacks syndrome)

6. Conditions simulating oculomotor nerve lesion

a) Thyrotoxicosis: Weakness of the superior and lateral rectus muscles due to an inflammatory myopathic process.

b) Myasthenia gravis: Diplopia, ptosis, varying eye signs or fatigability of eye movements should always raise this possibility.

c) Internuclear ophthalmoplegia: Diplopia without weakness of any eye movement, disruption of the conjugate eye movements, e.g., MS, brainstem infarction.

d) Latent strabismus: Diplopia under conditions of fatigue or drowsiness.

e) Progressive ocular myopathy (familial ptosis variant): Rare form of muscular dystrophy affecting the extraocular muscles.

7. Childhood causes of oculomotor nerve palsy
    a) Trauma
    b) Neoplasm
    c) Undetermined
    d) Ophthalmoplegic migraine
    e) Postoperative cause
    f) Meningitis/encephalitis
    g) Subdural hematoma
    h) Viral or post-upper-respiratory-tract infection
    i) Varicella zoster virus
    j) Aneurysm
    k) Orbital cellulitis
    l) Sinus disease
    m) Mesencephalic cyst
    n) Cyclic oculomotor nerve palsy
    o) Poison

4.2.2 Differential diagnosis

The diagnosis of CN III palsy includes the following conditions:
1. Anisocoria (pupillary dilatation)
    a) Cycloplegic eye drops
    b) Adie's syndrome
    c) Contralateral Horner's syndrome
    d) Traumatic mydriasis
2. Ocular motility findings and ptosis
    a) Progressive external ophthalmoplegia
    b) Early signs of thyroid disease
    c) Myasthenia gravis
    d) Orbital inflammatory disease
    e) Type II Duane's syndrome
    f) Congenital Blepharoptosis
    g) Generalized myopathic conditions

Kwan ESK, Laucella M, Hedges TR, III, Wolpert BM. A cliniconeuroradiologic approach to third cranial nerve palsies. Am J Neuroradiol 1987;8(3):459–468

Lazaridis C, Torabi A, Cannon S. Bilateral third nerve palsy and temporal arteritis. Arch Neurol 2005;62(11):1766–1768

Varma D, Tesha P, George N. Acute painful third nerve palsy: the sole presenting sign of a pituitary adenoma. Eye (Lond) 2002;16(6):792–793

Blake PY, Mark AS, Kattah J, Kolsky M. MR of oculomotor nerve palsy. AJNR Am J Neuroradiol 1995;16(8):1665–1672

Taw LB, Taw M. Oculomotor nerve palsy—An integrative East-West approach Proceedings of UCLA Healthcare 2015; 19

4.3 Trochlear Nerve Palsy

This condition may be clinically characterized by vertical diplopia, incomitant hypertropia that increases upon head tilt toward the paralyzed site (positive Biel-schowsky test), excyclotropia, and head tilt (▶ Fig. 4.2). This nerve controls the superior oblique muscle, which helps the eye to look downward and assists with eye rotation when one tilts his/her head sideways. A person with trochlear nerve palsy complains of *vertical double vision*, where objects look stacked on top of each other. The double vision may get worse when looking to the side or trying to read a book. Trochlear nerve palsies can be subtle and hard to detect as the eyes appear normal on casual inspection. There are many causes of trochlear nerve palsy. The number of cases with undetermined cause was 60%.

4.3.1 Causes of trochlear nerve palsy

1. Intra-axial (brain stem)
   a) Infarction
   b) Hemorrhage
   c) Trauma
   d) Demyelination
   e) Iatrogenic (neurosurgical complication)
   f) Congenital aplasia of CN IV nucleus
2. Subarachnoid space
   a) Trauma
   b) Mastoiditis
   c) Meningitis (infectious and neoplastic)
   d) Tumor (e.g., tentorial meningioma, germinoma, teratoma, gliomas, choriocarcinoma, trochlear schwannoma, metastases)
   e) Iatrogenic (neurosurgical complication)
3. Cavernous sinus and superior orbital fissure
   a) Diabetic infarction (this is the most common cause; reversible within 3 months)
   b) Aneurysm (e.g., congenital, aneurysmal dilatation of the intracavernous portion of the internal carotid artery (ICA) usually occurring in elderly hypertensive females)
   c) Carotico-cavernous fistula (e.g., traumatic, spontaneous)
   d) Cavernous sinus thrombosis (serious complication from sepsis of the skin over the upper face or in the paranasal sinuses)
   e) Tumor (e.g., pituitary adenoma, parasellar, tuberculum, or diaphragm sella meningioma, teratoma, dysgerminoma, metastases)

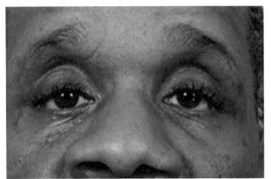

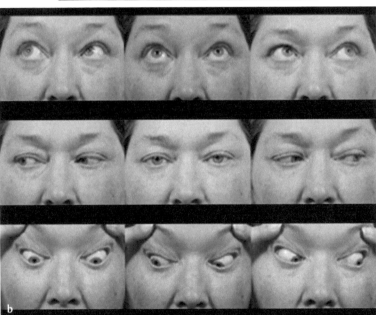

Fig. 4.2 CN IV palsy. (a) Traumatic left fourth nerve palsy showing left hypertropia in primary gaze. (b) Patient with left fourth nerve palsy. Note the left eye hypertropia and the limitation of the left eye to look down and in compared with the right eye. (Reproduced from 55.6 Cranial Nerve IV. In: Sekhar L, Fessler R, ed. Atlas of Neurosurgical Techniques: Brain, Volume 2. 2nd edition. Thieme; 2015.)

   f) Tolosa–Hunt syndrome
   g) Herpes zoster
4. Conditions simulating trochlear nerve palsy
   a) Thyrotoxicosis (myopathy of the extraocular muscles)
   b) Myasthenia gravis
   c) Latent strabismus
   d) Brown's syndrome: Mechanical impediment of the tendons of the
      superior oblique muscle in the trochlea characterized by sudden onset,
      transient, and recurrent inability to move the eye up and inward.

4.3.2 Differential diagnosis of trochlear nerve palsy

Fourth cranial nerve palsies must first be distinguished from other causes of vertical diplopia. These include oculomotor palsy, skew deviation, myasthenia gravis, and Grave's ophthalmopathy. These patients typically have other clinical findings that help differentiate them from isolated CN IV palsies. Furthermore, in time, these patients often develop other findings that unmask the diagnosis. (1) The differential diagnosis of a CN IV palsy can be subdivided into congenital and acquired. Congenital CN IV palsies are identified in several ways. First, the patient will often have very high vertical fusional amplitudes. Normal vertical fusional amplitudes are in the range of 1–3 prism diopters. Patients with a congenital CN IV palsy can often fuse 10–15 prism diopters. Also, old pictures can show whether or not there has been long-standing head tilt since childhood. This would give more evidence to suggest that a CN IV palsy was congenital. When a cause can be identified, the most common etiology of an acquired CN IV palsy is trauma (30%). Another common etiology is microvascular or ischemic, often in the setting of diabetes or hypertension (8%). (2) Other etiologies include compressive lesions such as tumors (6%) or aneurysms (8%), increased intracranial pressure, intrinsic neoplasms of the CN IV, and, very rarely, giant cell arteritis.

Bagheri A, Fallahi MR, Abrishami M, Salour H, Aletaha M. Clinical features and outcomes of treatment for fourth nerve palsy. J Ophthalmic Vis Res 2010;5(1):27–31
Brodsky MC. Pediatric Neuro-Ophthalmology. 3nd ed. Springer; 2006
Gentry LR, Mehta RC, Appen RE, Weinstein JM. MR imaging of primary trochlear nerve neoplasms. AJNR Am J Neuroradiol 1991;12(4):707–713

4.4 Abducens Nerve Palsy (Sixth Cranial Nerve)

This condition is a common cause of acquired horizontal diplopia. Signs pointing toward the diagnosis are an abduction deficit and an esotropia increasing with gaze toward the side of the deficit. The most important characteristic of the condition is double vision in which a patient sees two side-by-side images of any object. The diplopia is typically worse at distance. However, children may not complain of diplopia. In case of unilateral abducens nerve palsy, the distance between the two images appears to be greatest when the gaze is directed to the affected side. Measurements are made with the uninvolved eye fixing (primary deviation), and will be larger with the involved eye fixing (secondary deviation), A small vertical defect may accompany a CN VI palsy, which may raise the question of additional pathology, such as a CN IV palsy or skew deviation. (▶ Fig. 4.3)

Abducens nerve palsy is the most common encountered extraocular muscle palsy and its incidence is 11.3 in 100,000 people. In 35% of the cases, the patients had hypertension and/or, less frequently, diabetes, 26% were undetermined, 5% had a neoplasm, and 2% had an aneurysm.

Bilateral abduction deficit in the setting of trauma or subarachnoid hemorrhage often indicate increased intracranial pressure causing a bilateral CN VI palsy. This sudden rise in intracranial pressure can lead to downward displacement of the brain stem which can compress CN VI in the prepontine cistern as it makes a 90° bend and exits the pontomedullary junction to ascend along the clivus toward the cavernous sinus. Other causes of acquired bilateral abduction deficits include damage to the convergence pathway, thalamic esodeviation, or breakdown of a pre-existing phoria due to loss of conscious control, diabetes mellitus type II, Kearns–Sayre syndrome, cavernous sinus thrombosis, Wildervanck syndrome, thiamine deficiency, Tolosa–Hunt syndrome, Duane's ocular retraction syndrome, Moebius syndrome, Raymond Cestan syndrome, Gradenigo–Lannois syndrome.

4.4.1 Causes of abducens nerve palsy and differential diagnosis

1. Intra-axial (pons)
   a) Infarction: Paramedian and basal pontine infarction; e.g., Foville's syndrome, Gasperini's syndrome, and Millard–Gubler syndrome.
   b) Wernicke's encephalopathy: Serious complication of alcoholism and severe malnutrition; reversible following intravenous therapy with vitamin B1.

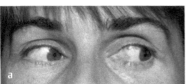 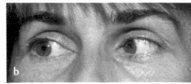

Fig. 4.3 Partial right abducens nerve palsy. **(a)** On leftward gaze, the eyes are parallel; **(b)** on rightward gaze, the right eye fails to abduct to the full extent. (Reproduced from 12.3 Disturbances of Ocular and Pupillary Motility. In: Mattle H, Mumenthaler M, Taub E, ed. Fundamentals of Neurology: An Illustrated Guide. 2nd edition. Thieme; 2017.)

    c) Moebius syndrome: Congenital absence of facial nerve nuclei and associated absence of the abducens nuclei.

    d) Pontine glioma: Many of these tumors start in the region of the abducens nerve nucleus; any combination of CN VI and VII palsy in a young child or a patient with neurofibromatosis should be regarded with suspicion.

    e) Demyelination (e.g., MS; internuclear ophthalmoplegia or isolated CN VI palsy is a common manifestation.)

    f) Duane's ocular retraction syndrome (abduction defect with palpebral fissure narrowing)

2. Basal subarachnoid space

    a) Trauma (16–17%) (e.g., severe head injury and movement of the brain stem)

    b) Raised intracranial pressure (causing downward displacement of the brain stem and stretching of the abducens nerve over the petrous tip leading to its paresis)

    c) Basal meningeal process (e.g., tuberculous, fungal, bacterial, and carcinomatous meningitis, meningovascular syphilis)

    d) Subarachnoid hemorrhage (obstruction of the cerebrospinal fluid at the aqueduct level causing obstructive hydrocephalus and raised ICP)

    e) Clival tumors (e.g., chordoma, chondroma, sarcoma, metastases, Paget's disease)

    f) Large cerebellopontine angle tumors (e.g., acoustic neurinoma, meningioma, epidermoid, metastases, giant aneurysm—AICA or BA aneurysm—arachnoid cyst)

    g) Gradenigo's syndrome (diffuse inflammation of the petrous bone and thrombosis of the petrosal sinus causing severe ear pain and a combination of CNs VI, VII, VIII, and occasionally CN V nerve lesions)

    h) Infiltration (e.g., carcinomas of the nasopharynx or the paranasal sinuses, leukemias, CNS lymphoma)

    i) Sarcoidosis

    j) Iatrogenic (neurosurgical complication)

3. Cavernous sinus and superior orbital fissure

    a) Aneurysm (e.g., congenital, aneurysmal dilatation of the intracavernous portion of the ICA usually occurring in elderly hypertensive females)

    b) Carotico-cavernous fistula (e.g., traumatic, spontaneous)

    c) Cavernous sinus thrombosis: Serious complication from sepsis of the skin over the upper face or in the paranasal sinuses

    d) Tumor (e.g., pituitary adenoma, parasellar, tuberculum, or diaphragm sella meningioma, metastases, nasopharyngeal carcinoma)

    e) Tolosa–Hunt syndrome

    f) Herpes zoster

    g) Diabetic infarction

4. Miscellaneous

    a) Nonspecific febrile illness (benign transient CN VI palsy, particularly in children

    b) Infectious (e.g., diphtheria, botulism intoxication) and parainfectious diseases: Spontaneous recovery of the CN VI palsy is almost the rule.

    c) Lumbar puncture: Differential pressure gradients between the supra and infratentorial compartments causes downward herniation resulting in a reversible CN VI palsy.

5. Conditions simulating abducens nerve palsy

    a) Thyrotoxicosis (myopathy of the extraocular muscles)
Thyroid eye disease and orbital inflammatory disease may result in restriction of extraocular muscles, but are typically accompanied by characteristic signs and symptoms, such as proptosis, injection over the rectus, muscle insertions, lid retraction, and lid lag. Forced duction testing may be helpful to rule out a restrictive etiology for an abduction deficit.

    b) Myasthenia gravis
This condition is always an etiologic consideration with the acute onset of strabismus. The ice test and rest test are useful office procedures to look for functional improvement in cases with myasthenia. Tensilon test may give a false-negative result. Single muscle fiber electromyography may be the best test for definitive diagnosis.

    c) Congenital esotropia

    d) Convergence spasm
Spasm of the near reflex can stimulate an abduction deficit. The convergence is associated with miotic pupils, and ductions are full with one eye occluded.

    e) Migraine

    f) Divergence paresis or divergence insufficiency with a comitant esodeviation greater at distance than near (or none at near), and with decreased divergence fusional amplitudes can also simulate a sixth nerve weakness. Divergence paresis has little localizing value.

Goodwin D. Differential diagnosis and management of acquired sixth cranial nerve palsy. Optometry 2006;77(11):534–539

Keane JR. Bilateral sixth nerve palsy. Analysis of 125 cases. Arch Neurol 1976;33(10):681–683

Durkin SR, Tennekoon S, Kleinschmidt A, Casson RJ, Selva D, Crompton JL. Bilateral sixth nerve palsy. Ophthalmology 2006;113(11):2108–2109

4.5 Trigeminal Neuropathy

1. Intra-axial (pons)
   a) Infarction: Distal pontine dorsolateral infarction may cause ipsilateral facial anesthesia because the lesion damages the entering and descending fibers of the CN V.
   b) Neoplastic (e.g., pontine glioma, metastases)
   c) Demyelination (e.g., MS; an attack of numbness of one side of the face in a young person occasionally following local anesthesia for dental work is quite a common symptom of MS.)
   d) Syringobulbia (congenital, e.g., Chiari malformations; secondary, e.g., trauma, ischemic necrosis, high cervical intramedullary tumor)
2. Cerebellopontine angle
   a) Acoustic neurinoma
   b) Meningioma: Usually associated with bony hyperostosis and/or calcification within the lesion.
   c) Ectodermal inclusions (e.g., epidermoid, dermoid)
   d) Metastases
   e) Trigeminal neurinoma
   f) Aneurysm
3. Lesions at the petrous tip
   a) Petrositis (e.g., diffuse inflammation of the petrous bone from mastoiditis or middle ear infection. This causes severe ear pain and a combination of CNs VI, VII, VIII, and V nerve lesions and is known as Gradenigo's syndrome.)
4. Cavernous sinus/orbital fissure
   a) Severe trauma
   b) Metastatic carcinomas (e.g., carcinomas of the nasopharynx or the paranasal sinuses)
   c) Cavernous sinus thrombosis
   d) Aneurysm: Dilatation of the intracavernous portion of the carotid artery at the posterior end of the sinus may irritate the ophthalmic division of the CN V.)
   e) Tumors arising in the orbit and optic foramina (e.g., meningioma 40%; hemangiomas 10%; pseudotumor 5%; glioma 5%; lacrimal duct carcinoma, neurofibroma, epidermoid, fibrous dysplasia of bone, sarcoma, melanoma, lipoma, Tolosa–Hunt syndrome, Hand–Schuller–Christian disease 40%)
5. Miscellaneous
   a) Diabetic vascular neuropathy
   b) Trigeminal neuralgia

c) Acute herpes zoster: In the elderly, the virus has a predilection for the first division of the CN VII nerve.

d) Systemic lupus erythematosus (vasculitic trigeminal neuropathy)

e) Scleroderma: Isolated trigeminal neuropathy may be the presenting sign in 10% of patients with neurologic manifestations of scleroderma and occurs in 4–5% of all patients with scleroderma.

f) Progressive systemic sclerosis: Fibrosis with nerve entrapment is the likely cause of trigeminal and other cranial neuropathies.

g) Sjögren syndrome (vasculitic trigeminal neuropathy)

h) Amyloidosis: Peripheral neuropathy with involvement of the Vth cranial nerve)

i) Arsenic neuropathy (peripheral and trigeminal neuropathy)

j) Trigeminal sensory neuropathy: A slowly progressing unilateral or bilateral facial numbness or paresthesia thought to be caused by vasculitis or fibrosis of the Gasserian ganglion; most frequently leads to the diagnosis of an underlying connective tissue disease, e.g., Sjogren's syndrome, systemic lupus erythematosus, and dermatomyositis.)

Hutchins LG, Harnsberger HR, Hardin CW Dillon WP Smoker WR Osborn AG. The radiologic assessment of trigeminal neuropathy. AJNR Am J Neuroradiol 1989;10:1031–1038

Zakrzewska JM. Diagnosis and differential diagnosis of trigeminal neuralgia. Clin J Pain 2002;18(1):14–21

Siccoli MM, Bassetti CL, Sándor PS. Facial pain: clinical differential diagnosis. Lancet Neurol 2006;5(3): 257–267

Krafft RM. Trigeminal neuralgia. Am Fam Physician 2008;77(9):1291–1296

Majoie CB, Verbeeten B, Jr, Dol JA, Peeters FL. Trigeminal neuropathy: evaluation with MR imaging. Radiographics 1995;15(4):795–811

4.6 Orbital Apex Syndrome(s)

An orbital apex syndrome (OAS) has been described to involve the oculomotor nerve (III), trochlear nerve (IV), abducens nerve (VI), and ophthalmic branch of the trigeminal nerve (VI) in association with optic nerve dysfunction.

The superior orbital fissure syndrome (SOFS) or Rochon-Duvigneaud syndrome is often applied to lesions located immediately anterior to the orbital apex, including the structures exiting the annulus of Zinn and often those external to the annulus. In this clinical setting, multiple cranial nerve palsies may be seen in the absence of optic nerve pathology.

Visual loss and ophthalmoplegia are often the initial manifestations of an OAS. Periorbital or facial pain may reflect involvement of the ophthalmic (V1) or maxillary (V2) branch of the trigeminal nerve. Periorbital pain is one of the diagnostic criteria for Tolosa–Hunt syndrome, an idiopathic inflammatory syndrome of the orbital apex. The periorbital skin and the corneal reflexes should be tested for asymmetry in sensation. Infectious, inflammatory, and neoplastic conditions may be associated with proptosis. Vascular causes of a CCS, such as a carotid-cavernous fistula, classically are associated with pulsatile proptosis. The assessment of the optic nerve dysfunction includes measurement of best corrected visual acuity, examination of the pupils for the presence of an afferent pupillary defect, color vision testing, and visual field testing with kinetic and static perimetry. Diplopia may be the presenting symptom in SOFS, OAS, or CSS. The pattern of an ocular deviation is especially important in evaluation of a single ocular motor nerve palsy; however, as multiple cranial nerves may be involved, a distinct pattern may be difficult to detect.

4.6.1 Etiology

The superior orbital fissure, orbital apex, and cavernous sinus are all contiguous, and although these terms define the precise anatomic locations of the disease process, the etiologies of these syndromes are similar.

1. Inflammatory
   a) Wegener's granulomatosis (both the systemic and limited form may involve the cavernous sinus)
   b) Sarcoidosis (CCS is the only manifestation of this inflammatory condition)
   c) Systemic lupus erythematosus
   d) Churg–Strauss syndrome (may involve the cavernous sinus and superior orbital fissure)
   e) Giant cell arteritis (may mimic an OAS and present with periorbital pain and ophthalmoplegia)
   f) Tolosa–Hunt syndrome (granulomatous inflammation within the cavernous sinus or orbital apex)
2. Infectious
   a) Fungi involving the CNS and the paranasal structures may lead to an OAS (e.g., mucormycosis, aspergillosis)
   b) Bacterial infection may result in cavernous sinus thrombosis from paranasal sinuses and cause CSS and OAS (e.g., *Streptococcus* spp, *Staphylococcus* spp, *Actinomyces* spp, *Mycobacterium tuberculosis*, Gram-negative bacilli, anaerobes)
   c) Viruses (herpes zoster)
   d) Spirochetes (*Treponema pallidum*)
3. Vascular
   a) Carotid cavernous aneurysm
   b) Carotid cavernous fistula (▶ Fig. 4.4)
   c) Cavernous sinus thrombosis
   d) Sickle cell anemia

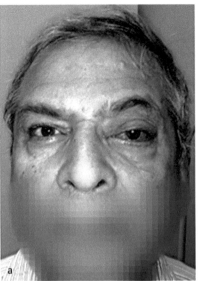
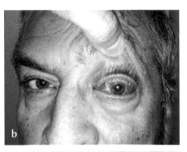
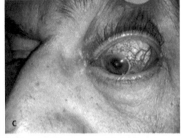

Fig. 4.4 Representative ocular findings in a patient with a carotid-cavernous fistula. Prominent proptosis, chemosis, and ophthalmoplegia are demonstrated. **(a)** Patient with spontaneous dural carotid-cavernous fistula. **(b)** Left eye abduction weakness from cranial nerve VI palsy. **(c)** Chemosis of affected eye. (Reproduced from Clinical Presentation. In: Spetzler R, Kalani M, Nakaji P, ed. Neurovascular Surgery. 2nd edition. Thieme; 2015.)

4. Neoplastic
   a) Head and neck tumors (nasopharyngeal carcinoma, adenoid cystic carcinoma, squamous-cell carcinoma)
   b) Neural tumors (neurofibroma, ciliary neurinoma, schwannoma)
   c) Metastatic lesion (lung, breast, renal cell, malignant melanoma)
   d) Hematologic (leukemia, non-Hodgkin lymphoma)
5. Trauma
   a) Penetrating/nonpenetrating injury
   b) Orbital apex fracture
   c) Retained foreign body
   d) Iatrogenic (sinusoidal surgery, orbital/facial surgery)
6. Miscellaneous
   a) Mucocele

Restman J. Diseases of the Orbit. A Multidisciplinary Approach. 2nd ed. Lippincott William and Wilkins; 2003
Bray WH, Giangiacomo J, Ide CH. Orbital apex syndrome. Surv Ophthalmol 1987;32(2):136–140
Yeh S, Foroozan R. Orbital apex syndrome. Curr Opin Ophthalmol 2004;15(6):490–498

4.7 Facial Nerve Palsy

The causes of facial nerve palsy (FNP) may be classified as a central type (upper motor neuron) or a peripheral type (lower motor neuron).

A central lesion interrupting the corticobulbar pathways results in paralysis only of the lower facial muscles on the *opposite* site of the lesion. This is explained by the fact that the corticobulbar fibers to the forehead and the upper half of the face are distributed bilaterally; however, the fibers to the lower half of the face are predominantly crossed. Commonly the etiology is vascular in origin (i.e., stroke) but can include masses (e.g., neoplasm, abscess) or neurodegenerative disease (e.g., facial apraxia in the absence of overt muscle weakness).

The peripheral-type lesion of the facial nerve occurs at the level of the pons or anywhere along the distal course of the nerve. This lesion produces total facial paralysis on the *same* side as the lesion. Acute lower motor neuron palsy can present at any age but is most frequently seen at age 20–50 years, affecting both sexes equally. Incidence is around 30 cases per 100,000 per year (45 per 100,000 in pregnant women). There is usually a rapid onset of unilateral facial paralysis. Aching pain below the ear or in the mastoid area is also common and may suggest middle ear or herpetic cause if severe. There may be hyperacusis and patients with lesions proximal to the geniculate ganglion may be unable to produce tears and have loss of taste (▶ Fig. 4.5).

A central lesion produces a less severe type of facial paralysis compared to the peripheral lesion, but its origin may represent a serious problem in the brain. To differentiate a central from a peripheral lesion in a patient with facial nerve paralysis, we ask the patient to wrinkle the forehead; if the patient can wrinkle the entire forehead, the lesion is centrally located. If the patient can wrinkle only half the forehead, the lesion is peripherally located.

1. Intra-axial (1%)
    a) Supranuclear
        i. Contralateral central motor neurons lesions: Either in the region of the precentral gyrus or its efferent pathways; e.g., vascular insults, trauma, tumor
        ii. Progressive supranuclear palsy: Marked neuronal loss in subcortical structures such as basal nucleus of Meynert, the pallidum, subthalamic nucleus, substantia nigra, locus coeruleus, and superior colliculi; patients have ophthalmoparesis of down gaze, parkinsonism, pseudobulbar palsy, and frontal lobe signs.
    b) Nuclear (pontine tegmentum)
        i. Vascular insults: Paramedian and basal infarction; e.g., Millard–Gubler syndrome, Gasperini syndrome, and Foville's syndrome)

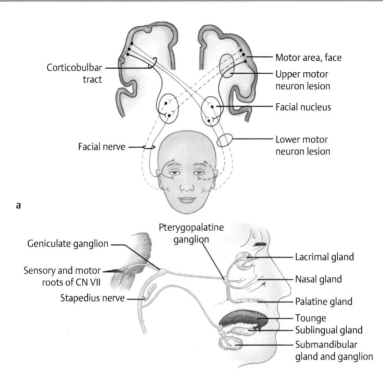

Fig. 4.5 (a, b) Facial nerve: central and peripheral anatomical course.

  ii. Pontine tumors (e.g., gliomas, metastases): Many of the pontine gliomas start in the region of the CNs VI and VII nuclei. Ipsilateral CN VI palsy may suggest a pontine lesion, whereas an absent ipsilateral corneal reflex is an early sign of cerebellopontine angle syndrome.

c) MS

d) Syringobulbia: Progression of the disease is marked by symptoms of long-track involvement and eventually by dissociated sensory loss in the face.

e) Poliomyelitis: Acute facial paralysis always associated with paralysis and atrophy of other nuclear muscles.

2. Cerebellopontine angle (e.g., tumors = 6%)
   Slowly progressing facial paralysis in combination with other cranial nerve involvement, particularly the statoacoustic, and eventually by CNS dysfunction.
   a) Acoustic neurinoma
   b) Meningioma: Usually associated with bony hyperostosis and/or calcification within the lesion.
   c) Ectodermal inclusions (e.g., epidermoid, dermoid)
   d) Metastases
   e) Trigeminal, facial, or other cranial nerve neurinoma
   f) Aneurysm
   g) Dolichoectasia of the basilar artery
3. Peripheral lesions
   a) Bell's palsy (57%)
      The most common cause of acute facial paralysis is Bell's palsy. It is an acute onset, idiopathic facial paralysis resulting from a dysfunction anywhere along the peripheral part of the facial nerve from the level of the pons distally. Retinal changes associated with diabetes and hypertension are predisposing factors of idiopathic FNP. Although herpes simplex virus type I is postulated to be the cause, Bell's palsy remains a diagnosis of exclusion. Misdiagnosis of other causes of facial paralysis as Bell's palsy may be as high as 28% of patients.
   b) Head trauma with basal fracture (17%)
      A fracture across the pyramid will also involve the statoacoustic nerve, whereas a longitudinal fracture usually does not involve it.
   c) Infections (4%) (e.g., herpes zoster virus, varicella zoster virus, cytomegalovirus, mumps, rubella, Epstein–Barr virus (EBV), Lyme disease, syphilis, human immunodeficiency virus, HIV)
   d) Ramsey Hunt syndrome
      Herpes zoster involving the CNs VII and VIII. Pain is often a prominent feature and vesicles are seen in the ipsilateral ear, on the hard palate and/or on the anterior two-thirds of the tongue. It can include deafness and vertigo and other cranial nerves can be affected. When the rash is absent it is known as zoster sine herpete. Immunodeficiency is a risk factor.
   e) Melkersson–Rosenthal syndrome
      Patients present recurrent episodes of facial weakness associated with chronic facial and lips edema, and hypertrophy/fissuring of the tongue.
   f) Heerfordt syndrome
      Facial diplegia associated with sarcoidosis, swelling of the parotid glands, and involvement of the optic apparatus.
   g) Otitis media, acute and chronic mastoiditis, and middle ear tumors are important causes of facial nerve paralysis (e.g., cholesteatoma, glomus tumor).

h) Mechanical lesions of the mandibular branch of the facial nerve
Pressure, facial trauma, or surgical trauma from procedures in the submandibular area, e.g., high cervical fusions, carotid endarterectomy, parotid surgery.

i) GBS
Proximal motor neuropathy with frequent involvement of the CN VIth and VIIth.

j) Porphyria
Peripheral neuropathies with involvement of mostly CN VIIth and Xth.

k) Neoplastic (fewer than 5% of all cases of facial nerve paralysis)
For example, parotid malignancies, schwannoma, parotid tumor, carcinoma, fibrous dysplasia, Von Recklinghausen's disease.

A tumor should be suspected if weakness progress over weeks, if a mass is present in the ear, neck, or parotid gland, and if no functional improvement is seen within 4–6 weeks.

May M, Klein SR. Differential diagnosis of facial nerve palsy. Otolaryngol Clin North Am 1991;24(3):613–645

James DG. Differential diagnosis of facial nerve palsy. Sarcoidosis Vasc Diffuse Lung Dis 1997;14(2):115–120

Evans AK, Licameli G, Brietzke S, Whittemore K, Kenna M. Pediatric facial nerve paralysis: patients, management and outcomes. Int J Pediatr Otorhinolaryngol 2005;69(11):1521–1528

Hohman MH, Hadlock TA. Etiology, diagnosis, and management of facial palsy: 2000 patients at a facial nerve center. Laryngoscope 2014;124:283–293

4.8 Bell's Palsy

This is the most common cause of facial paralysis, accounting for 70% of facial palsies, when other causes have been eliminated. Incidence is 20 per 100,000 between the ages of 10–40 years but 59 per 100,000 over the age of 65 years. The incidence is higher in people with diabetes. There may be a familial component. Recent work suggests that a large number of cases may be due to herpetic viral infection—particularly herpes simplex type 1 or varicella (herpes) zoster. The widely accepted mechanism is inflammation of the facial nerve during its course through the bony labyrinthine part of the facial canal which leads to compression and demyelination of the axons, and disruption of blood supply to the nerve itself.

Bell's palsy begins abruptly with paralysis of the entire half of the face (hemifacial paralysis) that evolves in a few hours. The most characteristic symptom is the loss of expression in half of the face with an inability to fully close the eyes, raise an eyebrow, frown, and smile. Other symptoms usually appear as decrease in the tearing of the eyes, increased sensitivity to sound in one ear, reduced sense of taste in two-thirds of the tongue, decreased salivation, and headache or pain around the jaw. Bell's palsy usually regresses spontaneously. About 7% of cases may recur within a 10-year interval.

4.8.1 Differential diagnosis

Bell's palsy is a diagnosis of exclusion. The following are some of the conditions that should be ruled out:

1. Ramsay Hunt syndrome: Varicella zoster virus infection of the geniculate ganglion, associated with facial weakness and a painful vesicular eruption of the external ear canal.
2. Infections of the middle ear, or mastoid
3. Neoplasms of the facial nerve
   a) *Benign tumors*: Schwannomas of the facial nerve can present with recurrent acute facial palsy. More rarely neurofibromas, glomus jugulare tumors, and hemangiomas may compress the facial nerve.
   b) *Malignant tumors*: Parotid malignancies, acute lymphoblastic leukemia, basal-cell carcinoma, squamous-cell carcinoma from the middle or external ear canal, adenocarcinoma of the ceruminous glands, and temporal bone metastases from the breast, lungs, and kidneys may cause facial paralysis.
4. Hemifacial spasm: No apparent association, although synkinesis of facial muscles may occur in both conditions.
5. Cerebellopontine angle tumors or aneurysms: Acoustic schwannomas, meningiomas, and glomus jugulare tumors may compress the CN VII at the cerebellopontine angle.
6. Lyme neuroborreliosis: Facial nerve paralysis is the most common neurologic complication of Lyme disease. It should be suspected in a patient who presents with isolated facial weakness and who has a history of tick bite, rash, or arthritis or who lives in an area where Lyme disease is endemic.
7. Demyelinating disorders: MS, acute inflammatory demyelinating polyneuropathy. Visual changes, vertigo, and weakness or numbness may suggest a brainstem lesion, such as demyelination.
8. Neurosarcoidosis: Association of the VIIth nerve palsy with uveitis, parotid gland enlargement, and fever.
9. Diabetes mellitus: It is an unusual cause of peripheral VIIth nerve neuropathy. However, 20% of patients in a large number of patients were found to be diabetic. Generally, the prognosis for recovery is worse in these patients compared to nondiabetic patients.
10. Syphilis and tuberculosis: Both are rare but treatable causes of facial nerve paralysis. Syphilitic gumma compress the nerve within the temporal bone, whereas tuberculosis of the middle ear causes inflammation of the tympanic segment.
11. Melkersson–Rosenthal syndrome: Alternating CN VII palsy occurring mainly in children. It is associated with a large fissured tongue and swelling of the face and lips.

Adour KK, Hilsinger RL, Jr, Callan EJ. Facial paralysis and Bell's palsy: a protocol for differential diagnosis. Am J Otol 1985(Suppl):68–73

Peitersen E. Bell's palsy: the spontaneous course of 2,500 peripheral facial nerve palsies of different etiologies. Acta Otolaryngol Suppl 2002;122(549):4–30

Sullivan FM, Swan IR, Donnan PT, et al. Early treatment with prednisolone or acyclovir in Bell's palsy. N Engl J Med 2007;357(16):1598–1607

4.9 Bilateral Facial Nerve Palsy

Bilateral FNP is exceedingly rare, representing less than 2% of all the facial palsy cases, and has an incidence of 1 per 5,000,000 population. Bell's palsy accounts for only 23% of bilateral facial paralysis.

The most common infectious cause of bilateral FNP is Lyme disease, whose carrier is a common tick. Bilateral FNP can be seen in about 30–35% of patients with Lyme disease.

GBS is an inflammatory postinfectious polyradiculopathy of uncertain etiology. Bilateral FNP can occur in up to 50% of the fatal cases.

Approximately 40% of the EBV-infection-associated FNP cases are bilateral. It has been well documented that EBV infections in the paediatric age group cause FNP, but few cases have been reported in the adult population.

Traumatic skull fractures, cerebellopontine angle tumors, and sarcoidosis are known causes of FNP. Diabetes has been noted to be present in 28.4% of patients with bilateral FNP and can be explained by the fact that diabetic patients are more prone to nerve degeneration.

Melkersson–Rosenthal syndrome is characterized by VIIth nerve palsy, facial edema, and tongue fissuring. Symptoms occur from teenage years and recurrent FNPs have been described.

Moebius syndrome is a rare neurological disease where children are born with facial nerve and abducens nerve underdevelopment leading to facial muscle weakness and inability to abduct the eyes.

4.9.1 Differential diagnosis

1. GBS
2. Multiple idiopathic cranial neuropathies
3. Lyme disease
4. Sarcoidosis
5. Meningitis (neoplastic or infectious)
6. Brainstem encephalitis
7. Benign intracranial hypertension
8. Leukemia

9. Melkersson–Rosenthal syndrome (rare neurological disorder characterized by facial palsy, granulomatous cheilitis, and fissured tongue)
10. Diabetes mellitus
11. HIV injection
12. Syphilis
13. Infectious mononucleosis
14. Malformations, such as Mobius syndrome
15. Vasculitis
16. Bilateral neurofibromas
17. Intrapontine and prepontine tumor should also be considered
18. Leprosy

Price T, Fife DG. Bilateral simultaneous facial nerve palsy. J Laryngol Otol 2002;116(1):46–48

Terada K, Niizuma T, Kosaka Y, Inoue M, Ogita S, Kataoka N. Bilateral facial nerve palsy associated with Epstein-Barr virus infection with a review of the literature. Scand J Infect Dis 2004;36(1):75–77

Jain V, Deshmukh A, Gollomp S. Bilateral facial paralysis: case presentation and discussion of differential diagnosis. J Gen Intern Med 2006;21(7):C7–C10

4.10 Dizziness

Dizziness is a nonspecific and very common complaint that includes a broad differential diagnosis. The incidence of dizziness in the general population ranges from 20 to 30%. The first challenge is to establish the presence or absence of vestibular disease, as it comprises approximately 50% of the presenting complaint. Once vestibular disease is confirmed, emphasis is on differentiating peripheral from central causes of dizziness. Most commonly, the ward is used to describe a variety of subjective symptoms, including vertigo, unsteadiness, generalized weakness, presyncope, syncope, or falling.

The distinction between vertigo and nonvertigo is critical in the medical history, as true vertigo is most likely due to vestibular organ dysfunction, whereas nonvertigo symptoms may be due to a variety of CNS, cardiovascular, or systemic diseases.

Most causes of dizziness are benign; however, a small percentage may represent a serious underlying disorder such as cerebrovascular disease or posterior fossa tumor.

4.10.1 Differential diagnosis

The causes of dizziness are as follows: peripheral vestibular dysfunction 40%, CNS lesions 10%, psychiatric disorders 25%, presyncope/dysequilibrium 25%, and nonspecific dizziness 10%.

Presyncope

Describes loss of consciousness as a result of temporary disruption to cerebral oxygenation due to interruption of blood flow to the brain. Common causes are orthostatic hypotension, cardiac arrhythmias, psychogenic disorders, and vasovagal syncope.

Dysequlibrium

It is a sense of unsteadiness and loss of balance involving the legs or trunk. Causes include peripheral neuropathy, vestibular disorder, musculoskeletal disorder, gait disorder, and Parkinson's disease.

Nonspecific dizziness

Designates patients with nonvertiginous dizziness, subjective imbalance, and hypersensitivity to motion cues in the absence of active vestibular deficits. Psychiatric disorders represent the primary cause, such as depression, generalized anxiety disorder, panic or phobic disorder, and conversion disorder.

4.10.2 Causes of vertigo

The vestibular system consists of a central and a vestibular component. (1) The peripheral parts include the semicircular canals, the utricle, the saccule, and the vestibular nerve. (2) The central part comprises the vestibular nuclear complex, vestibular cerebellum, brain stem, spinal cord, and vestibular cortex.

1. **Peripheral causes of vertigo**
   a) Benign paroxysmal positional vertigo (BPPV)
      Consists of brief vertiginous episodes lasting seconds with head movement. It is the most commonly recognized cause of vertigo assumed to be due to debris (canalithiasis) in the posterior (90–95%) or the lateral (5–10%) semicircular canal. The Dix–Hallpike maneuver is the test to confirm then diagnosis of posterior canal BPPV.
   b) Meniere's disease
      Characterized by discrete episodic vertigo lasting minutes to hours, fluctuating low-frequency sensorineural hearing loss, tinnitus, and aural fullness. The vertigo associated with Meniere's disease is often severe and associated with nausea, vomiting, and loss of balance. Believed to be related to excess endolymphatic fluid pressure (hydrops).
   c) Vestibular neuronitis or labyrinthitis
      Characterized by a rapid onset of severe vertigo, nausea, vomiting, and gait instability. The vertigo is present at rest and may be exacerbated by

position change. It is believed to be a viral inflammation of the vestibular portion of the CN VIII. Hearing loss may be present if the cochlear
portion of CN VIII is additionally involved (labyrinthitis).

2. **Central causes of vertigo**

The presence of pure vertical and multidirectional nystagmus with no optical fixation suppression is usually indicative of a central cause of vertigo.
Central vertigo is generally associated with severe vertigo with neurologic
signs and less prominent movement illusion.

a) Migrainous vertigo

Migraine headache is a cause of recurrent vertigo, associated with visual
aura, tinnitus, decreased hearing, diplopia, ataxia, dysarthria, photophobia during episodes. Three subtypes are recognized: basilar migraine,
benign recurrent vertigo of childhood, and vestibular migraine.

b) Cerebrovascular disorders

The vertebrobasilar arterial system provides blood supply to the inner
ear, brain stem, and cerebellum.

i. Brainstem ischemia: Episodic vertigo lasting minutes to hours with
concurrent diplopia, dysarthria, and ataxia.

ii. Wallenberg's syndrome (Lateral medullary infarction): Acute onset
vertigo, abnormal eye movements, ipsilateral Horner's syndrome,
ipsilateral limb ataxia, and loss of pain/temperature sensation on
ipsilateral face and contralateral trunk.

iii. Cerebellar infarction and hemorrhage: Older patients, vertigo associated with nausea, vomiting, limb ataxia, and impaired gait.

3. **Multiple sclerosis**

Vertigo occurs in 20–50% of MS patients lasting days to weeks and symptoms may resemble vestibular neuronitis. Dysfunction of adjacent CNs
(facial numbness, diplopia) or cerebellar signs (severe ataxia) may be present.

4. **Hereditary ataxia**

Post RE, Dickerson LM. Dizziness: a diagnostic approach. Am Fam Physician 2010;82(4):361–368, 369

Ozono Y, Kitahara T, Fukushima M, et al. Differential diagnosis of vertigo and dizziness in the emergency
department. Acta Otolaryngol 2014;134(2):140–145

Karatas M. Central vertigo and dizziness: epidemiology, differential diagnosis, and common causes. Neurologist 2008;14(6):355–364

4.11 Cranial Nerves IX, X, and XI Neuropathy

From their exit site at the ventral medulla, through the jugular foramen and to the
level of the hyoid bone, the CN IX, X, and XI are in close proximity to one another
and are thus often affected by the same pathology. The subjacent to the hyoid

bone, isolated vagal pathology (recurrent laryngeal nerve) can result in hoarseness and dysphagia, with sparing of the gag reflex and other oropharyngeal signs. In this situation, superior mediastinal pathology, such as infection, tumor, and aneurysm, must be included in the differential diagnosis and the imaging examination should be tailored to exclude such pathology.

The *glossopharyngeal* (CN IX) is sensory to the posterior one-third of tongue and the pharynx and middle ear. Glossopharyngeal paralysis only rarely causes throat and tongue sensory impairments, sometimes accompanied by parotid secretory dysfunction. However, motor symptoms are often not obvious, because of the compensation of the vagus nerve. This can be seen in the throat cancer. Irritation is manifested as glossopharyngeal neuralgia. The *vagus* (CN X) is motor to the muscles of the palate, pharynx, and larynx. The impact of the vagus nerve palsy is expressed on the dysfunction of the recurrent laryngeal nerve, which results in temporary (up to 1 year) or permanent hoarseness. The *accessory* (CN XI) provides motor innervation to the sternocleidomastoid and trapezius muscles. Injury of this nerve results in shoulder drop and inability to abduct the upper extremity. These lower CNs are commonly involved together in disease and their combined impairment results in a significant loss of function in the mouth, bulbar area, and the shoulder. If the site of the lesion is a lower motor neuron, then the disorder is termed a *bulbar palsy* and if the site of the lesion is an upper motor neuron, it is termed a *pseudobulbar palsy*. The main neurological causes of a bulbar palsy are motor neuron disease (MND) and myasthenia gravis, and of pseudobulbar palsy are stroke and MND. The main non-neurological cause is local malignancy.

4.11.1 Causes of CN IX, X, and XI neuropathy

1. Intra-axial (medulla)
    a) Dorsolateral infarction (lateral medullary or Wallenberg's syndrome)
    b) Hemorrhage (hypertensive, arteriovenous malformation)
    c) MS
    d) Central pontine myelinolysis: Demyelinating disease occurring in malnourished or alcoholic patients complicated by hyponatremia; rapid correction of the hyponatremia is implicated as a cause of the demyelination which presents with tetraparesis and lower CN involvement.
    e) Tumor (e.g., gliomas, metastases)
2. Jugular foramen
    a) Infection (e.g., meningitis, malignant external otitis media: destructive soft tissue mass in temporal bone that can mimic neoplasm)
    b) Vascular lesions (e.g., vertebral artery ectasia, vertebral artery aneurysm)
    c) Tumor

      i. Paraganglioma (Glomus jugulare or carotid body tumors)
      ii. Neural sheath (e.g., schwannoma, neurofibroma)
      iii. Nasopharyngeal carcinomas (80% squamous cell, 18% adenocarcinoma; latter are often from minor salivary glands)
      iv. Metastases (most common tumors affecting skull base; Source: lung, breast, prostate, or nasopharyngeal tumors)
      v. Miscellaneous neoplasms (e.g., non-Hodgkin's lymphoma, rhabdomyosarcoma in children)
      vi. Meningiomas
      vii. Epidermoid tumors (cholesteatomas)
  d) Trauma
      i. Extensive base of skull fractures
      ii. Penetrating wounds
      iii. Surgical wounds (e.g., radical dissection of the neck)
3. Other causes
  a) Polyneuritis cranialis
  Idiopathic entity consisting of multiple transient CN palsies; predilection in patients suffering from diabetes or syphilis. Rule out metastatic carcinoma. Irradiation without tissue diagnosis is not justified particularly since the prognosis is very good.
  b) Glossopharyngeal neuralgia
  Exploration often reveals aberrant vessels coursing across the nerve or unsuspected neurofibromas, leptomeningeal metastases, jugular foramen syndrome.
4. Extracranial neuropathy
  a) Vagal nerve
      i. Infection (e.g., mediastinum, carotid space)
      ii. Vascular (e.g., jugular vein thrombosis, left aortic arch aneurysm)
      iii. Surgical trauma (e.g., intubation, thyroidectomy, carotid endarterectomy, cardiovascular surgery, esophageal resection for carcinoma)
      iv. Tumor
        – Paraganglioma (glomus jugulare)
        – Neural sheath (e.g., schwannoma, neurofibroma)
        – Primary or nodular squamous-cell carcinoma; other metastases
        – Non-Hodgkin's lymphoma
        – Thyroid malignancies
        – Lung carcinoma
        – Mediastinal masses on the left
  b) Accessory nerve
      i. Iatrogenic
        – Lymph node biopsy in the posterior triangle of the neck

- Radical neck dissections
- Neck surgery
  - Excision of benign neck masses
  - Parotidectomy
  - Carotid vessel surgery (e.g., endarterectomy)
  - Internal jugular vein manipulation (e.g., vein cannulation)
  - Facelift

ii. Traumatic
- Penetrating injury (glass cut or gunshot injury)
- Blunt injury (e.g., wrestling, unsuccessful hanging, vigorous neck movements, "whiplash" injury)

iii. Neurologic
- Vernet syndrome (e.g., tumor near jugular foramen)
- Poliomyelitis
- Motor neuron disease
- Brachial neuritis
- Syringomyelia

iv. Miscellaneous: Spontaneous isolated nerve injury

Panisset M, Eidelman BH. Multiple cranial neuropathy as a feature of internal carotid artery dissection. Stroke 1990;21(1):141–147

Ebright J. Septic thrombosis of the cavernous sinuses Arch Intern Med 2001;161(22):2671–2676

Keane JR. Multiple cranial nerve palsies: analysis of 979 cases. Arch Neurol 2005;62(11):1714–1717

4.12 Hypoglossal Neuropathy

The hypoglossal nerve supplies the intrinsic and most of the extrinsic muscles of the tongue (the palatoglossus is supplied by CN X). Hypoglossal nerve injury results in atrophy of the ipsilateral intrinsic and extrinsic tongue musculature. It is examined by inspecting the tongue at rest, and on repeated protrusion in and out. On examination, fasciculations may be present along with ipsilateral tongue atrophy. With protrusion, the tongue deviates toward the side of the lesion due to unopposed function of the contralateral glossal muscles (supranuclear pathology manifests *contralateral* to the lesion); however, swallowing and speech usually present no difficulty. Bilateral hypoglossal nerve palsy results in incomplete paralysis of the tongue such that it cannot exercise in the floor of the mouth, causing difficulty eating and swallowing, dysphonia, especially when made retroflex. Lesions may affect the hypoglossal nerve at the level of the brain stem, cistern, skull base, or exocranial segments. Inflammatory, neoplastic, vascular, and degenerative/demyelinating diseases are the most common offenders (list below). In addition to the offending lesion, imaging studies may reveal the manifestations of denervation: tongue muscle atrophy and fat infiltration.

4.12.1 Causes of hypoglossal neuropathy

1. Intra-axial (medulla)
   a) Paramedian-basal medullary infarction (Dejerine's anterior bulbar syndrome)
   b) Brainstem hemorrhage, ischemia
   c) MS, ALS (with lesions affecting the intramedullary parts of the lower CNs)
   d) Glioma, metastases
   e) Syringobulbia
   f) Bulbar-type poliomyelitis
   g) Botulism, diphtheria (bilateral paralysis of the caudal cranial nerves)
   h) Degenerative process (e.g., true bulbar paralysis in association with amyotrophic lateral sclerosis; Shy–Drager syndrome: orthostatic hypotension of multiple system atrophy)
2. Subarachnoid space/base of skull
   a) Chiari malformation
   b) Basilar invagination
   c) Chronic meningitis or carcinomatous meningitis
   d) Sarcoidosis (may affect any CN either unilaterally or bilaterally)
   e) Vascular lesions (e.g., vertebrobasilar dolichoectasia, aneurysm, subarachnoid hemorrhage)
   f) Skull base neoplasms
      i. Meningioma
      ii. Neural sheath tumors (e.g., schwannoma, neurofibroma)
      iii. Metastases (e.g., lung, breast, prostate, nasopharyngeal carcinomas)
      iv. Primary osteocartilaginous tumors (e.g., chordoma, osteoma, sarcoma)
      v. Glomus jugulare or chemodectoma
   g) Trauma
      i. Extensive base of skull fractures
      ii. Penetrating wounds
      iii. Surgical wounds (e.g., radical dissection of the neck, carotid endarterectomy)
   h) Infection (e.g., malignant external otitis media, mucormycosis, aspergillosis)
3. Distal (nasopharynx/carotid space)
   a) Neoplasms (e.g., squamous-cell carcinoma, metastases, non-Hodgkin's lymphoma, glomus jugulare)
   b) Trauma (e.g., penetrating, surgical wounds)
   c) Infection (e.g., bacterial abscess, "cold" abscess)
   d) Vascular thrombosis

4. Miscellaneous
   a) Benign recurrent CN paralyses (predominantly affecting CN V, VII, VIII, and XII)
   b) Isolated benign unilateral palatal palsy (predominantly in boys preceded by a viral illness with spontaneous recovery)

Keane JR. Twelfth-nerve palsy. Analysis of 100 cases. Arch Neurol 1996;53(6):561–566

Boban M, Brinar VV, Habek M, Rados M. Isolated hypoglossal nerve palsy: a diagnostic challenge. Eur Neurol 2007;58(3):177–181

Lindsay FW, Mullin D, Keefe MA. Subacute hypoglossal nerve paresis with internal carotid artery dissection. Laryngoscope 2003;113(9):1530–1533

4.13 Multiple Cranial Nerve Palsies or Weakness of Multiple Ocular and Faciobulbar Muscles

Patients presenting with multiple cranial neuropathies are common in neurologic clinical practice. Dysfunction of the cranial nerves can occur anywhere in their course from intrinsic brainstem dysfunction to their peripheral course. According to Keane's series, the abducens nerve was the most commonly involved cranial nerve, followed by the facial nerve. The oculomotor and trigeminal nerves were the third and fourth most affected nerves. Oculomotor and trochlear dysfunction was the most common combination of cranial nerve dysfunction followed closely by trigeminal plus abducens as well as trigeminal plus facial palsies. Focal brainstem lesions are often characterized by "crossed" syndromes, consisting of ipsilateral cranial nerve dysfunction and contralateral long motor or sensory tract dysfunction. Due to the rich vestibular and cerebellar connections, patients with brainstem disease often complain of vertigo, gait unsteadiness, ataxia, discoordination, nausea, and vomiting.

1. Intra-axial (brainstem syndromes)
   In the current era, the vast majority of brainstem syndromes are the result of following factors:
   a) Vascular insults, mainly brainstem infarctions and hemorrhages
      The brainstem syndromes and the anatomic regions, the neural structures, and blood vessels involved are described in detail in the section "Brain Stem Vascular Syndromes" of the chapter "Cerebrovascular Disease."
   b) Nonvascular disorders
      i.   Demyelinating disease (MS)
      ii. Acute disseminating encephalomyelitis (ADEM)
      iii. Intramedullary neoplasms (brainstem gliomas/ependymomas)
      iv. Brainstem encephalitis (Bickerstaff's encephalitis)
      v.   Central pontine myelinolysis

        vi. Arnold–Chiari malformations
       vii. Syringobulbia
   c) Motor neuron disease
   d) Leigh's disease (subacute necrotizing encephalomyelopathy)
2. Subarachnoid
   a) Severe head trauma (e.g., sphenoid fractures, orbital apex fractures affect the orbital motor nerves, temporal bone fractures affect the CN VI and VII and uncal herniation the CN III)
   b) Meningeal infection (e.g., tuberculosis)
   c) Base of brain inflammation (e.g., sarcoidosis)
   d) Basal meningeal carcinomatosis
   e) Leukemic meningitis
   f) Tumor (e.g., clivus tumor or nasopharyngeal tumor invading the intracranial cavity)
   g) Giant ICA aneurysms
   h) Iatrogenic (posterior fossa and cerebellopontine angle explorations)
3. Cavernous sinus and orbital processes
   a) Tumor
   Neoplasms occurring at the base of the skull/clivus may be the cause of multiple cranial neuropathy in 30% of the patients, representing the most common group of etiologies.
      i. Nasopharyngeal carcinoma
        It occurs in younger patients and may be associated with an EBV infection. CN VI is most often involved, as well as CN II, V, and VII; CN XII particularly if radiotherapy involving the clivus has been used.
      ii. Chordoma
        Another rare tumor that commonly involves and causes cranial nerve dysfunction and even brainstem compression.
     iii. Other skull-based neoplasms
        Other neoplasms with similar results include metastasis, meningioma, lymphoma, myeloma, histiocytosis, neurinoma, giant cell tumor, hemangioblastoma, and various primary bone tumors.
     iv. Prepontine neoplasma
        Examples are exophytic gliomas, dermoid, and epidermoid tumors which often present with multiple cranial neuropathies, particularly CN III, V, and VI dysfunction.
      v. Neoplasms involving the temporal bone involve the facial and the lower cranial nerves by direct extension, include adenoid cystic carcinoma, adenocarcinoma, and mucoepidermoid carcinoma.
     vi. Other neoplasms include schwannomas, pituitary adenomas, fibrosarcomas, primitive neuroectodermal tumors, leukemias, craniopharyngiomas, cholesteatomas, and glomus jugulare tumors.

b) Extramedullary vascular disease may compress multiple cranial nerves with CN III, VI, and V most commonly involved.
   i. Vertebrobasilar dolichoectasia
   ii. Basilar artery ectasia
   iii. Giant or fusiform aneurysm
   iv. Carotid artery dissection (ipsilateral headache, Horner's syndrome, and lower cranial neuropathies)
   v. Diabetes mellitus (often causes isolated cranial neuropathies)
   vi. Sickle cell disease (rarely causing multiple cranial neuropathies, mainly CNs V and VII)
c) Cavernous sinus thrombosis
d) Carotico-cavernous fistula
e) Iatrogenic postsurgical complication
   Multiple craniopathies occur following carotid endarterectomies, posterior triangle lymph node biopsies, radical surgery of head and neck.
f) Orbital trauma with entrapment of connective tissue and muscles
   Accidental trauma is one of the most common causes of multiple cranial neuropathies representing 12% of the cases.
g) Fungal infections (e.g., actinomycosis, mucormycosis especially in elderly diabetic and immunosuppressed patients)
h) Pseudotumor (myositis)
i) Tolosa–Hunt syndrome
j) Thyroid orbitopathy
   Autoimmune disorder where the extraocular muscles are enlarged and infiltrated with inflammatory elements, eventually leading to a restrictive oculomyopathy and motility disorder. On the onset of the ensued painful exophthalmos and chemosis, diplopia and lid retraction are rapid. The clinical picture needs to be differentiated:
   i. In adults from idiopathic orbital inflammation, and
   ii. In children from rhabdomyosarcoma and orbital cellulitis
4. Miscellaneous
   a) Infection
      i. Specific viral infection (e.g., EBV or herpes zoster. This disorder has autoimmune features and seems to cause symptoms by demyelination.)
   b) Lambert–Eaton syndrome
   c) Metabolic
      i. Wernicke's encephalopathy
      ii. Leigh's syndrome
   d) Rare disorders
      i. Trichinosis
      ii. Amyloid

        iii. Arteritis (especially temporal arteritis)
        iv. Tumor infiltration of the muscles
  e) Paraproteinemia
        i. Bing–Neel syndrome
  f) Vasculitides
        i. Polyarteritis nodosa
        ii. Cogan's syndrome
        iii. Wegener's granulomatosis
  g) Bone disorders

Bone disorders can result in compressive cranial neuropathies at the base of skull exit neural foramina.

        i. Osteopetrosis (Albers-Schonberg or marble bone disease)
        ii. Fibrous dysplasia
        iii. Expansive lesions of the jugular foramen
        iv. Hyperostosis cranialis interna
  h) Peripheral polyneuropathies with cranial nerve involvement

Conditions that may present with prominent weakness of bulbar muscles and mimic brainstem dysfunction include peripheral neuropathies, neuromuscular junction disorders, and certain myopathies.

        i. Polyneuropathies with cranial neuropathies

Peripheral nerve localization represent 17% of cases, dominated by cases of:

- Guillain–Bare syndrome
- The Miller–Fisher syndrome (Postinflammatory neuropathy and variant of the GBS)
- Polyneuropathy cranialis (multiple cranial neuropathy attributed to Lyme disease, herpes zoster, and as a GBS variant)
- Lyme disease
- Diphtheria
- Diabetes mellitus
- HIV
- Sarcoidosis
- Certain chemotherapeutic agents (vincristine/vinblastine/cisplatinum)
- Idiopathic cranial neuropathy (speculated overlap with Tolosa–Hunt syndrome)
- Neuromuscular junction disease

        ii. Neuromuscular junction disease

- Myasthenia gravis
- Botulism

        iii. Myopathies with bulbar involvement

- Mitochondrial (chronic progressive external ophthalmoplegia)

- Fascioscapular humeral dystrophy
- Oculopharyngeal dystrophy

Hokkanen E, Haltia T, Myllylä VV. Recurrent multiple cranial neuropathies. Eur Neurol 1978;17(1):32–37
Keane JR. Multiple cranial nerve palsies: analysis of 979 cases Arch Neurol 2005;62:1714–1717

4.14 Lower Cranial Nerve Syndrome

The lower cranial nerve syndromes involve CNs IX–XII unilaterally in various combinations. These nerves exit the skull just above the foramen magnum. CNs IX–XI exit through the jugular foramen, and CN XII exits through the hypoglossal canal just inferiorly. The term *jugular foramen syndrome* is often used to refer to any combination of palsies affecting the lower four cranial nerves, which are associated with the symptoms of dysphasia, dysphonia, and dysarthria.

1. **Jugular foramen syndrome or Vernet's syndrome (Schmidt's syndrome)**
   Characterized by ipsilateral paralysis of CNs IX, X, and XI and contralateral hemiparesis. This syndrome is caused by a lesion at the jugular foramen or in the retroparotid space. Schmidt's syndrome is characterized by ipsilateral paralysis of CNs IX, X, XI, and XII with contralateral hemiparesis. Glomus tumors (paraganglioma) are common causes. They are benign, slow-growing tumors arising from the neural crest cells That erode through bone and extend into the jugular foramen or even into the hypoglossal canal. Other common lesions are schwannomas, meningiomas, and metastases. Rarer causes include retromastoid abscesses, chordomas, and thrombosis of the jugular bulb.

2. **Collet–Sicard syndrome or intercondylar space syndrome**
   Consists of jugular foramen syndrome (dysfunction of CNs IX, X, and XI) with additional involvement of CN XII.

3. **Villaret's syndrome**
   It is Collet–Sicard syndrome with the addition of sympathetic involvement (Horner's syndrome). This is also referred to as the retropharyngeal space syndrome. If the process extends into the retroparotid space, there may be additional CN VII involvement.

4. **The petrous apex syndrome or Gradenigo's syndrome**
   This syndrome is typically associated with suppurative otitis media affecting the petrous apex of the temporal bone. It typically presents with pain in the trigeminal nerve distribution combined with abducens palsy. If the infection spreads to the skull base, then features of jugular foramen syndrome may coexist.

Gutiérrez Ríos R, Castrillo Sanz A, Gil Polo C, Zamora García MI, Morollón Sánchez-Mateos N, Mendoza Rodríguez A. Collet-Sicard syndrome. Neurologia 2015;30(2):130–132
Tiliket C, Petiot P, Arpin D, et al. Clinical and radiological aspects of Villaret's syndrome. Clin Neurol Neurosurg 1996;98(2):194–196
Jo YR, Chung CW, Lee JS, Park HJ. Vernet syndrome by varicella-zoster virus. Ann Rehabil Med 2013;37(3):449–452

5 Neuro-Ophthalmology

5.1 Horner's Syndrome

Horner's syndrome is an interruption of the sympathetic supply to the eye. It is characterized by miosis with a pupil that is slow to dilate, a mild (1–2 mm) ptosis, ipsilateral anhidrosis, and apparent enophthalmos (affected eye appears to be sunken) as a result of a combination of the ptosis and slight elevation of the inferior eyelid. The irides may be of different colors if the lesion is congenital or long standing. This three-neuron oculosympathetic pathway runs from the brain to the pupil (▶ Fig. 5.1).

5.1.1 Causes of Horner's syndrome

1. **First-order (central) neuron**
   Central neurons pass from the posterior hypothalamus through the brain stem into the spinal cord, via the intermediolateral column, to synapse at the ciliospinal center of Budge at the C8–T2 level of the spinal cord.
   a) Cerebral hemispheric lesions (e.g., hemispherectomy, massive infarction may cause an ipsilateral Horner's syndrome)
   b) Brainstem lesions
      The sympathetic and spinothalamic pathways in the brain stem lie throughout their course next to each other; therefore, Horner's syndrome is frequently associated with contralateral pain and temperature loss.
      i. Infarction (e.g., dorsolateral pontine; lateral medullary or Wallenberg's syndrome)
      ii. Demyelinating diseases (e.g., multiple sclerosis (MS))

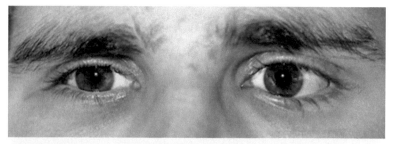

Fig. 5.1 Right Horner syndrome in a patient with right carotid artery dissection. The right pupil and eyelid gap are markedly narrower than on the left. (Reproduced from 12.3 Disturbances of Ocular and Pupillary Motility. In: Mattle H, Mumenthaler M, Taub E, ed. Fundamentals of Neurology: An Illustrated Guide. 2nd edition. Thieme; 2017.)

       iii. Pontine gliomas
       iv. Syringobulbia
       v. Bulbar poliomyelitis
       vi. Encephalitis (e.g., herpes zoster)
       vii. Basal meningitis (e.g., syphilis)
  c) Cervical cord lesions

    These lesions usually cause loss of pain and deep tendon reflexes in the arms and frequently a bilateral Horner's syndrome; ptosis usually draws attention to the condition.

       i. Trauma (particularly causing a central cord lesion)
       ii. Gliomas or ependymomas
       iii. Syringomyelia
       iv. Bulbar-type polio
       v. Amyotrophic lateral sclerosis or Lou Gehrig's disease
       vi. Arnold–Chiari malformation
       vii. Cervical vertebral dislocation or dissection of the vertebral artery

2. **Second-order (preganglionic) neuron**

Preganglionic axons exit the cord via ventral roots to pass over the apex of the lung to enter the sympathetic cervical chain. This sympathetic chain is associated with the carotid arteries. The second-order neurons synapse at the superior cervical ganglion located at the bifurcation of the cervical carotid artery.

  a) Trauma to the lower brachial plexus (e.g., D1 and C8 root avulsion known as Klumpke's paralysis)
  b) Lesions of the lower trunk of the brachial plexus (e.g., carcinoma of the lung apex extending through the apical pleura, also known as Pancoast's tumor; metastatic disease in the axillary glands from malignant disease from the breast or elsewhere; radiation damage to the lower plexus)
  c) Iatrogenic (e.g., surgical procedures on thyroid, larynx, pharynx, anterior cervical decompression, and fusion)
  d) Neck and paravertebral masses usually lymphadenopathy (impingement upon the paravertebral sympathetic chain, e.g., thyroid tumor, lymphoma, bacterial or tuberculous abscess, tumors of the posterior mediastinum, prevertebral hematoma)
  e) Neural sheath tumors (e.g., neurofibroma affecting the D1 nerve root)
  f) Cervical rib syndrome (usually in young females)
  g) Cervical disc (very rare; less than 2%)
  h) Apical lung tumors (e.g., Pancoast's tumors)
  i) Aneurysms of the aorta, subclavian, or common carotid disease
  j) Neuroblastoma
  k) Mandibular dental abscess

3. **Third-order (postganglionic) neuron**

The third-order (postganglionic) axons leave the superior cervical ganglion to accompany the internal and external carotid arteries. Most third-order axons pass with the internal carotid artery (ICA) to reach the ipsilateral cavernous sinus and then travel with fibers of the abducens (CN VI) nerve to pass to the nasociliary branch of the trigeminal nerve and enter the orbit through the superior orbital fissure. These long ciliary nerves pass through the ciliary ganglion (without synapsing) and enter the eye in the subarachnoid space to innervate the radially oriented iris dilator muscle. Both vasomotor (flushing) and sudomotor (sweating) sympathetic fibers of the face travel with the branches of the external carotid artery.

a) Cluster headaches or migraine (12% of cases; postganglionic oculosympathetic palsy)
b) Carotid artery lesions (e.g., trauma, dissection; associated with persistent facial pain and is an indication for further evaluation)
c) Cavernous sinus lesions
   Both the sympathetic and the parasympathetic nerves are usually damaged by these lesions leading to a semi-dilated and fixed pupil associated with other extraocular nerve palsies.
d) Superior orbital fissure lesions (ipsilateral partial dilatation and pupillary fixation with extraocular nerve palsies)
   i. Herpes zoster infection
   ii. Raeder's syndrome (paratrigeminal syndrome)

Mahoney NR, Liu GT, Menacker SJ, et al. Pediatric Horner's syndrome: Etiologies and role of Imaging and Urine studies to detect neuroblastoma and other responsible mass lesions. Am J Pathol 2006;142(4):651–659

Asch AJ. Turner's syndrome occurring with Horner's syndrome.Seen with coarctation of the aorta and aortic aneurysm Am J Dis Child 1999;133(8):827–830

Schievink WI. Spontaneous dissection of the carotid and vertebral arteries. N Engl J Med 2001;344(12):898–906

5.2 Abnormal Pupils

1. Anisocoria

This refers to unequal pupils. This is physiological in about 20% of people. However, if this is a new complaint, the steps to the underlying diagnosis lie in determining which of the pupils is abnormal and then look for associated signs. The first step is to compare the pupils in light and dim conditions.

a) If there is a poor reaction to light in one eye and the anisocoria is more evident in a well-lit room, then the affected pupil is abnormally large.
b) If there is a good reaction to light in both eyes but a poor dilation in the dark (i.e., the anisocoria is enhanced), then the affected pupil is abnormally small.

2. Large pupil
   There is poor constriction in a well-lit room.
   Differential diagnosis:
   a) Drugs (i.e., antipsychotic agents, atropine, cocaine, adrenaline)
   b) Traumatic iris damage
   c) CN III palsy
   d) Pharmacological dilation (i.e., dilating drops)
   e) Iris rubeosis
   f) Adie's pupil
   g) Serotonin syndrome (a toxic reaction to serotonin)
   h) Blood loss
3. Small pupil
   There is poor dilation in a dim light.
   Differential diagnosis:
   a) Drugs (i.e., Heroin, fentanyl, Codeine, tramadol and other narcotics)
   b) Physiologically small pupil
   c) Pilocarpine drops[1]
   d) Uveitis with synechiae (adhesions)
   e) Horner's syndrome
   f) Migraine
   g) Pancoast tumor (carcinoma of the lung apex)
   h) Corneal ulcer
4. Abnormally colored pupil
   Leukocoria: This refers to a white pupil and may be due to a number of conditions.
   Differential diagnosis:
   a) Congenital cataracts (must exclude the possibility of a retinoblastoma)
   b) Persistent fetal vasculature syndrome
   c) Coat's disease
   d) Retinopathy of prematurity
5. Abnormally shaped pupil
   A pupil should be round. Any deviation from this suggests abnormalities.
   Differential diagnosis:
   a) Congenital iris defects (e.g., colobomata)
   b) Iris inflammation
   c) Trauma
   d) Argyll Robertson pupil

---

[1]Drugs are by no means the single factor of pupil change, but depending on the type of drug involved they can cause pupils to constrict, dilate, or show a lack of reactivity. Drugs are often the first suspect in any pupil change where there has been no trauma and no history of an existing illness.

e) Acute angle closure glaucoma
   A fixed oval pupil in association with severe pain, a red eye, a cloudy cornea and systemic malaise.

6. Abnormally reacting pupil
   a) Light reflex test: Abnormalities arise as a result of severe optic nerve damage (e.g., transection). The patient will be blind in the affected eye; neither pupil reacts when the affected side is stimulated, but both pupils react normally when the fellow eye is stimulated.
   b) Swinging flashing test: When the pupil exhibits a relative afferent pupillary defect (RAPD), it is known as a Marcus Gunn pupil. It suggests optic nerve disease, central retinal artery or vein occlusions. A mild RAPD may also occur in amblyopia, with vitreous hemorrhage, retinal detachment, or advanced macular degeneration.
   c) Near-reflex test: There are several causes of light-near dissociation that can be grouped according to whether the problem is unilateral or bilateral.
      i. Unilateral light-near dissociation
         – Afferent conduction defect
         – Adie pupil
         – Herpes zoster ophthalmicus
         – Aberrant regeneration of the third cranial nerve
      ii. Bilateral light-near dissociation:
         – Neurosyphilis
         – Diabetes
         – Myotonic dystrophy
         – Parinaud dorsal midbrain syndrome
         – Familial amyloidosis
         – Encephalitis
         – Chronic alcoholism

5.3 Pupillary Syndromes

5.3.1 Argyll Robertson pupil

1. Loss of light reflex
   The pupil does not contract when the eye is exposed to bright light. Artificial light is better for testing than strong daylight. Best performed in a darkened room.
2. Retention of power of accommodation
   Strong and tonic contractions to near effort
3. Miosis is usually present
4. Imperfect dilatation of pupil after instillation of atropine

5. No ciliospinal reflex
When the neck is irritated or when cocaine is instilled into the eye the
pupil will dilate on the contralateral side.
6. Usually bilateral, asymmetrical, and irregular

Significance

The Argyle Robertson pupil is traditionally ascribed to damage of the central
parasympathetic pathway in the periaqueductal area.
1. It is a classical sign of meningovascular syphilis (e.g., neurosyphilis, tabes,
and general paresis).
2. Occasionally occurs in epidemic brainstem encephalitis, alcoholism,
pinealomas, and advanced diabetes.

5.3.2 Horner's syndrome

1. Ptosis of variable degree of the upper and lower eyelid
In its worst form, the lid may reach to the edge of the pupil, whereas in
mild cases the ptosis is barely detectable; isolated ptosis of the lower lid
may occur, known as "upside-down ptosis."
2. Narrowing of the palpebral fissure
This happens due to ptosis of the upper eyelid and slight elevation of the
lower lid: paresis of Müller's muscle
3. Miosis
The affected pupil is slightly smaller than its fellow; the resultant anisocoria is minimal in a bright light and exaggerated in darkness. Occasionally,
pupillary involvement can only be demonstrated on pharmacological
testing.
4. Transient increase in accommodation
5. Anhidrosis
Occurs in 5% patients, with preganglionic lesions; sudomotor and vasoconstrictor fibers to face travel with branches of the external carotid artery.
6. Transient vascular dilatation of face and conjunctiva
The conjunctiva may be slightly bloodshot due to the loss of vasoconstrictor
activity.
7. Enophthalmos
This sign is not easily detected; it is not a feature of oculosympathetic palsy.
8. Change in tear viscosity
9. Iris heterochromia
In congenital Horner's syndrome, the iris on the affected side fails to
become pigmented and remains a blue-grey color.

Significance

Horner's syndrome results from an interruption of the sympathetic supply to the eye. The pathway has three neurons. First-order fibers descend from the ipsilateral hypothalamus through the brain stem and cervical cord to T1–T2, and C8 (ciliospinal center of Budge). They synapse on ipsilateral preganglionic sympathetic fibers, exit the cord through the first and second anterior dorsal roots, ascend in the cervical sympathetic chain as second-order neurons to the superior cervical ganglion, and then they synapse on postganglionic sympathetic fibers. The third-order neurons travel via the ICA, pass to the Gasserian ganglion and through the first division of the trigeminal nerve to the orbit and innervate the radial smooth muscle of the iris pupil. The sudomotor and vasoconstrictor fibers travel to face separately with the external carotid artery branches. (See "Causes of Horner's syndrome.")

5.3.3 Holmes–Adie or "tonic" pupil

1. Widely dilated, circular pupil
2. Does not react to light
   Pupil may react very slowly, i.e., after prolonged exposure to very bright light.
3. Tonic accommodation
4. Strong and tonic contraction to near effort
5. Usually unilateral (80%) and more frequently found in females.
6. Often associated with loss of knee tendon reflexes and impairment of sweating.

Significance

The Holmes–Adie or tonic pupil is due to the degeneration of the nerve cells in the ciliary ganglion (▶ Fig. 5.2). The cause of this condition is not known but it often occurs after a viral illness (e.g., herpes zoster ophthalmicus).

The dissociation between the poor or absent light reaction and of the more definite response to accommodation are thought to be produced by slow inhibition of the sympathetic and not by any residual parasympathetic activity. Diagnosis is confirmed by the pupil's hypersensitivity to weak miotic drops (e.g., 0.05–0.125% pilocarpine) which cause the abnormal pupil to contract vigorously and the normal pupil minimally.

5.3.4 Afferent pupillary defect or Marcus Gunn pupil

The normal eye has a brisk pupillary constriction when exposed to light (the affected eye will also constrict consensually). When a light is shone into the normal eye it will cause a brisk pupillary constriction; the affected eye will also constrict consensually. When the light in turn is shone into the affected eye, the

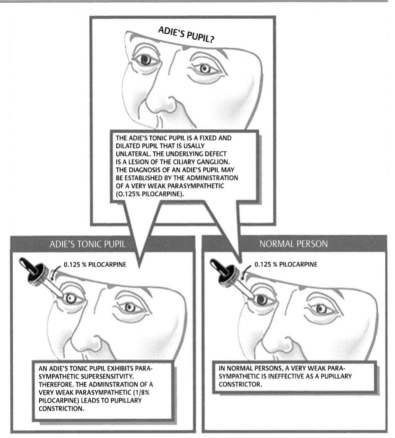

Fig. 5.2 Adie's tonic pupil. (Reproduced from Adie's Tonic Pupil. In: Alberstone C, Benzel E, Najm I, et al, ed. Anatomic Basis of Neurologic Diagnosis. 1st edition. Thieme; 2009.)

reaction is slower, less complete, and so brief that the pupil is slow to dilate again (the pupillary escape phenomena) (▶ Fig. 5.3). The reaction is best seen when:
- The light is moved rapidly from the normal to the affected eye and vice versa,
- Each stimulus lasting approximately 1 second with 2–3 seconds in between. The affected pupil will thus be dilating when the swinging light hits it.

Significance

The Marcus Gunn pupillary reaction is thought to be due to a reduction in the number of the fibers subserving the light reflex on the affected side. The lesion must be prechiasmal, and almost always involves the optic nerve often due to MS.

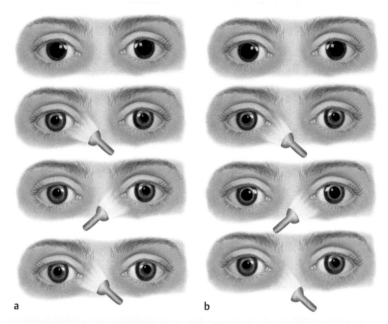

Fig. 5.3 (a) Normal pupillary reaction to swinging light without a change in the size of the pupils. **(b)** Loss of pupillary reaction to the left eye. The pupils constrict when the light is shone to the right eye, but when the light is directed to the left eye, both pupils are dilated.

5.3.5 Posttraumatic mydriasis or iridoplegia

1. Irregular pupillary dilatation
2. Poor or absent reaction to light

Significance

Disruption of the fine short ciliary nerve filaments in the sclera by blunt trauma results in a usually transient paralysis of the iris causing an irregularly dilated pupil with impairment of the light reaction. History of trauma and findings of local periorbital/orbital injuries in a conscious and mentally intact patient are diagnostic.

5.3.6 Hippus

Spontaneous, partially rhythmic and alternate contractions and dilatations of the pupil under uniform, constant illumination. The pupils present wide excursions visible to the naked eye, gradually decreasing. This phenomenon is called hippus.

Pupils normally exhibit fine movements, i.e., pupillary unrest, particularly under high magnification. Absence of pupillary unrest is indicative of organic disease.

Significance

Mostly seen in:
1. Normal individuals
2. Hysteria
3. Incipient cataracts, MS, meningitis, and contralateral cerebrovascular insults
4. Recovery from oculomotor paralysis

5.3.7 Unilateral pupillary dilatation (mydriasis)

1. Local mydriatic and cycloplegic drug agents
   a) Phenylephrine, epinephrine,
   b) Cocaine
   c) Hydroxyamphetamine
   d) Atropine, homa-eucatropine
   e) Scopolamine
   f) Cyclopentolate
2. Migraine (cluster headaches often lead to miosis with Horner's syndrome)
3. Holmes—Adie pupil
4. Oculomotor nerve paralysis
   a) Aneurysm (e.g., posterior communicating, posterior cerebral, superior cerebellar)
   b) Temporal lobe (uncal) herniation
5. Acute ciliary ganglionitis
   A large pupil nonreacting to initially to accommodation and to light or convergence, develops suddenly several days after an infection or trauma.
6. Ciliospinal reflex
   When the neck is irritated or when cocaine is instilled into the eye, the pupil will dilate on the ipsilateral side.
7. Pseudodilatation
   Contralateral pupillary constriction: for example, in Horner's syndrome

Significance

Unilateral pupillary dilatation is the most important physical sign in the unconscious patient, and until proven otherwise, a dilated pupil indicates that a herniated temporal lobe is compressing the ipsilateral oculomotor nerve and immediate surgical action is required.

5.3.8 Bilateral pupillary dilatation (mydriasis)

See ▶ Fig. 5.4.

1. Rostrocaudal deterioration from supratentorial masses leading to an almost irreversible cerebral damage and coma.
2. Systemic drug poisoning
   a) Anticholinergics (e.g., atropine, scopolamine, belladonna, propantheline)
   b) Tricyclic antidepressants
   c) Antihistamines (e.g., diphenhydramine, chlorpheniramine)

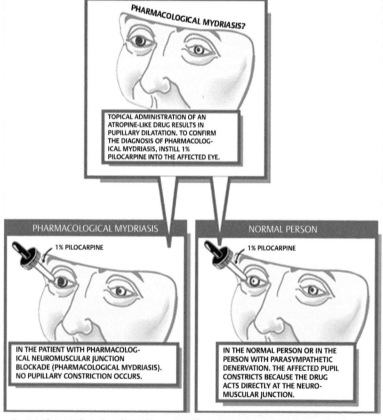

Fig. 5.4 Pharmacological mydriasis. (Reproduced from Pharmacological Mydriasis. In: Alberstone C, Benzel E, Najm I, et al, ed. Anatomic Basis of Neurologic Diagnosis. 1st edition. Thieme; 2009.)

   d) Phenothiazines
   e) Amphetamines
   f) Cocaine
   g) Epinephrine, norepinephrine
   h) Lysergic acid diethylamide
   i) Thiopental
3. Postictal (e.g., major seizures)
4. Bilateral optic nerve damage and blindness
5. Parinaud's syndrome
   Lesions within the tectum will interfere with the decussating light reflex
   fibers in the periaqueductal area and result in dilated and nonreacting
   pupils and paralysis of the upward gaze.
6. Thyrotoxicosis
7. Emotional state (sympathetic overdrive, e.g., fear, pain)

5.3.9 Unilateral pupillary constriction (miosis)

1. Horner's syndrome
2. Local miotic drugs
   a) Pilocarpine
   b) Neostigmine, physostigmine
   c) Carbachol
   d) Methacholine
3. Local affection of the anterior chamber of the eye

5.3.10 Bilateral pupillary constriction (miosis)

1. Systemic drug poisoning
   a) Narcotics (e.g., morphine and opiates, meperidine, methadone, propoxy-
      phene)
   b) Barbiturates
   c) Phentolamine
   d) Meprobamate
   e) Cholinergics (e.g., neostigmine, edrophonium, physostigmine,
      pyridostigmine)
   f) Marijuana
   g) Guanethidine
   h) Monoamine oxidase inhibitors, reserpine
2. Pontine lesions
   A massive intrapontine hemorrhage is usually associated with pin-point
   pupils, loss of consciousness, and a spastic tetraparesis with brisk reflexes.

3. Argyle Robertson pupils
4. Neurosyphilis (very rarely may cause unilateral miosis)
5. Advanced age

5.4 Diplopia

5.4.1 Monocular diplopia

This disorder is psychogenic or due to a refractive disturbance in the eye.

1. Astigmatism or opacity of the cornea or lens
2. Corneal dystrophy
3. Iridodialysis
4. Foreign body (e.g., air bubbles, glass, parasites)
5. Large retinal tear
6. Retinal macular cyst
7. Occipital lobe lesions
8. Tonic conjugate gaze deviation
9. Noncorrespondence between the frontal eye fields and occipital associative areas
10. Palinopsia

5.4.2 Binocular diplopia

Double vision is due to misalignment of the visual axes if it is relieved by occlusion of either eye.

1. Extraocular muscle disorders
   a) Myasthenia gravis
   b) Thyroid orbitopathy
   c) Orbital apex trauma with connective tissue and muscle entrapment
   d) Orbital myositis
   e) Tumors (e.g., pituitary adenoma and growth-hormone-secreting adenoma; they cause enlargement of the extraocular muscles.)
2. Ocular motor nerve disorders
   a) Severe head trauma (e.g., sphenoid fractures (orbital apex) affect the ocular motor nerves, temporal bone fractures (CNs VI and VII)
   b) Microvascular ischemia (associated with diabetes mellitus)
   c) Compression
      i. Tumor (meningioma, pituitary adenoma with apoplexy, metastases, particularly nasopharyngeal carcinoma)
      ii. Giant ICA aneurysm
   d) Increased intracranial pressure (ICP) (e.g., uncal and tonsillar herniation affecting the CNs III and VI)

  e) Meningeal infection, basal inflammation, and carcinomatosis
3. Central pathways disorders
    a) Internuclear ophthalmoplegia
       A lesion of the medial longitudinal fasciculus (MLF) between the CNs III and VI produces disconjugate eye movements and diplopia on lateral gaze.
    b) Skew deviation
       It is thought to represent damaged otolithic inputs and occurs frequently with unilateral MLF lesions, but may occur in many brainstem lesions. Usually, the higher eye is on the side of the lesion.
    c) Divergence insufficiency (e.g., bilateral CN VI palsies, increased ICP)
    d) Convergence insufficiency (e.g., convergence spasm suggested by associated miosis due to the near response)
    e) Decompensated strabismus (usually of no pathologic importance)
4. Eye optical system disorders
    a) Nuclear lens sclerosis
    b) Uncorrected refractory error
    c) Corneal disease
        i. Keratoconus (e.g., Gorlin–Goltz syndrome or focal dermal hypoplasia, Crouzon's disease)
       ii. Megalocornea (e.g., Marfan's syndrome, Pierre Robin's syndrome)
      iii. Microcornea (e.g., Bardet–Biedl syndrome)
    d) Peripheral iridectomy
    e) Disorders of the lens
        i. Dislocated lens (e.g., Alport's syndrome, Marfan's disease)
       ii. Spherophakia (e.g., hyperlysinemia, sulfite oxidase deficiency)
5. Unclear or combined disorders
    a) Chronic progressive external ophthalmoplegia
    b) Toxic ophthalmoplegia (e.g., Botulism and diphtheria)
    c) Miller-Fisher syndrome and Guillain–Barre syndrome (e.g., postviral neuropathy)
    d) Metabolic (e.g., Wernicke's encephalopathy)
    e) Eaton–Lambert myasthenic syndrome
    f) Myotonic dystrophy

5.4.3 Vertical binocular diplopia

1. Blowout fracture of orbital floor with entrapment of the inferior rectus muscle
2. Thyroid orbitopathy with tight inferior rectus muscle
3. Ocular myasthenia
4. CN III palsy
5. CN IV palsy
6. Skew deviation

5.4.4 Horizontal binocular diplopia

1. Blowout fracture of medial orbital wall and entrapment of the medial rectus muscle
2. Thyroid orbitopathy with tight medial rectus muscle
3. Ocular myasthenia
4. Internuclear ophthalmoplegia
5. Convergence insufficiency
6. Decompensated strabismus
7. CN III palsy
8. CN VI palsy

Rucker JC, Tomsak RL. Binocular diplopia. A practical approach. Neurologist 2005;11(2):98–110

Loong SC. The eye in neurology: evaluation of sudden visual loss and diplopia—diagnostic pointers and pitfalls. Ann Acad Med Singapore 2001;30(2):143–147

Pelak VS. Evaluation of diplopia: an anatomic systemic approach. Hosp Physician 2004;40(3):16–25

Brazis PW, Lee AG. Acquired binocular horizontal diplopia. Mayo Clin Proc 1999;74(9):907–916

5.5 Ptosis

1. Congenital
    a) Isolated (drooping is unilateral in 70% of congenital ptosis)
    b) Familial (very rare and bilateral)
    c) Sympathetic denervation (congenital Horner's syndrome)
    d) Anomalous synkinesis between CN III and V (Marcus Gunn phenomenon, jaw winking)
    e) Blepharophimosis syndromes
    f) Neonatal myasthenia
2. Neurogenic (e.g., due to third nerve lesions)
    a) Nuclear lesions (severe bilateral ptosis, medial rectus weakness, upgaze paresis, and pupillary dilatation if the lesion is complete)
    b) Peripheral lesions (unilateral ptosis, mydriasis, and ophthalmoplegia)
3. Myopathy
    a) Myasthenia gravis
    b) Oculopharyngeal muscular dystrophy
    c) Chronic progressive external ophthalmoplegia
    d) Polymyositis
    e) Chronic use of topical steroid eye drops/ointment
4. Orbit
    a) Inflammatory disease
        i. Thyroid orbitopathy
        ii. Idiopathic orbital inflammatory disease (orbital pseudotumor)
        iii. Tolosa–Hunt syndrome
        iv. Orbital apex syndrome (painful ophthalmoplegia)

b) Tumors
   i. Infantile rhabdomyosarcoma
   ii. Dermoid cyst
   iii. Hemangioma
   iv. Metastatic neuroblastoma
   v. Optic glioma
c) Trauma (iatrogenic especially following surgery for strabismus, retinal detachment, and cataract)

5. Pseudoptosis
   a) Secondary to ocular irritations, foreign body (e.g., protective)
   b) Blepharospasm
   c) Enophthalmos
   d) Pathologic contralateral lid retraction
   e) Contralateral exophthalmos
   f) Huntington's chorea (lid opening apraxia)
   g) Hysterical

Patten J. Neurological Differential Diagnosisnd ed. Springer; 2005

Victor M, Hayes R, Adams R. Oculopharyngeal muscular dystrophy—a familial disease of late life characterized by dysphagia and progressive ptosis of the eyelid N Engl J Med 1962;267:1267–1272

Chezzi A, Zaffarini Y. Neurological manifestations of gastrointestinal disorders, with particular reference to the differential diagnosis of multiple sclerosis. Neurol Sci 2001;22(2):117–122

5.6 Acute Ophthalmoplegia

5.6.1 Unilateral acute ophthalmoplegia

1. Aneurysm or anomalous vessels
   The nerve palsy is considered to be due to hemorrhage either within the aneurysmal sac to which the nerve is adherent or directly into the nerve.
   a) Oculomotor nerve palsy: Aneurysms at the junction of the posterior communicating and internal carotid artery
   b) Abducens nerve palsy: Aneurysm of the anterior inferior cerebellar artery and basilar artery
2. Small brainstem hemorrhages (e.g., emboli, leukemia, blood coagulopathies)
3. Ophthalmoplegic migraine
   Transitory palsy affecting the oculomotor nerve in 85% and only 15% the abducens and trochlear nerves.
4. Cavernous sinus thrombosis
   Originating almost exclusively from spread of infection from the mouth, nose, or face.

5. Inferior petrosal sinus thrombosis (Gradenigo's syndrome)
   Originating from infections of the middle ear and affecting the abducens nerve, the facial nerve, and the trigeminal ganglion.
6. Cavernous sinus fistula (traumatic in origin)
7. Brain tumors
   a) Brainstem glioma
   b) Craniopharyngioma
   c) Pituitary adenoma
   d) Nasopharyngeal carcinoma
   e) Lymphoma
   f) Pineal region tumors
8. Idiopathic cranial nerve palsy
   Transitory nerve palsy attributed to a viral infection and affecting the abducens nerve more commonly than the oculomotor or trochlear nerve.
9. Myasthenia gravis (and other pharmacologic or toxic causes of neuromuscular blockade)
10. Orbital
    a) Tumors
       i. Dermoid cyst
       ii. Hemangioma
       iii. Metastatic neuroblastoma
       iv. Optic glioma
       v. Rhabdomyosarcoma
    b) Inflammatory disease
       i. Tolosa–Hunt syndrome
       ii. Orbital pseudotumor
       iii. Sarcoid
11. Trauma (e.g., blowout fracture of the orbit with entrapment myopathy)
12. Increased ICP (e.g., uncal herniation, pseudotumor cerebri)
13. Demyelination (e.g., fascicular affecting all three nerves)

5.6.2 Bilateral acute ophthalmoplegia

Most of the conditions causing unilateral ophthalmoplegia may also produce bilateral ophthalmoplegia.
1. Botulism
2. Intoxications
   Ocular motility may be impaired by drugs, such as anticonvulsants, tricyclic antidepressants, and other psychotropic medications at toxic serum concentrations.
3. Encephalitis of the brain stem
   Caused by echoviruses, coxsackie viruses and adenoviruses.

4. Diphtheria
5. Cavernous sinus thrombosis
6. Carotico-cavernous fistula
7. Myasthenia gravis, thyrotoxicosis

Roy FH. Ocular Differential Diagnosis. Jaypee-Highlights Medical Publishers Inc; 2012

Lee SH, Lim GH, Kim JS, et al. Acute ophthalmoplegia (without ataxia) associated with anti-GQ1b antibody. Neurology 2008;71(6):426–429

Abrahamson IA Jr, Horwitz ID. Acute ophthalmoplegia: a differential diagnosis. Am J Ophthalmol 1954;38(6): 781–787

Smith J, Clarke L, Severn P, Boyce R. Unilateral external ophthalmoplegia in Miller Fisher syndrome: case report. BMC Ophthalmol 2007;7:7

5.7 Internuclear Ophthalmoplegia

A disorder of horizontal eye movements due to a lesion of the MLF in the mid pons between CNs III and VI. The MLF lesion produces disconjugate eye movements and diplopia on lateral gaze, because impulses to the lateral rectus travel normally, whereas those to the medial rectus are intact (▶ Fig. 5.5 and ▶ Fig. 5.6).

1. Brainstem infarction
   Most common in the older population, the syndrome is unilateral and caused by occlusion of the basilar artery or its paramedian branches.

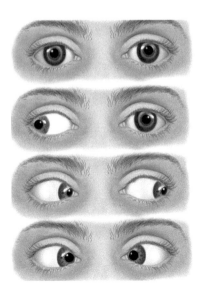

Fig. 5.5 Left internuclear ophthalmoplegia (Cogan posterior type). Convergence of the eyes denotes normal function of inner rectal muscle of the eye.

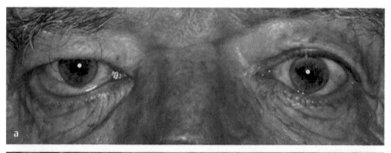

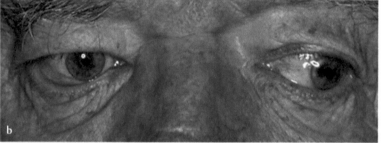

Fig. 5.6 Right internuclear ophthalmoplegia in a patient with a lacunar brainstem infarct. **(a)** When the patient looks straight ahead, the eyes are parallel. **(b)** On attempted leftward gaze, right eye adduction is impaired (weakness of the medial rectus muscle). (Reproduced from 12.3 Disturbances of Ocular and Pupillary Motility. In: Mattle H, Mumenthaler M, Taub E, ed. Fundamentals of Neurology: An Illustrated Guide. 2nd edition. Thieme; 2017.)

2. MS
   Most common in the young adults, especially when the syndrome is bilateral.
3. Intrinsic and extra-axial brain stem and 4th ventricular tumors (e.g., glioma, metastasis)
4. Brainstem encephalitis (e.g., viral or other forms of infection)
5. Drug intoxication (e.g., tricyclic antidepressants, phenothiazines, barbiturates, or phenytoin)
6. Metabolic encephalopathy (e.g., hepatic encephalopathy, maple syrup urine disease)
7. Lupus erythematosus
8. Head trauma
9. Degenerative conditions (e.g., progressive supranuclear palsy)
10. Syphilis

11. Chiari II and III malformation and associated syringobulbia
12. Pseudointernuclear ophthalmoplegia (as a feature of:)
    a) Myasthenia gravis
    b) Wernicke's encephalopathy
    c) Guillain–Barre syndrome
    d) Exotropia
    e) Fisher syndrome

Keane JR. Internuclear ophthalmoplegia: unusual causes in 114 of 410 patients. Arch Neurol 2005;62(5): 714–717

Bolaños I, Lozano D, Cantú C. Internuclear ophthalmoplegia: causes and long-term follow-up in 65 patients. Acta Neurol Scand 2004;110(3):161–165

5.8 Vertical Gaze Palsy

1. Tumors
   a) Pineal area
   b) Midbrain
   c) 3rd ventricle
2. Aqueduct stenosis and hydrocephalus
3. Infarction or hemorrhage of the dorsal midbrain
4. Head trauma
5. MS
6. Miller-Fisher syndrome
7. Vitamin B12 or B1 deficiency
8. Neurovisceral lipid storage diseases
   a) Gaucher disease
   b) Niemann–Pick disease, type C
9. Congenital vertical ocular motor apraxia
10. The syndrome can be mimicked by:
    a) Progressive supranuclear palsy
    b) Thyroid ophthalmopathy
    c) Myasthenia gravis
    d) Guillain–Barres syndrome
    e) Congenital upgaze limitation

Strupp M, Kremmyda O, Adamczyk C, et al. Central ocular motor disorders, including gaze palsy and nystagmus. J Neurol 2014;261(Suppl 2):S542–S558

Hommel M, Bogousslavsky J. The spectrum of vertical gaze palsy following unilateral brainstem stroke. Neurology 1991;41(8):1229–1234

5.9 Unilateral Sudden Visual Loss

1. Vascular disturbances
   a) Ischemic optic atrophy due to arteriosclerosis
   Pallor of the optic nerve head, pale retinas, pseudopapilledema, and incomplete blindness are the prominent diagnostic features.
   b) Transient monocular blindness or amaurosis fugax
   Stenosis of the ICA or cardiogenic emboli are mainly responsible.
   c) Temporal arteritis
   Affects elderly individuals and frequently leads to complete blindness; patients complain of headaches and the erythrocyte sedimentation rate is usually elevated.
2. Acute retrobulbar neuritis
   Acute inflammatory reaction of the optic nerve as a response to the following:
   a) MS (up to 50% of cases have other manifestations of MS)
   b) Metabolic and toxic insults
   c) Birth control pill
   Patients complain about impairment of central vision (e.g., "puff of smoke," "fluffy ball"). Examination reveals impaired visual acuity (20/200), a central scotoma, and occasionally papilledema (when the inflammation is just behind the nerve head).

Differential diagnosis from:
   a) Papilledema
   By the severe visual loss, as vision remains normal in the case of papilledema unless a hemorrhage or exudate occurs into the macula retinal area which may lead into rapid central visual loss.
   b) Optic chiasmal compression
   Central vision is served by the papillomacular bundle, which is more sensitive to external compression than the rest of the optic nerve fibers. The presence of optic atrophy and bitemporal field defects are the clues to the diagnosis.
   c) Trauma
   Fracture of the anterior cranial fossa extending into the optic foramen.
   d) Amblyopia with papilledema
   Short-lived attacks associated with increased ICP: e.g., benign intracranial hypertension.

5.10 Bilateral Sudden Visual Loss

1. Cortical blindness
   Loss of vision with preservation of the pupillary light reflex and normal ophthalmoscopic examination.

- a) Transient blindness
    - i. Mild head trauma
    - ii. Migraine
    - iii. Hypoglycemia
    - iv. Hypotension
- b) Permanent blindness
    - i. Anoxia
        - – Infarction: (1) Sudden and marked impairment of the basilar artery flow usually in elderly individuals. (2) Posttraumatic intracranial hypertension leading to tentorial herniation and causing compression of the posterior cerebral arteries.
        - – Hemorrhage (e.g., traumatic or rarely spontaneous)
    - ii. Multifocal metastatic tumors in the occipital lobes
    - iii. Multifocal primary tumors (e.g., malignant gliomas)
    - iv. Multifocal abscess in the occipital lobes
2. Optic nerve neuropathy
    - a) Ischemic neuropathy (e.g., infarction of the anterior portion of the optic nerve from systemic vascular disease or hypotension)
    - b) Traumatic neuropathy (e.g., severe head trauma with indirect optic neuropathy from nerve swelling, tear, or hemorrhage)
    - c) Toxic Nutritional neuropathy
        - i. Drugs (e.g., barbiturates, streptomycin, chloramphenicol, isoniazid, and sulfonamides)
        - ii. Alcohol (e.g., methyl alcohol: overnight visual loss; tobacco and ethyl alcohol: progressive visual loss)
        - iii. B1, B12, and folic acid deficiencies: progressive visual loss over weeks
    - d) Demyelinating neuropathy (binocular visual loss in more than 50% of children whereas in adults it is monocular as a rule)
3. Retinal disease
    - a) Retinal ischemia (e.g., central retinal artery occlusion)
        - i. Usually hemodynamic retinal ischemia with aortic arch syndrome following a sudden change from the recumbent to the upright position in elderly individuals.
        - ii. Retinal migraine (e.g., in one-third of the children and young adults)
        - iii. Coagulopathies (e.g., increased platelet activity and increased factor VIII)
        - iv. Miscellaneous risk factors (e.g., congenital heart disease, sickle cell disease, vasculitis, and pregnancy)
    - b) Blind trauma (e.g., retinal contusion, tear, or detachment)
4. Trauma to carotid or vertebral arteries (symptoms establish within several hours and sometimes days)

5. Pituitary apoplexy (hemorrhagic infarction of the pituitary gland occurring usually in preexisting pituitary tumor)
6. Psychogenic blindness
   Pupillary reaction to light is normal and fundoscopy is unremarkable; there is a nonalarming reaction of the patient to his/her sudden blindness and he/she has not experienced any of the described causes of blindness.

5.11 Slowly Progressing Visual Loss

1. Compressive optic nerve atrophy (e.g., mostly unilateral) (▶ Fig. 5.7)
   a) Aneurysm of the carotid artery
   b) Tumor
      i. Pituitary adenoma
      ii. Meningioma
      iii. Optic nerve and hypothalamic glioma in children
      iv. Craniopharyngioma
      v. Dermoid
2. Hereditary optic atrophy
   a) Macular degeneration
   b) Familial Leber's optic atrophy
   c) Wolfram syndrome (e.g., juvenile diabetes mellitus, optic atrophy, and bilateral hearing loss)
   d) Infantile Refsum's disease (e.g., blindness, deafness, dementia, ataxia)

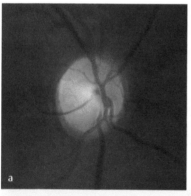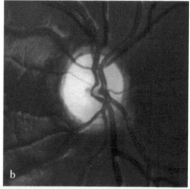

Fig. 5.7 Optic disc (papilla) of the right eye. **(a)** Normal disc. **(b)** Pale, atrophic disc. (These images are provided courtesy of the Department of Ophthalmology, University of Bern.) (Reproduced from 3.3 Head and Cranial Nerves. In: Mattle H, Mumenthaler M, Taub E, ed. Fundamentals of Neurology: An Illustrated Guide. 2nd edition. Thieme; 2017.)

3. Prolonged elevation of the ICP
   a) Pseudotumor cerebri
   b) Obstructive hydrocephalus
4. Intraocular tumors (e.g., retinoblastoma)
5. Toxic agents (e.g., industrial solvents)
6. Tapetoretinal degenerations
   a) Aminoacidopathies
   b) Abnormal lipid metabolism
   c) Abnormal carbohydrate metabolism
   d) Cockayne syndrome (primary pigmentary degeneration of the retina, ataxia, spasticity, deafness, peripheral neuropathy)

Khan J, Chong V. Sudden visual loss. Lancet 2007;370(9587):590

Jones RG, Peall A. Sudden unilateral visual field loss. J Emerg Trauma Shock 2009;2(3):211–212

Beran DI, Murphy-Lavoie H. Acute, painless vision loss. J La State Med Soc 2009;161(4):214–216, 218–223

Cormack G, Dhillon B. Sudden loss of vision. Practitioner 1998;242(1593):851–853

Levy J, Marcus M, Shelef I, Lifshitz T. Acute bilateral blindness in meningeal carcinomatosis. Eye (Lond) 2004;18(2):206–207, discussion 207–208

Trojano M, Paolicelli D. The differential diagnosis of multiple sclerosis: classification and clinical features of relapsing and progressive neurological syndromes. Neurol Sci 2001;22(Suppl 2):S98–S102

5.12 Transient Monocular Blindness

1. Embolic
   The duration is 3–5 minutes usually; quadratic, altitudinal, or total visual loss, corresponding in distribution of retinal arterioles; associated with contralateral hemiplegia with or without hemihypoesthesia. The most common type of embolus is a cholesterol embolus manifesting as a glistening, shiny, slightly irregular object with the narrowed retinal vessel corresponding to a field defect and in other retinal areas since the cholesterol emboli are often multiple. Fibrin platelet emboli manifest as creamy white molding to the arterial tree like an amorphous plug; they may coexist with the cholesterol emboli. The calcific emboli are the rarest and appear as jagged, bright white spots within the vessels originating exclusively from the heart valves.
   a) Carotid bifurcation thromboembolism (the most frequent source)
   b) Cardiogenic emboli (valve, mural thrombus, intracardial tumor)
   c) Great vessel or distal internal carotid atheroembolism
   d) Drug abuse-related intravascular emboli
2. Hemodynamic
   Binocular attacks of visual loss predominantly in the elderly that last few seconds to minutes, and are described as a graying out or dimming out of vision. They are related to posture and/or cardiac arrhythmias. They may be

associated with occasional tinnitus, diplopia, vertigo, and perioral paresthesias.
a) Extensive atheromatous occlusive disease
b) Inflammatory arteritis (Takayasu's disease)
c) Hypoperfusion (e.g., cardiac failure, acute hypovolemia, coagulopathy, blood viscosity)

3. Ocular
a) Anterior ischemic optic neuropathy (AION)
b) Central or branch retinal artery occlusion (often embolic)
c) Central retinal vein occlusion
d) Nonvascular causes (e.g., hemorrhage, pressure, tumor, congenital)

4. Neurologic
Extremely brief and secondary episodes of visual dimming affecting both eyes simultaneously or either eye alternatively; these episodes occur in association with papilledema.
a) Brain stem, vestibular, or oculomotor
b) Optic neuritis, compression of optic nerve or chiasm
c) Papilledema
d) MS
e) Migraine
f) Psychogenic

5. Idiopathic

The Amaurosis Fugax Study Group. Current management of amaurosis fugax. Stroke 1990;21(2):201–208
Biousse V, Newman NJ, Sternberg P Jr. Retinal vein occlusion and transient monocular visual loss associated with hyperhomocystinemia. Am J Ophthalmol 1997;124(2):257–260

5.13 Transient Visual Loss

1. Embolic
Usually uniocular, lasting 3–10 minutes. Mostly, source is ulcerated plaque at carotid bifurcation, but can also be at cardiac valves, mural thrombi, and atrial myxomas. Clinically, it produces a quadrantic, altitudinal, or total pattern of visual loss, corresponding to distribution of retinal arterioles. In case of a central transient ischemic attack, it is associated with contralateral hemiplegia, with or without hemihypoesthesia.
a) Cholesterol embolus or carotid bifurcation thromboembolism (50%)
The most common type of embolus is a cholesterol embolus most frequently from the ipsilateral carotid bifurcation and less frequently from the distal internal carotid and the great vessels. In fundoscopy, it manifests as a glistening, shiny, slightly irregular object with the vessel and sometimes at a bifurcation.

b) Fibrin platelet emboli or cardiogenic emboli (4%)
These emboli may come from thrombotic changes in ulcerated plaques, mural thrombi in the heart, abnormalities of the valves, or drug abuse-related intravascular emboli and intracranial tumor. In fundoscopy, they appear as soft and creamy and mold themselves to the arterial tree like an amorphous plug; they may coexist with the cholesterol emboli (79%).

c) Calcific emboli (9%)
Very rare, appear as bright, white spots within the vascular tree and originate almost exclusively from heart valves.

d) Other
Rarer emboli include cardiac myxomas, fat (Purtscher's retinopathy and pancreatitis), air, amniotic fluid, and particles injected by intravenous drug abusers.

2. Hemodynamic
Uniocular or binocular attacks of blindness described as usually total and rarely altitudinal graying out or dimming out of vision. The predominantly affected elderly patients may describe flickering to field like "TV snow", or may have attacks without complaining. These attacks last from few seconds to minutes and are occasionally associated with tinnitus, diplopia, vertigo, and rarely perioral paresthesias. These attacks of blindness are related to:

a) Hypoperfusion (cardiac failure, cardiac arrhythmia, compression of the vertebral artery, postural hypotension, acute hypovolemia, coagulopathy, blood viscosity)

b) Extensive vascular occlusive disease (example of the orbit or carotid distribution making the orbital circulation susceptible to slight decrease in perfusion that normally would not affect visual function)

c) Inflammatory arteritis (Takayasu's disease—"pulseless disease")

3. Ocular
a) Anterior ischemic optic neuropathy
Presents with sudden uniocular decrease in visual acuity and color vision on awakening, swelling of the optic head cup, an afferent pupillary defect, and microhemorrhages within the nerve fibers. The AION occurs with increased incidence in subjects with systemic diseases (e.g., diabetes mellitus, atherosclerosis, hypertension, hypotension, hypoxia, migraine, carotid occlusive disease), vasculitides (e.g., temporal arteritis, systemic lupus erythematosus, postviral vasculitis, radiation necrosis, postimmunization), hematological conditions (e.g., polycythemia vera, hyperviscosity, increased antiphospholipid antibodies, protein C deficiency, sickle cell disease), and infectious and inflammatory diseases (e.g., sarcoidosis, syphilis, Lyme's disease, CMV, herpes)

b) Central or branch retinal artery occlusion (often embolic)

About 20% of central artery occlusions are due to emboli; most others are arteriosclerotic and inflammatory in nature; contributing processes include hypertension, diabetes mellitus, sarcoidosis, fungi, temporal arteritis, hypercoagulable states. Clinically, there is a sudden severe visual loss and fundoscopy would show opaque posterior retina and cherry-red macula, whereas fovea and peripheral retina maintain a normal color.

c) Central retinal vein occlusion

Following a few hours or days of fluctuating visual acuity, it finally leads to very poor vision (20/200) and photopsia, with fundoscopy showing a massive retinal hemorrhage, tortuous and dark-distended veins and papilledema. Often spontaneous recovery of visual acuity occurs (up to 20/50 in half cases) 6–12 months later. Important factors in the pathogenesis of venous occlusions are: atherosclerosis and hypertension (75%), glaucoma (15%), diabetes, and hyper viscosity states.

d) Nonvascular causes (e.g., hemorrhage, pressure, tumor, congenital)

4. Neurologic

a) "Classic" migraine

By far, the most frequent cause of transient visual loss is "classic" migraine manifesting by a bilateral homonymous visual field loss, often followed by a scotoma. It is considered to be due to vascular spasm or arteriovenous shunting, which rarely leads to infarction and usually clears within 10–20 minutes. It is almost invariably is followed by headache, which lasts from hours to more than a day and may be accompanied with nausea and photophobia.

b) Optic neuritis, MS

Optic neuritis is the most frequent cause of neurogenic blindness in patients under the age of 50 years. Optic neuritis is often a manifestation of demyelination (e.g., idiopathic MS, Schilder's disease, or other leukodystrophy) and it is the first symptom in 20–75% of MS patients. Demyelination is the most frequent cause of optic neuritis, and MS is the most frequent cause of demyelination.

c) Brain stem, vestibular, or oculomotor

d) Papilledema

The only symptom with true papilledema may be obscuration or momentary episodes of visual blur usually unilateral on each occurrence, but either eye may be affected. True papilledema with equivocal disc swelling from generalized increased ICP is not associated with visual loss until the disc swelling has become chronic and atrophy begins. Visual loss can occur in association with papilledema secondary to compression of optic nerve or chiasma by intracranial tumors (e.g., craniopharyngioma, pituitary adenoma)

e) Psychogenic

Biousse V, Trobe JD. Transient monocular visual loss. Am J Ophthalmol 2005;140(4):717–721

Krieglstein GK, Weinreb RN. Pediatric Ophthalmology, Neuro-ophthalmology, Genetics. Lorenz R-Borruat FX, eds. Springer Verlag; 2008

Balmitgere T, Vighetto A. [Transient binocular visual loss: a diagnostic approach] J Fr Ophtalmol 2009;32(10): 770–774

Cohen AB, Ploss ML. Neuro-ophthalmology: Disorders of the afferent visual pathway. In Hospital Physician Board Review Manual 2007;1–16

5.14 Swollen Optic Discs (Papilledema)

The term papilledema is usually reserved for bilateral swelling of the optic disc associated with increased ICP. All other types should be described as a *swollen disc* or *disc swelling* and the majority are unilateral.

True papilledema with raised ICP is not associated with visual loss unless the disc swelling becomes chronic and atrophy sets in. Papilledema must also be distinguished from pseudopapilledema, such as optic disc drusen.

1. Pseudopapilledema
    a) Congenital disc elevation (▸ Fig. 5.8)
       False impression of papilledema usually caused by hyaline bodies (drusen) within the nerve head. Found in 4% of adults; children before the age of 10 years do not have optic nerve head drusen.
    b) "Small full disc"
       Slightly indistinct disc margins, late-branching central vessels, and no central cup; a true normal variant

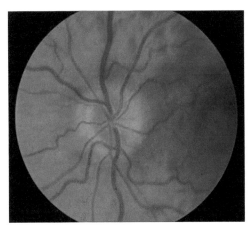

Fig. 5.8 Pseudopapilledema with slightly blurred disk margins but no retinal vessel obscuration or surface capillary dilation. (Reproduced from 21.4 The Optic Disk. In: Gasco J, Nader R, ed. The Essential Neurosurgery Companion. 1st edition. Thieme; 2012.)

2. True papilledema (almost always bilateral; ▸ Fig. 5.9)
   a) Increased ICP
      i. Intracranial mass lesion (e.g., tumor, abscess, hematoma)
      ii. Diffuse brain swelling (e.g., posttraumatic, infectious)
      iii. Acute obstructive hydrocephalus
      iv. Pseudotumor cerebri
   b) Perineuritis or neuritis or neuroretinitis
      i. Syphilitic
      ii. Sarcoid
      iii. Viral meningoencephalitis
      iv. Lyme disease
3. Unilateral disc swelling
   a) Without visual loss
      i. The big blind spot syndrome (? a viral optic meningitis)
      ii. Juvenile diabetes
   b) Associated with visual loss
      i. Papillitis (papilledema, central scotoma, profound decrease in color vision, afferent pupillary defect, and pain on movement)
      ii. AION (sudden decrease in visual acuity, optic nerve head swelling, afferent pupillary reflex, decrease in color vision, and altitudinal field defect)
      iii. Foster–Kennedy syndrome (optic atrophy in one eye and a swollen disc in the other associated with anosmia)
      iv. Pseudo-Foster–Kennedy syndrome (more common and refers to a swollen disc from an acute AION and atrophy of the other eye from a previous AION. May occur due to cocaine abuse or orbital groove meningiomas.
      v. Other ischemic optic neuropathies
         – Infectious and inflammatory diseases (e.g., sarcoidosis, syphilis, Lyme disease, cytomegalic, Epstein–Barr and herpes virus infections give rise to an ischemic appearance)
         – Systemic arteritis (e.g., SLE)
         – Invasion of the optic nerve head by tumor: (1) *Primary*, such as hemangioma, hemangioblastoma, melanocytomas); (2) *Metastatic*, such as leukemia, reticulum cell sarcoma, and meningeal carcinomatosis, breast Ca, lung Ca)
         – Tumors compressing the optic nerve in the orbit

Van Stavern GP. Optic desc edema. Scand Neurol 2007;2:233–243

Foroozan R, Buono LM, Savino PJ, Sergott RC. Acute demyelinating optic neuritis. Curr Opin Ophthalmol 2002;13(6):375–380

Jung JJ, Baek SH, Kim US. Analysis of the causes of optic disc swelling. Korean J Ophthalmol 2011;25(1):33–36

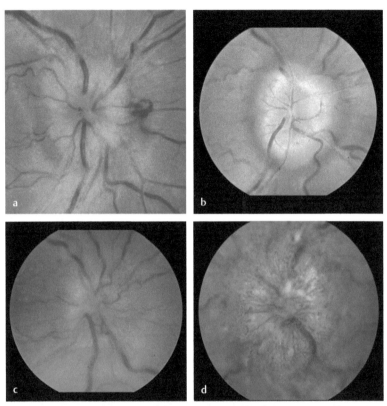

Fig. 5.9 (a) Acute papilledema in a patient with a brain tumor. The optic disc is swollen, with blurred margins and a small hemorrhage at 3 o'clock. (Reproduced from 12.2 Neurologic Disturbances of Vision (Optic Nerve). In: Mattle H, Mumenthaler M, Taub E, ed. Fundamentals of Neurology: An Illustrated Guide. 2nd edition. Thieme; 2017.) **(b)** Grade II papilledema with a 360-degree halo circumferential to blurred disk margins. (Reproduced from 21.4 The Optic Disk. In: Gasco J, Nader R, ed. The Essential Neurosurgery Companion. 1st edition. Thieme; 2012.) **(c)** Grade IV papilledema with obscuration of major vessels on the disk centrally. (Reproduced from 21.4 The Optic Disk. In: Gasco J, Nader R, ed. The Essential Neurosurgery Companion. 1st edition. Thieme; 2012.) **(d)** Grade V papilledema with total obscuration of vessels on the disk. (Reproduced from 21.4 The Optic Disk. In: Gasco J, Nader R, ed. The Essential Neurosurgery Companion. 1st edition. Thieme; 2012.)

5.15 Optic Nerve Enlargement

MRI scanning is able to differentiate most of the vascular lesions and helps to decrease the large number of confusing lesions within the orbit.

1. Tumors
   a) Optic nerve gliomas
      i. Astrocytic tumors of the anterior visual pathway
         They occur predominantly in prepubertal children and one-third of these tumors are associated with neurofibromatosis. Clinically present with unilateral visual loss, proptosis, disc pallor and/or swelling, and strabismus. Half of the childhood gliomas run a stable clinical course, particularly those associated with neurofibromatosis; the other half of the tumors continue to have progressive enlargement. Neuroimaging workup with CT and MRI scanning demonstrates a characteristic fusiform shape of the glioma, optic canal enlargement if the tumor extends out if the orbit, and associated abnormalities of the sphenoid ridge.
      ii. Malignant glioma or glioblastoma
         These are rare and affect the adult; may present as an optic neuritis with unilateral visual loss. The contralateral optic nerve becomes involved rapidly and in few months the disease progresses to total blindness and finally to death within a year.
   b) Meningiomas
      i. Primary meningiomas of the optic nerve sheaths
         Classically occur in middle-aged women with insidious and minor visual loss and with time proptosis. Neuroimaging will usually show a "railroad-track" enlargement of the optic nerve shadow, sometimes associated with calcification on both CT and MRI scanning.
      ii. Meningiomas originating intracranially
         These may involve the optic nerve, either by invasion along its sheaths or by compression. Intracranial meningiomas arise from the sphenoid ridge, the planum sphenoidale, and areas of the tuberculum sella. En plaque meningiomas originate from the outer third of the sphenoid wing, form a thin layer of tumor, spread medially and infiltrate the optic nerve. They produce massive hyperostosis, significant proptosis with chemosis, vascular engorgement, and enlargement of the extraocular muscles.
   c) Other tumors of neurogenic origin
      Example of this is plexiform neuroma causing massive enlargement of nerves within the orbit often coexistent with enlargement of nerves within the cavernous sinus and associated with neurofibromatosis.
   d) Metastases
      Most common of these are:

       i. In children
- Neuroblastoma
- Ewing's sarcoma

      ii. In adults
- Breast cancer in women
- Lung cancer in men
- Prostate cancer in men

  e) Leukemic infiltration

2. Idiopathic inflammatory pseudotumor
An inflammation acting like a tumor and histologically resembling orbital lymphomas.

3. Central retinal vein occlusion

4. Optic neuritis
Inflammation of the optic nerve causing an acute or subacute decrease in central vision; the latter ranging from 20/15 to no light perception over hours to days, contrast sensitivity in 98% and photopsia in 30%, diminution of color vision, pain during eye movement, and an afferent pupillary defect. Excellent prognosis for visual recovery over months.

  a) Idiopathic

  b) Demyelination
It is the most common cause of optic neuritis.

      i. MS
It is the most frequent cause of demyelination, and the first symptom of optic neuritis is observed in 20–75% of MS patients.

      ii. Devic's disease

      iii. Adrenoleukodystrophy (Schilder's disease)

  c) Viral (e.g., measles, mumps, rubella, polio, coxsackie, viral encephalitis, herpes zoster, infectious mononucleosis)

  d) Special infections (e.g., toxoplasmosis, cryptococcus, histoplasmosis, Lyme disease, syphilis, tuberculosis)

  e) Inflammatory (e.g., sarcoidosis may involve chiasmal, sellar/parasellar structures and is usually associated with meningeal thickening on contrast-enhanced CT or MRI scanning)

  f) Associated with systemic disease (e.g., Crohn's disease, ulcerative colitis, Whipple's disease, Reiter's syndrome, autoimmune disorders)

Turbin RE, Pokorny K. Diagnosis and treatment of orbital optic nerve sheath meningioma. Cancer Control 2004;11(5):334–341

Uccello G, Fedriga P, Tranfa F, et al. CT scan in the differential diagnosis of thickened optic nerve. Orbit 1986;5(4):255–258

Purvin V, Kawasaki A, Jacobson DM. Optic perineuritis: clinical and radiographic features. Arch Ophthalmol 2001;119(9):1299–1306

6 Intracranial Tumors

Brain tumors may originate from neural elements within the brain or they may represent spread of distant cancers. Gliomas, metastases, meningiomas, pituitary adenomas, and acoustic neuromas account for 95% of all brain tumors.

Presenting symptoms and signs of patients with an intracranial neoplasm tend to be similar for primary brain tumors and intracranial metastases. The onset of symptoms usually is insidious, but an acute episode may occur with bleeding into the tumor or when an intraventricular tumor suddenly occludes the third ventricle.

Manifestations may be nonspecific and include the following:
- Headache
- Altered mental status
- Ataxia
- Nausea/vomiting
- Weakness
- Gait disturbances

Headache characteristics of brain tumors:
- Usually nonspecific resembling tension-type headaches.
- Not an isolated finding, often is a late complaint.
- New onset headaches in middle-aged or older patients is worrisome.
- The location of headache reliably indicates the side of the head affected, but it does not indicate the precise site of the tumor.
- Headaches are more common with posterior fossa tumors.
- Headache is a more frequent symptom of intracranial tumor in children.

Prevailing inaccurate portrayals of a tumor headache include:
- Pain is worse in the early morning accompanied by vomiting (with or without nausea).
- Exacerbation with Valsalva maneuver, bending over, or rising from a recumbent position.

Brain tumors may also manifest as follows:
- Focal seizures
- Fixed visual changes
- Speech deficits
- Focal sensory abnormalities

More than one-third of patients with newly diagnosed brain tumors develop epileptic seizures. If the tumor involves the cerebral hemispheres, seizures occur in at least 50% of patients. Any brain tumor, benign or malignant, common or uncommon, can cause seizures. Patients with low-grade tumors may be more likely to develop epilepsy, possibly because their longer survival allows more time for seizures to develop.

The tumors that are highly associated with the development of epilepsy are:
- Melanoma
- Hemorrhagic lesions
- Multiple metastases
- Slowly growing primary tumors
- Tumors near the Rolandic fissure

The tumors most often presenting with seizures in adults are:
- Dysembryoplastic neuroepithelial tumors (DNETs)
- Gangliogliomas
- Glioblastoma multiforme (GBM)
- Low-grade astrocytomas
- Meningiomas
- Metastatic tumors
- Oligodendrogliomas

The tumors most often presenting with seizures in children are:
- Ganglioglioma
- Low-grade astrocytomas
- DNETs
- Oligodendrogliomas

No physical finding or pattern of findings unmistakably identifies a patient with a central nervous system (CNS) neoplasm. Based on their location, intracranial tumors may produce a focal or generalized deficit, but signs may be lacking (e.g., frontal lobe tumors) or even falsely localizing.
The findings may include:
- Papilledema, which is more prevalent with paediatric brain tumors, reflects an increase in intracranial pressure (ICP) for several days or longer.
- Diplopia may result from displacement or compression of the sixth cranial nerve at the base of the brain.
- Impaired upward gaze, called Parinaud's syndrome, may occur with pineal tumors.
- Tumors of the occipital lobe specifically may produce homonymous hemi-anopia or partial visual field deficits.
- Anosmia may occur in case of frontal lobe tumors.
- Brain stem and cerebellar tumors induce cranial nerve palsies, ataxia, incoordination, nystagmus, pyramidal signs, and sensory deficits on one or both sides of the body.

CT and MRI have complementary roles in the diagnosis of CNS neoplasms. The speed of CT is desirable for evaluating clinically unstable patients; it is superior for detecting calcification, skull lesions, and hyperacute hemorrhage (bleeding less than 24 hours old) and helps direct differential diagnosis as well as immediate management. MRI has superior soft-tissue resolution; it can better detect isodense lesions, tumor enhancement, and associated findings such as edema, all phases of hemorrhagic states (except hyperacute), and infarction. High-quality MRI is the diagnostic study of choice in the single-photon emission computed tomography (SPECT) and positron emission tomography (PET) may be useful in differentiating tumor recurrence from radiation necrosis.

Purdy RA, Kirby S. Headaches and brain tumors. Neurol Clin 2004; 22(1):39–53
DeAngelis LM. Brain tumors. N Engl J Med 2001; 344(2):114–123

World Health Organization (WHO) brain tumor grades

Grade	Characteristics	Tumor types
Low grade	WHO grade I	Least malignant (benign)
		Possibly curable via surgery alone
		Noninfiltrative
		Long-term survival
		Slow growing
		E.g., pilocytic astrocytoma, craniopharyngioma, gangliocytoma, ganglioglioma
	WHO grade II	Relatively slow growing
		Somewhat infiltrative
		May recur as higher grade
		E.g., "diffuse" astrocytoma, pineocytoma, pure oligodendroglioma
High grade	WHO grade III	Malignant
		Infiltrative
		Tend to recur as high grade
		E.g., anaplastic astrocytoma, anaplastic ependymoma, anaplastic oligodendroglioma
	WHO grade IV	Most malignant
		Rapidly growing, aggressive
		Widely infiltrative
		Rapid recurrence
		Prone to necrosis
		E.g., glioblastoma multiforme, pineoblastoma, medulloblastoma, ependymoblastoma

Source: Kleihues P, Burger PC, Scheithauer BW. The new WHO classification of brain tumours. Brain Pathol 1993;3(3):255–268

6.1 Intracranial Tumors Based on Their Anatomic Location

6.1.1 Cerebral hemisphere tumors

Adults:
1. Astrocytoma
   a) Anaplastic astrocytoma (10–30% of gliomas)
   b) GBM (45–50% of gliomas)
2. Meningioma
3. Metastases
4. Pituitary adenoma
5. Oligodendroglioma
6. Primary CNS lymphoma
7. Ependymoma
8. Ganglioglioma
9. Sarcoma

Young adults and children:
1. Glioblastoma
2. Ganglioglioma
3. Gangliosarcoma
4. Malignant astrocytoma
5. Meningioma
6. Meningiosarcoma
7. Oligodendroglioma
8. Juvenile pilocytic astrocytoma
9. Solitary metastasis
10. Pleomorphic xanthoastrocytoma
11. Fibrous histiocytoma
12. Fibrous xanthomas

Infants:
1. Primitive neuroectodermal tumor (PNET)
2. Supratentorial ependymomas
3. Astrocytoma
4. Desmoplastic infantile gangliogliomas
5. Dysembryoplastic neuroepithelial tumors

6.1.2 Intraventricular tumors

1. Lateral ventricles (LVs) (favored sites)
   a) Astrocytoma (anaplastic, glioblastoma)
   b) Subependymal giant cell astrocytoma (Foramen of Monro)
   c) Ependymoma (fourth ventricle)
   d) Subependymoma (fourth ventricle)
   e) Oligodendroglioma (neurocytoma) (septum pellucidum, LV)
   f) Choroid plexus cysts/xanthogranulomas (atrium of LV)
   g) Meningioma (atrium of LV)
   h) Metastases (all sites)
   i) Choroid plexus papilloma/carcinoma (atrium of LV)
   j) Epidermoid/dermoid
   k) Primary cerebral neuroblastoma
   l) Hamartomas (ependyma of LV)
   m) Cerebral hemangiomas (all sites)
   n) Spongioblastomas
   o) Neurinomas
   p) Cysticercosis (all sites)
   q) Ependymal cyst
   r) Choroidal xanthomas (Foramen of Monro)
2. Third ventricle
   a) Colloid cyst
   b) Pilocytic astrocytoma/Astrocytoma
   c) Oligodendroglioma
   d) Ependymoma
   e) Metastases
   f) Lymphoma
   g) Sarcoid
   h) Cysts (Glioependymal, choroid, or inflammatory)
   i) Extrinsic mass
      i. Pituitary adenoma
      ii. Vein of Galen AVM
      iii. Astrocytoma or other neoplasm arising from hypothalamus, quad-rigeminal body.
      iv. Pinealoma, teratoma
3. Fourth ventricle/aqueduct
   Adults:
   a) Metastases
   b) Hemangioblastoma
   c) Brain stem glioma
   d) Choroid plexus papilloma

e) Subependymoma
f) Dermoid/Epidermoid
g) Non-neoplastic masses (Inflammatory cysts, vascular malformations, cysticercosis)

Children:
a) Medulloblastoma
b) Astrocytoma
c) Ependymoma
d) Choroid plexus papilloma
e) Brain stem glioma
f) Dermoid cyst
g) Meningioma

Brenner AV, Linet MS, Fine HA, et al. History of allergies and autoimmune diseases and risk of brain tumors in adults. Int J Cancer 2002; 99(2):252–259

Chandana SR, Movva S, Arora M, et al. Primary brain tumors in adults. Am Fam Physician 2008; 77(10):1423–1430

Perkins A, Liu G. Primary brain tumors in adults: diagnosis and treatment. Am Fam Physician 2016; 93(3):211–217

Arora RS, Alston RD, Eden TOB, Estlin EJ, Moran A, Birch JM. Age-incidence patterns of primary CNS tumors in children, adolescents, and adults in England. Neuro-oncol 2009; 11(4):403–413

Morales H, Gaskill-Shipley M. Imaging of common adult and pediatric primary brain tumors. Semin Roentgenol 2010; 45(2):92–106.– Elsevier

al-Mefty O, Kersh JE, Routh A, Smith RR. The long-term side effects of radiation therapy for benign brain tumors in adults. J Neurosurg 1990; 73(4):502–512

Al-Okaili R, Krejza J, Wang S, et al. Advanced MR imaging techniques in the diagnosis of Intraaxial brain tumors in adults. Radio Graphics 2006; 26(Suppl 1)

6.2 Pineal Tumors

Pineal region tumors make up 0.4–1.0% of intracranial tumors in adults and 3.0–8.0% of brain tumors in children. Most children are aged 10–20 years at presentation, with the average age at presentation being 13 years. Adults typically are older than 30 years at presentation (▶ Fig. 6.1).

Most tumors are a result of displaced embryonic tissue, malignant transformation of pineal parenchymal cells, or transformation of surrounding astroglia. A complete differential diagnosis for masses in the pineal region should also include vascular anomalies, as well as metastatic tumor.

Mass lesions in the pineal region commonly present with headaches, nausea, and vomiting caused by aqueductal compression and resultant obstructive hydrocephalus, which if left untreated may lead progressively to lethargy, obtundation, and death. Compromise of the superior colliculus results in a syndrome of vertical gaze palsy (Parinaud's syndrome) that can be associated with pupillary or oculomotor nerve paresis. Further compression of the periaqueductal gray region may

233

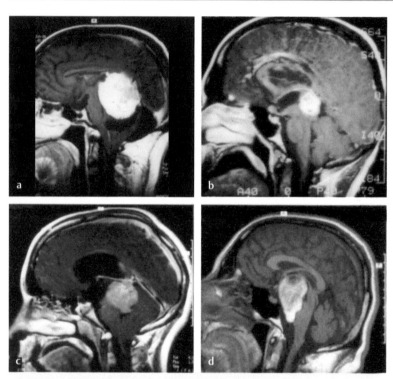

Fig. 6.1 Pineal lesions **(a)** Germinoma. Sagittal T1-WI with a large, solid space-occupying lesion originating from the pineal gland and a high postcontrast signal intensity causing compression of the brain stem and cerebellum with distortion of the fourth ventricle. There is also descent of the cerebellar tonsils. **(b)** Astrocytoma and suprasellar metastasis. Sagittal T1-WI shows a post-contrast enhancing mass in the pineal region producing compression of the quadrigeminal plate. A second suprasellar mass compresses the pituitary stalk. The patient presented clinical signs of diabetes insipidus. **(c)** Medulloblastoma. Sagittal T1-WI with a solid, multilobular space-occupying lesion, which presents an intermediate, heterogenous postcontrast enhancement and is housed in the upper region of the cerebellum and fourth ventricle. **(d)** Basilar aneurysm. Sagittal T1-WI demonstrates a partially thrombosed giant aneurysm of the basilar artery, which acts as a space-occupying mass and thus compresses the pons, the cerebral peduncles, and the third ventricle, extending retrochiasmatically into the suprasellar cisterns.

cause mydriasis, convergence spasm, pupillary inequality, and convergence of refractory nystagmus. Children may also present with endocrine malfunction (diabetes insipidus, pseudoprecocious puberty—93% of girls > 12 years had secondary amenorrhea and 33% of patients < 15 years had growth arrest).

1. Germ-cell tumors
   a) Pure germinoma
      The most common variant of germ neoplasm in this area, accounting for 50% of pineal neoplasms.
   b) Embryonal cell carcinoma
   c) Choriocarcinoma
   d) Teratoma
   e) Mixed germ-cell tumor
   f) Yolk sac tumor (endodermal sinus)
2. Pineal parenchymal (cell origin) tumors
   a) Pineoblastoma
   b) Pineocytoma
3. Tumors of supportive tissues and adjacent structures
   a) Astrocytomas
   b) Ependymomas
   c) Meningiomas
   d) Hemangiopericytomas
   e) Ganglioneuroma
   f) Ganglioglioma
   g) Chemodectomas
   h) Craniopharyngiomas
   i) Lipoma (quadrigeminal cistern)
4. Metastatic tumors of the pineal gland (extremely rare; 75 total reported cases)
   a) Lung
   b) Breast
   c) Stomach
   d) Kidney
5. Non-neoplastic tumor-like conditions
   a) Pineal cysts (degenerative cysts lined by fibrillary astrocytes)
   b) Arachnoid cysts
   c) Cysticercus cysts
   d) Vascular lesions (aneurysmal dilatation of the vein of Galen, vertebrobasilar dolichoectasia, basilar tip aneurysm)

Cho BK, Wang KC, Nam DH, et al. Pineal tumors: experience with 48 cases over 10 years. Childs Nerv Syst 1998; 14(1–2):53–58

Smith AB, Rushing EJ, Smirniotopoulos JG. From the archives of the AFIP: lesions of the pineal region: radiologic-pathologic correlation. Radiographics 2010; 30(7):2001–2020

Villano JL, Propp JM, Porter KR, et al. Malignant pineal germ-cell tumors: an analysis of cases from three tumor registries. Neuro Oncol 2008; 10(2):121–130

Chang T, Teng MM, Guo WY, Sheng WC. CT of pineal tumors and intracranial germ-cell tumors. Am J Neuroradiol 1989; 10(5):1039–1044

6.3 Cerebellopontine Angle Masses

Tumors of the cerebellopontine angle (CPA) constitute about 6–10% of all intracranial tumors. It is a disease common in adults and rare in children. There is a wide variety of conditions that can occur at this level, derived from both the structures forming the CPA, as well as lesions that grow near it and can secondarily invade this area of CPA (▶ Fig. 6.2 and ▶ Fig. 6.3).

The masses are the most commonly vestibular-cochlear schwannomas and meningiomas, representing approximately 85–90% of all tumors of the anterior pontine cistern (APC). Next in frequency are epidermoid cyst and schwannomas of other cranial nerves.

Masses of the CPA with their frequency are discussed below.

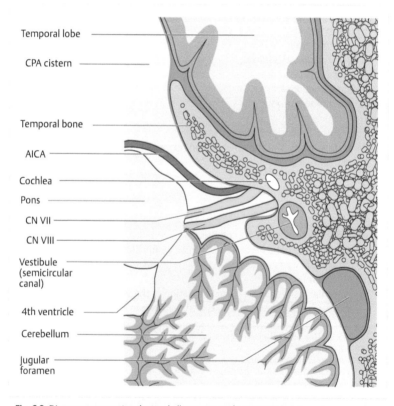

Temporal lobe

CPA cistern

Temporal bone

AICA

Cochlea

Pons

CN VII

CN VIII

Vestibule
(semicircular
canal)

4th ventricle

Cerebellum

Jugular
foramen

Fig. 6.2 Diagram representing the cerebellopontine angle anatomy.

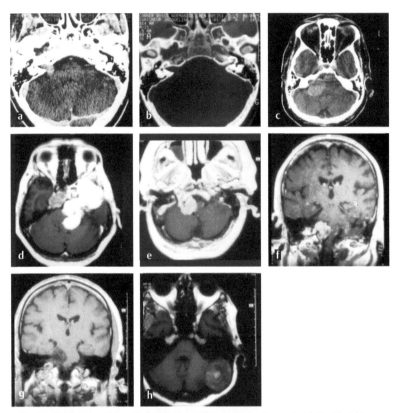

Fig. 6.3 Cerebellopontine angle (CPA) lesions. **(a)** Acoustic neurinoma. Axial CT with right acoustic neurinoma and erosion of the internal auditory meatus with a small protrusion of the tumor in the CPA. **(b)** Erosion of the auditory meatus. Bone windows of an axial CT of the same patient with an abnormal erosion of the right internal auditory meatus. **(c)** Acoustic neurinoma. A solid space-occupying mass with mild postcontrast enhancement producing erosion of the right acoustic meatus, protrusion into the right CPA, and compression of the pons and cerebellar peduncles. **(d)** Chordoma. Axial T1-WI shows a solid, space-occupying lesion with postcontrast enhancement occupying the left middle temporal fossa and ipsilateral CPA as well as erosion of the apex of the petrous and sphenoid bone. **(e, f)** Meningioma. Axial and coronal T1-WI with a postcontrast enhancing meningioma of the right CPA that extends into the right jugular foramen causing compression of the medulla oblongata and the right cerebellar hemisphere. **(g)** Epidermoid tumor. Coronal T1-WI with a cystic space-occupying, nonenhancing lesion in the right CPA with compression signs of the pons. **(h)** Epidermoid tumor. A solid and heterogeneous mass with smooth margins eroding the left occipital bone and compressing the left cerebellar hemisphere is seen on axial T1-WI.

6.3.1 Adult

1. Acoustic schwannoma
   Most common mass that comprises 60–92% of CPA lesions and involves the vestibular division of the CN VIII.
2. Meningioma
   Second most common lesion seen in up to 3–7% of cases. Usually arises from posterior surface of the petrous bone and does not extend into IAC. Broad-based against petrous bone.
3. Ectodermal inclusion tumors
   a) Epidermoid
      Also known as congenital cholesteatoma or pearly tumor; accounts for 2–6% of CPA masses. Congenital lesions of rest of ectodermal tissue containing stratified squamous linings and keratin. May arise within the temporal bone or in the CPA. Low attenuation (CT); lobulated mass (MRI) of signal similar to cerebrospinal fluid (CSF) on most sequences but increased signal on fluid-attenuated inversion recovery (FLAIR) and diffusion-weighted imaging (DWI). Grows surrounding vessels and nerves.
   b) Dermoid
4. Metastases
5. Paragangliomas (2–10%)
   Also known as glomus jugulare tumor; a chemodectoma arising from the jugular foramen (JF) and extending into the CPA.
   a) Glomus jugulare
   b) Glomus tympanicum
6. Other schwannomas (2–5%)
   Trigeminal and facial nerves are probably the most common sites of nonacoustic schwannomas. Other cranial nerves involved are CNs VI, IX, X, XI, and rarely XII.
7. Vascular (2–5%)
   a) Vertebrobasilar dolichoectasia (3–5%)
      Elongation and dilatation of the vertebrobasilar artery. Symptoms are fascial spasms, trigeminal neuralgia etc.
   b) Giant aneurysm (1–2%)
   c) Vascular malformation (1%)
   d) Anterior inferior cerebellar artery (AICA) loop: May loop over, under, or between CNs VII and VIII. Main symptom is vertigo.
8. Choroid plexus papilloma (1%; primary in the CPA or extension via the lateral foramina of Luschka)
9. Ependymoma (1%; extension from the fourth ventricle)

10. Skull base/temporal bone tumors (e.g., glomus tumors, metastases, cholesterol granuloma)
11. Skull base infection (e.g., osteomyelitis of the petrous apex = Gradenigo's syndrome, malignant otitis external)
12. Uncommon lesions (< 1% incidence)
    a) Arachnoid cyst
    b) Lipoma
    c) Exophytic brain stem or cerebellar astrocytoma
    d) Chordoma
    e) Osteocartilagenous tumors
    f) Cysticercosis
    g) Ganglioglioma
    h) DNET
    i) Hemangioblastoma
    j) Medulloblastoma
    k) Neurosarcoidosis
    l) Primary melanocytic neoplasm
    m) Brainstem glioma
    n) Lymphoma

6.3.2 Paediatric

1. Cerebellum/fourth ventricle
   a) Medulloblastoma
      Midline, vermian or roof; usually hyperdense on plain CT, often enhance homogeneously
   b) Pilocytic astrocytoma
      Usually two-third are cystic with mural nodule, cyst fluid denser than CSF due to protein
   c) Ependymoma (intraventricular, "cast" of lumen, 50% are calcified)
2. Brain stem
   a) Brainstem glioma
      Expands brain stem (infiltration without destruction), hydrocephalus (may be late)
3. Extra-axial fluid collection
   a) Large cisterna magna ("mega cisterna magna")
   b) Epidermoid inclusion cyst
   c) Arachnoid cyst (may bevel inner table of skull)
   d) Dandy–Walker cyst of fourth ventricle
   e) Vermian agenesis
   f) Chronic subdural hematoma

6.3.3 Differential diagnosis based on the MRI characteristics

1. Enhancing mass
   a) Acoustic schwannoma
   b) Meningioma
   c) Trigeminal schwannoma
   d) Facial nerve schwannoma
   e) Ependymoma
   f) Metastasis (e.g., breast, lung malignant melanoma)
2. High T1 signal mass
   a) Hemorrhagic acoustic schwannoma
   b) Neurenteric cyst (usually prepontine, but fluid may be proteinaceous and high on T1-WI)
   c) Thrombosed berry aneurysm (often will have calcified rim, and hemosiderin staining)
   d) White epidermoid (rare, and will restrict on DWI)
   e) CPA lipoma (usually has the facial nerve and vestibulocochlear nerve coursing through it; will saturate on fat suppressed sequences)
   f) Ruptured intracranial dermoid (often multiple droplets, and original midline lesion can be often seen)
3. Low T1 signal mass (CSF density mass)
   a) Epidermoid cyst (approx. 5% of CPA masses; third most common)
   b) Arachnoid cyst
   c) Neurocysticercosis

Smirniotopoulos JG, Yue NC, Rushing EJ. Cerebellopontine angle masses: radiologic-pathologic correlation. Radiographics 1993; 13(5):1131–1147

Bonneville F, Savatovsky J, Chiras J. Imaging of cerebellopontine angle lesions: an update. Part 1: enhancing extra-axial lesions. Eur Radiol 2007; 17(10):2472–2482

Holman MA, Schmitt WR, Carlson ML, Driscoll CL, Beatty CW, Link MJ. Pediatric cerebellopontine angle and internal auditory canal tumors: clinical article. J Neurosurg Pediatr 2013; 12(4):317–324

Press GA, Hesselink JR. MR imaging of cerebellopontine angle and internal auditory canal lesions at 1.5T. AJNR 1988; 150:1:371–1381

6.4 Internal Auditory Meatus Masses

1. Neoplastic masses
   a) Intracanalicular acoustic schwannoma
   b) Facial schwannoma
   c) Meningioma
   d) Metastases

  e) Lipoma
  f) Hemangioma
  g) Lymphoma
 2. Non-neoplastic masses
  a) Neuritis (Bell's palsy, Ramsay Hunt syndrome or herpes zoster otitis, and viral infections are benign conditions that can cause cranial nerve enlargement)
  b) Postoperative reactive dural fibrosis (second most common cause of enlargement of the internal auditory meatus)
  c) Meningitis
  d) Sarcoidosis
  e) Vascular (hemorrhage, vascular loop of AICA, arteriovenous malformations (AVM) or aneurysm)
  f) Langerhans' cell histiocytosis

Gupta S, Mends F, Hagiwara M, Fatterpekar G, Roehm PC. Imaging the facial nerve: a contemporary review. Radiol Res Pract 2013; 2013:248039

Swartz JD. Lesions of the cerebellopontine angle and internal auditory canal: diagnosis & differential diagnosis. U CT MRI 2004; 25(4):332–352

Fukui MB, Weissman JL, Curtin HD, Kanal E. T2-weighted MR characteristics of internal auditory canal masses. AJNR Am J Neuroradiol 1996; 17(7):1211–1218

Bohner PS, Chole RA. Unusual lesion of the internal auditory canal. Am J Otol 1996; 17(1):140–186

6.5 Foramen Magnum Masses

In cases of benign extramedullary tumors of the foramen magnum (e.g., commonly meningiomas, neurofibromas, and the less common teratomas, chordomas etc.), the most frequent presenting complaints were suboccipital neck pain, dysesthesias, gait disturbances, weakness, and hand clumsiness. The average time from initial symptoms to diagnosis was 2¼ years. The most common findings included hyperreflexia, arm or hand weakness, Babinski sign, spastic gait, sensory loss, and CN XI involvement. There is no clinical finding that is pathognomonic (▶ Fig. 6.4 and ▶ Fig. 6.5).

 1. Intra-axial cervicomedullary masses
  a) Non-neoplastic
   i. Syringomyelia (in 25% of Chiari I patients; secondary syrinxes due to trauma can be seen)
   ii. Demyelinating diseases
    – Multiple sclerosis
    – Acute transverse myelopathy
    – Miscellaneous (e.g., radiation, AIDS, vascular AVM)

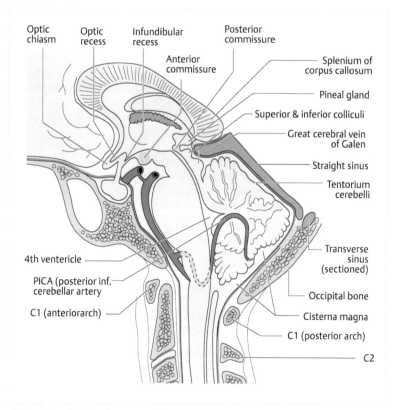

Fig. 6.4 Intracranial tumors. Midsagittal anatomic diagram of the pineal and foramen magnum regions.

b) Neoplastic
  i. Gliomas
     – Astrocytomas
       Commonly of low grade and 50% of them occur in the cervicomedullary junction. Extension of spinal cord glioma in this area is also common. Other types of gliomas, however, such as anaplastic astrocytoma, ganglioglioma, ependymoma are also found here.
  ii. Nonglial neoplasms
      Inferior extension of medulloblastoma in children and hemangioblastoma in adults are common in this area.
  iii. Metastases (rare)

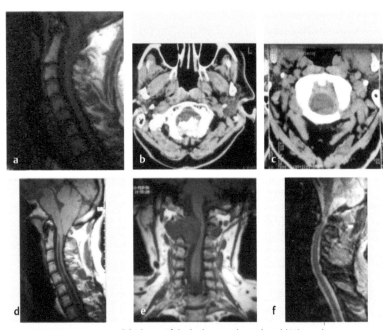

Fig. 6.5 Foramen magnum **(a)** Glioma of the high cervical spinal cord (C2), producing a focal expansion of the spinal cord, is seen on this midsagittal T1-WI. **(b)** Meningioma. Axial CT demonstrates a calcified meningioma of the posterior part of the foramen magnum compressing the medulla oblongata. **(c)** Epidermoid cyst. Axial CT with a cystic lesion of the foramen magnum causing compression of the medulla oblongata. **(d)** Chiari II malformation. Sagittal T1-WI shows a descent of the cerebellar tonsils and compression of the medulla oblongata and associated syringomyelia. **(e)** Osteolysis of C2 and a mass of soft tissues producing compression and displacement of the spinal cord is seen on coronal T1-WI. **(f)** Atlantoaxial subluxation. Sagittal T2-WI shows atlantoaxial subluxation with the development of inflammatory tissue around the dens of C2. This pathology causes stenosis of the foramen magnum and compression of the spinal cord and lower medulla. Focal myelinolysis is indicated by a high-intensity signal.

2. Anterior extramedullary intradural masses
   a) Ectatic vessel/aneurysm
      Most common mass anterior to the medulla is a tortuous, ectatic vertebral artery. Occasionally, aneurysms of the vertebral or the PICA are seen.
   b) Meningioma
      Most common primary neoplasm in this area.

    c) Schwannoma
       From CNs IX and XI. Neurofibromas from existing spinal nerve segments occur laterally.
    d) Epidermoid tumors
    e) Metastases (cisternal, perineural, and skull base)
    f) Paragangliomas
    g) Arachnoid, inflammatory, and neurenteric cysts
    h) Chordomas, rheumatoid nodules (extraosseous intradural)

3. Posterior extramedullary intradural masses
    a) Congenital/acquired tonsillar herniation (comprises 5–10% of all foramen magnum masses)
    b) Ependymoma and medulloblastoma (intra-axial caudal extension of posterior fossa neoplastic masses)

4. Extradural masses
    a) Trauma (odontoid fractures)
    b) Arthropathies
       i. Rheumatoid arthritis
          Affects 80% of cervical spine of the patients causing severe cord compression.
       ii. Osteoarthritis
       iii. Paget's disease
       iv. Osteomyelitis
    c) Congenital anomalies
       i. Os odontoideum
       ii. Vertebralization of occipital condyles
       iii. Odontoid hypoplasia
       iv. Arch hypoplasia or aplasia
    d) Neoplasms
       i. Primary
          – Chordoma
          – Osteocartilagenous tumors (chondroma and chondrosarcoma)
       ii. Metastases
          Hematogenous or local extensions from nasopharyngeal or skull base tumors.

Meyer FB, Ebersold MJ, Reese DF. Benign tumors of the foramen magnum. J Neurosurg 1984; 61(1):136–142

Benzel EC. Spine surgery. 3nd ed. Vol 1. Saunders-Elsevier; 2012

Bradley WG, Daroff RB, Fenichel CM, Jankovic J. Neurology in clinical practice. 4th ed. Butterworth-Heinemann; 2004

Epelman M, Daneman A, Blaser SI, et al. Differential diagnosis of intracranial cystic lesions at head US: correlation with CT and MR imaging. Radiographics 2006; 26(1):173–196

Davies ST. In Chapman & Nakielny's Aids to Radiological Differential Diagnosis. 6th ed. Sanders-Elsevier; 2014

6.6 Skull Base Tumors

Skull base tumors arise from the cranial base or reach it either from an intracranial or extracranial origin. These may originate from the neurovascular structures of the base of the brain and the basal meninges (e.g., meningioma, pituitary adenoma, schwannoma, paraganglioma, hemangiopericytoma), the cranial base itself (e.g., chordoma, chondrosarcoma, osteosarcoma, plasmacytoma, metastasis), or the subcranial structures of the head and neck (e.g., sinonasal carcinomas, olfactory neuroblastoma, juvenile angiofibroma, nasopharyngeal carcinoma, adenoid cystic carcinoma, primary sarcomas) (▶ Fig. 6.6 and ▶ Fig. 6.7).

1. Anterior skull base (orbital plates, frontal bones, cribriform plate, planum sphenoidale)
   a) Extracranial lesions
      i. Nasal/paranasal sinus malignant tumors
         Occur in up to 30% of anterior skull base cases

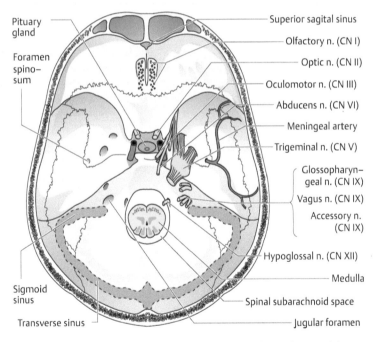

Fig. 6.6 Intracranial tumors. Anatomic drawing depicting the endocranial aspect of the skull base.

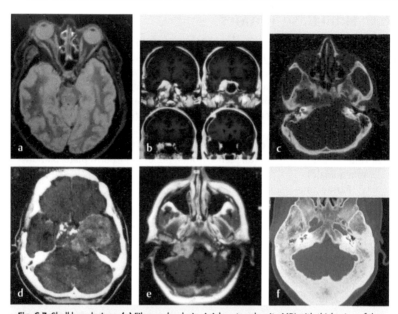

Fig. 6.7 Skull base lesions. **(a)** Fibrous dysplasia. Axial proton density MRI with thickening of the right sphenoid bone and reduction of the size of the orbit and associated exophthalmos. **(b)** Meningioma of the right cavernous sinus. Coronal T1-WI shows expansion of the right cavernous sinus and a very high signal intensity following contrast enhancement. **(c)** Metastasis. Axial CT demonstrating an osteolytic lesion of the sphenoid tip of the petrous bone. **(d)** Chordoma. Axial CT with a high-density space-occupying lesion of the left temporal fossa and the parasellar region. The mass is eroding the apex of the petrous bone and is extending to the cerebellopontine angle (CPA) of the same side. **(e)** Paraganglioma or glomus jugulare. Axial CT shows a space-occupying lesion of the right CPA that occupies the right jugular foramen and demonstrates intense, heterogeneous postcontrast enhancement. **(f)** Paget's disease. Axial CT shows a marked thickening of all bones of the skull base with reduction of the size of the posterior fossa.

- Carcinomas
  Comprise 98% of adult nasopharyngeal tumors.
  - Squamous-cell carcinomas (80%)
  - Adenocarcinomas (18%)
- Rhabdomyosarcoma
  The most common soft-tissue sarcoma in children; up to 35% of these lesions occur here.
- Esthesioneuroblastoma or olfactory neuroblastoma
  Arise from the bipolar sensory cells and are histologically similar to adrenal or sympathetic ganglionic neuroblastomas or retinoblastomas.

       ii. Bacterial or fungal sinusitis

      iii. Sarcoidosis

      iv. Lymphoma

       v. Granulomatoses
- Abuse of cocaine
- Wegener's granulomatosis

b) Intrinsic lesions

       i. Fibrous dysplasia

      ii. Paget's disease

      iii. Osteopetrosis

c) Intracranial lesions

       i. Meningioma

Planum sphenoidale and olfactory groove meningiomas account for 10–15% of all meningiomas.

      ii. Nasoethmoidal encephalocele

Most common anterior skull base lesion that originates from the brain; 15% of basal cephaloceles occur here.

      iii. Dermoid sinuses

      iv. Cerebral heterotopias

       v. Primary brain neoplasms

Rare lesions that may cause dural invasion or calvarial destruction.
- Ganglioglioma
- Anaplastic glioma or GBM

2. Central skull base lesions (upper clivus, sella turcica, cavernous sinuses, sphenoid alae)

a) Metastases

Arise from regional extension of head and neck malignancies or hematogenous spread from extracranial sites, such as prostate, lung, and breast carcinomas.

b) Infection and inflammatory disease

       i. Osteomyelitis

Immunocompromised states, diabetes, chronic mastoiditis, paranasal sinus infection, trauma, or necrotizing otitis externa

      ii. Bacterial sinusitis

From ethmoid or sphenoid sinuses, or intracranially via emissary veins and the cavernous sinus, resulting in cerebral infarction, meningitis, subdural empyema and brain abscess

      iii. Fungal sinusitis

Candidiasis, aspergillosis, histoplasmosis, rhinomucormycosis resulting in multiple cranial nerve palsies, internal carotid artery thrombosis, cavernous sinus thrombosis, cerebral infarction, and brain abscess of immunocompromised patients.

iv. Nonfungal granulomas
   - Wegener's granuloma
   - Sarcoidosis
   - Leprosy
   - Syphilis
   - Rhinoscleroma
   - Cocaine abuse granulomatosis
   - Lethal midline granuloma (variant to a T-cell lymphoma)
   - Eosinophilic granuloma

c) Primary benign neoplasms
   i. Pituitary adenoma
      May extend superiorly through the diaphragma sellae and laterally into the cavernous sinus.
   ii. Meningioma
      Located alongside the sphenoid wing, diaphragma sellae, clivus, and cavernous sinus.
   iii. Nerve sheath tumors
      - Plexiform neurofibromas
         Diffusely infiltrating masses originating primarily along the ophthalmic and the maxillary and mandibular divisions of the trigeminal nerve.
      - Schwannomas
         Cause one-third of primary trigeminal nerve and Meckel's cave tumors. Neurinomas of the CNs III, IV, and VI are rare.
   iv. Juvenile angiofibroma
      The most common benign nasopharyngeal tumor; highly vascular.
   v. Chordoma (is usually located in the midline)
   vi. Enchondroma
      Most common benign osteocartilaginous tumor in this area.
   vii. Epidermoid tumors
   viii. Lipomas
   ix. Cavernous hemangiomas

d) Primary malignant neoplasms
   i. Nasopharyngeal carcinoma
   ii. Rhabdomyosarcoma
   iii. Multiple myeloma
      The most common primary bone tumor originating in the central skull base
   iv. Solitary plasmacytoma
   v. Osteosarcoma
      The second most common primary bone tumor after multiple myeloma

vi. Chondrosarcomas

Usually arise off the midline; the differential diagnosis would include a metastasis and a paraganglioma

3. Posterior skull base/clivus (includes the clivus below the spheno-occipital synchondrosis, the petrous temporal bone, the pars lateralis and squamae of the occipital bones, and surrounds the foramen magnum)

a) Lesions in the temporal bone

b) Lesions in the foramen magnum

c) Clival and paraclival lesions

i. Chordoma

Chordomas or chondrosarcomas usually originate from the sacro-coccygeal region, the spheno-occipital region (40%) or the vertebrae. Both these tumors represent 6–7% of all primitive skull base lesions and are very rare representing only 0.2% of all intracranial tumors. Differential diagnosis of intracranial chordomas from other invasive and calcified tumors includes:

– Chromophobe adenoma
– Mucinous adenocarcinoma
– Meningioma
– Craniopharyngioma
– Schwannoma
– Nasopharyngeal carcinoma
– Salivary gland tumors

ii. Chondrosarcomas

iii. Metastasis

– Regional extension (e.g., nasopharyngeal squamous-cell carcinoma)
– Hematogenous extracranial sites (e.g., lung, prostate, breast)

iv. Meningioma

v. Osteomyelitis (including Gradenigo's syndrome)

vi. Multiple myeloma

vii. Plasmacytoma

viii. Histiocytosis

d) Jugular foramen lesions

i. Neoplastic masses

– Paragangliomas

Chemodectomas or glomus tumors; parasympathetic paragan-glia located in the jugular bulb adventitia and in various sites of the head and neck especially the carotid body, glomus jugulare and glomus tympanicum.

– Metastases

Retrograde perineural spread from malignancies of the face and oral cavity may give rise to JF metastases. Lymphoma,

melanoma, and squamous cell carcinoma show this type of tumors extension. The key concept that indicates perineural spread is effacement or obliteration of the normal fat pad that is present at the extracranial opening of JF.
- ○ Regional extension (e.g., nasopharyngeal carcinoma, lymph node metastatic disease)
- ○ Hematogenous extracranial sites (e.g., lung, prostate, breast)
- – Nerve sheath tumors (uncommon location)
  - ○ Schwannomas of CNs IX and XI
  - ○ Neurofibromas
- – Epidermoid tumor
- – Chondroid/chordoma lesions
- – Meningioma

  The pattern of spread allows differentiation between primary meningiomas (centered in the foramen magnum), neural sheath tumors (schwannomas), and paragangliomas within the JF. Paragangliomas typically involve the hypotympanum superolaterally with limited involvement of the carotid space inferiorly, only rarely extend medially into the jugular tubercle, hypoglossal canal, and clivus. Unlike paragangliomas, JF schwannomas follow the course of the CNs IX, X, and XI from the lateral aspect of the brain stem, with variable inferior spread into the nasopharynx and carotid space of the suprahyoid neck.
- – Primitive neuroectodermal tumor (PNET)
  Uncommon intrinsic tumor that usually presents with a progressive bulbar palsy.
- – Trauma and other rare intrinsic lesions
  Skull base fracture with or without a dural tear and CSF leak, localized bone destruction caused by bone diseases such as fibrous dysplasia, Paget's disease, histiocytosis X, and multiple myeloma.
- – Non-neoplastic masses
  - ○ Prominent jugular bulb ("pseudomass"; normal variant)
  - ○ Jugular vein thrombosis
  - ○ Osteomyelitis
4. Diffuse skull base lesions
   a) Neoplastic masses
      i. Metastases
      ii. Multiple myeloma/plasmacytoma
      iii. Meningioma

iv. Lymphoma

Primary or secondary; uncommon but increasing in incidence causing leptomeningeal disease and multiple cranial nerve palsies.

b) Non-neoplastic masses

   i. Fibrous dysplasia

The most common benign skeletal disorder in adolescents and young adults. In the most common monostotic type 25% of skull and facial bones are involved as compared to 40–60% in the polyostotic type causing facial deformities and cranial nerve palsies)

   ii. Paget's disease

   iii. Eosinophilic granuloma

5. Cavernous sinus lesions

a) Unilateral (▶ Fig. 6.8)

   i. Schwannoma (CNs III, IV, V, and VI)

   ii. Meningioma

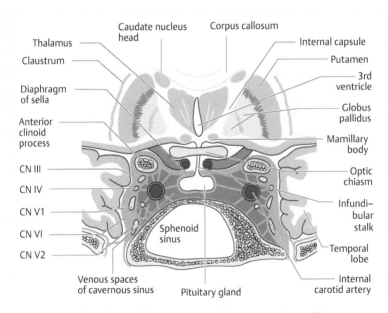

Fig. 6.8 Suprasellar and parasellar lesions. Diagram of the cavernous sinus and its contents; the sellar, suprasellar, and parasellar structures.

They tend to follow the lateral margin of the cavernous sinus and may extend posteriorly along the tentorial margin with a dovetail appearance on MRI. May encase or distort the cavernous portion of the ICA.

iii. Metastasis

Examples are adenoid cystic carcinoma, basal-cell carcinoma, lymphoma, mucoepidermoid carcinoma, melanoma, and schwannoma which demonstrate perineural spread through the basal skull foramen and into the brain.

iv. Vascular lesions (e.g., ectatic carotids, carotico-cavernous fistula, cavernous carotid aneurysm, cavernous hemangioma, and cavernous sinus thrombosis)

v. Chordoma

vi. Lymphoma

vii. Chondrosarcoma

viii. Lipoma

ix. Infection (e.g., actinomycosis, Lyme disease, and herpes zoster can also demonstrate perineural involvement)

x. Idiopathic inflammatory disease

Tolosa–Hunt syndrome: characterized by recurrent attacks of retro-orbital pain, defects of CNs III, IV, Va, and VI, spontaneous remission, and by prompt response to steroid therapy.

b) Bilateral

i. Extensive and aggressive pituitary adenoma

ii. Meningioma

iii. Metastases

iv. Thrombosis of the cavernous sinus

May occur as part of a septic process associated with spontaneous dural malformations or may result from an interventional or surgical procedure.

Kazner E, Wende S, Gramme T, et al. Computed tomography in intracranial tumors: differential diagnosis and clinical aspects; Springer-Verlag NY; 1982

Michael AS, Mafee MF, Valvassori GE, Tan WS. Dynamic computed tomography of the head and neck: differential diagnostic value. Radiology 1985; 154(2):413–419

Lui YW, Dasari SB, Young RJ. Sphenoid masses in children: radiologic differential diagnosis with pathologic correlation. AJNR Am J Neuroradiol 2011; 32(4):617–626

Lloret I, Server A, Taksdal I. Calvarial lesions: a radiological approach to diagnosis. Acta Radiol 2009; 50(5):531–542

Lustig LR, Holliday MJ, McCarthy F, Nager GT. Fibrous dysplasia involving the skull base and temporal bone. Arch Otoralyngol Head Neck Surg 2001; 127(10):1239–1247

6.7 Astrocytic Brain Tumors

Gliomas account for 50–60% of primary brain tumors. Low-grade glioma is most common in the first decade of a person's life and decreases progressively with age. Astrocytoma peaks in incidence in the third decade. Anaplastic astrocytoma has a bimodal peak in the first and third decades. GBM becomes progressively more frequent with age, representing only 1% of gliomas in the first decade but over 50% after the age of 60.

6.7.1 Differential diagnosis

Pathology	Findings	Investigation
Brain metastasis	May or may not have systemic disease and/or known cancer. Systemic symptoms include cachexia, respiratory problems, hemoptysis, chest pain, and bone pain	MRI: typically, more localized lesions that may be multiple, and with proportionally more vasogenic edema. Chest-abdominal CT scan, bone scan, and PET scan provide evidence of systemic disease (▶ Fig. 6.9). Histology provides a definitive diagnosis
Brain abscess	May or may not have systemic symptoms such as fever, chills, and cachexia. Risk factors differ and may include pulmonary abnormalities, congenital cyanotic heart diseases, bacterial endocarditis, and penetrating head injuries	MRI demonstrates a thinner capsule toward the ventricle, with restricted diffusion of pus and elevated lactate level; may show multiple lesions. Blood tests, such as ESR, CRP, and elevated WBC count, are suggestive of infection with sensitivity 90% and specificity 77%. Biopsy or aspiration provides the definitive diagnosis, demonstrating pus, not tumor cells, and a positive culture or bacterial agent or fungus
Multiple sclerosis	Typically presents in women aged 20–40 years with acute neurologic symptoms that wax and wane (dissemination in space and time), e.g., optic neuritis, transverse myelitis (spinal cord symptoms), and focal neurologic symptoms	MRI shows multiple lesions in the periventricular white matter, may or may not enhance. CSF shows oligoclonal bands. Histology provides the definitive diagnosis, demonstrating demyelinating lesions, inflammatory cells, and absence of tumor cells, but usually it is not necessary

(Continued)

► *(Continued)*

Pathology	Findings	Investigation
Necrosis	Known brain tumor treated with radiation therapy in the past. May present with progressive neurologic symptoms or no symptoms at all	PET scan is cold. Histology provides definitive diagnosis (no tumor cells and extensive necrosis)
Acute stroke	Acute onset of neurologic symptoms. Often in older patients with cerebrovascular risk factors. Rarely present with seizures (3–5% only)	MRI shows typical vasculature distribution and restricted diffusion
Encephalitis	Systemic symptoms present (fever and cachexia)	CSF shows leukocytosis, HSV antibodies, and/or RBCs. EEG is characteristic with periodic lateralizing epileptiform discharges. CT and MRI show edematous temporal lobes and hemorrhagic transformation. Brain biopsy is definitive with virus isolation
Oligodendroglioma	No specific differences in clinical presentation except that oligodendrogliomas are more prone to present with seizures	CT scan demonstrates calcification in 90% of cases. Cortical location on MRI. Histology provides definitive diagnosis with classic fried egg cytoplasm and chicken wire vasculature
Dysembryoplastic neuroepithelial tumor	Typically, occurs in patients < 20 years of age and presents with chronic seizures disorder	MRI demonstrates a cortical lesion with distinct margins. CT may show deformity over the calvaria. Histopathology provides definitive diagnosis
Ganglioglioma	Patients in the first 2 or 3 decades of life with seizure disorder	MRI commonly demonstrates medial temporal lobe lesion with cystic components and/or calcifications. Histology is definitive with characteristic cell types: ganglion and glial cells

Abbreviations: CRP, C-reactive protein; CSF, cerebrospinal fluid; EEG, electroencephalogram; ESR, erythrocyte sedimentation rate; HSV, herpes simplex virus; PET, positron emission tomography; RBCs, red blood cells; WBCs, white blood cells.
Source: BMJ group: Epocrates 2004.

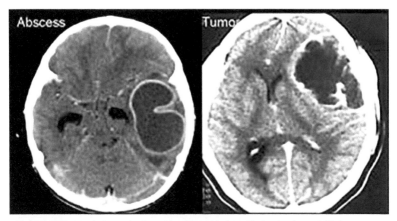

Fig. 6.9 Difference between benign and malignant lesions. Contrast-enhanced CT shows smooth, uniform, thin ring enhancement in abscess and irregular, undulating, thick wall enhancement in tumor.

Horská A, Barker PB. Imaging of brain tumors: MR spectroscopy and metabolic imaging. Neuroimaging Clin N Am 2010; 20(3):293–310

Hayashi T, Kumabe T, Jokura H, et al. Inflammatory demyelinating disease mimicking malignant glioma. J Nucl Med 2003; 44(4):565–569

Plotkin M, Amthauer H, Eisenacher J, et al. Value of 123I-IMT SPECT for diagnosis of recurrent non-astrocytic intracranial tumours. Neuroradiology 2005; 47(1):18–26

Cunliffe CH, Fischer I, Monoky D, et al. Intracranial lesions mimicking neoplasms. Arch Pathol Lab Med 2009; 133(1):101–123

Omuro AM, Leite CC, Mokhtari K, Delattre JY. Pitfalls in the diagnosis of brain tumours. Lancet Neurol 2006; 5(11):937–948

6.8 Intraventricular Masses

The ventricular system of the brain plays host to a variety of unique tumors, as well as tumors more frequently seen elsewhere (e.g., meningiomas). In addition, some intra-axial (parenchymal) masses can be mostly exophytic appearing mostly intraventricular. A systemic approach, taking into account location, patient demographics (age, gender), and imaging appearances, can often substantially narrow the differential, and in most cases suggest one diagnosis as by far the most likely. This is especially important if the mass is being and can be safely ignored/observed.

Neoplasms in the LVs frequently obstruct the ventricles producing hydrocephalus. Patients may be asymptomatic or may present with varied nonspecific symptoms.

The differential diagnosis in adults is glioma (astrocytoma, subependymoma, giant cell astrocytoma), meningioma, ependymoma, choroid plexus papilloma, metastasis, and neurocysticercosis; *in children, the differential diagnosis* is choroid plexus papilloma, ependymoma, PNET, teratoma, and astrocytoma.

Important features for differential diagnosis include the age of the patient, the tumor's location within the LV, and density on CT before intravenous administration of contrast material. Fifty percent of the tumors are in the ventricular atrium. All intraventricular tumor types (except subependymomas) show contrast enhancement. MRI is most useful in evaluating tumor location, size, and extend, but it does not help in eliminating alternative diagnoses.

Ependymomas are more common in children, and in the fourth ventricle these are typically calcified. *Subependymomas* and *central neurocytomas* have an affinity for the anterior portion of the LV. Subependymomas are more common in older adults (males) and usually do not enhance after contrast. Central neurocytomas are more common before 40 years of age. *Subependymal giant cell astrocytomas* always line the foramen of Monro, show intense enhancement, and frequent calcification. When a mass is centered on the choroid plexus, a highly vascular tumor (either *choroid plexus papilloma, choroid plexus carcinoma, meningioma, or metastases*) should be considered. In adults, *atrial meningiomas* are among the most common tumors seen in the LVs (most cases in the left LV of middle-aged women). The low signal intensity on T2-weighted imaging (T2-WI) is one of the features of the diagnosis. The atrium of the LV is also known site for the *metastatic spread of* renal cell carcinoma, lung carcinoma, melanoma, gastric carcinoma, colon carcinoma, and lymphoma. On MRI, metastatic disease occasionally may mimic the signal characteristics of an intraventricular meningioma. *Cysticercosis* may also manifest as an intraventricular mass/cyst, hyperintense compared to CSF on T1-weighted imaging (T1-WI) and similar high signal of CSF on T2-WI. *Central neurocytomas* are uncommon tumors of the CNS; they often mimic oligodendrogliomas.

The main lesions are discussed below.

1. Tumors
    a) Ependymoma
    b) Central neurocytoma
    c) Subependymoma
    d) Subependymal giant cell astrocytoma/subependymal hamartomas of tuberous sclerosis
    e) Intraventricular meningioma
    f) Choroid plexus papilloma/choroid plexus carcinoma
    g) Choroid plexus metastases
    h) Craniopharyngioma
    i) Oligodendroglioma

2. Cysts
    a) Colloid cyst (▶ Fig. 6.10)
    b) Intraventricular simple cyst (including arachnoid cysts, ependymal cysts, and large choroid plexus cysts)
    c) Choroid plexus xanthogranuloma
    d) Cavum septum pellucidum
    e) Cavum vergae
    f) Cavum velum interpositum
3. Infection
    a) Neurocysticercosis
    b) Intracranial tuberculoma
    c) Intracranial hydatid cyst (▶ Fig. 6.11)
4. Intraventricular hemorrhage
5. Periventricular parenchymal lesions
    a) GBM
    b) Primary intraventricular CNS lymphoma
    c) Medulloblastomas/PNET tumors
    d) Hemangioblastoma
    e) Pilocytic astrocytoma
    f) Atypical teratoid/rhabdoid tumor
    g) Pineal region masses
    h) Sarcoma

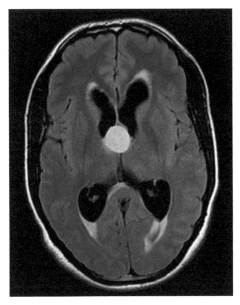

Fig. 6.10 Axial fluid-attenuated inversion recovery (FLAIR) magnetic resonance image demonstrating a colloid cyst of the third ventricle. (Reproduced from Neoplasms. In: Shaya M, Gragnaniello C, Nader R, ed. Neurosurgery Rounds: Questions and Answers. 2nd edition. Thieme; 2017.)

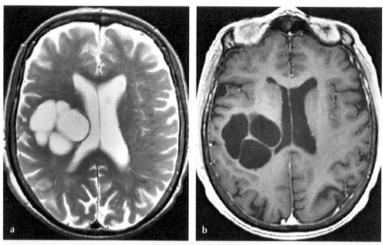

Fig. 6.11 Patient with intracranial hydatid cysts that are well-circumscribed lesions with **(a)** high signal on axial T2-weighted imaging and **(b)** low signal without gadolinium contrast enhancement on axial T1-weighted imaging. (Reproduced from Fetal Brain MRI. In: Meyers S, ed. Differential Diagnosis in Neuroimaging: Brain and Meninges. 1st edition. Thieme; 2016.)

Jelinek J, Smirniotopoulos JG, Parisi JE, Kanzer M. Lateral ventricular neoplasms of the brain: differential diagnosis based on clinical, CT, and MR findings. AJNR Am J Neuroradiol 1990; 11(3):567–574

Majós C, Coll S, Aguilera C, Acebes JJ, Pons LC. Intraventricular mass lesions of the brain. Eur Radiol 2000; 10(6):951–961

Anselem O, Mezzetta L, Grangé G, et al. Fetal tumors of the choroid plexus: is differential diagnosis between papilloma and carcinoma possible? Ultrasound Obstet Gynecol 2011; 38(2):229–232

Ginat DT, Meyers SP. Intracranial lesions with high signal intensity on T1-weighted MR images: differential diagnosis. Radiographics 2012; 32(2):499–516

Suh DY, Mapstone T. Pediatric supratentorial intraventricular tumors. Neurosurg 2001; 10(6)-E4

6.9 Choroid Plexus Disease

6.9.1 Differential diagnosis

1. Tumors
   a) Choroid plexus papilloma
   b) Choroid plexus carcinoma
   c) Meningioma
   d) Ependymoma/subependymoma
   e) Neurofibroma

    f) Glioblastoma/astrocytoma
    g) Oligodendroglioma
    h) Tuberous sclerosis/subependymal giant cell astrocytoma
    i) CNS lymphoma
    j) PNET (e.g., medulloblastomas, ependymoblastomas, pineoblastomas, cerebral neuroblastomas, medulloepitheliomas, melanotic vermian PNET of infancy)
    k) Metastases
2. Non-neoplastic tumorlike lesions
    a) Epidermoid tumor
    b) Dermoid tumor
3. Non-neoplastic cysts
    a) Colloid cyst
    b) Rathke's cleft cyst
    c) Neuroglial (neuroepithelial) cyst
4. Vascular malformations
    a) Choroid plexus angiomas
    b) Phakomatosis (e.g., Sturge–Weber syndrome)
5. Infection
    a) Choroid plexitis (e.g., pathogens include *Cryptococcus* and *Nocardia*)
    b) Other
6. Inflammation
    a) Sarcoidosis
    b) Xanthogranuloma

Naeini RM, Yoo JH, Hunter JV. Spectrum of choroid plexus lesions in children. AJR Am J Roentgenol 2009; 192(1):32–40

Netsky MG, Shaangshoti S, Collaborators. The choroid plexus in health and disease. Bristol: Wright; 2013

Osborn AG, Preece MT. Intracranial cysts: radiologic-pathologic correlation and imaging approach. Radiology 2006; 239(3):650–664

McLendon RE, Rosenblum MK, Binger DD. In Russell-Rubinstein Pathology of tumors of thenervous system. 7th ed. Hodder Arnold; 2006

6.10 Gliomatosis Cerebri or Astrocytosis Cerebri

A diffusely infiltrative neoplasm with variably undifferentiated astrocytes and without a necrotic center. Gliomatosis cerebri presents as a diffuse involvement of the cerebral hemispheres leading to progressive changes in personality, headaches, and impaired mental status. PET scanning with methionine show isotope accumulation in the diffusely infiltrative tumorous area with greater accuracy than CT or MRI. It can be extremely difficult to distinguish gliomatosis cerebri from a diffuse glioma presenting with widespread continuous tumor infiltration into adjacent brain regions. Oligodendroglioma shows necrosis, cysts, and calcifications but the main feature differentiating a conventional glioma from gliomatosis cerebri is mass effect in case of conventional glioma. Definitive diagnosis at autopsy. Prognosis is variable with median survival measured in 14.5 months.

6.10.1 Differential diagnosis

1. Low- or intermediate-grade glioma
2. Oligodendroglioma
3. Gliomatosis cerebri
4. Leptomeningeal gliomatosis
5. Encephalitis
6. Diffuse and demyelinating disease (such as Marburg's disease)
7. Pseudotumor cerebri
8. Infections (progressive multifocal leukoencephalopathy)
9. Metabolic disorders (posterior reversible encephalopathy syndrome)
10. Ischemic cerebrovascular diseases, vasculitis
11. Posttraumatic changes (brain radiotherapy)

Bendszus M, Warmuth-Metz M, Klein R, et al. MR spectroscopy in gliomatosis cerebri. AJNR Am J Neuroradiol 2000; 21(2):375–380

Yu A, Li K, Li H. Value of diagnosis and differential diagnosis of MRI and MR spectroscopy in gliomatosis cerebri. Eur J Radiol 2006; 59(2):216–221

6.11 Tolosa–Hunt Syndrome

(Idiopathic inflammatory disease of the cavernous sinus)

Painful ophthalmoplegia syndrome with typical onset in middle to late life. It is a noncaseating granulomatous disorder of unknown etiology, characterized by severe retro-orbital and supraorbital pain, diplopia, paralysis of CNs III, IV, and VI with less frequent involvement of CNs II, V1, and V2. Inflammation involves the superior orbital fissure and cavernous sinus region, visualized clearly on enhanced MRI scans, which help in the differential diagnosis of the Tolosa–Hunt syndrome from conditions such as meningioma, lymphoma, and sarcoidosis, as well as confirming the similarities of the Tolosa–Hunt syndrome and orbital pseudotumor (▶ Fig. 6.12).

As the diagnosis of Tolosa–Hunt syndrome can be made only after other disease processes have been excluded, it behoves the clinician to be familiar with the differential diagnosis of painful ophthalmoplegia. In fact, during the initial patient evaluation, there are often no clues in the history or physical examination to distinguish Tolosa–Hunt syndrome from other causes of painful ophthalmoplegia. Therefore, the clinician should be aware of: (1) causes of parasellar syndrome, and (2) other entities producing painful ophthalmoplegia.

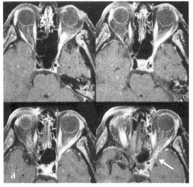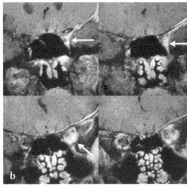

Fig. 6.12 Tolosa-Hunt syndrome. **(a)** Axial and **(b)** coronal fat-suppressed T1-weighted images show poorly defined gadolinium contrast enhancement in the left orbital apex extending posteriorly into the left superior orbital fissure and left cavernous sinus (*arrows*). (Reproduced from Table 2.3 Extraocular lesions involving the orbit. In: Meyers S, ed. Differential Diagnosis in Neuroimaging: Head and Neck. 1st edition. Thieme; 2016.)

6.11.1 Differential diagnosis

1. Iatrogenic
   a) Sinonasal surgery
   b) Orbital/facial surgery
2. Traumatic
   a) Penetrating/nonpenetrating injury
   b) Orbital apex fracture
   c) Retained foreign body
3. Vascular
   a) Intracavernous carotid artery aneurysm
   b) Posterior cerebral artery aneurysm
   c) Carotid cavernous fistula/thrombosis
   d) Sickle cell anemia
4. Inflammatory
   a) Sarcoidosis
   b) Systemic lupus erythematosus
   c) Churg–Strauss syndrome
   d) Wegener's granulomatosis
   e) Tolosa–Hunt syndrome
      Episodes of unilateral orbital pain associated paralysis of CNs III, IV, and/or VI, and/or demonstration of a granuloma by MRI or biopsy; pain resolves within 72 hours after adequate corticosteroid therapy.

    f) Giant cell arteritis

    g) Orbital inflammatory pseudotumor

    h) Thyroid orbitopathy

5. Infectious

    a) Bacterial (*Streptococcus* spp., *Staphylococcus* spp., *Actinomyces* spp., Gram-negative bacilli, anaerobes, *Mycobacterium tuberculosis*)

    b) Viruses (herpes zoster)

    c) Fungi (aspergillosis, mucormycosis)

    d) Spirochetes (*Treponema pallidum*)

6. Neoplastic

    a) Primary intracranial tumor (pituitary adenoma, meningioma, craniopharyngioma, sarcoma, neurofibroma, epidermoid)

    b) Primary cranial tumor (chordoma, chondroma, giant cell tumor)

    c) Local metastases (nasopharyngeal tumor, squamous-cell carcinoma, cylindroma, Adamantinoma)

    d) Distant metastases (lymphoma, multiple myeloma, lung, breast, renal cell malignant melanoma)

    e) Hematologic (Burkitt lymphoma, non-Hodgkin's lymphoma, leukemia)

    f) Perineural invasion of cutaneous malignancy

Schats NJ, Farmar P. Tolosa–Hunt syndrome: the pathology of painful ophthalmoplegia. In Neuro-ophthalmology. Symposium of the University of Miami and the Bascoam Palmer Eye Institute. Vol VI ed Smith JL (Mosby, St Louis) pp 102–112

Kline LB, Hoyt WF. The Tolosa–Hunt syndrome. J Neurol Neurosurg Psychiatry 2001; 71(5):577–582

6.12 Recurrence of Malignant Gliomas

An enlarging lesion at the site of a previously treated glioma represents most probably regrowth of an incompletely treated initial tumor and less likely the development of a new pathologic entity.

In the differential diagnosis of an enlarging lesion at the site of a previously eradicated malignant glioma, the clinician should consider the following factors:

1. The development of a distinctly new tumor

    In cases of genetic predisposition to tumor development shared by cells in the area.

    a) Multiple gliomas in patients with tuberous sclerosis

    b) Multiple neurofibromas developing along the same nerve root in patients with neurofibromatosis

2. Growth of a tumor with related pathology

    A tumor with related histopathology may supplant the original tumor.

a) The astrocytic component of a mixed glioma replacing its previously treated oligodendrocytic component

b) A gliosarcoma may arise from a previously treated glioblastoma

3. Growth of a secondary tumor

The initial therapy may induce a secondary tumor of a different type.

a) A parasellar sarcoma after irradiation for a pituitary adenoma

b) A glioblastoma in the radiation field of a meningioma

4. Metastatic tumor in the original tumor site

Example is a breast metastasis within a pituitary adenoma.

5. Non-neoplastic lesions

These non-neoplastic lesions may mimic tumor growth.

a) Radiation necrosis following focal high dose irradiation

b) Abscess formation at the site of tumor resection

6.13 Congenital Posterior Fossa Cysts and Anomalies

1. Dandy–Walker complex

In 70% of cases, this syndrome has a number of associated anomalies such as hydrocephalus, agenesis of the corpus callosum, nuclear dysplasia of the brain stem, and other cerebro-cerebellar heterotopias.

a) Dandy–Walker malformation

Large posterior fossa and CSF cyst, high transverse sinuses and tentorial insertion, vermian, cerebellar hemispheric and brainstem hypoplasia in 25% of cases.

b) Dandy–Walker variant

Mild vermian hypoplasia, moderately enlarged fourth ventricle although the posterior fossa is typically normal in size, the brain stem is normal and there is a variable degree vermian hypoplasia.

2. Other posterior fossa cysts

a) Arachnoid and neuroepithelial cysts

Arachnoid cysts are formed by splitting of the arachnoid membrane with layers of thickened fibroconnective tissue, whereas neuroepithelial or glioependymal cysts are lined with a low cuboidal-columnar epithelium.

b) Mega cisterna magna

The fourth ventricle appears normal, and the vermis and cerebellar hemispheres are normal but occasionally the posterior fossa can be enlarged with prominent scalloping of the occipital bones.

    c) Isolated fourth ventricle
       Post ventriculoperitoneal shunt leading to secondary aqueductal stenosis, but in addition the CSF outflow from the fourth ventricle is prohibited or its absorption prohibited. For example, in patients whose hydrocephalus is due to or associated with an inflammatory meningeal process such as infection or hemorrhage.

    d) Pulsion diverticulum
       In advanced hydrocephalus, the thin ventricular wall may dehisce into the adjacent subarachnoid space thus forming diverticula commonly in the inferomedial wall of the atria, the suprapineal recess, and through the incisura causing downward displacement of the cerebellum.

3. Miscellaneous cerebellar hypoplasia

    a) Chiari IV malformation (absent or severely hypoplastic cerebellum and small brain stem)

    b) Joubert's syndrome
       Split or segmented vermis transmitted by autosomal recessive genes.

    c) Rhombencephalosynapsis
       Agenesis of the vermis and midline fusion of the cerebellar hemispheres and peduncles.

    d) Tectocerebellar dysgraphia
       Vermian hypoplasia, occipital encephalocele and dorsal brainstem traction

    e) Lhermitte–Duclos disease or dysplastic cerebellar gangliocytoma
       Gross thickening of the cerebellar folia, hypertrophy of the granular cell layer, and axonal hypermyelination of the molecular cell layer.

6.14 Posterior Fossa Cysts

1. Dandy–Walker complex (▶ Fig. 6.13)
2. Mega cisterna magna
3. Arachnoid cyst
4. Non-neoplastic cysts
    a) Inflammatory
    b) Enterogenous
5. Neoplastic cysts
    a) Hemangioblastoma
    b) Pilocytic astrocytoma
6. Cyst-like tumors
    a) Dermoid
    b) Epidermoid

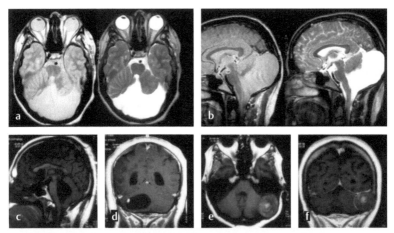

Fig. 6.13 Posterior fossa cysts. **(a)** Dandy–Walker cyst. Proton density axial MRI T2-WI presenting a cystic dilatation of the cisterna magna that communicates with the fourth ventricle. There is an associated atrophy of the cerebellar vermis and a smooth erosion of the occipital bone. **(b)** Dandy–Walker cyst. Proton density sagittal T2-WI (same case). The communication of the cyst with the fourth ventricle and the significant vermian atrophy are noted. There is also elevation of the confluence of sinuses and of the tentorium cerebelli.

Bosemani T, Orman G, Boltshauser E, Tekes A, Huisman TA, Poretti A. Congenital abnormalities of the posterior fossa. Radiographics 2015; 35(1):200–220

Kollias SS, Ball WS Jr, Prenger EC. Cystic malformations of the posterior fossa: differential diagnosis clarified through embryologic analysis. Radiographics 1993; 13(6):1211–1231

Barkovich AJ, Kjos BO, Norman D, Edwards MS. Revised classification of posterior fossa cysts and cystlike malformations based on the results of the MR images. Am J Roentgenol 1989; 153:1289–1300

6.15 Intracranial Cysts

Intracranial cysts and cyst-like intracerebral masses are common findings at routine cerebral imaging examinations. These findings might be accompanied by neurological focal signs or just completely incidental information in persons investigated by CT or MRI for trivial symptoms, such as chronic headaches.

6.15.1 Differential diagnosis

1. Metastatic cysts
   Detection of an intracerebral mass in patients with known malignant tumor strongly suggests the presence of brain metastases (multiple lesions in 70%

of cases). The most frequent carcinomas capable to metastasize to the brain are bronchogenic carcinoma, carcinoma of the breast, choriocarcinoma, and melanoma with melanoma metastasizing in up to 90% of patients. Only 5% of the intracranial metastases are from mucinous adenocarcinomas of gastrointestinal origin, and about 50% of those are located in the posterior fossa, particularly in the cerebellum.

Contrast cerebral CT and MRI evaluation increase the specificity of diagnosis but none of them can differentiate between the lesion types. Ring-enhancing necrotic or cystic neoplasms require differential diagnosis with brain abscess in their capsular stage. DW MRI and spectroscopy can be helpful in such cases. Reduced diffusion (restricted fluid of water molecules) occurs within abscesses because of the highly viscous purulent fluid. However, some cystic neoplasms (primary intracerebral or metastatic) may also show reduced diffusion, which raises another problem in differentiating them from abscesses. MRI spectroscopy of an abscess shows elevation of acetate, succinate, lactate, and amino acids such as valine, leucine, and isoleucine. These amino acids are not seen in MR spectra of brain tumors. Spectral changes have been observed after antibiotic therapy, therefore, the investigation must be performed before starting antibiotic treatment. This may also monitor the disease response to such therapies. Using these tests, the accuracy of diagnosis increases up to 94%.

2. Cerebral toxoplasma abscess

In patients with AIDS, toxoplasmosis is the most common opportunistic infection and the most common cause of focal brain lesion. Toxoplasmosis may generate focal brain lesions mostly localized to the basal ganglia, but sometimes these may also be in other brain regions. Dissemination in the spinal cord is infrequent.

Plain CT scan shows usually multiple low-density areas, and contrasted CT scan show no enhancement. MRI studies show hypointensity on T1-WI and variable intensity on T2-WI, due to presence of hemorrhage and/or calcification. Typical radiological findings comprise multiple ring-enhancing lesions in both cerebral hemispheres. On DW MRI, the center of the abscess is slightly hyperintense and the wall is relatively hypointense, with hyperintense surrounding edema. At MR spectroscopy, high lipid and lactate peaks, associated with a decrease in other metabolites, are characteristic for toxoplasmosis.

The most important differential diagnosis for cerebral toxoplasmosis is primary brain lymphoma, but pyogenic abscess and cystic metastasis can mimic it.

3. Neurocysticercosis

It is the most common form of parasitic disease of the brain in the world and occurs in 60–90% of all cases of systemic cysticercosis. Common locations in the brain are the grey–white matter junction and deep nuclei, and less common are the subarachnoid spaces and fourth ventricle; spinal involvement is rare.

Clinically presents with seizures (most common), headaches, signs of raised ICP, encephalitis, chronic meningitis, ischemic or hemorrhagic stroke, or spinal involvement.

Imaging findings in neurocysticercosis vary with the stage of cyst development. The early vesicular stage is typified by a smooth thin-walled cyst that is CSF-like cyst on CT and MRI images. Edema and contrast enhancement are rare. A mural nodule is often present (viable larval scolex), the "cyst with a dot" appearance. When the colloidal-vesicular stage (degeneration) begins and host inflammatory response ensues, pericystic edema and cyst wall enhancement are present. Cyst fluid is hyperintense to CSF on MRI, in this stage. In the granular, nodular (healing) stage nonenhanced CT scans show an isoattenuated cyst with a hyperattenuated calcified scolex. Surrounding edema is still present and enhancement to contrast material persists. The residual cyst is isointense to the brain on T1-WI and iso- to hypointense on T2-WI. Nodular or micro ring enhancement is common, suggesting granuloma. Occasionally, a "target" or "bull's eye" appearance is seen with the calcified scolex in the center of the mass.

The differential diagnosis includes abscess, tuberculosis, neoplasm (primary or metastatic), enlarged perivascular space (PVSs), and other parasitic infections (Echinococcosis, schistosomiasis, trichinosis, malaria, amebic encephalitis, sparganosis, trypanosomiasis). Abscesses have a T2-hypointense rim, whereas cysticercosis cysts are typically isointense except when they are in the ventricles where the rim is hyperintense in FLAIR images. Tuberculomas often occur with meningitis, are rarely cystic, and are often profoundly hypointense on T2-WI. Enlarged PVSs have the same appearance as CSF at all MR sequences. None of these cystic lesions has the characteristic "cyst with dot" appearance.

4. Hydatic cyst
   Echinococcosis is the larval stage of *Echinococcus granulosus* infection. The disease frequently involves the liver and lungs. Cerebral cysts are rare (2% of cases), and are usually solitary, spherical, and unilobular. When the infection involves the CNS, it is usually located in the brain parenchyma supplied by the middle cerebral artery and less commonly the LVs and cerebellum. Cysts contain clear fluid with daughter cysts and a granular deposit of scolices.

   The best diagnostic clue of a hydatid cyst is a single, large, thin-walled, spherical, nonenhancing CSF-attenuation cyst in the parietal region of the brain. The two visible imaging components are the cyst and the pericyst, which is a peripheral capsule of the cyst. While MRI is more sensitive in demonstrating the pericyst, CT is more sensitive in depicting cyst calcification.

Differential diagnosis: The identification of a single, large, unilocular cyst lesion without surrounding edema in the parietal brain area is most typically suggestive for hydatid cyst.

The main differential diagnosis includes other parasitic diseases involving CNS, such as neurocysticercosis, where usually more numerous lesions are found; cerebral abscesses, which are surrounded by prominent edema; arachnoid cysts, and epidermoid cyst, with characteristic features as described appropriately.

5. Other parasitic cysts

A number of parasites may occasionally infect the CNS and appear at least partially cystic. Amebiasis, paragonimiasis, schistosomiasis, and sparganosis can cause both unilocular and complex intraparenchymal cysts with or without accompanying meningoencephalitis. Perilesional edema and petechial hemorrhage are common.

Imaging: Complex conglomerate cysts with thick enhancing rims and striking edema are common.

Differential diagnosis: Complex conglomerate parasitic cysts of any origin may mimic primary or metastatic brain tumor. The patients' personal and travel history, as well as serologic findings, are key to the diagnosis.

6. Neoplasm-associated benign cysts

Extra-axial tumors (e.g., meningioma, schwannoma, craniopharyngioma, and pituitary macroadenoma) may be associated with large non-neoplastic cysts. These peritumoral cysts appear to contain CSF. Some, such as cysts that occur adjacent to vestibular schwannoma, are true arachnoid cysts. Others, such as meningioma, trap CSF within the cleft between the expanding tumor and the adjacent brain. Craniopharyngiomas and pituitary macroadenomas with extrasellar extension may obstruct and enlarge adjacent PVSs. Interstitial fluid is retained within the enlarged PVSs and may result in edema along the optic tracks.

Tumor-associated arachnoid cysts and cystic PVSs do not enhance. Most parallel CSF in signal intensity. If protein content is elevated within the trapped pools of CSF, the arachnoid cysts may appear slightly hyperintense to normal CSF on MRI.

Differential diagnosis: True arachnoid cyst associated with neoplasm may be impossible to distinguish from enlarged PVSs with trapped interstitial fluid unless biopsy is performed.

7. Arachnoid cysts

The arachnoid cyst is a benign, probably congenital lesion, localized in the intra-arachnoid space. Usually these cysts are supratentorial. They may occur in the sylvian fissure or interhemispheric fissure and more rarely in the cisterna magna and CPA. They generally do not communicate with the ventricles. Appear to be formed by splitting or duplication of the arachnoid membrane, active fluid secretion by the cyst wall, and slow and progressive distention caused by CSF pulsations and a "ball valve" mechanism hypothesis (one-way valve between arachnoid cysts and subarachnoid space leading to its expansion). Arachnoid cysts might be posttraumatic as well.

The cysts are well circumscribed, having the same signal intensity as CSF at CT scans and all MRI sequences and no contrast enhancement. Occasionally, signs of hemorrhage, high protein content within the cysts occur on MRI.

Differential diagnosis includes epidermoid cysts, chronic subdural hematoma, and porencephalic cysts. Epidermoid cysts are hyperintense on FLAIR MRI sequence and show increased signal intensity on diffusion sequences, while arachnoid cysts have low signal intensity on both FLAIR and DW sequences. The chronic subdural hematomas do not show the same signal intensity with CSF on MRI examinations. Porencephalic cysts are CSF-filled cavities with a thin wall and surrounded by gliotic or spongiotic white matter.

8. Colloid cysts

These are endodermal mucin-containing congenital malformations that account for 0.5–1.0% of primary brain tumors and 15–20% of intraventricular masses. More than 99% are found wedged in the foramen of Monro. They are usually asymptomatic due to their small size and found incidentally. Occasionally colloid cysts expand rapidly. Acute hydrocephalus may lead to sudden death.

The best diagnostic clue to a colloid cyst is its location at the foramen of Monro. The classic colloid cyst appears as a well-delineated hyperattenuated mass on plain CT scans. In T1-WI MRI two-thirds of colloid cysts are hyperintense. The majority are isointense to brain on T2-WI and some show peripheral rim enhancement.

Differential diagnosis includes arachnoid cysts, epidermoid and dermoid cysts, and choroid plexus cysts. The location of a colloid cyst is almost pathognomonic. A CSF flow artefact (MR pseudocyst) may be easily mistaken for a colloid cyst. The arachnoid and ependymal cysts are isointense relative to CSF in all sequences. The choroid plexus cysts are hyperintense in T2-WI. Epidermoid and dermoid cysts are very rarely seen in the third ventricle. Neoplasms, such as subependymomas or choroid plexus papilloma that may occur at the foramen of Monro, are much less common and typically enhance.

9. Epidermoid cysts

Intracranial epidermoid cysts are congenital inclusion cysts; they comprise 0.2–1.8% of primary intracranial tumors, and are 4–5 times as common as dermoid cysts. The most common location is the CPA (40–50%), the fourth ventricle (17%), and the sellar and/or parasellar regions (10–15%). Epidermoid cysts are well-demarcated, encapsulated lesions with a whitish capsule of a mother-of-pearl sheen (pearly tumor). Mostly asymptomatic, but depending on their location, they may simulate an acoustic neuroma, may cause involvement of the facial nerve followed by unilateral hearing loss, may also cause vertigo, imbalance, or trigeminal neuralgia. In case of rupture, they may produce intense chemical meningitis.

On CT scans, epidermoid cysts appear as well-demarcated hypodense lesions that resemble CSF and do not enhance with contrast. Most of them show low signal on T1-WI and high signal on T2-WI MRI sequences.

Differential diagnosis: The major differential consideration is an arachnoid cyst. Arachnoid cysts are isointense to CSF at all sequences, including FLAIR. They displace rather than invade structures such as the epidermoid. Other epidermoid cyst mimics include dermoid cysts, neurocysticercosis, and cystic neoplasm. Dermoid cysts are typically located along the midline and resemble fat, not CSF. Cystic neoplasms often enhance and do not resemble CSF. Neurocysticercosis cysts often enhance and demonstrate surrounding edema or gliosis.

10. Dermoid cysts

These cysts are congenital ectodermal inclusion cysts. They are extremely rare, comprising fewer than 0.5% of primary intracranial tumors and 4–5 times less common than epidermoid cysts. They tend to occur in the midline sellar, parasellar, or frontonasal regions. Other dermoid cysts are midline in the posterior fossa (vermian lesions, fourth ventricle). These cysts increase in size (glandular secretion and epithelial desquamation) and thus may rupture causing chemical meningitis that may lead to vasospasm, infarction, and even death. Malignant transformation into squamous-cell carcinoma may result from malignant transformation of both dermoid and epidermoid cysts.

Dermoid cysts appear as well-circumscribed, hypodense masses on CT scan as a result of their rich lipid content. On MRI, they are hyperintense on T1-WI and give a variable signal from hypo- to hyperintense on T2-WI sequences. The best diagnostic clue of a ruptured dermoid cyst is fatlike droplets in the subarachnoid cisterns, sulci, and ventricle, and pial enhancement from chemical meningitis.

Differential diagnosis includes epidermoid cysts, craniopharyngiomas, lipomas, and teratomas. Epidermoid cysts typically resemble CSF (not fat), lack dermal appendages, and are usually located off midline. Like dermoid cysts, craniopharyngiomas are suprasellar, with a midline location, and demonstrate nodular calcification. However, most craniopharyngiomas are strikingly hyperintense on T2-WI and enhance strongly. Teratomas may also have a similar location but usually occur in the pineal region. Lipomas demonstrate homogeneous fat attenuation and/or signal intensity and show a chemical shift artefact, which typically does not occur with dermoid cysts.

11. Ependymal cysts

    These are usually common benign cysts of the LVs and also in other sites (subarachnoid space, brain stem, spinal cord, and CPA). Ependyma cells secrete a clear fluid. Ependymal cysts are asymptomatic, but some might become manifest with headache, seizure, or obstructive hydrocephalus.

    The lesions are isointense with CSF on MRI T1-WI and T2-WI and have nonenhancing walls.

    Differential diagnosis includes choroid plexus cysts, but these are typically bilateral and other enhancing arachnoid cysts, but these occur in different locations (in subarachnoid spaces) and intraventricular neurocysticercosis which show a hyperintense rim and scolexes inside the masses on FLAIR images.

12. Neurenteric cysts

    These are rare, benign, congenital, endodermal lesions commonly located in the spine than in the brain (posterior fossa). The wall cyst is lined up by a single layer of epithelium resembling gastrointestinal or respiratory epithelium and contains mucoid and protein component. Patients may present with symptoms such as headache, dizziness, cranial nerve deficits (decreased sensation of the CN V, sensory neural hearing loss, or CN III palsy), or seizures.

    The classic mesenteric cysts are seen as well-circumscribed, nonenhancing, slightly hyperintense masses of the cerebral posterior fossa, usually located in front of the medulla. On CT scans, these are iso-/hypointense lesions. Most of them are iso-/slightly hyperintense compared with CSF on T1-WI and typically hyperintense on T2-WI on MRI.

    Differential diagnosis includes epidermoid cysts, dermoid cysts, arachnoid cysts, Rathke's cleft cysts, colloid cysts, and craniopharyngiomas. Epidermoid and dermoid cysts show moderate to intense diffusion restriction. Arachnoid cysts have the same signal intensity as CSF on all MRI sequences. Rathke's and colloid cysts have a different location than neurenteric cysts. Craniopharyngiomas are hyperintense in T2-WI MRI strongly enhancing in T1-WI with contrast agent examination.

13. Rathke's cleft cysts

    These cysts are congenital lesions arising from remnants of the embryonic Rathke's cleft. They are intra- and/or suprasellar cysts (13–33%) with intracystic nodules. The cyst content is mainly mucoid. The lesions are mainly asymptomatic but eventually can trigger symptoms due to compression of the optic chiasm, hypothalamus, or pituitary gland.

    Rathke's cysts might be difficult to differentiate from intra- or suprasellar masses on pure radiologic bases because of variable intensities of MRI sequences. Still, important aspects are the lack of enhancement and absence of calcifications of the cyst. Cystic fluid shows low signal intensity on T1-WI and isointensity to high signal intensity on T2-WI MRI sequences.

    Differential diagnosis: The most common lesion needing to be differentiated from Rathke's cysts are pituitary adenomas and craniopharyngiomas. The pituitary adenomas appear like solid, homogenous enhancing tumors. The craniopharyngiomas have mixed solid and cystic characteristics and show enhancement of the solid part. Epidermoid and dermoid cysts have already been discussed. However, the intracystic nodule of Rathke's cyst visible on both T1-WI and T2-WI sequences is very helpful in diagnosis.

14. Porencephalic cysts

    These cysts are congenital or acquired cavities within the cerebral hemispheres that usually (not invariably) communicate directly with the ventricular system. Congenital cysts originate from a fetal or perinatal process that results from intrauterine vascular or infectious injury. Acquired cysts are secondary to injury later in life usually due to trauma, surgery, ischemia, or infection.

    The cysts have the same appearance as CSF at all MRI sequences. Adjacent white matter typically shows hyperintensity on T2-WI and FLAIR MRI.

    Differential diagnosis includes arachnoid cyst, schizencephaly, ependymal cyst, encephalomalacia, and hydranencephaly. Arachnoid cysts are extra-axial and displace the brain cortex away from the adjacent skull. Schizencephaly is a CSF-filled cavity that is lined with heterotopic gray matter and extends all the way from the ventricle to the brain surface. Ependymal cysts are typically intraventricular with normal surrounding brain tissue.

Osborn AG, Preece MT. Intracranial cysts: radiologic–pathologic correlation and imaging approach. Radiology 2006; 239(3):650–664

Bannister CM, Russell SA, Rimmer S, Mowle DH. Fetal arachnoid cysts: their site, progress, prognosis and differential diagnosis. Eur J Pediatr Surg 1999; 9(Suppl 1):27–28

Preece MT, Osborn AG, Chin SS, Smirniotopoulos JG. Intracranial neurenteric cysts: imaging and pathology spectrum. AJNR Am J Neuroradiol 2006; 27(6):1211–1216

Taillibert S, Le Rhun E, Chamberlain MC. Intracranial cystic lesions: a review. Curr Neurol Neurosci Rep 2014; 14(9):481

6.16 Enhancing Lesions in Children and Young Adults

Imaging differential diagnoses for a peripheral enhancing lesion in a child or young adult include:

1. Glioblastoma
2. Ganglioglioma
3. Gangliosarcoma
4. Malignant astrocytoma
5. Meningioma
6. Meningiosarcoma
7. Oligodendroglioma
8. Juvenile pilocytic astrocytoma
9. Solitary metastasis
10. Pleomorphic xanthoastrocytoma
11. Fibrous histiocytoma
12. Fibrous xanthomas

6.16.1 Multiple ring-enhancing lesions of the brain

Multiple ring-enhancing lesions are one of the most commonly encountered neuroimaging abnormalities. A wide range of etiologies may present as cerebral multiple ring-enhancing lesions. On neuroimaging, these lesions appear as hypodense or isodense mass lesions on plain CT studies. After contrast administration, there is a ring- or a homogeneous disk-like enhancement within the region of hypodensity. The enhancing lesions are often of variable size and are usually surrounded by a varying amount of perifocal vasogenic edema. Typically, the ring-enhancing lesions are located at the junction of the grey and white matter, but they could be located in the subcortical area, deep in the brain parenchyma, or may even be superficial.

Clinically, they manifest as recurrent seizures, visual impairment, focal neurological deficit, and raised ICP (severe headache, vomiting, and papilledema). If cerebral edema is severe, patients may develop loss of sensorium and posturing of limbs, because of transtentorial brain herniation.

The *differential diagnosis* of multiple ring-enhancing lesions depends on the age and the immune status of the patient. In the immunocompetent host, malignancies (both primary and metastatic) and pyogenic abscesses remain the most likely diagnoses in patients with large-size lesions. Abscesses caused by atypical microorganisms and demyelinating disease should also be considered in the differential diagnosis of multiple ring-enhancing lesions of the brain. In tropical countries, cysticercus granuloma frequently needs to be differentiated from intracranial tuberculoma. Tuberculomas tend to be larger than 20 mm in diameter, have an irregular outline, cause more mass effect, and have a progressive focal neurologic deficit; whereas cysts tend to be smaller than 20 mm in diameter, have a smooth regular outline, and seldom cause progressive focal neurologic deficits. Attempts have been made to identify the lesion on the basis of distinctive neuro-imaging characteristics of ring-enhancing lesions. In general, abscesses are char-acterized by a thin, uniform ring, which is thinner on the medial border with a smoother outer margin; satellite lesions are often present. A thick, irregular, ring-like enhancement suggests a necrotic brain tumor. Some low-grade brain tumors are "fluid-secreting" and may form heterogeneously enhancing lesions. These low-grade brain tumors may present with an incomplete ring and may reveal the classic: "cyst-with-nodule" morphology. Multiple ring-enhancing lesions can be seen in patients with multifocal glioma. However, the presence of more than three distinct lesions is unusual for a patient with primary brain tumor. The radio-logical differential considerations for a cystic tumor with an enhancing mural nodule include pilocytic astrocytoma, hemangioblastoma, pleomorphic xantho-astrocytoma, meningioma, and ganglioglioma. These benign brain tumors rarely present as multiple enhancing lesions. Demyelinating lesions, including both clas-sic multiple sclerosis and tumefactive demyelination, may present with an open ring or incomplete ring sign and are often misdiagnosed as brain neoplasms.

In HIV-infected patients, the leading causes of multiple enhancing lesions are toxoplasmosis and primary CNS lymphoma. Imaging characteristics that are helpful in distinguishing toxoplasmosis from CNS lymphoma include subcortical gray matter location of toxoplasmosis lesions, their multiplicity, presence of eccentric target sign, and enhancing wall of the lesions thinner than that observed in lymphomas. Thick and irregular periventricular enhancement is typical for pri-mary CNS lymphoma. Corpus callosum involvement is infrequent in primary CNS lymphoma. Furthermore, the immunocompromised patients are at risk for abscesses, from both pyogenic and atypical organisms, and tumors. Tuberculomas and tuberculous brain abscesses should be considered in endemic regions in both immunocompetent and immunocompromised hosts. Due to the low sensitivity of *Mycobacterium tuberculosis* cultures or polymerase chain reaction detection of mycobacterial DNA from CSF, diagnosis of intracranial tuberculoma is often diffi-cult. Several patients may remain undiagnosed despite extensive evaluation.

Diseases causing multiple ring-enhancing lesions of the brain are infectious, neoplastic, inflammatory, or vascular in origin.

6.16.2 Differential diagnoses

In the list below, lesion sizes are denoted as: **S** = small (< 1–2 cm), **M** = medium, **L** = large.

1. Bacterial
   a) Pyogenic abscess (**L**)
   b) Tuberculoma and tuberculous abscess (**L, M, S**)
   c) Neurosyphilis
   d) Listeriosis
2. Fungal granuloma (**L, M**)
   a) Nocardiosis
   b) Actinomycosis
   c) Zygomycosis
   d) Histoplasmosis
   e) Coccidioidomycosis
   f) Aspergillosis
   g) Mucormycosis
   h) Cryptococcosis
3. Parasitic
   a) Neurocysticercosis (**S**)
   b) Toxoplasmosis (**M**)
   c) Amebic brain abscess
   d) Echinococcosis
   e) Chagas disease
4. Neoplastic
   a) Metastases (**M, S**)
   b) Primary brain tumor (**L, M**)
   c) Primary CNS lymphoma (in immunocompromised patients)
5. Inflammatory and demyelinating (**M**)
   a) Multiple sclerosis
   b) Tumefactive demyelination
   c) Acute disseminating encephalomyelitis (incomplete ring)
   d) Sarcoidosis (**M**)
   e) Neuro-Behcet's disease (**S**)
   f) Whipple's disease
   g) Systemic lupus erythematosus
6. Other
   a) Subacute infarcts
   b) Resolving hematoma
   c) Cavernous hemangioma
   d) Radiation necrosis
   e) Aneurysm with central thrombus
   f) Postoperative change

6.16.3 Radiologic features

No single feature is pathognomonic, although a cystic lesion that markedly restricts centrally (the fluid component) on DWI of MRI should be considered an abscess until proven otherwise. Many features of the lesion as well as clinical presentation and patient demographics need to be taken together to help narrow the differential.

Helpful rules of thumb include:

1. Enhancing wall characteristics
   a) Thick and nodular favors neoplasm
   b) Thin and regular favors abscess
   c) Incomplete ring often opened toward the cortex favors demyelination
   d) Intermediate to low T2 signal capsule favors abscess
   e) Restricted diffusion of enhancing wall favors GBM or demyelination
2. Surrounding edema
   a) Extensive edema relative to lesion size favors abscess
   b) Increased perfusion favors neoplasm (metastases or primary cerebral malignancy)
3. Central fluid content
   a) Restricted diffusion favors abscess
   b) Absence of diffusion restriction favors a tumor with a central necrotic component (classically a metastasis)
4. Number of lesions
   a) Similar size rounded lesions at grey–white junction favor metastases or abscess
   b) Irregular mass with adjacent secondary lesions embedded in the same region of "edema" favors GBM
   c) Small (< 1–2 cm) lesions with thin walls, especially if other calcific foci are present, suggest neurocysticercosis

Garg RK, Sinha MK. Multiple ring-enhancing lesions of the brain. J Postgrad Med 2010; 56(4):307–316

Smirniotopoulos JG, Murphy FM, Rushing EJ, Rees JH, Schroeder JW. Patterns of contrast enhancement in the brain and meninges. Radiographics 2007; 27(2):525–551

Hartmann M, Jansen O, Heiland S, Sommer C, Münkel K, Sartor K. Restricted diffusion within ring enhancement is not pathognomonic for brain abscess. AJNR Am J Neuroradiol 2001; 22(9):1738–1742

6.17 Tumoral Hemorrhage

Intratumoral hemorrhage is suspected under clinical circumstances such as in patients who have known malignancy, in elderly non-hypertensive persons, and in patients who had progressive symptoms before the hemorrhage ictus.

Hemorrhage has been noted in about 1% of brain tumors, whereas underlying tumors have been reported up to 10% of cases with intracranial hemorrhage.

Metastatic lesions are usually seen as well-defined, round masses located around the gray–white junction and demonstrate contrast enhancement and moderate edema. Hemorrhagic metastases are usually seen as areas of high signal intensity on T1-WI and T2-WI with a relative absence of hemosiderin deposition. Brain tumors associated with hemorrhage include:

1. Primary brain tumors
   a) Malignant astrocytoma
      i. Anaplastic astrocytoma
      ii. GBM
         Of the adult gliomas, GBM is the most common to have intratumoral hemorrhage and subarachnoid seeding.
   b) Oligodendroglioma (neurocytoma)
      Although the intraventricular neurocytomas have a more benign course, they hemorrhage more frequent than oligodendrogliomas, which may suggest that diagnosis.
   c) Meningioma
   d) Pituitary adenoma
   e) Hemangioblastoma
   f) Acoustic neurinoma
   g) Lymphomas (hemorrhage is rare in lymphomas)
2. Metastatic brain tumors
   a) Lung cancer
      Bronchial carcinomas spread to the CNS in 30% of cases; the oat cell carcinoma is the most frequent, whereas the squamous carcinoma is the least frequent subtype to metastasize to the brain.
   b) Breast cancer
      It is estimated that 18–30% of patients with breast cancer will develop brain metastases.
   c) Malignant melanoma
      Third most common neoplasm with a propensity for metastatic spread to the brain after lung and breast cancer.
   d) Renal cell carcinoma
   e) Thyroid cancer
   f) Gastrointestinal primary tumors
   g) Choriocarcinoma
   h) Retinoblastoma

Zeng C, Tang S, Jiang Y, Xiong X, Zhou S. Seven patients diagnosed as intracranial hemorrhage combined with intracranial tumor: case description and literature review. Int J Clin Exp Med 2015; 8(10): 19621–19625

Rumboldt Z, et al. Brain Imaging with MRI and CT: An image Pattern Approach. Cambridge University Press; 2012

6.18 Brain Metastasis

Approximately 60% of patients with brain metastases have subacute symptoms. Symptoms are usually related to the location of the tumor. About 85% of the lesions are in the cerebrum, 15% are in the cerebellum, and 5% are in the brain stem. Morning headaches with nausea and vomiting along with papilledema are suggestive of intracranial hypertension. Features such as headache, nuchal rigidity, and photophobia indicate meninges involvement. The timing of the onset of these symptoms is subacute rather than acute.

Acute onset of symptoms suggests vascular or electrical etiology such as bleeding or seizure. Dementia and cognitive deficits of a gradual onset most likely indicate a demyelination problem, radiation necrosis. Paraneoplastic syndromes include limbic encephalopathy and cerebellar degeneration. The latter is commonly associated with ovarian cancer. Progressive weight loss and general fatigue can be ominous and highly suggestive of recurrent systemic cancer. Similarly, neurologic problems such as polyneuropathy or myopathy can be sinister.

A known history of systemic cancer and the presence of multiple lesions on MRI make the diagnosis of metastatic brain tumor probable. Even a typical scan only suggests, but does not prove, that the lesion is a brain metastasis and not another lesion, like a primary brain tumor or a cerebral abscess. The stereotactic needle biopsy is required to make the diagnosis definitive.

6.18.1 Differential diagnosis

1. Primary brain tumors
   a) Meningioma
      Meningiomas show a homogeneous contrast enhancement, relative lack of peritumoral edema, and attachment to the dura. Metastatic cancers may also arise from the dura, and can even be supplied by the external carotid artery, making the distinction between metastasis and meningioma impossible except by biopsy. If the neurologic symptoms have developed very slowly or if the MRI suggests a lesion neighboring the falx or the inner skull table, the diagnosis is in favor of a meningioma. One should also bear in mind that breast cancer may metastasize to a meningioma.
   b) Astrocytoma
      Brain metastasis presents as a spherical mass, whereas primary gliomas are usually irregular, and present finger-like extensions of contrast-enhancing tumor running along white matter tracts and bundles.
   c) Primary brain lymphoma
      Often present as uniform, multiple, periventricular lesions on MRI with irregular and indiscrete margins.

- d) Acoustic neurinoma and pituitary adenoma
  Almost impossible to distinguish from metastatic brain tumors in the same areas.
2. Vascular disorders
   - a) Cerebral infarction
     Acute infarctions do not enhance and MRI findings may be entirely normal for 24–48 hours after the event. Contrast enhancement of the pial surface of the overlying cortical gyri develops 1–3 weeks after the ictus, unlike the ring-like enhancing lesion of a brain metastasis. Several weeks postictal, the contrast enhancement in an infarct diminished and gradually disappears, and the ischemic area becomes hypointense.
   - b) Cerebral hemorrhage
     Acute hemorrhage is hyperdense on a plain CT scan, but may show normal on MRI. Contrast enhancement 3–6 weeks postictal demonstrates an isodense clot with a ring enhancement, resembling a metastasis or an abscess. Early enhancement suggests tumoral hemorrhage.
3. Infections
   Cerebral abscess occurs usually in patients with depressed immunity and particularly in those suffering from Hodgkin's disease and other lymphomas, conditions in which brain abscesses are more common than metastatic brain tumors.
   - a) Toxoplasma abscess is the most common parasitic CNS infection and has a predilection to lodge in the basal ganglia as a single mass.
   - b) Multiple nocardia abscesses develop in 50% of the immunosuppressed patients with nocardia pulmonary infection.
   - c) Progressive multifocal leukoencephalopathy (PML)
     An infection of the oligodendrocytes caused by the JC papovavirus, affecting patients with depressed cellular immunity from lymphoma or chronic lymphocytic leukemia or prolonged chemotherapy.
     Differential features:
     - i. CT scanning and MRI help to identify brain abscesses. The enhancing ring of an abscess is generally thinner and more uniform than the ring of a tumor. The capsule of an abscess is characteristically thicker near the cortex, where oxygenation is better, and somewhat thinner near the ventricular surface.
     - ii. With suspected toxoplasma abscesses, a therapeutic trial with sulfadiazine and pyrimethamine has a rapid response and by that the diagnosis is established without biopsy. With other suspected abscesses, stereotactically directed needle biopsy performed early in the diagnostic work-up establishes both the diagnosis and reveals the involved organism for the appropriate antibiotic therapy.

      iii. CT and MRI in PML reveal multifocal, punched-out lesions of the white matter, no mass effect and usually no contrast enhancement. Nonenhancing lymphomas may be similar. A definitive diagnosis is secured only by biopsy.

4. Radiation necrosis

   CT and MRI reveal hypodense or isodense ring-enhancing brain lesion surrounded by edema. Differentiation between radiation necrosis and recurrent brain metastases in a patient previously irradiated for a brain metastasis may be impossible without needle biopsy.

5. Methotrexate leukoencephalopathy

   This will cause bilateral white matter lesions and ventricular enlargement. These lesions present a decreased density on CT scanning and hyperintense on T2-WI MR without enhancement, a feature that distinguishes it from a brain metastasis.

6. Multiple sclerosis

   MS lesions may be single or multiple and contrast enhancing, which makes them indistinguishable from brain tumors. MS lesions, however, do not enhance after 6–8 weeks, and other new nonenhancing lesions may be present, something unlikely with brain metastases.

7. Miscellaneous

   Transient changes in CT or MRI sometimes follow focal or generalized epilepsy in the absence of underlying primary or metastatic brain tumor. These lesions disappear within a few weeks after control of seizures.

Stark AM, Eichmann T, Mehdorn HM. Skull metastases: clinical features, differential diagnosis, and review of the literature. Surg Neurol 2003; 60(3):219–225, discussion 225–226

Fink KR, Fink JR. Imaging of brain metastases. Surg Neurol Int 2013; 4(Suppl 4):S209–S219

Szu G, Milano E, Johnson C, Hgeier L. Detection of brain metastases: comparison of contrast-enhanced MR with unenhanced MR and enhanced CT. AJNR Am J Neuroradiol 1990; 11:785–791

6.19 Subarachnoid Space Metastases

Between 6 and 18% of CNS metastases involve the arachnoid/subarachnoid space, pia, or both. The subarachnoid space can be diffusely or focally involved by spread from a primary CNS tumor or by an extraneural malignancy. The typical locations of the seedings are identified at the basal cisterns, CPA cistern, the suprasellar cisterns, along the course of cranial nerves, and over the convexities. Subtle leptomeningeal and subarachnoid space metastatic disease is identified up to 45% by the contrast-enhanced MRI scans. CSF cytology provides definitive diagnosis of leptomeningeal carcinomatosis, with abnormal CSF noted in up to 55% of cases after the first spinal tap and in up to 90% after the third. When the lumbar puncture is contraindicated or the CSF cytology is equivocal, the MRI with gadolinium is a useful diagnostic tool.

6.19.1 Sources of subarachnoid metastases

1. Children
   a) Primary brain tumors
      i. Primary neuroectodermal tumors (PNET)
         - Medulloblastoma
         - Ependymoblastoma
      ii. Pineal tumors (germinoma, pineoblastoma)
      iii. Choroid plexus carcinoma
   b) Primary extracranial tumors
      i. Neuroblastoma
      ii. Lymphoma
      iii. Leukemia
2. Adults
   a) Primary brain tumors
      i. GBM/anaplastic astrocytoma
      ii. Oligodendroglioma
      iii. Primary lymphoma
   b) Primary extracranial tumors
      i. Lung cancer
      ii. Breast cancer
      iii. Malignant melanoma
      iv. Gastrointestinal carcinoma
      v. Ovary
      vi. Lymphoma
      vii. Leukemia

6.19.2 Differential diagnosis

1. Cranial meningeal carcinomatosis
2. Meningitis
   a) Acute bacterial meningitis
   b) Chronic meningitis (Fungal and granulomatous meningitis)
      Chronic meningitides have a predilection to invade the basal cisterns.
      i. Tuberculous meningitis
      ii. Coccidioidomycosis imitans meningitis
      iii. Cryptococcus neoformans meningitis
      iv. Neurocysticercosis
3. Noninfectious inflammatory diseases
   a) Sarcoidosis
4. Lymphoma
5. Leukemia

6. Posttraumatic basal cranial adhesions
7. Intrathecal chemotherapy/radiation
8. Idiopathic pachymeningitis

Atlas SC. Magnetic Resonance Imaging of the Brain and Spine. 4th ed. Wolters Kluwer Lippincott; 2009
Haber-Gattuso-Spitz-David: Differential Diagnosis in Surgical Pathology. Saunders; 2002

6.20 Hyperprolactinemia

Hyperprolactinemia in women leads to amenorrhea, galactorrhea, and osteoporosis, while in men it may result in diminished sexual drive and impotence or it may be asymptomatic.

The degree of hyperprolactinemia is directly related to the functionality of the prolactin-secreting tumor. Serum prolactin levels greater than 200 ng/ml correlate well with the presence of a prolactinoma. Normal prolactin levels range from 1–20 ng/ml in men, and 1–25 ng/ml in women.

6.20.1 Differential diagnosis

1. Nonpathologic causes
   a) Pregnancy
   b) Early nursing periods
   c) Nipple stimulation
   d) Coitus
   e) Sleep
   f) Stress
   g) Exercise
2. Diseases
   a) True prolactinomas
   b) Pituitary traumatic stalk section
   c) Pituitary stalk compression from chromophobe macroadenomas
   d) Empty sella syndrome
   e) Hypothalamic disorders
      i. Tumors (e.g., craniopharyngiomas)
      ii. Histiocytosis X
      iii. Sarcoidosis
   f) Primary hypothyroidism
   g) Chiari–Frommel syndrome
   h) Renal failure
   i) Liver cirrhosis

3. Drugs
   a) Dopamine antagonists (e.g., phenothiazine-like drugs)
   b) Reserpine
      i. α-methyl
      ii. dopa
   c) Opiate derivatives (e.g., Morphine)
   d) Prostaglandin F2α
   e) Thyrotropin-releasing hormone
   f) Estrogens

Serri O, Chik CL, Ur E, Ezzat S. Diagnosis and management of hyperprolactinemia. CMAJ 2003; 169(6):575–581
Jameson JL, De Groot LG, et al. Endocrinology: Adult and Pediatric. 7th ed. Elsevier; 2015

7 Demyelinating Disease and Brain Atrophy

7.1 Multiple Sclerosis

(Synonym: Disseminated sclerosis)

Multiple sclerosis (MS) is a chronic inflammatory autoimmune disease of unknown etiology that involves demyelination of the central nervous system (CNS) with resultant neurologic dysfunction. The clinical manifestations are extremely variable in type and severity. Its onset is usually between 10 and 59 years (between 20 and 40 years approximately for 70% of patients). Prevalence is higher in Caucasians/Northern Europeans with female-to-male ratio of 2:1.

Most cases are sporadic; 25% concordance rate in monozygotic twin studies and studies of first-degree relatives (children of patients with MS have 30 to 50 times increased risk). Risk factors that are considered are the temperate latitudes, the family history, and the female preponderance.

MS is associated with conditions such as optic neuritis, trigeminal neuralgia, Bell's palsy, uveitis, transverse myelitis, and Devic's syndrome.

The clinical course of MS:
1. In 20% of patients with MS, the disease has a benign clinical course.
2. In 30% patients, the disease is relapsing (loss or deterioration of a neurologic function) and remitting (return to or toward normal function).
3. In other 50% patients, the disease is primarily progressive and secondarily progressive with relapse.

MS is sometimes classified as *clinically* definite, *laboratory* supported, probable, and possible depending on the history of attacks, signs on examination, and laboratory abnormalities (MRI, oligoclonal banding) supporting the diagnosis.

In the absence of a pathognomonic biomarker, MS remains a *clinical diagnosis*. An abnormal MRI without convincing clinical symptoms or signs cannot be used to make the diagnosis. Conversely, a normal MRI of the brain and spinal cord with a compatible history or examination *does not* exclude the diagnosis.

The laboratory tests are useful for diagnosing MS in the proper setting and with proper caution. The diagnosis of MD is seldom made without some laboratory support, especially in patients who do not quite meet all of the clinical criteria. However, no one test proves the diagnosis, and all laboratory data have sufficient problems with sensitivity and specificity to impair their usefulness.

Prospective studies have shown that two factors most reliably identify patients who *do not have* MS. The first is their lack of typical symptoms: no optic neuritis, Lhermitte's sign, sensory level, neurogenic bladder, or other common deficits. The second is their lack of typical findings on MRI and cerebrospinal fluid (CSF) examination. Very few patients with MS have a normal MRI of the brain or normal CSF.

When to doubt the clinical diagnosis of MS:
1. Dementia
2. Aphasia
3. Seizure
4. Pain (except trigeminal neuralgia)
5. Movement disorders

7.1.1 Symptoms and signs of MS

Any symptom/sign appropriate to a lesion in more than one area of CNS (brain and spinal cord) may raise the suspicion for MS. Gray matter signs, such as seizures and altered mental state, occur rarely.

Common symptoms of MS are as follows:
1. Sensory (numbness, tingling, heaviness in an extremity, sensory level)
2. Visual (visual loss, color vision change, field defects)
3. Brain stem (diplopia, dizziness, difficulty swallowing or speaking)
4. Motor (weakness, spasticity, cramping)
5. Bowel and bladder dysfunction: urinary urgency and incontinence
   The usual bladder dysfunction is sphincter dyssynergia: simultaneous contraction of the urinary bladder detrusor smooth muscle and the voluntary muscles of the pelvic floor.
6. cerebellar (ataxia of gait or of an extremity)
7. Cognitive complaints
8. Fatigue (midday loss of energy unrelated to other MS signs or symptoms)

Following are the common signs:
1. Corticospinal tract (weakness, spasticity, hyperreflexia, asymmetric reflexes, Babinski sign)
2. Sensory (vibration loss, decreased pin sense, sensory level, Lhermitte's sign which is an electric sensation descending the vertebrae with neck flexion. In addition to MS, another cause of this is cervical stenosis or other mechanical irritation to posterior column)
3. Brain stem (nystagmus, internuclear ophthalmoplegia. Internuclear ophthalmoplegia (INO) [Inability to adduct the eye with voluntary lateral gaze, but with preservation of adduction on convergence], facial weakness)
4. Optic nerve (loss of visual acuity, central scotomas, loss of color vision, optic nerve atrophy, afferent papillary defect/Marcus Gunn pupil, optic disc appearance: Pink, swollen with indistinct margin if papilla is involved; normal if involvement is retrobulbar. In optic atrophy pallor especially temporal area, distinct margin.)

5. Charcot's triad (intention tremor, nystagmus, scanning speech)
6. Uhthoff's phenomenon (worsening of symptoms and signs after exposure to heat or exercise)

7.1.2 Differential diagnosis

1. **Postinfectious encephalomyelitis**
   This is a subacute syndrome caused by autoimmune response or a viral infection. Patients complain of acute or subacute onset of gait abnormalities, confusion, disorientation, problems with bladder or bowel control, muscle weakness, and other symptoms. Abnormalities consistent with demyelinating lesions can be seen on MRI. This condition may or may not be reversible. Typically, however, it presents itself as a monophasic illness, but chronic cases do occur and require long-term treatment.

2. **Primary CNS vasculitis**
   Primary CNS vasculitis may result in syndromes resembling MS. Most notable symptoms include severe headaches, confusion, and sudden stroke-like episodes. High protein levels can be seen in CSF, as well as high erythrocyte sedimentation rate (ESR). Patients may have abnormal angiogram of cerebral vessels. Antinuclear or antiphospholipid antibodies may be present. Patients with vasculitis-related disorders, such as meningovascular syphilis, Sjogren's syndrome, lupus erythematosus, Bechet's disease, Wagener's granulomatosis, and isolated CNS vasculitis, may present with an MS-like picture. Asking about the features of the systemic disease and watching for atypical MRI or clinical appearance are helpful in diagnosis.

3. **Lyme disease and brucellosis**
   Sometimes infections of the CNS may present like MS, but usually they have a different CSF and clinical picture. Lyme disease is known to cause intermittent neurologic events. Some of the most frequent problems include Bell's palsy, nonspecific symptoms of numbness, fatigue, and amnesia. CSF findings may resemble those found in the MS and MRI may show a white matter disease. History of tick bites, rashes (erythema chronicum migrans), and arthralgia should be sought after. Screening for Lyme titer and/or a Lyme polymerase chain reaction (PCR) in the CSF or blood should help in diagnosis; predominantly axonal neuropathy on electromyography (EMG).

4. **Systemic lupus erythematosus (SLE)**
   This condition may cause multiple neurologic pathology such as optic abnormalities, encephalopathy, transverse myelitis, and strokes. One needs

to look for systemic abnormalities, such as elevated antinuclear antibody (ANA), leukopenia, hematuria, elevated ESR. On some occasions, lupus erythematosus and MS may be found in the same patient.

5. **Tropical spastic paraparesis**
It is a retroviral disease caused by human T-cell leukemia virus (HTLV)-1 virus. It is uncommon in the continental United States, but may be seen infrequently in patients who reside for some time around the Caribbean Sea Basin. The major clinical manifestations are progressive spastic paraparesis or generalized white matter disease.

6. **Bechet's syndrome**
This syndrome can result in MRI findings that are very similar to MS. However, the main distinguishing features of this condition are oral and genital ulcers, and uveitis, as well as possible involvement of lungs, joints, intestines, and heart. This group of patients may present with either quadriparesis, pseudobulbar palsy, cranial neuropathy, cerebellar ataxia or cerebral venous thrombosis.

7. **Sarcoidosis and Sjogren's syndrome**
Sarcoidosis and Sjogren's syndrome may show lesions on MRI that resemble those found in MS. These are autoimmune conditions that affect multiple organ systems and should not be confused with MS. A chest X-ray may show granulomatous disease of the lungs, and meningeal enhancement is seen in patients with CNS involvement. Oligoclonal bands and IgG are raised in CSF of patients with sarcoidosis; peripheral facial palsy is common; reduced glucose is seen in CSF. CNS involvement and the course of the disease may show striking similarity to MS. Angiotensin-converting enzyme determination may be used for further differential diagnosis. It may be elevated in either serum or CSF but it is not reliably abnormal.

8. **Vitamin B-12 deficiency and tertiary syphilis**
Vitamin B-12 deficiency and tertiary syphilis may result in dorsal column abnormalities and dementia. These two conditions need to be ruled out when patients present with the abovementioned symptoms as their chief complaints. Serum and CSF VDRL test and the reflex loss in tabes dorsalis are discriminating features of neurosyphilis.

9. **Leukodystrophies of adulthood**
Leukodystrophies of adulthood (metachromatic leukodystrophy, Krabbe disease, and adrenal leukodystrophy) show large areas of involvement on the MRI scan where no normal white matter can be found.

10. **Spinocerebellar degenerations**
These are hereditary degenerative disorders (olivopontocerebellar degeneration, spinocerebellar degeneration, etc.). Pedigree analysis; insidiously

progressive course; progressive involvement; atrophy without demyelination. Initially may resemble chronic-progressive MS. However, characteristic white matter lesions on the MRI scan are usually absent and the CSF is normal in these patients.

11. **Progressive multifocal leukoencephalopathy**
    CT and MRI lesions are nonenhancing; no oligoclonal banding; prominent dementia and aphasia; underlying immunosuppression always present (e.g., HIV, post-transplantation chemotherapy). HIV antibody positive; subcortical dementia; diffuse subcortical gray and white matter involvement on MRI.

12. **Compressive myelopathy**
    Revealed by MRI of spinal cord and craniovertebral junction (e.g., cervical spondylosis, Chiari malformations). Lower motor neuron signs in upper limbs, lower cranial nerve palsies.

13. **Intracranial tumors (gliomas, lymphomas)**
    Course gradually increasing in severity; recurrent seizures; normal evoked responses or lumbar puncture.

14. **Craniocervical-junction anomalies**

15. **Central pontine myelinolysis**
    Dysarthria; dysphagia; ophthalmoparesis; quadriparesis; rapidly corrected hyponatremia.

16. **Motor neuron disease**
    Lower motor neuron signs; abnormal EMGs; cerebral, sensory, or sphincter involvement against this diagnosis.

17. **Inborn errors of myelin metabolism**
    Usually presenting in childhood.
    a) Metachromatic leukodystrophy, a deficiency of the enzyme aryl sulfatase
    b) Adrenoleukodystrophy, a defect in metabolism of very-long-chain fatty acids
    c) Krabbe globoid leukodystrophy, a deficiency of the enzyme galactosyl-ceramidase

18. **Psychiatric disease**
    By far the most important disease confused with MS is psychiatric illness (45–76%). Most patients referred to a neurologist for a possible MS who do not have the disease instead suffer from some of psychiatric disorder: somatization, hypochondriasis, malingering, depression, anxiety or similar problems. There are seven conditions that account for almost all the alternative diagnoses at three MS centers in the United States as listed in the following table.

Conditions that account for almost all the alternative diagnoses at three MS centers in the United States

Disorder	Colorado (N = 139)	Dalhousie (N = 2)	Marshfield (N = 70)
Psychiatric disease	63 (45%)	14 (27%)	53 (76%)
Migraine headaches	29 (21%)	7 (14%)	2 (3%)
Stroke or TIA	7 (5%)	3 (6%)	2 (3%)
Peripheral neuropathy	6 (4%)	3 (6%)	1 (1%)
Cervical stenosis	4 (3%)	1 (2%)	1 (1%)
Benign sensory symptoms	0	11 (22%)	8 (11%)
Vertigo	0	3 (6%)	0

Abbreviation: TIA, transient ischemic attack.

Katzan I, Rudick RA. Guidelines to avoid errors in the diagnosis of multiple sclerosis Ann Neurol 1996;40:554
Rolak LA. The diagnosis of multiple sclerosis. Neurol Clin 1996;14(1):27–43
Rolak LA, Fleming JO. The differential diagnosis of multiple sclerosis. Neurologist 2007;13(2):57–72

7.1.3 Differential diagnosis based on the pathogenesis of MS

1. Autoimmune
   a) SLE
   b) Sjogren's syndrome
   c) Bechet's syndrome
   d) Neurosarcoidosis
   e) Chronic inflammatory demyelinating polyneuropathy
   f) Antiphospholipid antibody syndrome
   g) Hashimoto autoimmune encephalopathy
2. Genetic disorders
   a) Hereditary spinocerebellar ataxia
   b) Hereditary paraplegia
   c) Leber's optic atrophy and other mitochondrial cytopathies
3. Infections
   a) HIV-related myelopathy
   b) Lyme disease
   c) Meningovascular syphilis
   d) Viral myelitis
   e) Progressive multifocal leukoencephalopathy (PML)
   f) Postinfectious (postvaccination) encephalomyelitis

g) Subacute sclerosing panencephalitis

h) Whipple's disease

4. Metabolic and nutritional
   a) Vitamin B12 deficiency
   b) Leukodystrophies (metachromatic leukodystrophy, adrenoleukodystrophy and globoid cell (Krabbe's disease), and Pelizaeus–Merzbacher disease)
   c) Reversible posterior leukoencephalopathy
   d) Central pontine and extrapontine myelinolysis

5. MS-related
   a) Acute disseminated encephalomyelitis (ADEM)
   b) Optic neuritis
   c) Transverse myelitis
   d) Devic's syndrome (neuromyelitis optica)

6. Neoplastic
   a) Primary CNS lymphoma
   b) Spinal cord tumors
   c) Paraneoplastic syndromes (limbic and brainstem encephalitis, progressive spasticity, and dementia associated with anti-amphiphysin antibodies)
   d) Posterior fossa/foramen magnum neoplasms
   e) Gliomatosis cerebri
   f) Chemotherapy and radiation-induced CNS syndromes

7. Posterior fossa/spinal cord
   a) Chiari malformations
   b) Cervical spondylotic myelopathy (important in differential diagnosis with progressive MS)

8. Psychiatric disorders
   a) Conversion reaction
   b) Malingering

9. Vascular
   a) CNS vasculitis (e.g., periarteritis nodosa, primary CNS angiitis, drug-induced and infection-associated vasculitis, retinocochlear vasculopathy of Susac)
   b) Spinal and brainstem arteriovenous malformations
   c) Cavernous hemangiomas
   d) Moyamoya vasculopathy
   e) Thromboembolic stroke
   f) Cerebral autosomal dominant arteriopathy with subcortical infarcts and leukoencephalopathy (CADASIL)
   g) Takayasu disease
   h) Carotid and vertebral artery dissection

7.1.4 Laboratory diagnostic procedures for MS

There is no definitive laboratory test that is conclusive for MS.

1. Blood studies: (to exclude other disorders)
   a) ANA (can be positive in low titer in up to 80% of MS patients)
   b) Anti-SSA antibody (if sicca symptoms)
   c) HLTV-1 antibody (if spastic paraparesis appears)
   d) Vitamin B-12 level
   e) Fluorescent treponemal antibody absorption (FTA-ABS) test
   f) Serum Lyme antibody titer
2. CSF studies: If cranial MRI findings are not typical or diagnostic, CSF examination may provide additional support for diagnosis of MS.
   a) WBC: normal or slight lymphocytosis (< 50 cell/mm)
   b) Total protein should be normal or mildly increased in 25% of patients (> 54 mg/dl)
   c) Protein electrophoresis:
      i. Two or more oligoclonal bands (OCBs) in CSF, *in the absence* of corresponding serum OCBs. OCBs are not directed against specific antigens and are not involved in pathogenesis of disease. They are present in 30–40% of possible and 90–97% of definitive MS patients. OCBs are also observed in other chronic inflammatory diseases of the CNS, in infectious disorders, and in 7% normal controls.
      ii. Elevated IgG index (CSF IgG/CSF albumin)/(serum IgG/serum albumin) reflects activation of immune cells within CNS, present in 80% with definite MS (values > 0.68 support the diagnosis).
      iii. Increased IgG synthesis rate (> 3 mg/day)
      iv. Kappa light chains
      v. The sensitivity of these tests is improved during acute exacerbations
   d) The appearance of the CSF and the opening pressure are normal
      Differential diagnosis of increased CSF IgG:
      i. Guillain–Barre and other inflammatory neuropathies
      ii. CNS neoplasms
      iii. CNS lupus, sarcoidosis, Behcet's disease
      iv. Subacute sclerosing panencephalitis
      v. Encephalitides
      vi. Fungal meningitis
3. Neuroimaging
   a) *Cranial CT scan* is not sensitive enough to detect most MS lesions.
   b) *MRI* is the most powerful diagnostic tool. It shows abnormalities in 90% of patients with clinically definite MS, 60–70% probable MS, 30–50% possible MS.

Cranial MRI: Common locations include periventricular white (Dawson's fingers), corpus callosum, tapetum, brain stem, and spinal cord (especially posterior cervical cord). Active lesions tend to enhance with gadolinium. Characteristic lesions are ovoid, multifocal, and of varying ages (and intensities). Serial MRI scans can be useful to demonstrate dissemination in time by the appearance of new T2 (and proton density) or gadolinium-enhancing lesions at least 3 months after an initial scan without a second clinical exacerbation.

T2-weighted lesions are nonspecific and can be related to edema, inflammation, demyelination, gliosis, remyelination, or axonal loss. T1-weighted lesions without gadolinium enhancement ("black holes") are more specifically indicative of axonal loss or gliosis and correlate better with physical disability measures. (+)

Spinal MRI (cervical and/or thoracic levels): It is useful to rule out compressive lesions in cases of myelopathic presentation and may show either cord hypersensitivities when cranial MRI is not diagnostic, or cord atrophy in chronic cases. Fluid-attenuated inversion recovery (FLAIR) images enhance T2 lesion resolution, especially in the spinal cord. The contribution of myelin loss versus axonal loss to brain atrophy in MS is not differentiated by current MRI measures.

4. Neurophysiologic tests

Evoked potentials identify clinically silent white matter lesions and document dissemination in space (e.g., whether different parts of the CNS are affected). Patients may have significant defects along visual evoked response (VER), somatosensory evoked response (SSER), and brainstem auditory evoked response (BAERs) pathways without clinical symptoms or signs. In uncooperative patients and patients in whom MRI cannot be performed (e.g., due to pacemaker), measuring evoked potentials is an alternative. The sensitivity of evoked potential testing is high but its specificity is low.

Visual evoked potentials (VEP) are the most helpful; these record the electrical response from the visual cortex in the occipital lobe. Normally, a response appears approximately 100 milliseconds after the stimulus is presented to the eye, and a delay implies demyelination in the visual pathways.

VEPs are abnormal in approximately 40, 60, and 85% of possible, probable, and definite MS patients, respectively. Somatosensory evoked potentials (SSEPs) are abnormal in approximately 50, 70, and 80% of possible, probable, and definite MS patients, respectively. BAERs are abnormal in approximately 30, 40, and 70% of possible, probable, and definite MS patients, respectively (see the following table).

Wallace CJ, Sevick RJ. Multifocal white matter lesions. Semin Ultrasound CT MR 1996;17(3):251–264

Francis GS, Evans AC, Arnold DL. Neuroimaging in multiple sclerosis. Neurol Clin 1995;13(1):147–171

Gronseth GS, Ashman EJ. Practice parameter: the usefulness of evoked potentials in identifying clinically silent lesions in patients with suspected multiple sclerosis (an evidence-based review): Report of the Quality Standards Subcommittee of the American Academy of Neurology. Neurology 2000;54(9): 1720–1725

Lee KH, Hashimoto SA, Hodge JP, et al. MRI of the head in the diagnosis of multiple sclerosis. A prospective 2-year follow-up with comparison with clinical evaluation, evoked potentials, oligoclonal banding, and CT. Neurology 1991;41:657–660

7.1.5 Diagnostic criteria for MS

Clinical presentation	Additional data needed
= / > attacks (relapses)	None; clinical evidence will suffice (additional evidence desirable but must be consistent with MS)
= / > objective clinical lesions	
= / > attacks 1 objective clinical lesion	Dissemination in space demonstrated by MRI **OR** Positive CSF and = / > MRI lesions consistent with MS, **OR** Further clinical attack involving different site
1 attack = / > objective clinical lesions	Dissemination in time demonstrated by MRI **OR** Second clinical attack
1 attack 1 objective clinical lesion (monosymptomatic presentation)	Dissemination in space demonstrated by MRI **OR** positive CSF and = / > 2 MRI lesions consistent With MS **AND** Dissemination in time demonstrated by MRI **OR** Second clinical attack
Insidious neurologic progression Suggestive of MS (primary progressive MS)	Positive CSF **AND** Dissemination in space demonstrated my MRI Evidence of = / > T2 brain lesions, **OR** = / > spinal cord lesions, **OR** 4–8 brain and 1 spinal cord lesion, **OR** positive VEP with 4–8 MRI lesions, **OR** positive VEP with 4–8 brain lesions + 1 spinal cord lesion **AND** Dissemination in time demonstrated by MRI **OR** Continued progression for 1 year

Source: McDonald WI, Compston A, Edan G, etal. Recommended diagnostic criteria for multiple sclerosis: guidelines from the International Panel on the diagnosis of multiple sclerosis. Ann Neurol 2001;50(1)1:121–127

McDonald criteria for definite MS

The McDonald criteria make use of the clinical presentation and the advances of MRI.

When a patient presents with two or more attacks with clinical evidence of two or more neurological deficits, there is no need for additional requirements to make the diagnosis of MS, because there is dissemination in place and time (▶ Fig. 7.1).

In all other cases (less than two attacks or less than two clinical lesions), there is a role for MRI to fulfil the diagnostic criteria be demonstrating dissemination in space (DIS), in time, or both.

The McDonald criteria are very specific, because if you want to use MRI for the diagnosis of MS, you have to make sure that the patient really has MS.

For dissemination in space (DIS), lesions in two out of four typical areas of the CNS are required:

- Periventricular
- Juxtocortical
- Infratentorial
- Spinal cord

For dissemination in time (DIT), there are two possibilities:

- New T2 and/or gadolinium-enhancing lesion(s) on follow-up MRI, with reference to a baseline scan, irrespective of the timing of the baseline MRI.
- Simultaneous presence of asymptomatic gadolinium-enhancing and nonenhancing lesions at any time.

Schumacher criteria for definite MS

1. Two separate CNS symptoms
2. Two separate attacks—onset of symptoms is separated by at least 1 month
3. Symptoms must involve the white matter
4. Age 10–50 (although usually 20–40)
5. Objective deficits are present on the neurologic examination
6. No other medical problem can be found to explain the patient's condition

The key to the Schumacher criteria for the clinical diagnosis of MS is the first two features, i.e., two separate symptoms at two separate times or lesions disseminated in space and in time.

Noseworthy JH, Lucchinetti C, Rodriguez M, Weinshenker BG. Multiple sclerosis. N Engl J Med 2000;343(13): 938–952

Lucchinetti C, Brück W, Noseworthy J. Multiple sclerosis: recent developments in neuropathology, pathogenesis, magnetic resonance imaging studies and treatment. Curr Opin Neurol 2001;14(3):259–269

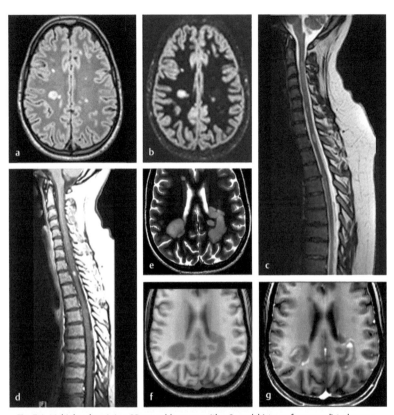

Fig. 7.1 Multiple sclerosis in a 22-year-old woman with a 6-week history of sensory disturbances in her right arm. No other symptoms were present. CSF was positive for oligoclonal bands. **(a)** Axial FLAIR sequence of the brain demonstrates multiple hyperintense lesions. **(b)** Axial DIR sequence of the brain. The lesions are depicted in higher contrast. **(c)** Sagittal T2w image of the cervical spine demonstrates multiple hyperintense lesions. Each of the lesions spans no more than one vertebral body height. **(d)** Sagittal T1w sequence after contrast administration. Individual lesions show marked enhancement. (Reproduced from Intramedullary Space. In: Forsting M, Jansen O, ed. MR Neuroimaging: Brain, Spine, Peripheral Nerves. 1st edition. Thieme; 2016.) Multifocal large confluent lesions demonstrating T2-hyperintensity **(e)**, T1-hypointensity **(f)**, and heterogeneous enhancement **(g)** in the periventricular white matter bilaterally. **(h)** The susceptibility-weighted image demonstrates the normal periventricular white matter venules (arrows) crossing through these confluent active MS plaques, a finding not usually seen with brain neoplasms. (Reproduced from Case 86. In: Tsiouris A, Sanelli P, Comunale J, ed. Case-Based Brain Imaging. 2nd edition. Thieme; 2013.) Tumefactive demyelinating lesions (TDLs). TDLs are demyelinating lesions > 2 cm in diameter, frequently showing mass effect and surrounding edema. (*Continued*)

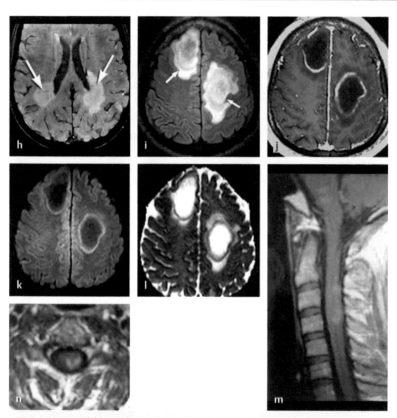

Fig 7.1 *(Continued)* **(i)** Axial fluid-attenuated inversion recovery image show two examples (arrows). **(j)** Axial enhanced T1-weighted image shows the enhancing edges that represent areas of increased inflammatory activity. **(k)** The lesion periphery frequently shows restricted water diffusion, with hyperintensity on diffusion weighted imaging **(l)** and hypointensity on the apparent diffusion coefficient map. (Reproduced from Diffusion Weighted Imaging and Diffusion Tensor Imaging in Demyelinating Diseases. In: Leite C, Castillo M, ed. Diffusion Weighted and Diffusion Tensor Imaging. A Clinical Guide. 1st edition. Thieme; 2015.) **(l)** Sagittal T1-weighted MRI of the cervical spinal cord following the administration of gadolinium-DTPA in a patient with acute multiple sclerosis showing slight enhancement at the C2-C3 level. There is virtually no widening of the spinal cord. **(m)** Axial T1-weighted MRI following the administration of gadolinium-DTPA shows characteristic quadrantic location of enhancement in the dorsolateral region of the cervical spinal cord. (Reproduced from Diagnostic Imaging Studies. In: Dickman C, Fehlings M, Gokaslan Z, ed. Spinal Cord and Spinal Column Tumors. 1st edition. Thieme; 2006.)

7.2 Isolated Idiopathic Optic Neuritis

(Synonyms: retrobulbar optic neuritis, optic papillitis, inflammatory optic neuropathy)

Optic neuritis is a common disorder, the pathogenesis of which refers to inflammation of the optic nerve with variable demyelination affecting individuals between the ages of 15 and 45, with a white (85%) predominance. Women are affected approximately three times more frequently than men. Optic neuritis occurs as the initial symptom of MS in 35–62% patients and is likely a forme fruste of MS in its isolated form. In pregnant women with MS, there is a diminished risk of new exacerbations including optic neuritis, especially during the third trimester.

Optic neuritis may be classified as follows:

1. *Anatomically* (retrobulbar optic neuritis, papillitis, neuroretinitis)
2. *By incidence* (retrobulbar being the most common, followed by papillitis, and neuroretinitis)
3. *Related to etiology:*
   a) MS
      Patients with known MS are at significant risk of optic neuritis. It is the first symptom in 20% of MS patients and occurs in 70% of patients sometimes during the course of the illness. In patients presenting with isolated optic neuritis, the risk of developing MS is approximately 30% after 5–7 years. In long term follow-up studies, 75% of women and 34% of men developed clinically definite MS.
   b) Viral and parainfectious causes
      Adenovirus, coxsackie, cytomegalovirus, HIV, hepatitis A, Epstein–Barr virus, measles, mumps, rubella, varicella zoster, herpes zoster
   c) Post vaccination
   d) Vasculitides (SLE, Wegener's granulomatosis)
   e) Syphilis
   f) Sarcoidosis
   g) Lyme disease
   h) Tuberculosis
   i) *Mycobacterium pneumoniae*
   j) Autoimmune
   k) Sinus infection
   l) Toxoplasmosis

7.2.1 Clinical features

Isolated idiopathic optic neuritis is characterized by the following:

1. Acute onset of orbital pain, particularly eye pain on an eye movement test
2. Central or paracentral scotoma
3. Color desaturation (dyschromatopsia)
4. Progressive, often unilateral vision loss over hours or days
5. Diminished contrast sensitivity (98%); photopsia (30%)
6. Excellent prognosis for visual recovery over months

On examination, a patient with isolated idiopathic optic neuritis will exhibit:

1. Decreased visual acuity
2. Impaired visual field. Central visual scotoma is the hallmark of optic neuritis, accounting for over 90% of the visual field defects, whereas the optic disc may appear normal in retrobulbar neuritis (two-thirds of patients), inspiring the adage "the patient sees nothing and the physician sees nothing." In anterior optic neuritis (or papillitis), the disc may be swollen, and in less than 6% of patients hemorrhage may occur at the disc margin. The optic disc may become pale weeks after the initial episode.
3. Impaired color perception
4. Afferent pupillary defect (Marcus Gunn pupil)

7.2.2 Differential diagnosis

Acute optic neuritis can usually be distinguished from other conditions on clinical grounds. History is usually suggestive with compressive optic neuropathy from intracranial tumors, anterior ischemic optic neuropathy, sinus disease, autoimmune optic neuropathies, radiation-induced optic neuropathies, and central serous choroidopathy.

Optic nerve diseases that may be confused with optic neuritis/papillitis include:

1. Leber's hereditary optic neuropathy
2. Diabetic papillopathy
3. Venous stasis retinopathy
4. Impending central retinal vein occlusion
5. Ischemic optic neuropathy
6. Optic nerve drusen
7. Carcinomatous meningitis
8. Infiltrating neoplasm (lymphoma)
9. Paraneoplastic disorder

7.2.3 Investigations

Special testing

A complete neuro-ophthalmologic examination emphasizing visual acuity at near and far distances, a search for the relative afferent pupillary defect (Marcus Gunn pupil), color vision testing, and careful perimetry are essential in evaluating optic neuritis.

Optic neuritis typically causes prolongation of the latency and decreased amplitude of the P100 of the VEPs, the first large positive peak occurring approximately 100 milliseconds after stimulus. Pattern reversal stimulus presentation yields more reproducible results. Abnormalities of the VEP indicate dysfunction at any point along the visual pathways from the retina to the striate cortex, and are not pathognomonic for demyelinating optic neuropathy. Other disorders, such as compressive lesions, glaucoma, hereditary and toxic optic neuropathy, and papilledema, can also cause VEP disturbances.

Imaging studies

Gadolinium enhancement on MRI is demonstrated in the optic nerves of the majority of patients with acute optic neuritis and correlates with recovery of visual acuity and improvement of VEP amplitudes. The incidence of white matter lesions found with MRI was 48.7%. However, more recent information showed that 36% of placebo-group patients with two or more periventricular lesions of at least 3 mm in size, identified by MRI developed definite MS within 2 years, compared with only 3% of those in whom MRI was normal (▸ Fig. 7.2).

Blood testing

Initial analysis of the Optic Neuritis Treatment Trial led to the conclusion that the use of the ancillary studies, (e.g., ANA, fluorescent treponemal antibody absorption test, Lyme titer, serum and/or CSF angiotensin-converting enzyme level, CSF studies including IgG index and synthesis rate, oligoclonal bands, cryptococcal antigen, cytology, and hypercoagulable studies in selected patients, such as anticardiolipin antibodies, protein C & S, antithrombin III, activated CRP, factor V Leiden, plasma viscosity, fibrinogen, and homocysteine) was limited for defining a cause for visual loss other than optic neuritis associated with demyelinating disease.

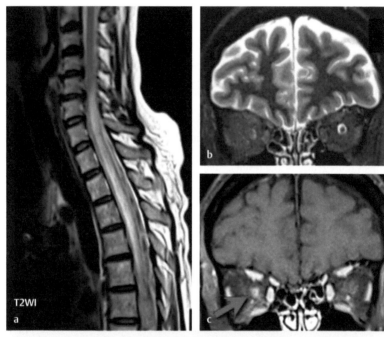

Fig. 7.2 **(a–c)** Idiopathic optic neuritis or Devic's disease. The optic nerves and the spinal cord are usually involved. Often there are few T2 lesions in the brain (*thick arrow*). There are extensive spinal cord lesions (> 3 vertebral segments) involving most of the cord with low T1 and high T2 signal intensity and swelling of the cord. Unlikely in MS the lesions are usually smaller and peripherally located.

Optic Neuritis Study Group. The five-year risk of multiple sclerosis after optic neuritis; experience of the Optic Neuritis Treatment Trial. Neurology 1997;49:1404–1413

Beck RW. Optic neuritis. In MIller NR, ed. Walsh and Hoyt's Clinical Neuro-ophthalmology. 5th ed. Baltimore: Williams & Wilkins;1998

Sedwick LA. Optic neuritis. Neurol Clin 1991;9(1):97–114

7.3 Acute Disseminated Encephalomyelitis

Acute disseminated encephalomyelitis (ADEM) is an acute, monophasic postin-fectious or parainfectious (occurs after a viral illness or vaccination) encephalitis. In 50–75% of cases, the beginning of the disease is preceded by a viral or bacterial infection, usually a sore throat or cough (upper respiratory tract infection 7–14 days prior). Occasionally, ADEC occurs 3 months after a vaccination (most commonly after measles, mumps, and rubella vaccination). It is more common in children than in adults (more than 80% of childhood cases occur in patients younger than 10 years, the ratio of boys to girls is 1.3:1) and is believed to be caused by an immune response triggered by an antigen (viral or vaccine). ADEM is found in all ethnic groups and races. The prognosis for recovery is generally good; recovery is usually spontaneous. Mortality has been estimated as high as 10–20% and as low as less than 2%). Morbidity usually involves visual, motor, autonomic, or intellectual deficits, and epilepsy if grey matter is affected. Deficits may persist for several weeks; however, most deficits resolve within 1 year. Mental retardation is possible, especially in children younger than 2 years of age at disease onset.

7.3.1 Signs and symptoms

Early physical manifestations:
1. Irritability and lethargy are common first signs.
2. Fever returns nearly in half of cases.
3. Headache is reported in 45–65% of the cases.
4. Meningism is detected in 20–30% of cases.

Neurologic abnormalities:
May occur over hours to 6 weeks from onset of early symptoms.
1. Visual disturbances
   a) Visual field defects
   b) Ophthalmoparesis
   c) Optic neuritis (10–30%)
2. Cranial nerve palsies (35–40%)
3. Language disturbances (10%)
4. Psychiatric abnormalities
   a) Irritability
   b) Depression
   c) Personality changes
   d) Psychosis
5. Seizures, focal or generalized (25%)
6. Weakness (50–75%)
7. Sensory changes (15–20%)
   a) Posterior column/hemisensory changes
   b) Band or girdle dysesthesia or Lhermitte's sign
8. Extrapyramidal disorders
   a) Choreoathetosis
   b) Dystonia

7.3.2 Diagnosis

Criteria that facilitate diagnosis include:
1. History of recent infection (although it may have been clinically silent)
2. Monophasic disease course
3. Disseminated CNS disease with neurologic findings
4. Absence of metabolic or infectious disorders

The history of events is the single most important part of the diagnostic criteria. In many cases, especially in the absence of preceding illness or recent vaccination, ADEM is a diagnosis of exclusion. ADEM tends to have neurologic signs and symptoms not typically present in MS, such as headache, nausea, vomiting, drowsiness, and meningismus.

Neither MRI nor CSF results alone are adequate for diagnosing ADEM. MRI is useful in highlighting the disseminated involvement of the white matter and identifying extend and location. MRI findings are virtually impossible to distinguish from MS lesions.

MRI of the brain typically shows multiple high-signal intensity lesions involving white matter. The lesions usually are symmetric, and occipital head regions are predominantly involved. The lesions can affect gray matter and basal ganglia as well. In contrast to MS plaques, the lesions are usually of the same age (i.e., they show more uniform enhancement). If the spinal cord is involved, ADEM lesions are continuous affecting multiple levels, whereas a typical MS lesion is confined to one spinal cord level. The typical MS lesions are also posterior in location on axial, cross-sectional views of the spinal cord, whereas in the ADEM lesions tend to be more diffused throughout the entire cord.

In regard to ADEM, the CSF can be normal or, more likely, show nonspecific changes including an elevated protein and pleocytosis with lymphocytic predominance, a normal glucose, and negative cultures. Electroencephalogram (EEG) is also often performed, eliciting abnormal, yet nonspecific results including generalized and focal slowing and epileptiform discharges (▶ Fig. 7.3).

7.3.3 Differential diagnosis

There is a close diagnostic association between MS and ADEM that is difficult to differentiate on the basis of a single clinical encounter or radiographic image alone. See the following table.

It is also important to differentiate between ADEM and viral encephalitis. The striking feature of ADEM is the prodromal illness or history of recent vaccination, the visual loss in one or both eyes, and spinal cord involvement which are uncommon in encephalitis. A history of recent travel abroad or to areas of high risk for arboviruses is useful information for the diagnosis of encephalitis.

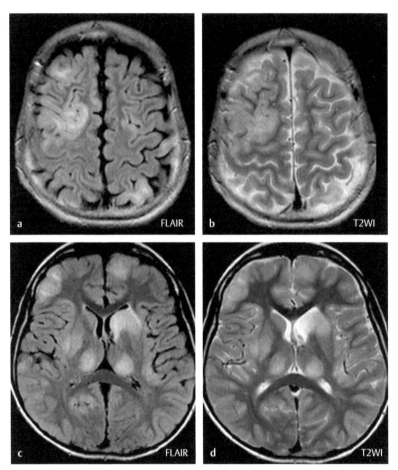

Fig. 7.3 (a–d) Young patient with acute disseminated encephalomyelitis (ADEM). On MRI, there are often diffuse and relatively symmetrical lesions in the supra and infratentorial white matter which may enhance simultaneously. There almost always is preferential involvement of the cortical gray matter and the deep gray matter of the basal ganglia and thalami.

Differentiation between acute disseminated encephalomyelitis and multiple sclerosis

Features	ADEM	Multiple sclerosis
Age	< 12 Years	Adolescents and adults
Provoking factor	Preceding infection	None
CSF oligoclonal IgG	Normal	Positive
Recurrence	Uncommon	Common
MRI	Plaques more amorphous, less sharply defined particularly at gray–white matter junction Thalamus involved	Rounded, elongated plaques with sharp margins in periventricular white matter Thalamus not involved
Clinical features	Accompanied by fever, lethargy, and disturbances of consciousness, seizures, or movement disorders	No other constitutional symptoms

List of differentials

1. MS
2. Acute inflammatory demyelinating polyradiculoneuropathy
3. Guillain–Barre syndrome
4. Aseptic meningitis
5. Cardioembolic stroke
6. Lymphoma
7. Toxic/metabolic encephalopathy
8. Infectious encephalitis (herpes simplex, Lyme disease)
9. Vasculitis (polyarteritis nodosa)
10. Post-malarial neurological syndrome
11. HIV-1-associated CNS complications
12. Metastatic tumor
13. Glioblastoma multiforme
14. Antiphospholipid antibody syndrome
15. Neurosarcoidosis
16. Cavernous sinus syndromes
17. Cerebral venous sinus thrombosis
18. Neurosyphilis
19. Systemic lupus erythematosus
20. Wagener's granulomatosis
21. Brucellosis
22. Spinal cord infarction
23. Spinal epidural abscess

Gabis LV, Panasci DJ, Andriola MR, Huang W. Acute disseminated encephalomyelitis: an MRI/MRS longitudinal study. Pediatr Neurol 2004;30(5):324–329

Höllinger P, Sturzenegger M, Mathis J, Schroth G, Hess CW. Acute disseminated encephalomyelitis in adults: a reappraisal of clinical, CSF, EEG, and MRI findings. J Neurol 2002;249(3):320–329

Petzold GC, Stiepani H, Klingebiel R, Zschenderlein R. Diffusion-weighted magnetic resonance imaging of acute disseminated encephalomyelitis. Eur J Neurol 2005;12(9):735–736

7.4 Transverse Myelitis

(Transverse myelopathy: The term doesn't imply any etiological factor, whereas "myelitis" refers to inflammatory diseases of spinal cord)

This is a neurologic syndrome caused by inflammation of the spinal cord that is localized over several segments of the cord and functionally transects one level of the cord. Transverse myelitis (TM) is uncommon with an incidence of 1–5 cases per million. It occurs in both adults and children. TM is generally a monophasic illness (one-time occurrence), but a small percentage of patients with a predisposing underlying illness may suffer a recurrence.

7.4.1 Etiology

TM may occur in isolation or in the setting of another illness. When it occurs without apparent underlying cause, it is referred to as *idiopathic*. Idiopathic TM is assumed to be a result of abnormal activation of the immune system against the spinal cord which causes inflammation and tissue damage. TM often develops in the setting of viral and bacterial infections, especially those which may be associated with a rash (e.g., rubeola, varicella, variola, rubella, influenza, mycoplasma, Epstein–Barr virus, cytomegalovirus, and mumps). Approximately one-third of patients with TM report a febrile illness (flu-like illness with fever) in close temporal relationship to the onset of neurologic symptoms. In some cases, there is evidence that there is a direct invasion and injury to the cord by the infectious agent (especially poliomyelitis, herpes zoster, and AIDS). A bacterial abscess can also develop around the spinal cord and injure the cord through compression, bacterial invasion, and inflammation.

7.4.2 List of illnesses associated with transverse myelitis

1. **Parainfectious:** occurring at the time of and in association with an acute infection or an episode of infection.
   a) *Viral:* herpes simplex, herpes zoster, cytomegalovirus, Epstein–Barr virus, enteroviruses (poliomyelitis, coxsackie virus, echovirus), human T cell leukemia virus, human immunodeficiency virus, influenza, rabies
   b) *Bacterial: Mycoplasma pneumoniae*, Lyme borreliosis, syphilis, tuberculosis

2. **Postvaccinal** (rabies, cowpox)
3. **Systemic autoimmune disease**
   a) Systemic lupus erythematosus
   b) Sjogren's syndrome
   c) Sarcoidosis
4. **MS**
5. **Paraneoplastic syndrome** (uncommon; the immune system produces an antibody to fight off the cancer and this cross-reacts with the molecules in the spinal cord neurons)
6. **Vascular** (primarily due to inadequate blood flow to the spinal cord instead of actual inflammation)
   a) Thrombosis of spinal arteries
   b) Vasculitis secondary to heroin abuse
   c) Spinal arteriovenous malformation

7.4.3 Signs and symptoms

Signs and symptoms of TM may develop rapidly over several hours to several days or more slowly over 1–2 weeks. Typical symptoms include:

1. Pain
   TM-associated pain often begins in the neck or back. Sharp, shooting sensations may also move down the legs or arms or around the abdomen.
2. Abnormal sensations
   Some patients with TM report numbness, tingling, coldness, or burning sensations below the affected area of the spinal cord. These patients are especially sensitive to the light touch of clothing, or the extreme heat or cold.
3. Weakness in arms or legs
   Some patients with mild weakness notice that they are stumbling, dragging one foot, or that their legs feel heavy as they move, where others may develop severe paralysis.
4. Bladder and bowel problems
   Increased urinary urgency, difficult micturition and constipation.
5. Muscle spasms (e.g., especially in the legs)
6. Headache
7. Fever
8. Loss of appetite

7.4.4 Screening and diagnosis

The general history and physical examination do not give clues about the cause of spinal cord injury. The first step concerning a patient with complaints and examination suggestive of a spinal cord disorder, is to rule out a mass lesion which might be compressing the spinal cord (e.g., tumor, herniated disc, spinal stenosis, and abscess). This is important because early surgery to remove the compression may sometimes reverse neurologic injury to the spinal cord. The easiest test to rule out such a compressive lesion is an MRI of the cord. If MRI is not available or the images are equivocal, myelography must be performed.

1. MRI

   T2-weighted MRI and contrast enhancement should be performed for complete spinal cord urgently. MRI also gives information about inflammation of the spinal cord and may suggest MS, intramedullary tumor, or abscess. Lesions with hyperintense signal on T2-weighted images over several cord segments are often found in TM. Sometimes the cord is swollen. An MRI of the brain is often performed to screen for lesions suggestive of MS (▶ Fig. 7.4).

2. CSF

   Some patients with TM may have abnormally high numbers of white blood cells (lymphocytic pleocytosis) with normal or elevated total protein level suggesting an infection or an inflammation. Oligoclonal bands are present in 20–40% of patients with TM.

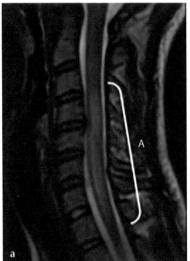
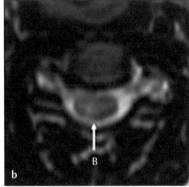

Fig. 7.4 (a, b) Transverse myelitis of cervical cord. Sagittal and axial T2 images. The T2 signal abnormality extends to 3 or more cord segments **(A)** and the lesion is centrally located **(B)**.

3. Blood work

   There are no specific blood tests to diagnose TM. The following work-up should be done to identify potential underlying causes: complete blood count (CBC)/differential, rapid plasma regain (RPR), ANA, double-stranded DNA, anti-SSA and anti-SSB antibodies, serum vitamin B12 level, HTLV-1 antibody, and serum angiotensin-converting enzyme.

7.4.5 Differential diagnosis

1. Extrinsic cord compression
   a) Spinal disc herniation
   b) Benign tumors (e.g., meningioma, neurofibroma)
   c) Metastatic disease of the spine (e.g., epidural-subdural metastases)
   d) Severe stenosis of spinal canal
2. Vascular disorders
   a) Spinal arteriovenous malformations
   b) Spinal cord infarction
   c) Vasculitis secondary to opiate abuse
3. Infectious/parainfectious
   a) Viral (e.g., herpes simplex-zoster, cytomegalovirus, influenza, rabies, Epstein–Barr virus, poliomyelitis, Coxsackie virus, echovirus, HTLV-1, HIV)
   b) Bacterial (e.g., *Mycoplasma pneumoniae*, Lyme borreliosis, syphilis, tuberculosis)
   c) Fungal and parasitic
4. Postvaccinal
   a) Rabies
   b) Cowpox
5. Autoimmune disorders
   a) SLE
   b) Sjogren's syndrome
   c) MS
   d) Neurosarcoidosis
   e) Paraneoplastic

7.4.6 Differential diagnosis of acute and subacute nontraumatic paraplegic syndromes (+)

1. Vascular disorders of the spinal cord
   a) Ischemic disorders of the spinal cord
   b) Primary ischemia (e.g., atherosclerosis, vasculitis)

    c) Secondary ischemia (e.g., vascular compression from mass lesions, aortic disorders)

    d) Decompression sickness

    e) Spinal hemorrhages (e.g., epidural-subdural hematoma, subarachnoid-intraparenchymal hemorrhage)

    f) Vascular malformations (e.g., dural arteriovenous fistula, perimedullar fistula, cavernoma, intramedullary arteriovenous angioma)

2. Inflammatory disorders of the spinal cord

    a) Without compression of the medulla

    b) Acute TM

    c) Myelitis in chronic inflammatory disorders of the CNS (e.g., MS, Lyme disease)

    d) Myelitis in systemic diseases (e.g., Behcet's disease)

    e) With medullary compression

    f) Epidural-subdural abscess

    g) Spondylodiscitis

3. Toxic or allergic disorders of the spinal cord

    a) Subacute myelo-optic neuropathy caused by clioquinol

    b) Late myelopathy after chemonucleolysis

4. Noninflammatory spinal space-occupying lesions

    a) Disc prolapses

    b) Neoplasms

5. Nonspinal disorders

    a) Acute polyradiculitis of Guillain Barre

    b) Hyperkalemic or hypokalemic paralysis

    c) Parasagittal cortical syndrome (e.g., bilateral infarction of the anterior cerebral arteries)

    d) Psychogenic paraplegic syndromes

Transverse Myelitis Consortium Working Group. Proposed diagnostic criteria and nosology of acute transverse myelitis. Neurology 2002;59(4):499–505

Stone LA. Transverse myelitis. In Rolak LA, Harati Y, eds. Neuroimmunology for the clinician. Boston MA: Butterworth-Heinemann; 1977:155–165

Schwenkreis P, Pennekamp W, Tegentheff M. Differential Diagnosis of Acute and Subacute Non-Traumatic Paraplegia Dtsch Arztebl 2006;103(44):A2948–A2954

Jacob A, Weinshenker BG. An approach to the diagnosis of acute transverse myelitis. Semin Neurol 2008;28(1):105–120

7.5 Progressive Multifocal Leukoencephalopathy

This is a fatal subacute progressive demyelinating disease of the CNS caused by reactivation of a latent papovavirus (the JC virus—this virus was isolated from the brain of a patient whose initials were J.C.) infection. It affects immunocompromised patients and is usually seen with patients having AIDS. Approximately 50–80% of all PML cases occur in patients with HIV infection, whereas cases are rare in patients with organ transplantation. Before the AIDS epidemic, PML was rare and associated with immunocompromised conditions, such as leukemia, lymphoma, sarcoidosis, SLE, organ transplantation (multiple immunosuppressive drugs), Wiskott–Aldrich syndrome, and severe combined immunodeficiency. Although reactivation of JC virus may be necessary, this by itself is insufficient to cause PML. A specific deficiency in cellular immune response to the JC viral antigen is probably required in addition to the general cellular immunodeficiency in persons with PML. It has been described in immunocompetent individuals.

The JC virus is believed to produce infection after it enters the tonsillar tissue during an upper respiratory tract infection. After infection, the virus becomes latent in the spleen, the reticuloendothelial system, and the medulla of the kidney. Reactivation of the JC virus occurs in the kidney and bone marrow immunocompromised persons. Infected lymphocytes (B cells) then cross the blood–brain barrier and pass the infection to astrocytes and eventually to adjacent oligodendrocytes that are responsible for forming and maintaining the myelin sheath. Infection of the oligodendrocytes causes destruction of the cells and loss of the myelin sheath. The axons are usually spared.

PML chiefly affects homosexual or bisexual men aged 25–50 years, with a male-to-female ratio of 7:1. The median survival of patients with PML as a complication of AIDS is 6 months. In 10% of patients, survival exceeds 12 months. Anatomically, lesions of PML may occur anywhere in brain, but the frontal lobes and parieto-occipital regions are commonly affected.

7.5.1 Diagnosis

Symptoms and signs

Progressive focal neurologic deficit is the *clinical hallmark*. Weakness and disturbance of speech are most common symptoms. Other symptoms include cognitive abnormalities, headaches, gait disorders, visual impairment, and sensory loss.

Headaches are most common in the HIV-infected population, and visual disturbances are most common in those without HIV infection. About 10% of patients have seizures. Cognitive deficits do not persist in isolation for long and distinguish PLM from HIV dementia. PML seems to have a more aggressive course in persons with other predisposing conditions.

Most common physical sign is limb weakness, which occurs in more than 50% of patients. Cognitive disturbances and gait disorders affect 25–33%, and diplopia affects 9% of the patients. Optic nerve disease does not occur with PML, and spinal cord involvement is rare.

Laboratory tests

1. Blood work
   There are no specific blood tests to diagnose PML, but the following tests should be considered to rule out other possible etiologies: ESR, coagulation profile, HIV, RPR, vitamin 12, BUN, creatinine, and toxoplasmosis titers. Severe cellular immunosuppression (CD4 lymphocyte count < 200 cells/µL)

2. CSF
   Other than helping in excluding other diagnoses, CSF study is not helpful in diagnosis. Cell counts are usually less than 20 cells/µl; protein level is normal or slightly elevated. Glucose, Gram stain, bacterial-fungal cultures, AFB, VDRL, and viral screen should be done to rule out other possible causes of white matter lesions. Measurement of an antibody to the major structural protein of the JP virus is known as VPI. PCR study of the CSF has high sensitivity (95%) and specificity (100%) for JP virus in PML, and should be done to aid in diagnosis.

3. Tissue biopsy
   The criterion standard for the diagnosis remains histological confirmation by means of tissue biopsy.
   However, with a characteristic clinical and MRI pattern accompanied by a positive PCR result for JC virus DNA in the CSF, brain biopsy is often avoided.

4. Imaging studies
   a) CT
      It is often the first neuroimaging technique used. CT scans usually show several bilateral, asymmetric hypoattenuating foci of various sizes without mass effect or enhancement. The lesions may involve the periventricular white matter, subcortical white matter usually seen in the frontal and parieto-occipital areas, or both.

   b) MRI
      MRI scan has far greater sensitivity than other studies in detecting the lesions of PML, and in defining their extent of involvement. On T2-Weighted MRI, lesions appear hyperintense and typically involve the periventricular and subcortical white matter, having a characteristic scalloped lateral margin when they involve the subcortical white matter. Lesions are more conspicuous on FLAIR images, appearing hyperintense against a background of suppressed CSF signal intensity. The lesions typically do not enhance and do not have mass effect; however, some reports describe lesions with faint peripheral enhancement or diffuse enhancement with mass effect, especially in the early stages, suggesting a probable relatively good immune response to an improved prognosis.

   c) MRI spectroscopy
      It reveals reduced N-acetylaspartate (NAA) and creatine levels, increased choline levels, and an excess of lipids and sometimes of myoinositol, in

PML patients. In some cases, lactate is present. The elevation of choline and myoinositol values is seen in the early phase of the disease. In the later phase, all the metabolites are decreased. These metabolic abnormalities are not specific for PML and may be similar in other lesions complicating HIV disease.

d) Magnetization transfer imaging

PML lesions appear to have strongly reduced magnetization transfer ratios. These features may help in distinguishing lesions from white matter lesions of HIV leukoencephalopathy (▶ Fig. 7.5).

PML must be distinguished from HIV leukoencephalopathy:

PML	HIV leukoencephalopathy
MRI	
Tends to be multifocal, with bilateral, asymmetric, and predominantly subcortical involvement	Tends to produce lesions that are usually diffuse, bilateral, and symmetric, in the periventricular area
	Diffuse cortical atrophy and ventricular dilatation
In T1-W images lesions appear well defined and hypointense	In T1-W images lesions appear isointense and poorly defined
Clinical features	
Progressive focal motor and sensory neurologic deficits	Global cognitive changes and dementia

7.5.2 Differential diagnosis

1. CNS toxoplasmosis
2. HIV demyelination
3. MS
4. Encephalomalacia
5. Chronic infarcts
6. ADEM
7. CNS lymphoma
8. White matter demyelination due to chemotherapy and/or radiotherapy
9. Focal cerebritis
10. Neurosyphilis
11. CNS opportunistic infection (e.g., tuberculosis, cryptococcosis, and cytomegalovirus)
12. Other (non-HIV) forms of dementia
13. Glioma
14. Central pontine myelinolysis

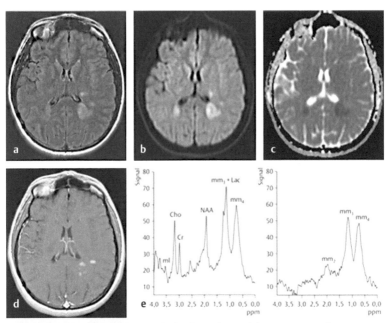

Fig. 7.5 Subacute and florid foci in multiple sclerosis lesions. **(a)** FLAIR sequence does not differentiate between subacute and florid lesions. **(b)** DWI sequence. The bilateral periventricular lesions show restricted diffusion. **(c)** ADC map shows a corresponding decrease in the ADC value. **(d)** Contrast-enhanced T1w sequence. Only portions of the left periventricular lesion show enhancement consistent with florid inflammation. **(e)** *Left:* Metabolite spectrum acquired from the posterior florid part of the lesion at a short echo time (TE = 30 ms) charts the levels of the principal metabolites *N*-acetylaspartate, choline, creatinine, and myo-inositol. The *N*-acetylaspartate level is slightly decreased while the choline level is slightly elevated. Positive lactate detection and especially the greatly increased macromolecule resonances at 0.9 and 1.3 ppm are signs of fulminant demyelination. *Right:* selective plot of macromolecule resonances. Cho = choline; Cr = creatinine; Lac = lactate; ml = myo-inositol; mm = macromolecules; NAA = *N*-acetylaspartate (Reproduced from Magnetic Resonance Imaging. In: Forsting M, Jansen O, ed. MR Neuroimaging: Brain, Spine, Peripheral Nerves. 1st edition. Thieme; 2016.)

Bradley WG, Daroff RB, Fenichel GM, et al. Neurology in clinical practice. Boston: Butterworth-Heinemann;2000:1369–1370

Dworkin MS. A review of progressive multifocal leukoencephalopathy in persons with and without AIDS. Curr Clin Top Infect Dis 2002;22:181–195

Chang L, Ernst T, Tornatore C, et al. Metabolite abnormalities in progressive multifocal leukoencephalopathy by proton magnetic resonance spectroscopy. Neurology 1997;48(4):836–845

Mader I, Herrlinger U, Klose U, Schmidt F, Küker W. Progressive multifocal leukoencephalopathy: analysis of lesion development with diffusion-weighted MRI. Neuroradiology 2003;45(10):717–721

7.6 Central Pontine Myelinolysis

(Osmotic demyelination syndrome)

Central pontine myelinolysis (CPM) is a rare neurologic disorder characterized by demyelination that affects the central portion of the base of the pons. There are no inflammatory changes, and blood vessels are normal. Clinical features usually reflect damage to the descending motor tracts and include spastic tetraparesis, pseudobulbar paralysis, and the locked-in syndrome. CPM is most commonly seen in alcoholics and malnourished patients.

7.6.1 Epidemiology

The exact incidence of CPM is unknown. Autopsy data suggest a prevalence of approximately 0.25%. A study demonstrated that CPM was present in 29% of postmortem examinations of liver transplant patients. Two-thirds of these patients had serum sodium fluctuations of only ± 15–20 mEq/l. No reports exist of CPM in African Americans. CPM occurs more frequently in females than in males.

7.6.2 Causes

The pathogenesis underlying CPM remains unknown, but the disorder is most commonly associated with rapid correction of hyponatremia. Conditions predisposing patients to CPM include *alcoholism, liver disease, malnutrition,* and *hyponatremia.*

7.6.3 Risk factors

Risk factors for CPM in the hyponatremic patient include the following:
1. Serum sodium of less than 120 mEq/l for more than 48 hours
2. Aggressive IV fluid therapy with hypertonic saline solutions
   The general recommendation is that sodium correction rates should not exceed 12 mEq/l within the first 24 hours or 20 mEq/l within the first 48 hours. Some argue that a greater risk of CMP occurs with chronic hyponatremia and that rates of sodium replacement should depend on the chronicity of the deficit. They recommend a minimum rate of correction of 1 mmol/l/h for acute hyponatremia and a maximum rate of correction of 0.5 mmol/l/h for chronic hyponatremia.
3. Development of hypernatremia during treatment
4. Hypokalemia is an additional risk factor for CPM, and should be addressed prior to treatment of hyponatremia

7.6.4 Associated conditions

1. Alcoholism (39.4–78%)
   Alcohol blocks antidiuretic hormone (ADH). During alcohol withdrawal, ADH function may be overactive, resulting in hyponatremia.
2. Rapid correction of hyponatremia (21.5–61%)
   Many patients who have hyponatremia that is corrected rapidly do not develop CPM. Thus, other less obvious risk factors probably exist. Patients with an acute episode of hyponatremia that is treated promptly are unlikely to develop CPM.
   CPM reportedly occurs occasionally in patients who are treated for hypernatremia.
3. CPM may complicate liver transplantation surgery (17.4%):
   a) Consider CPM when confusion and/or weakness complicate the liver transplant patient's postoperative recovery.
   b) Liver transplant patients may develop CPM and critical illness neuromyopathy.
      Liver transplant-associated CMP occurs more commonly in children and those with sepsis, metabolic disorders, hepatic encephalopathy, hypoxia, and use of cyclosporine (cyclosporine neurotoxicity).
4. Other liver disease, including cirrhosis (4.8%) and Wilson's disease (WD)
5. Burn patients with a prolonged period of serum hyperosmolality are prone to developing CPM (7%)
6. Diabetes (2%)
7. AIDS (1.4%)
8. Pregnancy (0.5%) and hyperemesis gravidarum (1.4%)
9. Other electrolyte disturbances and abnormalities in osmolality (0.7%), including hypernatremia, hypokalemia, lithium toxicity, and correction of hypoglycemia
10. Neoplasms (0.5%), particularly of lung or GI tract; Hodgkin's lymphoma
11. Cerebral infarct (0.5%), brainstem hemorrhage, and other CNS diseases
12. Schizophrenia (0.5%), acute porphyria (0.5%), pulmonary infections, hypoxia, sepsis, trauma, Sjogren's syndrome, and adrenal insufficiency
13. Extrapontine myelinolysis (EPM) occurs in 10–15% of patients with CPM. The demyelinating lesions, in order of frequency, occur in the cerebellum, lateral geniculate body, thalamus, putamen, and cerebral cortex or subcortex.

7.6.5 Clinical features

The most consistent examination findings are those of pseudobulbar palsy, spastic tetraparesis, and alterations in consciousness caused by demyelination of corticospinal and corticobulbar tracts within the pons. *Pseudobulbar paralysis* is characterized by head and neck weakness, dysphagia, and dysarthria occurs in approximately 40% of cases. Increased limb tone, limb weakness, hyperactive reflexes, and Babinski sign are typical features of *spastic tetraparesis* (occurs in 33% of patients) or lesions that involve upper motor neurons or the corticospinal tracts. Lesions within the pons cause *horizontal gaze paralysis. Vertical ophthalmoparesis* is caused by demyelination extending through the midbrain. *Alterations in consciousness* occur in 70% of cases, and can range from lethargy to coma. A large basis pontis lesion may cause a *"locked-in-syndrome,"* which includes paralysis of lower cranial nerves and limb musculature, whereas vertical eye movements, blinking, breathing, and alertness may remain intact. Abnormalities in *sensory modalities* usually *are not* observed. Patients may also present with *seizures* (25% of patients), *hyporeflexia, hypotension, respiratory depression,* and *bowel or bladder dysfunction.* In 25% of patients, the only manifestations of CPM are *psychiatric*, such as pseudobulbar laughing and crying, agitated delirium, akinetic mutism, or catatonia.

7.6.6 Laboratory studies

Lab studies

1. CSF studies are probably is not necessary when the etiology and diagnosis are obvious.
2. CSF studies may demonstrate increased opening pressure, elevated protein, or mononuclear pleocytosis.

Imaging studies

1. MRI is the imaging modality of choice. Characteristic images show an area of prolonged T1- and T2-relaxation in the central pons, sparing the tegmentum of pons and the ventrolateral pons. The lesion is often triangular on axial images and has a bat's wing configuration in coronal images. Typically, T2-weighted MRI images demonstrate hyperintense or bright areas where demyelination has occurred caused by relatively increased water content in those areas (▶ Fig. 7.6).
2. The CT finding is usually a symmetric, non-space-occupying, hypodense lesion in the central pons, similar to that demonstrated on MRI. CT is not as sensitive as MRI.
3. MRI or CT scan of the brain stem may not reveal an obvious anatomic disturbance. Hence, a thorough neurologic examination is indispensable. It is recommended, therefore, to repeat imaging in suspicious cases in

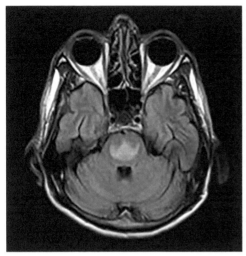

Fig. 7.6 Axial T2 FLAIR image demonstrates a symmetric hyperintensity imaging the central pontine region, sparing the tegmentum and corticospinal tracts resulting in a characteristic Mexican hat or bat wing configuration or hyperintensity.

10–14 days, if early scans are unrevealing. Some propose that early CT and MRI changes are secondary to edema and will often resolve, while later changes are secondary to demyelination itself and are more likely to be permanent.

4. Positron emission tomography (PET) studies have shown the demyelinating patches to have increased metabolic activity in early phase and decreased metabolic activity as CPM progresses. PET, however, is not routinely used in the evaluation of CPM.

Other tests

1. EEG in CPM may demonstrate diffuse bihemispheric slowing.
2. Brainstem-evoked potentials may reveal abnormalities, such as prolongation of the latency period between waves I and V, secondary to demyelination of auditory pathways in the pons. This finding, however, is nonspecific and inconsistent.

Pathology findings

A single, symmetric region of demyelination in the central basis pontis. Relative preservation of axons, blood vessels, and surrounding neurons within areas of demyelination and an associated reduction in oligodendroglia is present. Evidence of inflammation in notably absent.

7.6.7 Differential diagnosis

The differential diagnosis includes any acute neurological process that localizes to the pons:

1. MS
2. ADEM
3. Brainstem gliomas
4. Alcohol (ethanol) related neuropathy
5. Lacunar syndromes
6. Leptomeningeal carcinomatosis
7. Uremic encephalopathy
8. Hepatic encephalopathy
9. Wernicke's encephalopathy

Martin RJ. Central pontine and extrapontine myelinolysis: the osmotic demyelination syndromes. J Neurol Neurosurg Psychiatry 2004;75(Suppl 3):iii22–iii28

Lampl C, Yazdi K. Central pontine myelinolysis. Eur Neurol 2002;47(1):3–10

Laubenberger J, Schneider B, Ansorge O, et al. Central pontine myelinolysis: clinical presentation and radiologic findings. Eur Radiol 1996;6(2):177–183

Pirzada NA, Ali II. Central pontine myelinolysis. Mayo Clin Proc 2001;76(5):559–562

7.7 Multiple Sclerosis-Like Lesions

(Differentiation on MRI findings)

MS is a clinical diagnosis that should never be made on neuroimaging alone. In 78–95% of clinically diagnosed MS patients, the gadolinium-enhanced MRI features include usually ovoid periventricular, infratentorial, temporal lobe, and corpus callosum white matter lesions of isointensity to hypointensity on T1-weighted images, and high intensity on proton density and T2-weighted images.

Many processes must be considered in the differential diagnosis of multiple white matter high-signal abnormalities on PD-WI/T2-WI. These conditions manifest lesions with or without enhancement and occur in a similar patient population to that with MS. In the list of diseases with clinical and neuroimaging features similar to MS one may include the following:

1. Neurosarcoidosis

    The granulomatous process invades and thromboses affected blood vessels and produces a granulomatous angiitis similar to primary angiitis of the CNS. High-intensity white matter in sarcoid can be indistinguishable from MS.

2. Lyme disease (neuroberylliosis)

    Approximately 10–15% of patients with Lyme disease have CNS involvement. High-signal contrast-enhancing subcortical abnormalities on PD-WI/T2-WI on MRI in the frontal and parietal lobes, the basal ganglia and pons, cranial nerves (facial CN).

3. Vasculitides
   Multisystem immune-related vasculitis, with CNS involvement in 10–49% of cases, e.g., SLE and Behcet's disease may resemble MS clinically and by their white matter lesional pattern in the brain and spinal cord.

4. Neurosyphilis
   Contrast-enhanced MR images show patchy enhancement involving the basal ganglia or the middle cerebral artery territories.

5. Tuberculosis
   Single or multiple lesions located in the cerebral hemisphere and basal ganglia in adults and the cerebellum in children. In MR images with gadolinium injection, there is a hypodense rim that may separate the hyperintense center from the peripheral hyperintense edema on T2-WI and on T1-WI often show nodular enhancement.

6. Viral infection

7. Devic's disease or neuromyelitis optica

8. Diffuse sclerosis (Schilder's disease)
   An acute, rapidly progressing form of MS with bilateral, relatively symmetric, and large areas of demyelination often involving the centrum semiovale and the occipital lobes, seen usually in childhood and rarely after the age of 40 years.

9. Myelopathy

10. ADEM
    Acute monophasic inflammatory demyelination distinguished from MS by its clinical course: e.g., a single acute episode including fever and headache. The locations and characteristics of the lesions on the MRI may be indistinguishable from MS.

11. Balo's disease (concentric sclerosis)
    Represents a histologic MS lesion with alternating concentric regions of demyelination and normal brain.

12. Hypertension and ischemic white matter lesions
    In elderly patients with malignant hypertension high-signal patchy or diffuse bilateral periventricular white matter abnormalities, most likely representing the presence of small vessel disease manifested by the presence of lacunar, deep white matter infarctions.

13. Virchow–Robin spaces
    Dilated perivascular spaces that enlarge with age and hypertension and occur in characteristic locations, typically in the basal ganglia, around the ventricular atria, centrum semiovale, and brain stem. The perivascular spaces remain isodense to CSF whereas lesions are hypodense on PD-WI MR sequence.

14. Lesions associated with migraine
    High-intensity abnormalities in the centrum semiovale and the frontal white matter of young patients under 40 years of age, which appear to be a

diffuse process possibly the result of platelet microembolism or the consequence of primary neuronal damage related to the pathophysiology of migraine.

15. Multi-infarct dementia, leukoaraiosis, and Binswanger's disease
It affects the elderly population and the predominant clinical manifestations are the cognitive and behavioral disorders. The MRI shows periventricular white matter and centrum ovale watershed infarcts similar in appearance with the demyelinating lesions of MS; however, contrary to the MS lesions there are no associated lesions in the basal ganglia, brain stem, occipital horns and there is sparing of the subcortical U fibers.

16. Normal aging
In healthy individuals of 52–72 years of age, atrophic periventricular demyelination has been found in 53.4% and white matter infarcts in 13.4%. Incidental white matter T2 hyperintensities occur frequently in the elderly people.

17. Metastases and brain abscesses
Rarely produce lesional patterns quite similar to MS. The presence of mass effect and the clinical history suggesting a remote source for the lesions is important.

18. Motor neuron disease

19. Intracranial tumor (especially brain stem, cerebellum)

20. Vitamin B12 deficiency (gastrectomy, gastric carcinoma, malabsorption syndromes)

Rinker JR, Cross AH. Diagnosis and Differential Diagnosis of Multiple Sclerosis. Continuum Lifelong Learning Neurol 2007;13(5):13–34

Miller DH, Weinshenker BG, Filippi M, et al. Differential diagnosis of suspected multiple sclerosis: a consensus approach. Mult Scler 2008;14(9):1157–1174

Ferreira S, D'Cruz DP, Hughes GR. Multiple sclerosis, neuropsychiatric lupus and antiphospholipid syndrome: where do we stand? Rheumatology (Oxford) 2005;44(4):434–442

7.8 Cerebellar Atrophy

(Cerebellar cortical atrophy syndrome, cerebellar degenerations, late cortical cerebellar atrophy of Marie–Foix–Alajouanine)

7.8.1 Differential diagnosis

1. Toxic/metabolic
   a) *Chronic alcohol abuse* (alcoholic cerebellar degeneration)
   The most common cause, with predominant involvement of the dorsal vermis and the adjacent cerebellar lobes. It is thought to be due to

a combination of nutritional deficiency and alcohol neurotoxicity, likely involving glutamate. It remains largely a clinical diagnosis and is clinically characterized by ataxia of the trunk and lower limbs. The patient has difficulty in walking and may sway or fall while standing upright. Typically, the disease develops after more than 10 years of heavy drinking, though there is no direct relation between the "dose" of alcohol and severity of symptoms. Symptoms evolve in weeks or months and eventually stabilize, sometimes even with continued drinking and poor nutrition. Genetics probably play a significant role in the cause of this disorder. Clinical suspicion can be confirmed by brain imaging, which can, in some cases, display distinct cerebellar shrinkage. Unlike in *Wernicke's encephalopathy,* cognition remains intact, and the thalami and periaqueductal gray matter look normal on MRI.

b) *Wernicke–Korsakoff syndrome*

The triad of acute ophthalmoplegia, ataxia, and confusion is classic and appears in only 19% of patients, and is characteristic of the Wernicke's syndrome. If untreated, results in Korsakoff's psychosis which is diagnosed in the presence of appropriate risk factors, and a defect in learning new material (anterograde amnesia) and a loss of prior memories (retrograde amnesia). Signs of peripheral neuropathy and postural hypotension and syncope are common.

c) *Anticonvulsants*

Cerebellar toxins such as *phenytoin* and *carbamazepine* produce hemispheric cerebellar syndromes characterized by incoordination of the limbs.

d) *Chemotherapeutic agents*

Certain types of cancer chemotherapeutic agents, such as *cytosine arabinoside, 5-fluorouracil, procarbazine, vincristine* are cerebellar toxins. *Lithium,* given for manic-depressive disorder, is a cerebellar toxin.

e) *Mercury (organic), organophosphate insecticides, and solvents*

f) *Radiation necrosis*

A few months (6–8) following radiation, demyelination is seen histologically, associated with proliferation of the glial elements and mononuclear cells, endothelial hyperplasia resulting in reduced cerebral blood flow. These pathological changes continue to evolve for more than 2–3 years after the initial radiation. The amount of injury is related to the radiation dose, fractionation methods, and the portals used; although there is relative sparing of the posterior fossa (also basal ganglia and internal capsule), but in more severe cases these structures are also involved. MRI detects more lesions than CT and the changes parallel those seen in ischemia (high-signal foci on T2-WI).

2. Systemic diseases
    a) *Endocrine disorder*
       This involves thyroid or the pituitary gland. A common genetic mechanism is responsible for the Gordon–Holmes syndrome characterized by a progressive hypogonadotropic hypogonadism and cerebellar ataxia.
    b) *Gastrointestinal disorders*
        i. Celiac disease (Celiac disease/gluten-sensitive enteropathy/tropical sprue)
        ii. Other causes of vitamin E malabsorption
    c) *CNS vasculitis* (on pathogenetic mechanism)
        i. Immunological injury
            – Cell-mediated inflammation (Takayasu arteritis, giant cell arteritis, primary angiitis of the CNS)
            – Immune complex-mediated inflammation (SLE, polyarteritis nodosa, Bechet's syndrome, infection-malignancy-drug induced vasculitides, systemic sclerosis)
            – Antineutrophil cytoplasmic antibody-mediated inflammation (Wagener's granulomatosis, Churg–Strauss syndrome)
            – Mixed immunological disorder (Sjogren's syndrome)
        ii. Direct infection of blood vessels
            – Bacterial, viral (varicella zoster virus, Epstein–Barr virus), other (fungal, protozoal, mycoplasmal, rickettsial)
3. Autoantibodies
    a) *Paraneoplastic cerebellar degeneration*
       The cerebellum may be injured by antibodies, e.g., in the paraneoplastic cerebellar degenerations and in celiac disease (gluten enteropathy). These syndromes are accompanied by abnormal blood tests for antibodies directed against neurons about 50% of the time. The most common tumors are of the ovary, gastrointestinal tract, lung and breast.
    b) *Autoimmune disorders (MS)*
       MS is another fairly common source of cerebellar disorder. MS often involves the cerebellar connections in the brain stem, and particularly the middle cerebellar peduncles.
4. Inherited cerebellar degenerations
    a) *Olivopontocerebellar atrophy (OPCA)*
       (Synonyms: autosomal dominant cerebellar cortical atrophy, multiple system atrophy, Metzel ataxia, Schut–Haymaker ataxia, Dejerine–Thomas ataxia, Holmes ataxia, Sanger–Brown ataxia, Wadia–Swami ataxia, Marie ataxia, Nonne syndrome)
       The OPCAs are progressive neurodegenerative conditions that can be passed down through families (inherited forms), or they may affect

people without a known family history (sporadic). Sporadic forms involve abnormalities of alpha-synuclein, but that does not fully explain the abnormality involving many other yet unknown details. Many specific genes have been identified for the genetic forms, although how the genetic abnormalities cause the clinical findings remains uncertain.

b) *Friedreich's ataxia, and other spinocerebellar ataxia (SCAs)*
One of the most common forms of autosomal recessive ataxia, in which the spinocerebellar tracts, dorsal columns, pyramidal tracts, and, to a lesser extent, the cerebellum and medulla are involved. Friedreich's ataxia is caused by a defect in a gene called frataxin (*FXN*), which is located on chromosome 9.

c) *Transmissible spongiform encephalopathies*
The known human transmissible spongiform encephalopathies are Kuru, Creutzfeldt–Jakob disease (CJD), Gerstmann–Straussler–Scheinker disease, and fatal familial insomnia. Familial progressive subcortical gliosis and some inherited dementias may also be transmissible spongiform encephalopathies. PrP, in conjunction with proteins found in Alzheimer's disease (AD), is present in muscle fibers in inclusion-body myopathy.

d) *Cerebellar degeneration due to respiratory chain or mitochondrial disorders*
Predominant cerebellar involvement can be found in various respiratory chain defects or mitochondrial disorders of energy metabolism that can present at any age with a wide and nonspecific range of clinical symptoms and with any mode of inheritance, originating from any organ or tissue with high energy requirements, e.g., brain, skeletal muscle, and heart. The diagnostic work-up in patients with neuromuscular features whose brain MRI exhibit cerebellar volume loss should include the evaluation for mitochondrial encephalomyopathies.

5. Aging
Atrophy of vermis may occur selectively with aging without atrophy of the cerebral cortex, and without clinical manifestations. There was no other atrophy of infratentorial structures except for occasional enlargement of the cisterna magna and cerebellopontine angle cisterns.

6. Trauma
a) Immediate injury
b) Delayed injury

7. Structural lesions
a) Acute and hemorrhagic stroke
b) Ischemia (chronic vertebrobasilar atherosclerotic disease)
As the cerebellum is supplied by three major arteries on each side (SCA or superior cerebellar artery, AICA or anterior inferior cerebellar artery, and PICA or posterior inferior cerebellar artery), there are many

potential stroke syndromes to consider. The most common syndrome is that of the PICA, also called Wallenberg's syndrome or lateral medullary syndrome. The second most common is the AICA syndrome, and the least frequent is SCA. Vascular malformations such as cerebellar hemangioblastoma are also fairly common.

Strokes that bleed into the cerebellum, usually hypertensive, can be life threatening and may require surgical decompression.

8. Congenital anomalies
    a) *Chiari malformation*
    The most common congenital condition where the cerebellar tonsils are displaced downward with respect to the skull. Probably second most common are various types of agenesis syndromes.

    b) *Dandy–Walker syndrome*
    There is partial or complete agenesis of the cerebellar vermis, cystic formation of the posterior fossa communication with the fourth ventricle, and hydrocephalus. About 80% of the diagnoses of Dandy–Walker syndrome are made by the age of 1 year. It is often accompanied by other malformations, the most common of which is agenesis of the corpus callosum.

Pinheiro L, Freitas J, Lucas M, Victorino RM. Cerebellar atrophy in systemic sclerosis. J R Soc Med 2004;97(11):537–538

Bastos Leite AJ, van der Flier WM, van Straaten EC, Scheltens P, Barkhof F. Infratentorial abnormalities in vascular dementia. Stroke 2006;37(1):105–110

Greenlee JE. Cytotoxic T cells in paraneoplastic cerebellar degeneration. Ann Neurol 2000;47(1):4–5

Bang OY, Huh K, Lee PH, Kim HJ. Clinical and neuroradiological features of patients with spinocerebellar ataxias from Korean kindreds. Arch Neurol 2003;60(11):1566–1574

7.9 Friedreich's Ataxia

(Also known as: Familial ataxia, Friedreich's disease, Friedreich's tabes, hereditary ataxia-Friedreich's type, spinal ataxia-hereditofamilial or SCA)

Friedreich's ataxia is one of the most common forms of autosomal recessive ataxia, in which the spinocerebellar tracts, dorsal columns, pyramidal tracts, and, to a lesser extent, the cerebellum and medulla are involved. The peripheral nerves and the heart are also affected. Carbohydrate metabolism is also altered. It has an early onset, before age 20, and a rapidly progressive course. Males and females are affected equally.

About 1 in every 22,000–29,000 develops this disease. Family history of the condition raises the risk. Particularly high frequency of this disease was found in Cyprus and among the French Canadian population, whereas it does not exist in the Far East.

7.9.1 Etiology—genetics

Friedreich's ataxia is an autosomal recessive congenital ataxia caused by a mutation (2% of cases) in gene *X25* that codes for frataxin, located on chromosome 9. This protein is essential in neuronal and muscle cells for proper functioning of mitochondria. This protein has been associated with the removal of iron from the cytoplasm surrounding the mitochondria, and in the absence of frataxin, the iron builds up and causes free radical degenerative damage to the cells within the tissues of the spinal cord and its brain connections, the heart and pancreas, thereby reducing nerve signals to the muscles. The classic form (98% of cases) has been mapped to 9q13-q21; the mutant gene contains expanded GAA triplet repeats in the first intron of "*FXN* gene." This mutation does not result in the production of abnormal frataxin proteins, because the defect is located on an intron (which is removed from the mRNA transcript between transcription and translation).

Friedreich's ataxia and *muscular dystrophy*, though often compared, are completely different diseases. Muscular dystrophy is the result of muscle tissue degeneration whereas Friedreich's ataxia is the result of nerve tissue degeneration caused by a trinucleotide repeat expansion mutation.

7.9.2 Associated conditions

1. Enlargement of the heart, irregular heartbeat, or other symptoms of heart trouble (*hypertrophic cardiomyopathy*) occur in many individuals. Heart problems range from mild to severe. Approximately half of 82 fatal cases of Friedreich's ataxia died of heart failure or dysrhythmias that do not respond to treatment.
2. *Diabetes mellitus* was present in 23% in later stages of the disease.
3. *Scoliosis* or *Kyphoscoliosis* is a well-known complication and can cause secondary pulmonary complications.
4. *Partial deafness* and *loss of visual acuity* occur in a few patients.

7.9.3 Diagnosis

Diagnosis is based on a person's medical history, family history, and a complete neurological evaluation which includes an EMG. To supplement the evaluation, various tests may be performed which assist in the diagnosis and rule out other possible disorders that may present similar symptoms.

1. Clinical features
   a) The initial presentation is frequently gait ataxia (frequent falls). Difficulty in a steady standing and running are early symptoms, whereas arm

ataxia and slurred speech (dysarthria) also may be significant symptoms, but appear later.

b) Peripheral neuropathy, mixed sensory and cerebellar ataxia.

c) Pes cavus, muscle weakness and atrophy, kyphoscoliosis. Most patients are confined to a wheelchair by early adulthood.

d) Hypertrophic cardiomyopathy, jerky eye movements, diabetes, and deafness.

e) Loss of all tendon reflexes, loss of vibration and position sense, and extensor plantar responses, positive Romberg's test, ataxia and dysarthria are typical during a physical examination.

2. Laboratory tests

a) ECG

b) Genetic DNA testing for GAA repeats of the frataxin gene

c) X-ray of the spine and chest

d) Electrophysiological studies: sensory nerve responses absent in lower extremities, slowed in upper extremities. Motor nerve conductions usually are normal or show a mild reduction.

e) Muscle biopsy

f) CT scan and MRI are not helpful for making a diagnosis.

7.9.4 Differential diagnosis

1. Cerebellum-brainstem ataxias

a) *OPCA*

It is a neurodegenerative disease, which is characterized by cerebellar atrophy and mainly brainstem lesions. There are both familial and sporadic cases. For the most part, however, OPCA is a sporadic condition. The symptoms mostly become obvious at the age of 50 years. Patients often have limb ataxia, ataxia of brainstem muscles, Parkinsonism, motor disorders. Both forms of OPCA are characterized by progressive degeneration of certain structures of the brain, especially the cerebellum (loss of Purkinje cells), pons (loss of neurons in the pontine nuclei, and atrophy of the transverse fibers of the pons and middle cerebellar peduncles), and inferior olive.

Sporadic OPCA is frequently combined with *striatonigral degeneration* which causes Parkinsonian symptoms, and degeneration of sympathetic neurons of the spinal cord *(Shy–Drager syndrome)*, which causes orthostatic hypotension and other autonomic dysfunction. The combined degeneration is called *multiple system atrophy (MSA)*. In addition to loss of neurons in the affected nuclei, MSA shows oligodendroglial inclusions containing alpha-synuclein and ubiquitin. In this regard, MSA resembles Parkinson's disease. Hereditary OPCA refers to the group of disorders that overlap with SCA.

b) *Dentatorubropallidoluysian atrophy*

Dentatorubral and pallidoluysian atrophy (DRPLA) maps to chromosome 12p, and a gene designated "atrophin-1." and remains rare outside of Asia. Young adults and children display progressive chorea, cerebellar ataxia, oculomotor function, and dementia. This disorder has an unstable CAG repeat. Purkinje cells are intact, unlike SCA1, but there is degeneration of the cerebellar dentate nucleus. Autosomal dominant cerebellar ataxia associated with pigmentary macular dystrophy maps to chromosome 3p.

c) *Machado–Joseph disease*

A rare hereditary ataxia with highest prevalence among people of Portuguese/Azorean descent. The Machado–Joseph disease (MJD) is a progressive, adult-onset, neurodegenerative disorder transmitted in an autosomal dominant manner that affects the CNS. Its manifestations include cerebellar ataxia and progressive external ophthalmoplegia associated in a variable degree with pyramidal signs, extrapyramidal signs (dystonia or rigidity), amyotrophy, and peripheral neuropathy. The diagnosis is made by recognizing the symptoms and taking a family history. A definitive diagnosis of MJD can only be made with a genetic test. The gene associated with this disease, *MJD1*, was cloned in 1994, and the causative mutation was shown to be the expansion of a (CAG)n tract within its coding region. This tract contains 12–44 triplets in healthy individuals and from 61 to 87 in patients of diverse ethnic origin.

2. Predominantly cerebellar

a) Drug induced (phenytoin)

b) Alcohol

c) Paraneoplastic

d) Late cortical cerebellar atrophy of Marie–Foix–Alazouanine syndrome
Ataxia of the cerebellum in advanced age; frequently due to abuse of alcohol. A genetic subgroup is inherited as an autosomal dominant trait.

e) Holmes familial cortical cerebellar atrophy

f) Systemic sclerosis
Progressive subacute cerebellar degeneration can be part of a paraneoplastic syndrome, but there was no evidence of neoplasia on investigation or subsequent follow-up. CNS disease in systemic sclerosis is rare and apparently unrelated to systemic vascular damage, possibly related to a manifestation of autoimmunity. Patients present typical systemic sclerosis with skin and esophageal involvement and progressive pulmonary hypertension and ataxia due to cerebellar atrophy.

3. Spinocerebellar ataxia

A group of autosomal dominant ataxias (ADSCAs)—25 entities SCA:1–25 at last count—caused by CAG repeats on multiple chromosomal loci. All of these diseases have a common underlying molecular defect, i.e., CAG triplet expansion. CSAs exhibit gradually progressive pancerebellar dysfunction, usually beginning in childhood. Ataxia is caused by lesions that interrupt the sensory input to the cerebellum (*spinal or sensory ataxia*), pathology of the cerebellar cortex resulting in incorrect execution of cortical signals (*cerebellar ataxia*), or by a combination of both (*spinocerebellar ataxia*). In addition to ataxia, the ADSCAs cause Parkinsonism and other extrapyramidal manifestations, weakness and fasciculations, spasticity, ophthalmoplegia, retinal degeneration and optic atrophy, cognitive impairment, dementia, and peripheral neuropathy.

4. Cerebellar–brain stem–spinal ataxias
   A group of diverse sporadic diseases that cause cerebellar degeneration and degeneration of other anatomical systems.
   a) *Carbohydrate-deficient glycoprotein syndrome*
      An autosomal recessive OPCA in infants and children that is associated with a defect in glycosylation of proteins.
   b) *Ataxia-telangiectasia (Louis–Bar syndrome)*
      A childhood disease characterized by ataxia, extrapyramidal dysfunction, peripheral neuropathy and other neurologic deficits, vascular dilatation, and immunodeficiency. It is caused by mutations of a gene that regulates the cell cycle. These mutations result in defective DNA repair. In addition to cerebellar degeneration, there is loss of anterior horns, degeneration of brainstem nuclei, substantia nigra, and other neuronal groups, and loss of dorsal root ganglionic neurons with dorsal column degeneration. These patients frequently develop opportunistic infections and B-cell lymphomas.

Berciano J, Tolosa E. Olivopontocerebeller Atrophy. In: Jankovic J, Tolosa E, eds. Parkinson's Disease and Movement Disorders. Baltimore, MD: Williams& Wilkins;1993;163–169

Pinheiro L, Freitas J, Lucas M, Victorino RM. Cerebellar atrophy in systemic sclerosis. J R Soc Med 2004;97(11):537–538

Lynch DR, Farmer JM, Balcer LJ, Wilson RB. Friedreich ataxia: effects of genetic understanding on clinical evaluation and therapy. Arch Neurol 2002;59(5):743–747

Ackroyd RS, Finnegan JA, Green SH. Friedreich's ataxia. A clinical review with neurophysiological and echocardiographic findings. Arch Dis Child 1984;59(3):217–221

Marie P, Foix C, Alazouanine T. De l' atrophie cerebelleuse tardive a predominance corticale. Rev Neurol (Paris) 1922;38:849–885, 1082–1111

7.10 Inherited Cerebellar Diseases

(Hereditary ataxias)

The classification of inherited cerebellar diseases is not uniform and often very confusing. They usually cause progressive degeneration and atrophy of the cerebellum and their common manifestations are ataxia and incoordination of movement.

The most common ones are listed below:

1. Friedreich's ataxia

   Friedreich's ataxia is a relatively common autosomal recessive genetic disorder, and about 1 in every 22,000–29,000 develop this disease.

2. Syndromes associated with an autosomal recessive defect of DNA repair

   a) *Ataxia-telangiectasia*

      Autosomal recessive disorder characterized by mutations of ATM gene on chromosome 11q22–23 resulting in dysfunction of DNA repair process and impaired cell cycle control. Incidence of malignancies is estimated at 15–20%, especially leukemias and lymphomas. Clinical manifestations include truncal ataxia, delayed motor development, dysarthria, conjunctival and cutaneous telangiectasias, immune dysfunction with reduced concentrations of IgA and IgG2, recurrent respiratory and cutaneous infections, growth retardation, premature aging, and delayed sexual development, mild mental retardation, oculomotor abnormalities, myoclonus, and peripheral neuropathy.

   b) *Xeroderma pigmentosum (XP)* or DeSanctis–Cacchione syndrome

      Autosomal dominant disorder characterized by loss of genes required for excision of damaged DNA and for replication past regions of damaged DNA; depending on type of XP, mutations can occur in genes of different loci (*9q34.1, 2q21, 3q25.1* etc.). Cells are hypersensitive to ultraviolet light and chemical carcinogens. Clinical manifestations include dermal blistering and erythema, dwarfism, high risk of skin cancer, mental retardation, microcephaly, chorea, ataxia, spasticity, peripheral motor neuropathy, hearing loss, and supranuclear ophthalmoplegia.

3. Mitochondrial encephalopathies

   a) *Leigh's disease* (Leigh's necrotizing encephalopathy, Leigh's syndrome, subacute necrotizing encephalomyelopathy of Leigh's, subacute necrotizing encephalomyelopathy)

      Leigh's disease is a rare genetic neurometabolic disorder caused by isolated or combined defects of the mitochondrial respiratory chain resulting in impaired oxidative energy production. Male predominance related to mitochondrial DNA mutations (maternal inheritance) can be found in up to two-thirds of patients.

      Genomic DNA:
      i. Pyruvate dehydrogenase complex E1a in chromosome X
      ii. Complex I, NADH in chromosome 11q13
      iii. SURF1 in chromosome 9
      iv. Nuclear encoded flavoprotein gene (complex II) in chromosome 5

Mitochondrial DNA:

Several ATPase 6 and mitochondrial tRNA mutations. The symptoms usually begin between the ages of 3 months and 2 years. Symptoms are associated with progressive neurological deterioration and may include a variable combination of retarded motor and intellectual development, seizures, dystonia, swallowing and feeding difficulties, vomiting, ataxia, external ophthalmoplegia, impaired hearing and vision, and peripheral neuropathy. MRI scan is the most useful tool for premortem diagnosis of the disease. Increased signal intensity and edema are commonly found in the substantia nigra, caudate, putamen, and globus pallidus bilaterally and sometimes in tectum, tegmentum, and medullary olive. Postmortem neuropathologic findings are especially useful to confirm the diagnosis in affected siblings.

b) *Kearns–Sayre syndrome* (ophthalmoplegia-plus syndrome, mitochondrial cytopathy/encephalopathy, oculocraniosomatic syndrome, progressive ophthalmoplegia, Pearson syndrome).

Kearns–Sayre (K-S) syndrome occurs secondary to deletions in mtDNA, most of which are sporadic and believed to occur as germ cell mutations or very early in new embryo development. Deletions vary in size and position, whereas the 4.9-kb mutation accounts for one-third of cases. The K-S syndrome is characterized by a triad of features including: (1) onset before 20 years of age; (2) chronic, progressive, external ophthalmoplegia; and (3) pigmentary degeneration of the retina. The K-S syndrome may include signs of: muscle weakness (ptosis, decreased skeletal muscle power), CNS dysfunction (cerebellar ataxia, decreased higher mental function, cataracts), cardiac (bradycardia, congestive heart failure), and endocrine disorders (short stature in 38%, hypogonadism in 20% of affected individuals). In CSF the lactate and protein levels are elevated (> 100 mg/dl). MRI of the brain has limited diagnostic use. Although PCR test performed on DNA from blood samples can reveal deletions in mtDNA, the best means of achieving *definitive diagnosis* is via analysis of a muscle biopsy specimen, with quantification of the level of deletion using Southern blot analysis.

Differentials of K-S syndrome:

   i. Atrioventricular block (2nd and 3rd degree)
   ii. Failure to thrive
   iii. MELAS syndrome
   iv. Pearson syndrome

4. Syndromes of known metabolic disorder

a) *Hypo- or abetalipoproteinemia* (Bassen–Kornzweig syndrome)
Abetalipoproteinemia and hypolipoproteinemia is an autosomal recessive disorder of lipid metabolism. It is caused by a deficiency of micro-

somal triglyceride transfer protein and impairment of apolipoprotein B metabolism. This leads to failure of chylomicron formation and impaired absorption, and absorption of dietary lipids and fat-soluble vitamins.

Affected patients develop steatorrhea and failure to thrive within the first two decades of life. Neurologic complications occur primarily in infants. Typically, there is a sensory polyneuropathy associated with posterior column and spinocerebellar tract dysfunction. Impaired night vision, secondary to retinitis pigmentosa, develops in older children. More severely affected individuals may become nonambulant by their mid-20s.

During infancy, the diagnosis is suggested by clinical evidence of fat malabsorption or fat intolerance associated with extremely low total cholesterol levels, 20–50 mg/dL, with triglyceride levels less than 20 mg/dL. There is also a concomitant absence of apolipoprotein B, LDLs, VLDLs, and chylomicrons. Vitamin E and other fat-soluble vitamin levels are low. Anemia is common. However, the abnormal erythrocyte morphology (acanthocytosis) provides one of the major laboratory clues to the diagnosis. Nerve conduction studies show low-amplitude sensory action potential amplitudes with slight slowing of sensory conduction velocities. Motor nerve conduction is usually normal.

b) *Wilson's disease or hepatolenticular degeneration* (low or absent copper ceruloplasmin)

WD (autosomal recessive) and Menkes disease (X-linked) represent the most well-recognized and understood disorders of copper homeostasis. The WD P-type ATP7B and the Menkes P-type ATP7P are functionally homologous and share 67% protein identity. These copper transport proteins differ in tissue and developmental expression only. In WD, a genetic mutation of chromosome 13 affects ATP7B, a protein that helps transport copper into the bile. ATP7B is also involved in incorporating copper into ceruloplasmin, a protein that carries the mineral through the bloodstream. Ceruloplasmin contains 95% of copper found in serum. The defects in the ATP7B gene mean that copper is not eliminated properly, and instead builds up in the hepatocyte and results in cirrhosis and hepatic fibrosis. In time, excess copper spills out of the liver and begins accumulating in and damaging other organs, especially the brain, eyes, kidneys, and joints. Although copper accumulation begins at birth, symptoms of the disorder appear later in life. The most characteristic symptom of WD is liver disease with Kayser–Fleischer ring—a rusty brown ring around the cornea (▶ Fig. 7.7). The primary consequence of most of those with WD is liver disease, appearing in late childhood or early adolescence as acute hepatitis, liver failure, or progressive chronic liver disease in the form of chronic active hepatitis or cirrhosis of the liver. In others, the first

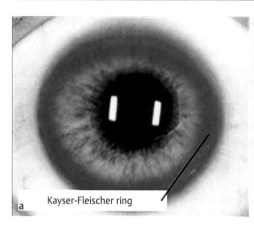

Fig. 7.7 (a) Kayser–Fleischer ring. This image is provided courtesy of The Wilson Disease Association 2009.

Kayser-Fleischer ring

a

symptoms occur later in adulthood and most commonly include slurred speech, difficulty swallowing, and drooling. Other symptoms may include tremor of the head, arms, or legs; impaired muscle tone, and sustained muscle contractions that produce abnormal postures, twisting, and repetitive movements (dystonia), and bradykinesia. Individuals may also experience ataxia and loss of fine motor skills. One-third of those with WD will also experience psychiatric symptoms such as an abrupt personality change, bizarre and inappropriate behavior, depression accompanied by suicidal thoughts, neurosis, or psychosis.

No single test—not even genetic tests—can diagnose WD by itself. Symptoms of WD are often indistinguishable from those of hepatitis, alcoholic cirrhosis, and other chronic liver diseases. Laboratory analysis reveals absent serum ceruloplasmin, mild anemia, low serum iron, low transferring saturation, and an elevated ferritin. Kayser–Fleischer ring can be viewed using an ophthalmologist's slit lamp. Needle or laparoscopic biopsies are remarkable for normal hepatic architecture without evidence of fibrosis or cirrhosis. Because more than 200 mutations of ATP7B exist, there isn't a simple genetic test that can help screen or diagnose WD in the general population.

c) *Refsum's disease* (heredopathia atactica polyneuritiformis)
Autosomal recessive lipidosis with deficiency of phytanoyl-coenzyme A hydroxylase and accumulation of phytanic acid, which is exclusively of dietary origin. Usually is manifested in childhood by progressive night blindness (granular pigmentary retinopathy), limb weakness, gait ataxia, peripheral neuropathy, loss of reflexes, and muscle wasting. Less common features include deafness, cataracts, miosis, pes cavus, cardiac arrythmias, and bone deformities.

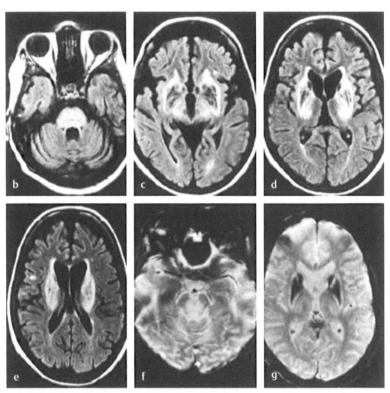

Fig. 7.7 (*Continued*) **(b)** Wilson disease. The signal abnormalities, consisting of a mix of increased and decreased signal intensities, primarily affect the basal ganglia, midbrain, and pons. **(b–e)** Axial MRI (FLAIR) shows mild ventricular dilatation and bilateral, symmetrical hyperintensity in the pons **(b)**, around the basal ganglia and internal capsule as far as the thalamus and hypothalamus **(c, d)**, and in the caudate nucleus **(e)**. **(f, g)** T2*-weighted MRI at the level of the midbrain **(f)** and basal ganglia **(g)** shows increased signal intensity in the midbrain and at the periphery of the lentiform nuclei on both sides and decreased signal intensity in the putamen, globus pallidus, and head of the caudate nucleus. (Reproduced from Degenerative Diseases with Primary Involvement of the Deep Gray Matter. In: Sartor K, ed. Diagnostic and Interventional Neuroradiology. 1st edition. Thieme; 2002.)

d) *Hartnup disease* (Hartnup aminoaciduria, Hartnup syndrome)
   Hartnup disease is an autosomal recessive disorder caused by defective transport of neutral (i.e., monoamino monocarboxylic) amino acids in the small intestine and the kidneys. Hartnup defect ranks among the

most common amino acid disorders in humans (1 case per 18,000–42,000 population). A causative gene *SLC6A19*, was located on band 5p15.33. *SLC6A19* is a sodium-dependent and chloride independent neutral amino acid transporter, expressed predominantly in the kidneys and intestine. Amino acids are retained within the intestinal lumen, where they are converted by bacteria to *indolic compounds* that can be toxic to the CNS. Tubular renal transport is also defective, contributing to gross aminoaciduria. Hartnup disease is manifested by a wide clinical spectrum. Most patients remain asymptomatic, but in a minority of patients, *skin photosensitivity* (dry, scaly, weel-marginated eruptions on the forehead, cheeks, periorbital regions, the dorsal surfaces of the hands, and other light exposed areas), *neurologic* (intermittent cerebellar ataxia, a wide-based gait, spasticity, delayed motor development, and tremulousness) and *psychiatric* symptoms may have a considerable influence on their quality of life. Rarely, severe CNS involvement may lead to death. Mental retardation and short stature have been described in a few patients. Ocular manifestations include diplopia, nystagmus, photophobia, and strabismus.

Gingivitis, stomatitis, and glossitis suggest niacin deficiency. Exacerbations are seen most frequently in the spring or early summer after exposure to light. Urine chromatography gives following results:

i. Increased levels of neutral amino acids (i.e., glutamine, valine, phenylalanine, leucine, asparagine, citrulline, isoleucine, threonine, alanine, serine, histidine, tyrosine, tryptophan) and indicant are found in the urine.

ii. Urine excretion of proline, hydroxyproline, and arginine remains normal, which differentiates Hartnup disease from other causes of gross aminoaciduria.

iii. Urine indoxyl derivatives (i.e., 5-hydroxyindoleacetic acid) may be demonstrated following an oral tryptophan load.

iv. Urine chromatography excludes a nutritional pellagra.

v. Plasma concentrations of amino acids are usually normal.

Differentials:

i. Ataxia-telangiectasia (especially in patients with mild skin involvement)

ii. Xeroderma pigmentosum

iii. SLE (can be confused if photosensitivity-malar rash with neuropsychiatric symptoms is present)

iv. Pityriasis alba

v. Nutritional pellagra (misdiagnosis can be avoided by performing urine chromatography)

vi. Congenital poikilodermas with photosensitivity (i.e., Cockayne syndrome)

vii. Infantile atopic eczema

viii. Seborrheic eczema

e) *Metabolic acidosis* (disorders of pyruvate and lactate metabolism)

f) *Hyperammonemia* (urea cycle enzyme defects)

Ammonia is a toxic compound produced in the body from catabolism of amino acids and protein. Hyperammonemia can damage muscle and brain. The body converts ammonia to urea in the liver by means of the urea cycle enzymes, and the urea so generated is subsequently eliminated in the urine as nitrogenous waste. Hyperammonemia is a dangerous condition that may lead to encephalopathy and death; the survivors of coma have a high incidence of intellectual impairment. It may be primary or secondary.

i. Primary:
   - Urea cycle defects:
     ◦ Carbamoyl phosphate synthetase (CPS) deficiency
     ◦ Ornithine transcarbamylase (OTC) deficiency
     ◦ Citrullinemia
     ◦ Argininosuccinic aciduria
     ◦ Argininemia
   - Transient hyperammonemia of the newborn

ii. Secondary:
   - Organic acidopathies
   - Fatty acid oxidation defects
   - Reye's syndrome

Diagnosis:

Assessment of hyperammonemia due to cycle defect begins with the assessment of the third enzyme in the urea cycle (argininosuccinate synthetase). A defect in this enzyme will result in an elevation of citrulline. Then follows the assessment of the fourth and fifth enzymes of the urea cycle (argininosuccinate lyase, arginase), a defect of which will result in a moderate elevation of citrulline. An assessment of the first and second enzymes (carbamoyl phosphate synthetase, ornithine transcarbamylase) is last; a defect of these enzymes will result normal or low citrulline levels.

Clinical features:

i. Newborn:
   - Neurological (lethargy to coma, infantile hypotonia, seizures)
   - Gastrointestinal (persistent vomiting, poor feeding, hepatomegaly)
   - Others (hyperventilation due to respiratory alkalosis, hypothermia)

      ii. Children: Usually present after a sudden protein load or an inter-current infection with recurrent episodes of:
- Neurological (lethargy to coma, acute ataxia, hyperactivity)
- Gastrointestinal (persistent vomiting, hepatomegaly)

g) *Biotinidase deficiency* (infantile/juvenile multiple carboxylase deficiency, deficiency of free biotin)

The primary function of biotinidase is to cleave biotin from biocytin, pre-serving the pool of free biotin for use as a cofactor for biotin-dependent enzymes, namely the four human carboxylases (pyruvate, propionyl-coenzyme A, beta-methylcrotonyl-CoA, and acetyl-CoA carboxylase). The carboxylases serve important roles in intermediary metabolism and im-pairment causes abnormalities in fatty acid synthesis, amino acid catabo-lism, and gluconeogenesis. Incidence of profound deficiency is estimated at 1 per 137,401 population. The gene mutation that encodes biotinidase is localized at *3p25*, and less common at Arg538 to Cys. Sudden death is reported due to seizures or brainstem dysfunction. The spectrum of clinical signs and symptoms is varied. Consider biotinidase deficiency at presentation of intractable seizures, acidosis, eczematous, scaly perioral/fascial rash, alopecia with loss of hair color, unexplained hearing or visual loss, spastic paraparesis or hypotonia, and failure to thrive.

Differential diagnosis:
      i. Consider sepsis, meningitis, or toxic exposure in a child with in-tractable epilepsy or severe metabolic disruption
      ii. Other inborn errors of metabolism, if laboratory testing indicates hyperammonemia and/or acidosis
      iii. Neonatal-onset symptoms of biotinidase deficiency may be difficult to differentiate from holocarboxylase synthetase deficiency

h) *Hexosaminidase deficiency* (GM2 gangliosidosis, Tay–Sachs disease)

Gm2-gangliosidosis type I; infantile variant of storage disease with deficiency of hexosaminidase A; autosomal recessive inheritance pattern; normal development until onset of symptoms by 6 months of age; clinical features include irritability and hyperexcitability, exaggerated startle response, delayed cognitive development, motor retardation with hypoto-nia, hyperactive reflexes, clonus, extensor plantar responses, progressive visual impairment, complete *blindness* by 1 year in most cases, presence of macular cherry-red spot, and occasional myoclonic seizures. Vegetative state occurs by the second year. Pathology reveals ballooned neurons in brain, cerebellum, and spinal cord. Supportive care, no specific treatment.

i) *Krabbe's leukodystrophy* (*metachromatic* leukodystrophy)

Lysosomal storage disease with deficiency of galactocerebrosidase and accumulation of galactocerebroside and psychosine in affected tissues of infants (rarely juvenile or adult years). Normal at birth, patients develop progressive irritability, inexplicable crying, fevers, limb stiffness, seizures, feeding difficulty, vomiting, mental slowing and psychomotor retardation, marked hypertonia, extensor *posturing*, optic nerve atrophy, flaccidity, and loss of tendon reflexes. Death usually occurs by 2 years.

j) *Ceroid lipofuscinoses* (*neuronal* ceroid lipofuscinosis)

The neuronal ceroid lipofuscinoses (NCL or CLN) are a mixed group of neurodegenerative disorders. They are considered *the* most common of the neurogenetic storage diseases with a prevalence of 1 in 12,500 in some populations, especially in the Scandinavian countries (Finland 1%), where most cases have infantile onset. Only 50% of the CLN1 cases have an infantile onset in the United States, and the other cases have late infantile, juvenile, or adult onset. These heterogenous disorders, genetically classified as CLN1 to CLN8, share similar symptoms and signs such as retinopathy with loss of vision, epilepsy, dementia, and accumulation of unusual waxy material termed ceroid lipofuscin in brain and other tissues. Their pathophysiology is poorly understood and involves the combination of an intracellular storage process and a progressive loss of nerve cells. Two CLN disorders are caused by deficient lysosomal enzymes, namely palmitoyl-protein thioesterase in CLN1 and tripeptidyl-peptidase in CLN2. In some others, it has been found that membrane proteins with unknown function are deficient. The genetic defect can be identified in most cases and forms the basis for family counselling and prenatal diagnosis.

The NCLs are defined by their age of onset and symptoms:

   i. Infantile NCL (Santavuori-Haltia disease)
   ii. Late infantile NCL (Jansky–Bielschowsky type)
   iii. Juvenile NCL (Batten disease or Spieimeyer–Vogt disease)
   iv. Adult NCL (Kufs disease or Parry disease)

NCLs are diagnosed on the basis of the symptoms the child or young adult is experiencing. In addition, in the early course of the disease, the EEG can be helpful by showing posterior spikes on slow photic stimulation. In addition, there may be an increase in evoked potentials. Brain MRI findings are mainly nonspecific, showing pronounced cerebral atrophy in the infratentorial region and some white matter changes. MRI changes may help to differentiate between classical and variant forms of late infantile NCLs. Electron microscopy of isolated lymphocytes, skin biopsy specimens, or other tissues reveals mainly "fingerprint-like" l curvilinear cell inclusion bodies.

Differential diagnosis:

   i. Benign childhood epilepsy
   ii. Complex partial seizures
   iii. Epilepsy in children or adults with mental retardation

  iv. Diseases of carbohydrate metabolism
  v. Frontal lobe epilepsy
  vi. Temporal lobe epilepsy
  vii. Friedreich's ataxia
 viii. Hallervorden–Spatz disease
  ix. Huntington's disease
  x. Lysosomal storage disease
  xi. Peroxisomal disorders
  xii. Inherited metabolic disorders
 xiii. Gangliosidosis
 xiv. Leber's optic atrophy
  xv. Mitochondrial disease
 xvi. Retinitis pigmentosa

k) *Niemann–Pick disease* (acid sphingomyelinase deficiency)

Niemann–Pick disease (NPD) is a lipid storage disorder. The original description of NPD referred to what is currently termed NPD type A. Since then six subtypes of NPD have been described, including type B and other rarer forms, all of which are inherited as autosomal recessive traits. NPD types A and B result from deficient activity of spingomyelinase, a lysosomal enzyme encoded by a gene located on chromosome bands 11p15.1–p15.4. The enzymatic defect results in pathologic accumulation of sphingomyelin and other lipids in the monocyte–macrophage system. Type A disease is fatal in early childhood particularly affecting the individuals of Ashkenazi Jewish descent (carrier frequency 1:80). All NPD subtypes display variable clinical features:

 i. NPD type A:
  – Cherry-red spot on ophthalmologic examination
  – Massive hepatosplenomegaly
  – Progressive neurodegeneration, and attainment of milestones does not progress beyond 10 months in any domain. Neurodegeneration is relentless leading to a spastic state. Seizures are not common.

 ii. NPD type B:
  – Up to 50% of case have a cherry-red spot or macular haloes
  – Hepatosplenomegaly can be quite variable
  – Most patients have normal neurological examination, although some patients presented with peripheral neuropathy and learning disabilities. Some patients present loss of language skills and onset of ataxia beginning around the third year of life.
  – Growth retardation in childhood
  – Skin may reveal extensive bruising and petechiae

Lab studies:
  i. The diagnosis is confirmed with measurement of the enzyme in peripheral white blood cells or in cultured fibroblasts.
  ii. Acid spingomyelinase mutation analysis: Sequencing of the gene in research labs permits the identification of precise gene mutations.
  iii. The pathologic hallmark in NPD type A and B is the histochemically characteristic lipid-laden foam cell, often termed the Niemann–Pick cell.

  Differential diagnosis:
  i. Gaucher disease
  ii. GM1 Gangliosidosis

5. Other syndromes
   a) Autosomal dominant diseases
      i. Olivopontocerebellar atrophy (ataxia, ophthalmoplegia, optic atrophy)
      ii. Spinocerebellar ataxia (ataxia, dysarthria, sensory loss)
      iii. Machado–Joseph disease (cerebellar, extrapyramidal and pyramidal deficits)
   b) Autosomal recessive diseases
      i. *Ramsay-Hunt syndrome I (dyssynergia cerebellaris myoclonica)*
         Early-onset ataxia syndrome: etiologically heterogenous, consists of progressive ataxia in combination with myoclonus (action or intention). In most patients, progressive ataxia develops first, followed by onset of myoclonus. In other patients, myoclonus may be the initial manifestation. The myoclonus may be a manifestation of another disease, such as mitochondrial encephalomyopathy with ragged red fibers (MERFF), Unverricht–Lundborg disease, or progressive myoclonus epilepsy. MERFF, the most common cause, consists of ataxia, myoclonus, seizure activity, myopathy, and hearing loss.

         The above syndrome should not be confused with what is called Ramsay Hunt syndrome II (Herpes zoster oticus), a common complication of shingles that is an infection caused by the varicella zoster virus which caused chickenpox. The spread of the reactivated varicella zoster virus into the fascial nerves causes the Ramsay Hunt syndrome II, which is characterized by intense ear pain, a rash around the ear, mouth, face, neck, and scalp, and paralysis of the fascial nerve. Further features may include vertigo, hearing loss, tinnitus, taste loss in the tongue, dry mouth and eyes.
      ii. *Behr's syndrome (ataxia, optic atrophy, and mental retardation)*
         Behr syndrome is a variant of familial spastic paraplegia in which the cardinal features are optic atrophy, ataxia, spasticity, and mental retardation. The syndrome is transmitted as an autosomal

recessive trait, but genetic heterogeneity is very likely. The symptoms appear in infancy and progress slowly. The features are bilateral optic atrophy, with field defects, generally temporal and rarely complete; neurologic signs (increased tendon reflexes, Babinski sign, slight inco-ordination with ataxia and spastic gait, mental deficiency, nystagmus). Additional features are speech defect, high arches of feet (pes cavus), muscle atrophy, leukodystrophy or demyelination, and cerebellar hemisphere hypoplasia.

c) X-linked spinocerebellar ataxia (rare)

Albert DM, et al. Phakomatoses-Ataxia Telangiectasia (Louis-Bar Syndrome). In Principles and Practice of Ophthalmology Clinical Practice. Philadelphia: EWB Saundersd;1994

Robbins JH, Brumback RA, Mendiones M, et al. Neurological disease in xeroderma pigmentosum. Documentation of a late onset type of the juvenile onset form. Brain 1991;114(Pt 3):1335–1361

Rahman S, Blok RB, Dahl HH, et al. Leigh syndrome: clinical features and biochemical and DNA abnormalities. Ann Neurol 1996;39(3):343–351

Bosbach S, Kornblum C, Schröder R, Wagner M. Executive and visuospatial deficits in patients with chronic progressive external ophthalmoplegia and Kearns-Sayre syndrome. Brain 2003;126(Pt 5):1231–1240

Rader DJ, Brewer HB Jr. Abetalipoproteinemia. New insights into lipoprotein assembly and vitamin E metabolism from a rare genetic disease. JAMA 1993;270(7):865–869

Waggoner DJ, Bartnikas TB, Gitlin JD. The role of copper in neurodegenerative disease. Neurobiol Dis 1999;6(4):221–230

Razvani J, Rosenblatt DS. Defects in metabolism of amino acids. In: Nelson WE, Bergmann RE, Klingmann RM, et al. eds. Nelson's Textbook of Pediatrics. Philadelphia: WB Saunders Co.; 1996:338–340

Batshaw ML. Hyperammonemia. Curr Probl Pediatr 1984;14(11):1–69

Weber P, Scholl S, Baumgartner ER. Outcome in patients with profound biotinidase deficiency: relevance of newborn screening. Dev Med Child Neurol 2004;46(7):481–484

ACOG Committee Opinion. Screening for Tay-Sachs disease Obstet Gynecol 2005;106:893–894

Goebel HH, Sharp JD. The neuronal ceroid-lipofuscinoses. Recent advances. Brain Pathol 1998;8(1):151–162

Schuchman EH, Desnick RJ. Niemann-Pick disease types A and B: acid sphingomyelinase deficiency. In: Metabolic and Molecular Bases of Inherited Disease. 7th ed. McGraw-Hill; 1977

Tassinari CA, Michelucci R, Genton P, Pellissier JF, Roger J. Dyssynergia cerebellaris myoclonica (Ramsay Hunt syndrome): a condition unrelated to mitochondrial encephalomyopathies. J Neurol Neurosurg Psychiatry 1989;52(2):262–265

Farah S, Sabry MA, Qasrawi B, et al. Behr syndrome with X-linked mode of inheritance. J Med Genet 1996;33(Suppl 1):S26

7.11 Cerebral Atrophy

1. Dementia Alzheimer's type
   Diffuse cortical atrophy especially in the temporal lobes and hippocampal/parahippocampal area and dilatation of more than 3 mm in diameter and dilatation of the choroidal–hippocampal fissure complex and temporal horns.

2. Pick's disease
   Severe atrophy of the anterior frontal and temporal lobes with swollen nerve cells and intracytoplasmic inclusions (Pick's bodies).

3. Parkinson's disease
   Substantia nigra small and basal ganglia intensity changed.
4. Progressive supranuclear palsy (Steele–Richardson–Olszewski syndrome)
   Third ventricular dilatation, midbrain atrophy, and enlargement of the interpeduncular cistern.
5. CJD
   Frontal predominance atrophy, abnormal intensity of the basal ganglia.
6. Multi-infarct dementia
   White matter and deep gray lacunae, central pontine infarcts, and strokes of different ages.
7. Dyke–Davidoff–Masson syndrome (e.g., hemiatrophy of one hemisphere)
8. Porencephaly (e.g., from trauma, infection, and perinatal ischemia)
9. Miscellaneous causes
   a) Previous infections
   b) Long-standing MS
   c) Extensive traumatic brain injury
   d) Chronic use of steroids
   e) Radiation injury
   f) Intrathecal chemotherapy
   g) Starvation/anorexia
   h) Dehydration

7.12 Dementia

7.12.1 General

Dementia is a clinical syndrome that is characterized by impairment of short- and long-term memory associated with impairment in abstract thinking and judgment, and other disturbances of higher cortical function (aphasia, apraxia, agnosia, executive function). These must represent a decline from previous level of function and be severe enough to interfere with work or usual social activities or relationships with others. Although AD is the most common type of dementia, there are many other types that can be diagnosed premorbidly by careful clinical evaluation. The major dementia syndromes include:

1. AD
2. Vascular dementia (VaD)
3. Dementia with Lewy bodies (DLB)
4. Parkinson's disease with dementia (PDD)
5. Frontotemporal dementia (FTD)
6. Reversible dementias

Most elderly patients with chronic dementia have AD (approximately 60–80%). The VaDs account for 10–20% and PDD for about 5%. The prevalence of VaD is relatively high in blacks, hypertensive persons, and patients with diabetes. DLB may be as prevalent as VaD in older cohorts of patients. Some of the reversible dementias (e.g., metabolic dementias) tend to occur in young individuals.

7.12.2 Causes

Dementia can occur due to numerous pathological states that affect the brain.

1. Drugs/toxin: Medications (beta-blockers, antidepressants, anticonvulsants, neuroleptics, opiate analgesics, adrenocortical steroids, anticholinergic preparations such as used in allergic reactions, movement disorders); substance abuse (virtually all of the chemicals used from heroin, glue sniffing, alcohol, marijuana, phencyclidine can produce dementing illness); exogenous toxins (carbon monoxide, carbon disulfide, lead, mercury, arsenic, and manganese).
2. Infections/inflammations: Any infection involving the brain can produce dementing illness. Focal cerebritis/abscess; leptomeningitis and encephalitis from chronic infections caused by bacteria (tuberculosis, Whipple's disease of the brain), protozoa (neurosyphilis), or fungi (cryptococcus), Lyme encephalopathy; certain chronic viral illnesses (HIV dementia and other opportunistic infections); CJD; progressive multifocal encephalopathy; neurosarcoidosis; postinfectious encephalomyelitis such as follows the viral exanthems, post herpes simplex encephalitis.
3. Metabolic disorders: Hypothyroidism, uremia/dialysis dementia, chronic hepatic encephalopathy, chronic hypoglycemia encephalopathy, Addison's/Cushing's diseases, pulmonary diseases causing hypercapnia, hypoxemia, hyperviscosity. A number of hereditary metabolic diseases are associated with dementia (hepatolenticular degeneration/WD, metachromatic leukodystrophy, the adrenoleukodystrophies, and the neuronal storage diseases.
4. Nutritional disorders: Vitamin B12 deficiency, vitamin B1 deficiency (Wernicke–Korsakoff's encephalopathy), vitamin E deficiency, nicotinic acid deficiency.
5. Vascular: Severe hypertension is one of the most frequent causes of dementia. Cerebral infarction, large and small, is the most common cause of multi-infarct dementia. Binswanger's disease (subcortical arteriosclerotic encephalopathy), strokes in certain brain areas (thalamic, bifrontal, infratemporal), amyloid dementia, transient ischemic attack (TIA)'s mitochondrial, encephalopathy, lactic acidosis, and stroke-like episodes (MELAS) syndrome, CADASIL; vasculitis (SLE, polyarteritis nodosa, CNS granulomatous angiitis, Bechet's disease).
6. Space-occupying lesions: Chronic subdural hematoma may produce dementia or complicate and add to the effects of other causes. Benign tumors of the brain produce dementia depending on their size and

location (subfrontal/orbital lobe or on the medial temporal lobe). Obstructive hydrocephalus due to benign lesions such as cerebellopontine angle neurofibroma. Malignant tumors of brain frequently produce dementia.

7. Normal pressure hydrocephalus: It produces dementia associated with gait disturbance and urinary/fecal incontinence with dramatic response to CSF shunting.

8. Psychiatric dementia: Pseudodementia as depression (reversible with successful treatment), chronic schizophrenia, hysteria, mania. Depression is commonly present with other causes of dementia, especially AD.

9. Trauma: Dementia pugilistica, diffuse axonal injury, hemorrhage, postconcussion syndrome.

10. Progressive degenerate diseases—adult: The most frequent of the dementing diseases are not arrestable or reversible. AD, Pick's disease, Parkinson's disease, Huntington's disease, FTD, progressive supranuclear palsy, diffuse cortical Lewy body disease, multisystem atrophy/spinocerebellar ataxias, corticobasal degeneration, progressive subcortical gliosis, dementia complex of Guam, familial or acquired hepatolenticular degeneration (WD), Hallervorden–Spatz disease.

11. Autoimmune/miscellaneous: MS, Schilder's disease, Balo's sclerosis, SLE, isolated angiitis of the CNS, tuberous sclerosis.

Frequency of dementia causes from 32 studies

1	Alzheimer's disease (AD)	57.0%
2	Vascular dementia (VD)	13.0%
3	Depression	4.5%
4	Alcohol	4.0%
5	Normal pressure hydrocephalus	1.6%
6	Metabolic	1.5%
7	Medications	1.5%
8	Parkinson's disease	1.2%
9	Huntington's disease	0.9%
10	Mixed AD and VD	0.8%
11	Infection	0.6%
12	Subdural hematoma	0.4%
13	Post trauma	0.4%
14	Anoxia	0.2%
15	Miscellaneous	6.9%
16	Not demented	3.7%

7.12.3 Signs and symptoms

Once the criteria of a patient for dementia are established, the history of present illness should be directed toward soliciting presenting symptoms and associated medical conditions that suggest a specific diagnosis. These include the symptoms noted below, as well as speed of progression, mode of onset, associated focal neurological deficits, presence or absence of headache, and incontinence. A thorough review of the patient's medications, assessment of patient's vascular and HIV risk factors, alcohol use, and family history of dementia should be obtained. Symptoms vary depending on the cause of dementia.

Dementia is characterized primarily by a gradual onset of following progressive symptoms:

1. Memory loss and changes in personality
2. Noticeable decline in cognitive abilities (including speech and understanding)
3. Loss of decision-making function
4. Impairment of daily living activities (dressing, eating, toileting, etc.)

Diagnostic and Statistical Manual of Mental Disorder (DSM-IV) diagnosis of dementia requires following criteria to be met:

1. Memory impairment
2. At least one of the following: aphasia, apraxia, agnosia, or disturbance in decision-making functioning
3. Impairment of social or occupational function
4. Diagnosis should not be made during the course of a delirium

Early signs of possible dementia include:

1. Memory loss that affects home or job skills
2. Difficulty performing familiar tasks
3. Problems with language
4. Disorientation to time and place
5. Poor or decreased judgement
6. Problems with complex and abstract tasks
7. Misplacing things
8. Changes in mood or behavior
9. Changes in personality
10. Loss of initiative

7.12.4 Laboratory tests

1. All patients with new onset of dementia should have several basic and standard diagnostic studies. Most of the reversible metabolic, endocrine, deficiency, and infectious states, whether causative or complications will be

revealed by these simple investigations, when combined with history and physical examination.

a) Initial evaluation should include CBC, liver function tests, sodium, calcium, thyroid-stimulating hormone, RPR, vitamin B12 level.

b) In appropriate circumstances, consider HIV testing or Lyme serology.

c) Atypical cases of dementia may require one of the following: ceruloplasmin and copper levels (WD), plasma levels of very-long-chain fatty acids (adrenoleukodystrophy), WBC arylsulfatase A (metachromatic leukodystrophy), vitamin E and B1 levels, porphyrins, blood gas, hemoglobin A1C, tumor markers (anti-Hu/Yo/Ri), ANA/vasculitis workup, urinary heavy metals, thyroid antibodies, toxicology screen.

2. Other ancillary studies are appropriate in certain circumstances:

a) CT scan of brain without contrast (in the presence of brain mass or focal neurologic signs, or in dementia of brief duration). MRI is more sensitive for detecting small infarcts, mass lesions, atrophy of the brainstem, and other structures.

b) EEG and cerebral angiography are appropriate in certain circumstances, such as CJD and CNS vasculitis respectively.

c) Formal psychiatric assessment is desirable when depression is suspected.

d) Bedside neuropsychological assessment including the Mini Mental Status Exam and the Clinical Dementia Rating Scale. These provide objective, reproducible scores for future comparison.

e) PET/SPECT can be helpful in diagnosing Alzheimer's and Huntington's disease.

f) Biological markers for progressive degenerative dementing diseases are still in the investigative stage:

  i. Genetic tests such as serum apoE-4, and tests for the presenilin gene

  ii. CSF analysis for the A beta form of the amyloid precursor protein and tau

g) Lumbar puncture is not routinely required in the initial evaluation of dementia, but it should be considered in the following circumstances:

  i. CNS bacterial or viral infection

  ii. Systemic infection

  iii. Immunocompromised patient

  iv. Rapid progression of symptoms

  v. Cancer

  vi. CNS vasculitis

h) Brain biopsy should be considered in unusual cases as follows:

  i. Focal, relevant lesions of undetermined cause, after extensive evaluation

    ii. CNS vasculitis

    iii. Subacute sclerosing panencephalitis

    iv. PML, where lymphoma cannot be conclusively ruled out by neuro-imaging or spinal fluid analysis

    v. Degenerative neurologic illnesses such as Kuf's disease, Alexander's disease

 i) Muscle biopsy in suspected mitochondrial disorders

7.12.5 Differential diagnosis

When assessing someone who has memory problems, it is important for the clinician to remember that *not all people with memory problems have dementia.* Diagnosing dementia is a two-stage process. The first stage is to establish a diagnosis of dementia, since 13% of all dementias are potentially reversible. The second is to elucidate the cause of dementia and the coexisting medical conditions ("co-morbidity" such as Parkinson's disease, depression, infection, congestive heart failure, and chronic obstructive pulmonary disease) which may worsen the dementia.

1. *Alzheimer's disease*

   AD is progressive, resulting in impairment in cognitive function. The clinical symptoms associated with this disease include memory loss, language disorders, visual-spatial impairment, and behavioral disturbances.

   Differentials:

   a) Aphasia

   b) Cortical basal ganglionic degeneration

   c) Dementia in motor neuron disease

   d) DLB

   e) Frontal and temporal lobe dementia

   f) Lyme disease

   g) Neurosyphilis

   h) Parkinson's disease and Parkinson-Plus syndromes

   i) Prion-related diseases

   j) Thyroid disease

   k) WD

   For a diagnosis of probable AD, the criteria are:

   a) Dementia established by examination and objective testing

   b) Deficits in two or more cognitive areas

   c) Progressive worsening of memory and other cognitive functions

   d) No disturbance in consciousness

   e) Onset between ages 40 and 90 years

   f) Absence of systemic disorders or other brain diseases, which could account for the deficits in memory and cognition

g) The classic neuropathology findings are neurofibrillary tangles and neuritic plaques

h) Detecting an e4 allele of the APOE gene on chromosome 19 can add confidence to the clinical diagnosis of late-onset and sporadic AD

i) Tests of CSF for abnormal levels on indicator proteins (Ab42 and tau) come slowest to fulfilling the criteria for a useful biomarker

j) The CSF 14–3-3 protein and neuron-specific enolase is useful for confirming or rejecting the diagnosis of CJD.

k) EEG can help in ruling out other diseases that cause dementia, such as prion-related diseases (e.g., CJD)

2. *Vascular dementia*

VaD may arise as a sequel to any form of cerebrovascular disease (CVD). As a co-morbid condition, VaD may worsen the dementia of AD. Patients have patchy cognitive impairment, often with focal neurologic signs and symptoms. Onset may be abrupt, with a step-wise decline.

Differentials:

a) Dementia due to head trauma

Patients have memory impairment, and other cognitive deficits associated with a history of head trauma. Dementia is not usually progressive and the symptoms depend on the location of injury.

b) Dementia due to HIV disease

Patients have cognitive changes with neurologic signs and a positive result from an HIV test.

c) Depression

In the case of cognitive symptoms secondary to depression, the onset is acute compared with the insidious onset in most other types of dementia. Patients with depression usually report their cognitive difficulties, which is unusual for patients with dementia. Patients with depression tend to state that they do not know the answers to questions, and they appear to not try very hard during neuropsychologic evaluations. Mood symptoms are prominent with dementia of depression.

d) Huntington's disease dementia

It is an autosomal dominant disease with an onset of cognitive changes as early as the third decade of life, with physical signs of choreoathetosis

e) PDD

Patients have cognitive slowing with extrapyramidal signs such as rigidity, bradykinesia, tremor, and gait disturbances. Usually dementia is seen in later stages of the disease.

f) AD

Patients with AD have early language and visuospatial deficits. The deficits of short-term memory are severe, and clues do not help in retrieving information. The onset of the disease is gradual with a slow progression. Usually, no motor findings are present until the middle or late stages of the disease.

g) Brain tumor

h) CJD

By far the most common human prion disease (about 85%) is CJD. Onset is between the 4th and 6th decades of life and is characterized by a rapid progressive dementia associated with signs such as myoclonus, seizures, and ataxia. The EEG findings show distinctive changes of high voltage (1–2 Hz) and sharp wave complexes on an increasingly slow and low-voltage background.

i) Neurosyphilis

j) Normal pressure hydrocephalus

The classical triad of mental deterioration, ataxia with characteristic spasticity of the lower limbs, and incontinence in well-established pathology is well characteristic finding.

k) FTD

Type of cortical dementia characterized by behavioral and personality disorders more than cognitive issues. Three distinct types are seen: FTD, semantic dementia, and progressive nonfluent aphasia.

l) Pick's disease

Patients have memory problems, personality changes, and deterioration of social skills. Onset is usually between the 5th and 6th decades of life. On examination patient has frontal release signs such as snout and grasp reflex.

m) DLB

Patients have recurrent visual hallucinations, fluctuating cognitive impairment, and parkinsonism features. Also, the frequency of adverse reactions to antipsychotic medications is high.

Diagnosis of probable VaD is supported from the following criteria:

a) Sudden onset of dysfunction in one or more cognitive domains

b) Stepwise deteriorating course

c) Presence of focal signs on neurologic examination such as: hemiparesis, fascial weakness, Babinski sign, sensory deficit, or hemianopia

d) History of previous strokes

e) Evidence of stroke risk factors and of systemic vascular disease

f) Evidence of relevant CVD by brain imaging, including multiple large-vessel infarcts, multiple basal ganglia and white matter lacune or extensive periventricular white matter lesions or combinations of these. Any combination of onset of dementia within 3 months following a recognized stroke; abrupt deterioration in cognitive functions; or fluctuating, stepwise progression of cognitive deficits.

g) The Hachinski ischemic index is probably the most widely used set of criteria for VaD. The scale is easy to apply in clinical practice and has reliably distinguished between possible atherosclerotic causes of dementia and AD.

3. *Frontotemporal dementia*

Patients with FTD have dysfunction of the brain's prefrontal regions, temporal lobes, or both. In many cases, there may be significant atrophy easily visible with MRI specific to the affected areas; in other instances, the abnormalities may be functional rather than structural. Although some patients (25%) have Pick's bodies, most do not. Clinical features include initial mild memory impairment, with more pronounced dysphasia (reduced speech output, severe naming difficulty, and problem with word meaning), personality changes (apathy, inattentiveness), and extrapyramidal motor dysfunction; dementia becomes severe in later stages of the disease. These deficits are not due to other nervous system conditions (e.g., CVD), systemic conditions (e.g., hypothyroidism), or substance-induced conditions. Pathology reveals Pick's bodies (argyrophilic intraneuronal inclusion bodies) and gliosis in affected areas, associated with mutations in tau gene on chromosome 17, with accumulation of abnormal tau proteins in Pick's bodies.

4. *Medication-induced dementia*

This type of dementia is the most frequent cause of "reversible" dementia. Many medications can cause memory problems and there should be a high suspicion if the memory symptoms appeared to start soon after a new medication is commenced. Drugs which are particularly associated with memory impairment are those that are known to affect the CNS, such as medication for epilepsy and Parkinson's disease, sleeping medication, anti-anxiety drugs, and barbiturates. Chronic alcohol abuse or the use of illicit drugs can also affect the memory function. A period without the suspected drug may prove its influence on the person's cognitive ability.

5. *Metabolic–endocrine–nutritional–systemic disorders*

Disorders such as hyponatremia, hypercalcemia, chronic hepatic failure, renal failure, hypo- or hyperthyroidism, Cushing's disease, Addison's disease, vitamin B12, B1, and B6 deficiencies are additional causes of "reversible" dementias. Most patients with dementia also have hematological impairment or myelopathy. 12–14% of all elderly patients have vitamin B12 deficiency but only a small number have dementia related to it and systemic infections. Routine laboratory tests, such as blood count, sedimentation rate (if indicated), electrolytes (including calcium), liver and renal function tests, urinalysis, syphilis serology, B12 levels, thyroid function tests, and a toxin and drug screen, are employed for the diagnosis.

6. *HIV*

   It is well known that HIV-1 DNA is present in the brains of both asymptomatic and symptomatic individuals. The virus has been shown to pass the blood–brain barrier early in the course of infection. Immune activation is associated with neuronal damage.

   HIV-1-associated dementia (HAD): HAD is generally thought to be a subcortical dementia. Diagnostic criteria include:

   a) Cognitive dysfunction in at least two cognitive functions for at least 1 month by self-report with objective verification by neuropsychological testing or by clinical neurological examination

   b) Moderate to severe functional status decrements

   c) Exclusion of other causes of cognitive–motor impairment

7. *HIV-associated conditions*

   a) Viral infection

      i. PML

         It occurs in 5% of all AIDS patients and is caused by papovavirus (JCV). Lesions are white matter demyelination without mass effect. Most common presentations are focal weakness, visual deficits (50% of cases), and cognitive abnormalities. Cerebellar involvement with limb and trunk ataxia (10%). Dementia is rapidly advancing unlike HAD. Death within 4 months is common and 80% die within one year.

      ii. Other common viral infections include: CMV and herpes simplex and varicella zoster infections.

   b) Neoplasms

      i. Lymphoma (1–4% on AIDS patients)

         Present with memory loss, seizures, cranial nerve deficits (10%). Tumors are B cell in origin (95%) and have an aggressive histologic type (large cell or large cell immunoblastic) as opposed to the intermediate- to high-grade subtypes seen in non-AIDS cases. Almost always associated with EBV infection. Neuroimaging show homogeneously enhancing lesions found most frequently in the periventricular deep gray matter area or corpus callosum. Two thirds of will have multiple lesions on scanning. CSF shows pleocytosis, elevated protein. Diagnosis is by brain biopsy.

      ii. Metastatic or primary tumors, paraneoplastic limbic encephalitis

   c) Opportunistic infections (OInfs)

      These opportunistic complications usually develop once the CD4 cell count is < 200/mm. Treatment with anti-retrovirals (protease inhibitors) has reduced the incidence of OInfs.

i. Parasitic
   - CNS toxoplasmosis (5 and 15% in AIDS cases with CD4
     < 100/mm) Cerebral toxoplasmosis results from reactivation of a
     dormant acquired *Toxoplasma gondii* infection during immuno-
     compromise (CD4 cell counts < 100/mm). Subacute presentation
     over days to weeks with lethargy, fever, headache, confusion, and
     focal signs (up to 75%). Seizures in up to 30% cases. Typical signs
     are hemiparesis, hemianesthesia, apraxia, aphasia, and move-
     ment disorders (hemichorea and hemiballismus). Cerebellar
     and brainstem abnormalities are less common. Measurement of
     serum antitoxoplasma immunoglobulin G (IgG) antibodies oc-
     curs in less than 50% cases. CSF has mild elevation of protein and
     mild pleocytosis. MRI is extremely useful. Lesions (multiple in
     66%) demonstrate ring or nodular enhancement in 90% of cases,
     and usually some surrounding mass effect is observed. Typical
     location is corticomedullary junction or in the basal ganglia.
ii. Fungal infections
   - CNS cryptococcus (5 and 15% in AIDS cases with CD4 < 100/mm)
     Yeast infection acquired through the respiratory tract. Meningi-
     tis is the chief clinical CNS event presenting with headache and
     fever (85%); nausea, vomiting, photophobia, blurred vision, stiff
     neck, and confusion and lethargy (about 30%). Focal neurologic
     deficits and seizures in about 10%. CSF with elevated opening
     pressure, increased protein, decreased glucose level, monocytic
     pleocytosis. Indian ink staining positive in more than 70% cases,
     positive cryptococcal antigen in 90% cases. Neuroimaging is
     frequently negative.
   - Other fungal infections
     ○ Candida (microabscesses, meningitis, and meningoencepha-
       litis)
     ○ Aspergillosis (subacute fever, altered mental status, and focal
       neurologic signs, abscess and vasculitic occlusive strokes
       occur)
     ○ Mucormycosis (extensive cerebral lesions)
     ○ Histoplasmosis, coccidioidomycosis, and blastomycosis
       (encephalopathy, meningitis, and focal abscesses)
iii. Bacterial infections
   - Syphilis
     Syphilitic meningitis during the course of secondary syphilis,
     late manifestations of meningovascular syphilis (meningitis,

cranial nerve abnormalities, and hydrocephalus). Tabes dorsalis (sensory loss, ataxia, lancinating pains to the lower extremities, sphincter abnormalities); strokes, general paresis (forgetfulness, dementia, psychiatric symptoms, changes in personality, papillary abnormalities); meningomyelitis, syphilitic polyradiculopathy, and cerebral gummata. CSF shows mononuclear pleocytosis, increased protein, and IgG. Positive FTA-ABS and VDRL.

– Tuberculosis

Tuberculous meningitis is the most frequent neurologic manifestation (preceded by a period of 2–8 weeks on nonspecific symptoms, including malaise, anorexia, fatigue, fever, chills, and headache). Later signs are worsening headache, altered mentation, seizures, and focal deficits when associated with intracerebral mass lesions (tuberculomas or abscesses). Cranial nerve abnormalities can occur. Fewer than 10% of cases may develop radiculomyelitis, transverse myelitis, or anterior spinal artery syndromes. CSF of mononuclear pleocytosis, low glucose, increased protein (generally between 100 and 200 mg/dl). CSF cultures positive (about 33%) and positive acid-fast staining to about 80% by the fourth spinal tap.

8. *Other conditions*

Normal pressure hydrocephalus (dementia, gait disturbance, and incontinence), brain tumors, and subdural hematoma, are the most common of the structural brain lesions presenting with dementia. Confirmation or exclusion of their presence usually requires a CT or MRI scan.

9. *Depression*

The most common cause of "reversible" dementia in the geriatric population is perhaps depression. Unlike younger individuals, elderly depressed patients may present with cognitive impairment, i.e., confusion, memory disturbance, attention deficits, all of which can be mistaken for dementia. Depression may also coexist with dementia and worsen the problem.

It can be problematic to differentiate between depression and dementia, but there are salient features which help to tell them apart. People with depression are more likely to complain of the memory problems themselves, while it is often the relatives and carers of people with dementia who notice the memory difficulties first. Both conditions can cause memory impairment and poor concentration, but people with depression can also experience sleep and appetite disturbances, reduced enjoyment, and loss of energy. They are also low in their mood and are often tearful. Unlike people with dementia, people with depression have negative thoughts about themselves, expressing guilty feelings, worthlessness, hopelessness, and sometimes thoughts about death. The duration of symptoms is usually shorter for depression than dementia and a past or family history of depression also makes depression the more likely diagnosis. It is however, unusual for depression to present for the first time after the age of 60 in the absence of a precipitant such as a loved one dying.

Depression can impair performance on memory tests in people of all ages, but especially the elderly. People with depression have particular problems learning new information and recalling it. Their memory deficits are at least partially related to poor attention and distractibility. On memory tests, the depressed person often cooperates poorly or exhibits poor effort, producing incomplete answers or frequent answering, "I don't know."

10. *Normal age-associated memory changes*
    It is now widely accepted that cognitive performance declines with age. Specifically, it has been reported that the ability to learn new information declines, but recall following prompts remains stable. It is, however, also accepted that age-related declines are not inevitable and when it does occur, it is age-related diseases that are often responsible. It is imperative for all people with memory complaints to undergo careful evaluation and it is not appropriate to assume that memory problems, at any age, are just a normal part of growing older.

11. *Mild cognitive impairment*
    Mild cognitive impairment (MCI) is a relatively new concept. It describes people with memory complaints who have significant objective memory impairment but are still able to function at the same level that they always have done. As their activities of daily living are intact, they do not meet the criteria for dementia. MCI is considered to be a transitional stage from normal ageing to dementia. As people with MCI are at increased risk of developing dementia, they should be monitored closely for any deterioration of their cognitive or functional abilities.

7.12.6 Differential diagnosis (in short)

1. Degenerative disorders
   a) Presenile dementia
      i. AD
      ii. Pick's disease
      iii. Cortical Lewy body disease
      iv. Prion disease
      v. Huntington's chorea
   b) Senile dementia

2. Cerebrovascular disease
   a) Multi-infarct dementia
      A series of relatively large infarcts that damage a sufficient volume of brain resulting in dementia. Neuropathological calculations indicate that infarct volumes which total over 50 ml are often associated with dementia, and that a total infarct volume over 100 ml is always associated with dementia. VaD may coexist with AD in 20% of cases, thus smaller volumes of infarct could contribute significantly to the dementing symptoms.
   b) Cerebral embolism
   c) Cerebral hemorrhage
   d) Subarachnoid hemorrhage
   e) Disseminated lupus erythematosus
   f) Transient ischemic attacks
3. Head injury
   a) Acute head injury
   b) Subdural hematoma
   c) Posttraumatic dementia
4. Hypoxia
   a) Post-cardiac arrest
      i. Heart failure
      ii. Myocardial infarction
   b) Respiratory disorders
   c) Carbon monoxide poisoning
5. Intracranial tumors
6. Infections
   a) Intracranial
      i. Encephalitis
      ii. Meningitis
      iii. Meningoencephalitis (e.g., general paresis)
      iv. AIDS dementia
   b) General (e.g., urinary tract, bronchopneumonia, topical infection)
7. Epilepsy
8. Toxic disorders
   a) Drugs (e.g., alcohol, barbiturates, opiates, amphetamines, LSD, cocaine, tricyclic antidepressants, steroids, lithium, L-dopa, cycloserine, digoxin, MAOIs, isoniazid)
   b) Heavy metals (e.g., lead, mercury, manganese)

9. Metabolic disorders
    a) Acute
        i. Electrolyte disturbance
        ii. Uremia
        iii. Hepatic encephalopathy
        iv. Hypoglycemia
        v. Porphyria
        vi. Endocrine diseases (e.g., thyrotoxicosis, diabetes mellitus, Addison's disease, parathyroid disorder, hypopituitarism)
        vii. Vitamin deficiencies (e.g., thiamine, B12, nicotinic acid)
    b) Chronic
        i. Chronic alcoholic dementia
        ii. Heavy metals
        iii. Myxedema, hypoglycemia, hypopituitarism
        iv. Vitamin deficiency (e.g., thiamine—Korsakoff's psychosis, nicotinic acid—pellagra, vitamin B12 and folic acid)
10. Other disorders affecting the CNS
    a) MS
    b) Parkinson's disease
    c) Normal pressure hydrocephalus

Walters RJL, Fox NC, Schott JM, et al. Transient ischaemic attacks are associated with increased rates of global cerebral atrophy. J Neurol Neurosurg Psychiatry 2003;74(2):213–216

Knopman DS, DeKosky ST, Cummings JL, et al. Practice parameter: diagnosis of dementia (an evidence-based review). Report of the Quality Standards Subcommittee of the American Academy of Neurology. Neurology 2001;56:1143–1153

Morris JC. The nosology of dementia. Neurol Clin 2000;18(4):773–788

Kertesz A, Nadkarni N, Davidson W, Thomas AW. The Frontal Behavioral Inventory in the differential diagnosis of frontotemporal dementia. J Int Neuropsychol Soc 2000;6(4):460–468

Diehl J, Monsch AU, Aebi C, et al. Frontotemporal dementia, semantic dementia, and Alzheimer's disease: the contribution of standard neuropsychological tests to differential diagnosis. J Geriatr Psychiatry Neurol 2005;18(1):39–44

American Psychiatric Association. Diagnostic and Statistical Manual Mental Disorders. 4th ed. Washington, DC: American Psychiatric Association; 1994

Ross GW, Bowen JD. The diagnosis and differential diagnosis of dementia. Med Clin North Am 2002;86(3):455–476

8 Cerebrovascular Disease (Stroke)

The diagnosis of acute ischemic stroke is often straight forward. The sudden onset of a focal neurologic deficit, such as hemiparesis, focal weakness, and aphasia, in a recognizable vascular pattern identifies a common syndrome of acute stroke. However, differential diagnostic problems remain because there are several subtypes of stroke and also because some nonvascular disorders may have clinical features identical to those of strokes.

8.1 Cerebral Infarction in Young Adults

Stroke affects mainly people aged over 65 years and atherosclerosis predominates as the main etiologic factor in ischemic stroke. On the other hand, cardiac embolism and arterial dissection are the most frequent causes of ischemic stroke in patients aged less than 45 years. However, inappropriate control of traditional vascular risk factors in young people may be causing a significant increase of atherosclerosis-related ischemic stroke. In endemic regions, neurocysticercosis and Chagas disease deserve consideration. Undetermined cause has been still reported in as many as one-third of young stroke patients.

1. Cerebrovascular atherosclerosis (thrombotic or embolic)
2. Embolism
    a) Cardiac source
        i. Valvular (mitral stenosis, prosthetic valve, infective endocarditis, marantic endocarditis, Libman–Sacks endocarditis, mitral annulus calcification, mitral valve prolapse, calcific aortic stenosis)
        ii. Atrial fibrillation and sick sinus syndrome
        iii. Acute myocardial infarction and/or left ventricular aneurysm
        iv. Left atrial myxoma
        v. Cardiomyopathy
    b) Paradoxical embolism or pulmonary source
        i. Pulmonary arteriovenous malformation (including Osler–Weber–Rendu disease)
        ii. Atrial and ventricular septal defects with right to left shunt
        iii. Patent foramen ovale (PFO) with shunt
        iv. Pulmonary vein thrombosis
        v. Pulmonary and mediastinal tumors
    c) Other
        i. Aortic cholesterol embolism
        ii. Transient embologenic aortitis
        iii. Emboli distal to unruptured aneurysm
        iv. Fat embolism syndrome

3. Arteriopathy
   a) Inflammatory (see also vasculitis classification discussed later in the chapter)
      i. Takayasu's disease
      ii. Allergic (Churg–Strauss syndrome) and granulomatous
      iii. Infective
          – Specific: syphilis, mucormycosis, ophthalmic zoster, TB, malaria
          – Nonspecific: severe tonsillitis or lymphadenitis
      iv. Associated with drug use (e.g., amphetamine, cocaine, phenylpropanolamine)
      v. Associated with systemic disease (lupus, Wegener's granulomatosis, polyarteritis nodosa, rheumatoid arthritis, Sjogren's syndrome, scleroderma, Degos disease, Behcet's syndrome, acute rheumatic fever, inflammatory bowel disease)
   b) Noninflammatory
      i. Spontaneous dissection
      ii. Post-therapeutic irradiation
      iii. Fibromuscular hyperplasia
      iv. Moyamoya disease and progressive arterial occlusion syndrome
      v. Congophilic (amyloid) angiopathy
      vi. Thromboangiitis obliterans
      vii. Familial: homocystinuria, Fabrys disease, pseudoxanthoma elasticum
4. Vasospasm associated with
   a) Migraine
   b) Subarachnoid hemorrhage
   c) Hypertensive encephalopathy
   d) Cerebral arteriography
5. Hematological disease and coagulopathy
   a) Hyperviscosity
      i. Polycythemia and myeloproliferative dysproteinemia myeloma, Waldenstrom's macroglobulinemia, cryoglobulinemia
   b) Coagulopathy
      i. Thrombotic thrombocytopenia purpura
      ii. Chronic diffuse intravascular coagulation
      iii. Paroxysmal nocturnal hemoglobinuria
      iv. Oral contraceptive use/peripartum/pregnancy
      v. Thrombocythemia
      vi. Sickle cell and hemoglobin C disease
      vii. Lupus anticoagulant
      viii. Nephrotic syndrome
      ix. C2 complement deficiency (familial)
      x. Protein C deficiency (familial)

c) Controversial associations
  i. Platelet hyperaggregability
  ii. Fibrinolytic insufficiency
  iii. Increased factor VIII
  iv. Antithrombin III deficiency
  v. Vitamin K and antifibrinolytic therapy
  vi. Acute alcohol intoxication

6. Miscellaneous
  a) Trauma (direct, indirect, rotation, and extension injuries)
  b) Mechanical (cervical rib, atlantoaxial subluxation)
  c) Related to systemic hypotension
  d) Iatrogenic (perioperative and periprocedural, including air and foreign particle embolism)
  e) Cortical sinus or vein thrombosis

8.1.1 Causes of infarction in young adults

Causes	Total (%)
Cerebrovascular atherosclerosis	18

Cerebral embolism
• Previously known cardiac disease (23%)
  – Rheumatic valvular heart disease
  – Valve prosthesis
• Previously unrecognized source (8%)
  – Left atrial myxoma
  – Pulmonary arteriovenous malformation
  – Atrial septal defect—patent foramen ovale (PFO): The presence of PFO in patients < 55 years is significantly associated with cryptogenic stroke, and associated prothrombotic state or concurrent atrial septal aneurysm seems to increase their stroke risk.
  – Occult mitral stenosis
  – Idiopathic cardiomyopathy
  – Chagas disease (CD) is an independent risk factor and dilated cardiomyopathy and arrhythmias cause cardioembolism in most patients with CD and stroke
	31

Nonatherosclerotic cerebral vasculopathy (angiographic diagnosis) • Spontaneous cervicocephalic dissections by far the most common cause of ischemic stroke (IS) within the nonatherosclerotic angiopathies, and rank first or second of all etiologies of IS in young adults. Angiographic evidence of fibromuscular dysplasia (FMD) is found in about 15% of this group of patients.	10

▶ (*Continued*)

Causes	Total (%)

• Moyamoya disease affects mainly Asian people
• Following neck irradiation
• Idiopathic venous sinus thrombosis
• Cerebral vasculitis
• Vertebral artery injury secondary to neck turning
• Neurocysticercosis must be considered in young adults in small or large vessel angiitis in endemic areas
• Genetic and hereditary disease
• Fabrys disease
   – Cerebral autosomal dominant arteriopathy with subcortical infarcts and leukoencephalopathy (CADASIL)
   – Mitochondrial encephalopathy with lactic acidosis and stroke-like episodes (MELAS) syndrome
   – Hereditary endotheliopathy with retinopathy, neuropathy and stroke (HERNS) syndrome
• Susac's syndrome (retinocochleocerebral vasculopathy) and Sneddon's syndrome (livedo reticularis associated with cerebrovascular events), with or without antiphospholipid antibodies, are other rare noninflammatory angiopathies that occur predominantly in young adults	

Coagulopathy and systemic inflammation (serological diagnosis) Acquired and genetic thrombophilia seems higher in young adults. The most common acquired thrombophilia in young adults is antiphospholipid syndrome. Antiphospholipid antibodies, particularly lupus anticoagulant, are an independent risk factor of ischemic stroke in young adults • Systemic lupus erythematosus (SLE) with/without lupus anticoagulant • Lupus anticoagulant without SLE • Homocystinuria • Systemic vasculitis • Coagulopathy with thrombocytopenia • Severe Crohn's disease	9
Peripartum • Call–Fleming syndrome or postpartum angiopathy secondary to vasoactive substances and to the postpartum state. – Ischemic stroke and transient ischemic attacks occur later than hemorrhagic strokes, mainly during the second week.	5
Migraine Migrainous infarction occur during a typical attack of migraine with aura mainly in the area of posterior cerebral artery. However, these patients disclose multiple related vascular risk factors as smoking, oral contraceptive use, and vasoconstrictive drugs (ergot alkaloids) that might trigger a migrainous infarct. The increased risk in migraineurs, especially young women with aura, probably has multifactorial basis, including migrainous infarctions, arterial dissection, fibromuscular dysplasia, PFO, drug-induced infarcts, prothrombotic states, and genetic factors	15

(*Continued*)

▶ *(Continued)*

Causes	Total (%)
Uncertain etiology (cryptogenic stroke)	12
• "Idiopathic" (no association)	
• Oral contraceptive use	
• Mitral valve prolapse	
• Associated with oral contraceptive use only	

Hart RG, Miller VT. Cerebral infarction in young adults: a practical approach. Stroke 1983;14(1):110–114

Hindfelt B, Nilsson O. Brain infarction in young adults (with particular reference to pathogenesis). Acta Neurol Scand 1977;55(2):145–157

Martin PJ, Enevoldson TP, Humphrey PR. Causes of ischemic stroke in the young Postgrad Med J 1997;73(855):8–16

Kittner SJ, Stern J,, Wozniak M. Cerebral infarction in young adults: the Baltimore-Washington Cooperative Young Stroke Study Neurology 1998;50(4):890–894

Adams HP Jr, Butler MJ, Biller J, Toffol GJ. Nonhemorrhagic cerebral infarction in young adults. Arch Neurol 1986;43(8):793–796

Griffiths D, Sturm J. Epidemiology and etiology of young stroke. Stroke Res Treat 2011;2011:209370

Ferro JM, Massaro AR, Mas J-L. Aetiological diagnosis of ischaemic stroke in young adults. Lancet Neurol 2010;9(11):1085–1096

Yew KS, Cheng EM. Diagnosis of acute stroke. Am Fam Physician 2015;91(8):528–536

Jordan LC, Hillis AE. Challenges in the diagnosis and treatment of pediatric stroke. Nat Rev Neurol 2011;7(4):199–208

8.2 Stroke Differential Diagnosis

1. **Stroke mimics:** Nonvascular conditions that simulate stroke are as follows:
   a) Most common
      i. Complicated migraine (especially younger women)
      ii. Hemorrhagic stroke (intracerebral hemorrhage)
      iii. Hypoglycemia
      iv. Hypertensive encephalopathy
      v. Seizures (postictal paralysis or Todd's paralysis)
      vi. Small vessel stroke/penetrating vessel stroke (comprise 20–25% of all strokes)
   b) Less common
      i. Head trauma
         – Diffuse axonal injury
         – Subdural hematoma
         – Epidural hematoma
      ii. CNS problems
         – Seizure/postictal
         – Generalized convulsive with postictal confusion or focal neurologic signs

- – Nonconvulsive status epilepticus
- – Meningitis
- – Encephalitis
- – Fat embolism
- – Hemiplegic migraine (Todd's paralysis)
- – Intracranial tumors (primary CNS, metastatic)
- – Hypertensive encephalopathy
- – Multiple sclerosis
- – Susac's syndrome (small vessel disease of brain, retina, and inner ear)

iii. Metabolic abnormality
- – Nonketotic hyperosmolar coma (hyperglycemia)
- – Postcardiac arrest ischemia
- – Toxin ingestion
  - ○ Metronidazole toxicity
  - ○ Methotrexate toxicity
  - ○ Vigabatrin toxicity
- – Antiepileptic drugs
- – Myxedema
- – Venous infarction (accounts for 1% of all strokes)
- – Uremia
- – Hepatic encephalopathy
- – Wernicke's encephalopathy
- – Carbon monoxide poisoning
- – Osmotic myelinolysis
- – Mitochondrial encephalopathy, lactic acidosis, and stroke-like events (MELAS)

iv. Systemic infection
- – Respiratory infection
- – Urosepsis

v. Miscellaneous
- – Psychiatric problems (factitious disorders)
- – Hypotension, shock state, or syncope
- – Hyperperfusion syndrome
- – Moyamoya disease
- – Radiation therapy

2. **Stroke "chameleons":** Strokes with atypical presentations that take on the appearance of other diseases.
   a) Acute confusional states
   Confusional states, agitation, and delirium have all been reported as a consequence of focal neurologic injury, involving the limbic cortex of the temporal lobes and the orbitofrontal regions. These states must be

distinguished from the neglect syndromes and fluent aphasias, but careful examination demonstrates a clear focal deficit (e.g., in syndromes of visual neglect, visual field testing will reveal a dramatic field cut).

b) Seizures with acute stroke

Any witnesses that suggest a convulsive episode should raise suspicion of the presence of an ictal or postictal phenomena.

c) Sensory symptoms

Sensory complaints of either unusual sensations or loss of sensation are common in parietal and thalamic strokes. They may take on a characteristic of another clinical condition, e.g., chest pain and limb pain that mimicked that of a myocardial infarction. Cortical involvement is usually accompanied by other neurological deficits such as hemiparesis, aphasia, hemineglect, or visual field abnormalities. Cortical blindness (Anton's syndrome) is unusual but may occur and may be distinguished from bilateral ocular disease by the normal pupillary light response and normal optic disks.

d) Movement disorders

Uncommonly, movement disorders will present from a focal lesion such as ischemic stroke or hemorrhage. Acute hemiballismus or unilateral dyskinesis often result from acute vascular lesions in the subthalamic nucleus or connections. The key to diagnosis is an abrupt onset of symptoms and risk factors for cerebrovascular disease.

8.2.1 Radiology (CT/MRI) characteristics of stroke mimics

See ▶ Fig. 8.1 for radiological characteristics of stroke mimics.

8.3 Stroke Risk Factors

1. Age

Most important stroke risk factor is age. About 30% of strokes occur before the age of 65; 70% occur in those over 65 years of age. Stroke risk approximately doubles for every decade of age greater than 55 years.

2. Hypertension

The risk of stroke relates to the level of systolic hypertension. This applies to both sexes, to all ages, and to risk for hemorrhagic, atherothrombotic, and lacunar stroke. Interestingly, the risk of stroke at a given level of systolic hypertension is less with advancing age, so it becomes a less powerful, albeit still important and treatable, risk factor in the elderly.

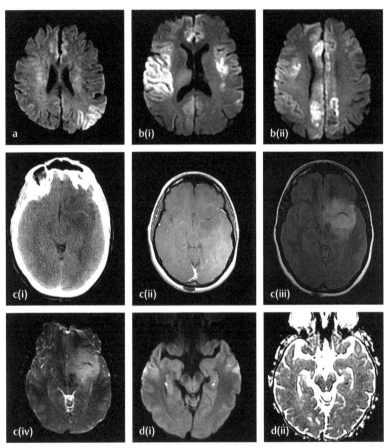

Fig. 8.1 Stroke radiological differential diagnosis and mimics. **(a)** Seizures: Restricted diffusion and edema in left parieto-occipital area. **(b)** HSV encephalitis: Initially diagnosed with bilateral anterior cerebral artery (ACA) and middle cerebral artery (MCA) infarction. Ultimately diagnosed with HSV encephalitis. MRI showed asymmetric multifocal regions of restricted diffusion in the bilateral temporal lobes, frontal lobes, insula, cingulate gyri, and thalamus. **(c)** Anaplastic astrocytoma: **(i, ii)** Plain and enhanced CT initially interpreted as an infarction with left MCA territory hypodensity and a hyperdensity. **(iii, iv)** MRI showed a nonenhancing expansible lesion with elevated diffusion. **(d)** Transient global amnesia: The diffusion-weighted imaging 4 days after the ictus shows punctate foci of restricted diffusion in bilateral hippocampi. (*Continued*)

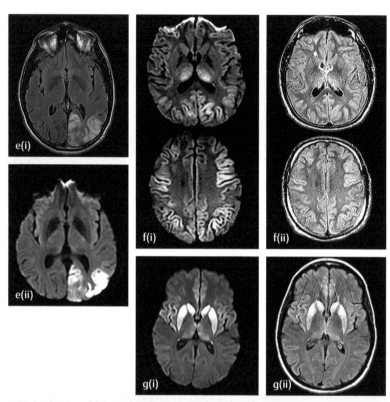

Fig. 8.1 (*Continued*) (**e**) Mitochondrial encephalopathy, lactic acidosis, and stroke-like events (MELAS). FLAIR imaging showed nonvascular distribution of cortical swelling in the left posterior parieto-temporal-occipital region with areas of both restricted and increased diffusion. (**f**) Global hypoxic injury: Hypoxic-ischemic encephalopathy following pulseless electrical activity (PEA) arrest. MRI demonstrated diffuse restricted diffusion with associated T2-FLAIR hyperintensity in the bilateral parieto-occipital and frontal lobes, bilateral thalami. The cerebellum is usually spared. (**g**) Creutzfeldt–Jakob disease: MRI showed restricted diffusion (**i**) and T2-FLAIR (**ii**) hyperintensity in the bilateral basal ganglia, thalami, and cortex.

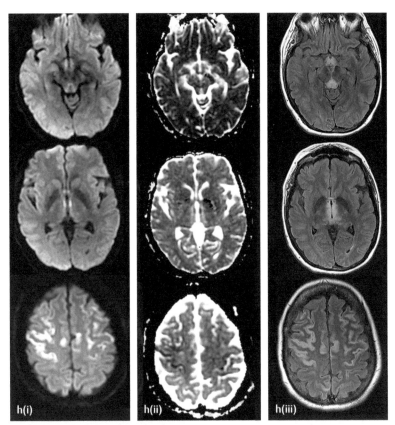

Fig. 8.1 (*Continued*) **(h)** Wernicke's encephalopathy: Diagnosis of Wernicke's disease was made due to malnutrition with a thiamine level of 35 nmol (normal 70–180 nmol). MRI showed variable diffusion with FLAIR hyperintensity in quadrigeminal plate, periaqueductal gray matter, hypothalamus, and bilateral superior colliculi.

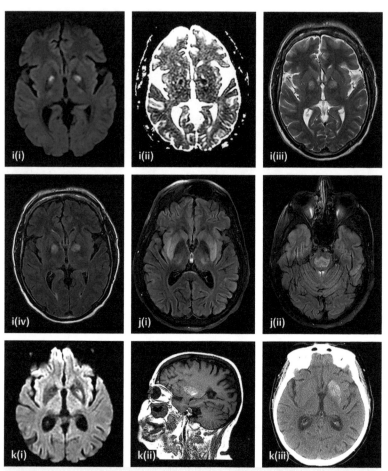

Fig. 8.1 (*Continued*) **(i)** Carbon monoxide poisoning: Camper found awake, staring, and foaming at the mouth with a respiratory rate of 6/min and a carboxy hemoglobin level of 22.9. MRI demonstrates symmetric restricted diffusion **(i, ii)** and T2-FLAIR hyperintensity **(iii, iv)** in the bilateral globus pallidi. **(j)** Osmotic myelinolysis: Alcoholic with severe hyponatremia who developed seizures and poor swallowing after correction of hyponatremia. MRI demonstrates T2 hyperintensity within the central pons, sparing the periphery and cortico-spinal tracts and bilateral putamen, caudate nuclei, thalami, external capsules, and central pons.
(k) Nonketotic hyperglycemia: MRI revealed restricted diffusion **(i)** and T1 hyperintensity **(ii)** within the lentiform nucleus. CT shows hyperintensity of the left lentiform nucleus and caudate head **(iii)**.

3. Gender (male > female)

   Brain infarcts and stroke occur some 30% more frequently in men than women; the gender differential is even greater before age 65.

4. Family history

   A fivefold increase in stroke prevalence among monozygotic compared to dizygotic male twin pairs suggests a genetic predisposition to stroke. The 1913 Swedish birth cohort study demonstrated a threefold increase in the incidence of stroke in men whose mothers died of stroke compared with men without such a maternal history. Family history also seems to play a role in stroke mortality among the upper middle-class Caucasian population in California.

5. Diabetes mellitus

   After controlling for other stroke risk factors, diabetes increases the risk of thromboembolic stroke by approximately two- to threefold relative to persons without diabetes. Diabetes may predispose an individual to cerebral ischemia via acceleration of atherosclerosis of the large vessels such as coronary artery, carotid tree or by local effects on the cerebral microcirculation.

6. Cardiac disease

   Individuals with heart disease of any type have more than twice the risk of stroke compared to those with normal cardiac function. *Coronary artery disease* is a strong indicator of both the presence of diffuse atherosclerotic vascular disease, and a potential source of emboli from mural thrombi due to myocardial infarction. *Congestive heart failure* and *hypertensive heart disease* are associated with increased stroke. *Atrial fibrillation* is strongly associated with embolic stroke and atrial fibrillation due to rheumatic valvular disease greatly increases the stroke risk by 17 times. Various other cardiac lesions have been associated with stroke, such as *mitral valve prolapse, PFO, atrial septal defect, atrial septal aneurysm,* and *atherosclerotic/thrombotic lesions of the ascending aorta.*

7. Carotid bruits

   A carotid bruit does indicate an increased risk of a future stroke, although the risk is for stroke in general, and not for stroke specifically in the distribution of the artery with the bruit.

8. Smoking

   Several reports including a meta-analysis of a number of studies have shown that cigarette smoking clearly confers an increased risk for stroke off all ages and both sexes, that the degree of risk correlates with the number of cigarettes smoked, and that smoking cessation decreases the risk and reverts to the risk of nonsmokers by 5 years after smoking cessation.

9. Increased hematocrit

   Heightened viscosity causes stroke symptoms when hematocrit exceeds 55%. The major determinant of whole blood viscosity is the red blood cell content; plasma proteins, particularly fibrinogen, play a contributing role. When heightened viscosity results from polycythemia, hyperfibrinogenemia, or paraproteinemia, it usually causes generalized symptoms, such as headache, lethargy, tinnitus, and blurred vision. Focal cerebral infarction and retinal vein occlusion is much less common and may follow platelet dysfunction due to thrombocytosis. Intracerebral and subarachnoid hemorrhages may occur occasionally.

10. Elevated fibrinogen level and other clotting system abnormalities

    A hypercoagulable state accounts for 1–2% of all strokes and 2–7% of stroke in younger patients, less than 50 years. The inherited thrombophilia i.e., protein C, S, and antithrombin deficiencies are relatively common at 1:200 to 1:2000 in the heterozygous form. Similarly, activated protein C resistance, including, but not limited to factor V Leiden mutation, are important genetic risk factors for venous thromboembolic disease. Elevated fibrinogen level constitutes a risk factor for thrombotic stroke. Rare abnormalities of the blood clotting system have also been noted, such as antithrombin III deficiency, and deficiencies of protein C and protein S and are associated with venous thrombotic events. Also, heparin is lowering antithrombin levels, and warfarin lowers functional levels of protein C and S.

11. Hemoglobinopathy

    Sickle cell disease can cause ischemic/hemorrhagic infarction, intracerebral and subarachnoid hemorrhages, venous sinus, and cortical vein thrombosis. The overall incidence of stroke in sickle cell disease is 6–15%. *Paroxysmal nocturnal hemoglobinuria* may result in cerebral venous thrombosis.

12. Drug abuse

    Up to 14% of ischemic and hemorrhagic brain infarcts in individuals aged 18–44 years were caused by substance abuse. Drugs that have been associated with stroke include methamphetamines, norepinephrine, lysergic acid diethylamide (LSD), heroin, and cocaine; also, over-the-counter sympatheticomimetics (phenylpropanolamine, ephedrine, and pseudoephedrine), phencyclidine, marijuana have been associated with stroke. The amphetamines induce a necrotizing vasculitis that may result in diffuse petechial hemorrhages or focal areas of ischemia and infarction. The heroin may produce allergic vascular hypersensitivity leading to infarction. Subarachnoid hemorrhage and cerebral infarction have been reported after the use of cocaine.

13. Hyperlipidemia

    Although elevated cholesterol clearly has been related to coronary heart disease, its relation to stroke has been less clear. Elevated cholesterol does appear to be a risk factor for carotid atherosclerosis, especially in males under 55 years of age. The significance of hypercholesterolemia diminishes as age advances. Cholesterol below 160 is related to intracerebral hemorrhage or subarachnoid hemorrhage. There is no apparent relationship of cholesterol level to lacunar infarction.

14. Oral contraceptives

The early high-estrogen oral contraceptives were reported to increase the risk of stroke in young women. Lowering the estrogen content has decreased this problem but not eliminated it altogether. This risk factor is strongest in women over 35 years who are also smokers. The presumed mechanism is an increased coagulation by estrogen stimulation of liver protein production or rarely an autoimmune one.

15. Diet

16. Alcohol consumption

Increased risk of cerebral infarction and subarachnoid hemorrhage has been associated with alcohol abuse in young adults. Mechanisms by which ethanol may produce stroke include effects on blood pressure, platelets, plasma osmolality, hematocrit, and red blood cells. Furthermore, alcohol-induced myocardiopathy, arrhythmias, changes in cerebral blood flow and autoregulation are also some of the effects of alcohol.

17. Obesity

Obesity (measured as relative weight or body mass index) consistently predicted subsequent strokes. Its association with stroke could be explained partly by the presence of hypertension and diabetes. Relative weight more than 30% above average was an independent contributor to a subsequent atherosclerotic brain infarction.

18. Peripheral vascular disease

19. Infection

Infection (particularly chlamydia pneumonia and HIV) and acute and chronic inflammation have been attributed to raising stroke risk in younger patients. The relative risk was higher in the injection-drug abuse, HIV-infected individuals, particularly for hemorrhagic stroke. High stroke risk was associated with low CD4 cell count before antiviral treatment. Meningeal infection can result in cerebral infarction through the development of inflammatory changes in vessel walls. Diagnostic considerations in the infection setting include meningovascular syphilis; nonbacterial thrombotic endocarditis with cardiogenic embolism; vasculopathies associated with cryptococcal, tuberculous, and lymphomatous meningitis; toxoplasmosis; and herpes zoster. Mucormycosis may cause cerebral arteritis and infarction.

20. Homocysteinemia or homocystinuria (homozygous form)

It predisposes to cerebral arterial or venous thromboses. The estimated risk of stroke at a young age is 10–16%.

21. Migraine

    Migrainous infarction accounts for 13.7% of ischemia in young adults, especially women with a long standing (mean of 13 years) history of severe migraine and prolonged aura symptoms persisting for more than 60 minutes, visual and cortical symptoms, cigarette smoking, use of oral contraceptives, and posterior circulation infarct on brain imaging are factors that raise suspicion for migrainous stroke.

22. Race

    African-Americans have disproportionately higher stroke rates than other ethnic or racial groups.

23. Geographic location

    In the United States and most European countries, stroke is the third most frequent cause of death after heart diseases and cancers. Most often strokes are caused by atherosclerotic changes rather than by hemorrhage. Middle-aged black women are exception, in whom hemorrhage leads the list. In Japan, stroke is the leading cause of death in adults and hemorrhage is more common than atherosclerosis.

24. Circadian and seasonal factors

    The circadian variation of ischemic strokes peaking between 10:00 a.m. and 12:00 noon has led to hypothesis that diurnal changes in platelet function and fibrinolysis may be relevant to stroke. A relationship between seasonal climatic variation and ischemic stroke occurrence has been postulated. An increase in referral for cerebral infarction was observed during the warmer months in Iowa. The mean ambient temperature negatively correlated with the incidence of cerebral infarction in Japan. Seasonality has been correlated with a higher risk of cerebral infarction in 40 to 64-year-old individuals who are nonhypertensive and individuals with serum cholesterol below 160 mg/dl.

25. Conditions with hematologic changes leading to stroke

    Include pregnancy, cancer, nephrotic syndrome, leukemia, inflammatory bowel disease, acute infection, paroxysmal nocturnal hemoglobinuria, and Bechet's syndrome.

Go AS, Hylek EM, Phillips KA, et al. Prevalence of diagnosed atrial fibrillation in adults: national implications for rhythm management and stroke prevention: the AnTicoagulation and Risk Factors in Atrial Fibrillation (ATRIA) Study. JAMA 2001;285(18):2370–2375

Hughes M, Lip GY. Stroke and thromboembolism in atrial fibrillation: A systematic review of stroke risk factors, stratification schema and cost effectiveness data Molecules to Medicine (Part 1). Stuttgart: Schattauer GmbH; 2008:295–304

Duken ML. Stroke risk factors. Chapter 6. In: JW Norris, et al. eds. Prevention of stroke Springer Science 1991:83

Feigin VL, Roth GA, Naghavi M, et al; Global Burden of Diseases, Injuries and Risk Factors Study 2013 and Stroke Experts Writing Group. Global burden of stroke and risk factors in 188 countries, during 1990–2013: a systematic analysis for the Global Burden of Disease Study 2013. Lancet Neurol 2016;15(9):913–924

8.4 Common Cardiac Disorders Associated with Cerebral Infarction

Cerebral embolism arising from the heart and leading to infarction may be the presenting symptom of previously unidentified cardiac disease. Most cerebral emboli, including those of cardiac origin, will lodge in the branches of the middle cerebral artery; no more than 6.8% will affect the anterior cerebral artery, and 10% of emboli occlude the vertebral or basilar arteries and their branches.

1. **Dysrhythmias**
   a) Chronic nonvalvular atrial fibrillation (CNVAF)
   It is recognized as a frequent cause of embolic cerebral ischemia, and is associated with some 15% of all ischemic strokes. Patients with NVAF have a fivefold risk of ischemic stroke compared with age-matched individuals, facing a 35% lifetime risk of ischemic stroke and a yearly stroke risk of 5%. NVAF with comorbid states can further increase the risk of embolic stroke. Risk of cerebral embolism in thyrotoxic NVAF averages 12% yearly, while associated congestive heart failure or coronary heart disease will increase the stroke risk slightly above the baseline. Other cardiac dysrhythmias carry a higher stroke rate than NVAF but are less common and do not pose the same challenge to population-based disease management. Patients with NVAF associated with rheumatic heart disease have a 17-fold increased risk of stroke compared with age-matched controls, but constitute no more than 25% of the entire atrial fibrillation population.
      i. Associated with rheumatic fever
      ii. Without rheumatic fever
   b) Sick sinus syndrome
   c) Prolonged QT intervals
2. **Valvular defects**
   a) Mitral valve prolapse
   A common disorder observed in 6–8% of the general population that could be associated with embolic infarction involving the brain or the retina. The incidence of cerebral infarction associated with this disorder is low—approximately 1 in 6,000 known cases.
   b) Prosthetic heart valves
   c) Infection
   The most common neurological complication of infective endocarditis was cerebral embolism, occurring in 17% of patients in a study. Cerebral embolism was associated with a high mortality rate killing 30 of the 37

patients of the study; brain abscess was discovered in 4.1% and mycotic aneurysm was detected in 1.8% cases.

- i. Bacterial
    - – *Streptococcus viridans* (acute or subacute bacterial endocarditis)
    - – Typically seen in elderly individuals who had rheumatic heart disease and were infected with *S. viridans.*
    - – *Staphylococcus aureus*
    - – Patients are more typically younger individuals, most frequently intravenous drug abusers, and the organism is the more virulent *S. aureus.*
- ii. Fungal
- d) Thrombotic endocarditis

    It is a clinical disorder consisting of aseptic cardiac valvular vegetations that may cause cerebral or systemic emboli. Abnormal coagulation profiles in cancer patients with cerebral ischemia should prompt consideration not only of embolic arterial occlusion observed in thrombotic endocarditis, but also of microvascular thrombosis associated with disseminated intravascular coagulation (DIC).

    - i. Associated with chronic systemic illnesses
    - ii. Associated with mucin-secreting tumors (7.4%)
        - – Adenocarcinoma *of the lung*
        - – *Gastrointestinal CA*
        - – *Breast CA*
        - – *Lymphoma*
        - – *Leukemia*
        - – *Misce*llaneous solid tumors
- e) Myxomatous degeneration caused by Libman–Sacks endocarditis

3. **Abnormalities of the myocardial wall**
    - a) Atrial myxoma
    - b) Mural thrombi associated with cardiac wall dyskinesia or aneurysm

        Approximately, 45% (range: 17–83%) of lethal myocardial infarctions have associated mural thrombi. These patients showed an overall stroke rate of 4.7%.

Lynch JK, Hirtz DG, DeVeber G, Nelson KB. Report of the National Institute of Neurological Disorders and Stroke workshop on perinatal and childhood stroke. Pediatrics 2002;109(1):116–123

Wolf PA, Dawbar TR, Thomas E, et al. Epidemiologic assessment of chronic atrial fibrillation and risk of stroke: the Framingham study. Neurology 1978;28(10):973

Arboix A, Alió J. Cardioembolic stroke: clinical features, specific cardiac disorders and prognosis. Curr Cardiol Rev 2010;6(3):150–161

8.5 Transient Ischemic Attack

A transient ischemic attack (TIA) is a temporary inadequacy of the circulation in part of the brain (a cerebral or retinal deficit) that gives a clinical picture similar to a stroke except that it is transient and reversible. Hence, TIA is a retrospective diagnosis. The duration is no more than 24 hours, and the majority of TIAs last for less than 30 minutes. Features that do not fully fit for TIA are called transient neurological attacks (TNAs); the risk of subsequent stroke is not as high as for TIA.

8.5.1 Incidence

TIAs affect 35 people per 100,000 of the population each year; they affect men more than women and black races are at greater risk. About 15% of first stroke victims have had a preceding TIA.

Disorder	Incidence (%)
Postural hypotension	14.6
Seizure disorder	14.6
Syncope	13.1
Dizziness	11.4
Anxiety	11.4
Cardiac arrhythmia and myocardial infarction	7.3
Mental confusion	5.7
Migraine headache	4.0
Brain tumor	4.0
Visual disturbances	3.3
Miscellaneous conditions	10.6

8.5.2 Differential diagnosis (the "three Bs")

Beware of diagnosing TIA if there has been loss of consciousness, or convulsion. Todd's paralysis follows a seizure and is characterized by a temporary, usually unilateral, paralysis. It may also affect speech or vision and usually resolves within 48 hours.

Before there is full recovery it is impossible to differentiate from a stroke. It is usually embolic, may be thrombotic, and occasionally hemorrhagic (unlikely to

produce a reversible lesion). It affects the carotid area in about 80% and the vertebrobasilar area in about 20% of the cases. The most common source of emboli is
the carotid bifurcation. They can originate in the heart with atrial fibrillation
particularly, with mitral valve disease, or aortic valve disease, or from a mural
thrombus forming on a myocardial infarct or a cardiac tumor, usually atrial
myxoma.

1. **Brain**
   a) Brain tumor
   b) Seizures
   c) Subdural hematoma
2. **Blood vessels**
   a) Atherosclerotic disease (extracranial, intracranial, aorta)
   b) Arteritides (giant cell arteritis, CNS angiitis, polyarteritis nodosa, etc.)
   c) Migraine or migrainous aura
   d) Dissection
   e) Fibromuscular dysplasia
   f) Moyamoya disease
   g) Hypercalcemia
   h) Arterial kinking
   i) Neck extension/rotation
   j) Venous occlusive disease
   k) Syncope due to cardiac arrhythmia
3. **Blood elements**
   a) Erythrocyte disorders (polycythemia vera, sickle cell disease)
   b) Platelet dysfunction (thrombocytosis)
   c) Protein abnormalities (anticardiolipin/antiphospholipid antibodies,
      protein C and S deficiency, lupus anticoagulant)
   d) Emboli (cardiogenic sources, infective endocarditis, atrial myxoma,
      mitral valve prolapse, lupus, paradoxical emboli etc.)

Easton JD, Sarer JL, Albers GW, et al. Definition and evaluation of transient ischemic attack Stroke
    2009;40:2276–2293
Wu CM, McLaughlin K, Lorenzetti DL, et al. Early risk of stroke after TIA: A systematic review and Meta-anal-
    ysis. Arc Intern Med 2007;67(22):2417–2422

8.6 "Cryptogenic Strokes" (Embolic Stroke of Undetermined Source—ESUS)

Despite efforts to arrive at a diagnosis, the cause of stroke remains undetermined in 25–40% of patients. Factors that contribute to undermined causes of

stroke include inadequate information about the underlying vascular pathology, ill-timed diagnostic workup, and incomplete evaluation. As a consequence, patients with unknown stroke causes are lumped together in a category called *cryptogenic*. The new definition of "embolic stroke of undetermined source" postulates an embolic mechanism of ischemic stroke. It is based on the exclusion of lacunar infarction by brain imaging, arterial stenosis in more than 50% cases, or dissection of the respective brain-supplying artery by CT/MR-angiography-ultrasound, atrial fibrillation by at least 24-hour electrocardiography (ECG) monitoring, as well as some rare etiologies such as vasculitis, drug abuse, or coagulopathies. However, it still comprises many patients with atherosclerotic etiologies (but < 50% stenosis) as well as covert paroxysmal atrial fibrillation which can be detected by repeated Holter ECG or an implantable device. A PFO can be found in up to 58% of cryptogenic stroke patients, but causality in an individual patient remains uncertain and can only be statistically inferred.

8.6.1 Diagnostic criteria of an ESUS

1. Stroke detected by CT or MRI that is not lacunar, i.e., 1.5 cm or less (<= 2.0 cm on MRI diffusion images) in largest dimension, including on MRI diffusion-weighted images, and in the distribution of the small, penetrating cerebral arteries; visualization by CT usually requires delayed imaging for more than 24–48 hours after stroke onset.
2. Absence of extracranial or intracranial atherosclerosis causing at least 50% luminal stenosis in arteries supplying the area of ischemia.
3. No major risk cardioembolic source of embolism, defined as: permanent or paroxysmal atrial fibrillation, sick sinus syndrome/atrial systole, intracardiac thrombus, prosthetic cardiac valve, atrial myxoma or other cardiac tumors, mitral stenosis, recent (< 4 weeks) myocardial infarction, left ventricular ejection fraction less than 30%, valvular vegetations, or infective endocarditis.
4. No other specific cause of stroke identified (e.g., arteritis, dissection, migraine/vasospasm, and drug abuse).

DeBaun MR, Armstrong FD, McKinstry RC, Ware RE, Vichinsky E, Kirkham FJ. Silent cerebral infarcts: a review on a prevalent and progressive cause of neurologic injury in sickle cell anemia. Blood 2012;119(20):4587–4596

Sanna T, Diener H-C, Passman RS, et al; CRYSTAL AF Investigators. Cryptogenic stroke and underlying atrial fibrillation. N Engl J Med 2014;370(26):2478–2486

Hart RG, Diener HC, Coutts SB, et al; Cryptogenic Stroke/ESUS International Working Group. Embolic strokes of undetermined source: the case for a new clinical construct. Lancet Neurol 2014;13(4):429–438

8.7 Recurrent Stroke in Patients Who Are under Preventive Therapy

A common problem in the diagnosis of stroke is that of the patient who has an acute recurrent stroke despite taking antithrombotic therapy (in the form of an antiplatelet agent or anticoagulation) or after having undergone carotid endarterectomy.

There are several reasons why the patient taking antithrombotic therapy may present with recurrent stroke:

1. The antithrombotic therapy may be not addressing specifically the pathogenic mechanism which caused the recurrent stroke. This may be due to inadequate or incomplete diagnosis at the time it was prescribed or to a new disease state, which appeared later after the patient was initially assessed.
2. The dose of the antithrombotic therapy involving anticoagulant or antiplatelet agents may have been inadequate or improperly monitored and therefore ineffective in this particular individual.
3. The patient may have developed resistance to the antithrombotic agent due to some unknown reason.
4. The patient may be noncompliant in taking the medication. In fact, in some circumstances where the antithrombotic therapy has been recently stopped, a rebound hypercoagulable state may occur.
5. The patient may have a recurrent stroke due to the anticoagulant therapy itself, i.e., a complication that may arise due to the therapy such as intracranial hemorrhage. Alternatively, an intracranial hemorrhage may have occurred unrelated to the anticoagulant therapy.

The same thinking applies to patients with previous carotid endarterectomy. The recurrent stroke may be unrelated to the previous carotid artery disease and be of cardiac or aortic-embolic source. This latter may have developed since the patient was last assesed or have been missed at the time of the first stroke due to inadequate diagnostic evaluation.

Likewise a hypercoagulable state may have developed since the time of the first stroke. In this regard, it is important fact that the hypercoagulable state can fluctuate. This has been shown for anticardiolipin antibody as well as for those titers of antithrombin III, protein C, and protein S.

Finally, restenosis of the carotid artery may have occurred, although the relationship of restenosis to recurrent stroke is not known for certain at this time.

8.8 Cervical/Carotid Bruit

Asymptomatic carotid bruit suggests the presence of an atherosclerotic lesion that has narrowed the lumen by at least 50%, i.e., to less than 3 mm. The pitch of the bruit increases with the severity of stenosis. Prolonged, very high-pitched bruits suggest a residual lumen of less than 1.5 mm (> 75% stenosis). Most atherosclerotic lesions causing bruits tend to be located on the posterior wall of the common carotid artery of the bifurcation, compromising flow at the origin of the internal carotid artery.

When stenosis is tight and flow is reduced, a mural thrombus may form distally in the proximal internal carotid artery worsening occlusion and serving as a source of emboli.

The annual incidence of stroke in the territory of a carotid bruit is 1.7% per year and increases to 5.5% per year as stenosis exceeds 75%. The risk of death (usually cardiac) in a patient with a carotid bruit is 4% per year.

Arterial bruit in the neck can be divided into supraclavicular, vertebral, and carotid. *Venous cervical murmurs* ("hums") are common in children but may occur in up to 27% of normal adults. Venous hums are usually heard at the base of the neck, their sound is low-pitched, roaring, usually continuous, maximal during diastole, loudest in the upright position, and decreased or abolished by the Valsalva maneuver.

8.8.1 The source of neck bruit

1. Carotid bifurcation arterial bruit
   a) Internal carotid artery stenosis
   b) External carotid artery stenosis
2. Supraclavicular arterial bruit
   a) Subclavian artery stenosis
   b) Vertebral artery origin stenosis
   c) Can be normal in young adults
3. Diffuse neck bruit
   a) Thyrotoxicosis
   b) Hyperdynamic circulation (pregnancy, anemia, fever, hemodialysis)
4. Transmitted bruit from the heart and great vessels
   a) Aortic valve stenosis
   b) Aortic arch atheroma
   c) Mitral valve regurgitation
   d) Patent ductus arteriosus
   e) Coarctation of the aorta

8.8.2 Differential diagnosis

1. Atherosclerotic stenosis
   a) Internal carotid artery

b) External carotid artery
c) Common carotid artery
d) Subclavian artery
2. Augmentation bruit (contralateral carotid occlusion)
3. Fibromuscular dysplasia
4. Arterial kink or loop
5. Transmitted cardiac murmur
6. Venous hum
7. High-flow states
8. Hyperthyroidism
9. Anemia
10. Intracranial arteriovenous malformation
11. Carotid cavernous fistula
12. Vascular fistula in the arm (hemodialysis)

Pessin MS, Panis W, Prager RJ, Millan VG, Scott RM. Auscultation of cervical and ocular bruits in extracranial carotid occlusive disease: a clinical and angiographic study. Stroke 1983;14(2):246–249

Sandok BA, Whisnant JP, Furlan AJ, Mickell JL. Carotid artery bruits: prevalence survey and differential diagnosis. Mayo Clin Proc 1982;57(4):227–230

Ingall TJ, Homer D, Whisnant JP, Baker HL Jr, O'Fallon WM. Predictive value of carotid bruit for carotid atherosclerosis. Arch Neurol 1989;46(4):418–422

Van Ruiswyk J, Noble H, Sigmann P. The natural history of carotid bruits in elderly persons. Ann Intern Med 1990;112(5):340–343

8.9 Cerebral Arteritis

Conditions associated with arteritis probably account for some portion of the (approximately 25%) strokes that are of undetermined etiology. Cranial arteritis is the most frequent form of vasculitis affecting persons over 50 years of age. In Europe, prevalence of 15–30 per 100,000 and incidence of 18 per 100,000 have been reported. A myriad of neurological symptoms, signs or syndromes can occur in CNS vasculitis reflecting the potential for infarction and ischemia, which may be micro- or macroscopic, focal, multifocal or diffuse, and affect any part of the brain. Three broad categories are recognized:

• Acute or subacute encephalopathy, commonly presenting as an acute confusional state, progressing to drowsiness and coma.
• Superficially resembling atypical multiple sclerosis ("MS-plus") in phenotype with a relapsing-remitting course, and features such as optic neuropathy and brainstem episodes, but also accompanied by other features less common in multiple sclerosis, such as seizures, severe and persisting headaches, encephalopathic episodes, or hemispheric stroke-like episodes.
• Intracranial mass lesions with headache, drowsiness, focal signs, and often raised intracranial pressure.

Causes for cerebral arteritis are as follows:

1. Infection
   a) Syphilis
   b) AIDS
   c) Lyme disease (borreliosis)
   d) Tuberculous meningitis
   e) Mycoplasma angiitis
   f) Herpes simplex virus
   g) Cytomegalovirus
   h) Bacterial meningitis
   i) Fungal meningitis (aspergillosis, candidiasis, coccidioidomycosis, and mucormycosis)
2. Drug abuse
   a) Amphetamines
   b) Heroin
   c) LSD
   d) Cocaine
   e) Neo-synephrine
   f) Ephedrine
   g) Oral use of methylphenidate
3. Diseases of altered immunity (including hypersensitive states)
   a) Hodgkin's disease with CNS vasculitis
   b) Non-Hodgkin's lymphoma with CNS vasculitis
   c) Serum sickness
4. Systemic necrotizing vasculitides
   Each of the systemic vasculitides may be complicated by cerebral involvement; often they carry their own defining characteristics. In contrast to primary angiitis of the CNS, constitutional disturbances—fever, night sweats, severe malaise, weight loss—are common and may be accompanied by a rash or arthropathy.
   a) Giant cell arteritis
   b) Polyarteritis nodosa
   c) Takayasu's arteritis
   d) Wegener's granulomatosis
   e) Henoch–Schönlein purpura
   f) Churg–Strauss syndrome
   g) Bechet's disease
   h) Primary angiitis of the central nervous system (PACNS)
   i) Vasculitis in collagen vascular disease
5. Connective tissue diseases
   a) Sjogren's syndrome

   b) Progressive systemic sclerosis
   c) Polymyositis/dermatomyositis
   d) Systemic lupus erythematosus
   e) Rheumatoid disease
   f) Bechet's syndrome
   g) Cryoglobulinemia
   h) Sarcoidosis
6. Primary (isolated) angiitis of the CNS
   There are no uniform diagnostic criteria for this condition and it appears to be unassociated with systemic illness, and yields evidence by cerebral angiography or biopsy of CNS tissue of vasculitis confined to the CNS. There is no typical and specific clinical presentation and this makes a high degree of suspicion the key to successful diagnosis. Suspicion should be greater if multifocal symptoms and signs develop in a stepwise progression accompanied by headache or altered mental status.
7. Malignancy and cerebral vasculitis (▶ Fig. 8.2)
   a) Lymphomatoid granulomatosis
      A premalignant lymphomatous disorder; inflammatory infiltration of T-lymphocyte-derived cells cause a true vasculitis; cutaneous and pulmonary involvement common; neurological syndromes occur in 25–30% of cases.
   b) Intravascular lymphoma (malignant angioendotheliosis)
      Rare disorder; the B-cell-derived neoplastic cells remain within the affected vessel. The neurological features may mimic vasculitis; skin manifestations predominating; lung involvement is unusual.

8.9.1 Differential diagnosis of cerebral vasculitis

The progressive bilateral narrowing of the terminal internal carotid artery and the proximal segments of the middle and anterior cerebral arteries of Moyamoya syndrome associated with strokes and headache may be mistaken for cerebral vasculitis. The main pathologic finding in this disease is endothelial thickening due to cellular fibrous tissue which leads to progressive stenosis. There are no inflammatory signs in the vessel wall. As soon as the typical collateral network of small leptomeningeal and transdural vessel occurs, the diagnosis can be made based on digital subtraction angiography (DSA) findings, but it may be difficult in early stages. Vessel biopsies may be necessary to verify the diagnosis and rule out vasculitis.

The diagnosis of Sneddon syndrome is based on the presence of fixed deep bluish-red reticular skin lesions on the legs and body in association with

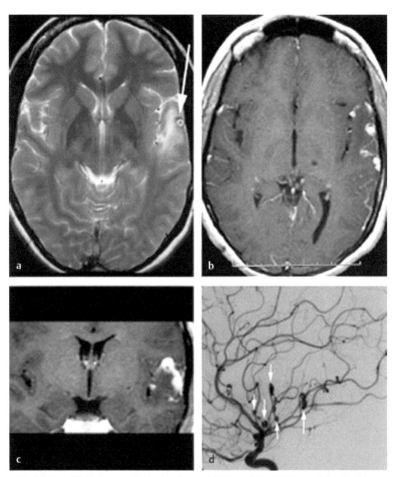

Fig. 8.2 Vasculitis in circumscribed scleroderma. Axial T2-weighted MR image **(a)** and axial T1-weighted MR image after contrast administration **(b)**. Coronal T1-weighted MR image after contrast administration **(c)**. Lateral DSA after injection into left internal carotid artery **(d)**. Broad area of hyperintensity in the left temporal operculum involving the cerebral cortex and subcortical white matter, consistent with a cerebral edema with inflammatory infiltrate **(a**, *arrow***)**. Enhancing thickened leptomeninges **(b, c)**. Enhancement is also due in part to the slow blood flow in aneurysmal branches of the middle cerebral artery **(b, c)**. DSA demonstrates multiple, primarily fusiform aneurysms in numerous branches of the left middle cerebral artery **(d**, *arrows***)**. (Reproduced from Cerebral Vasculitis. In: Sartor K, Hähnel S, Kress B, ed. Direct Diagnosis in Radiology. Brain Imaging. 1st edition. Thieme; 2007.)

strokes. Histologic studies reveal a thrombotic arterial vasculopathy of medium- and small-sized arteries. In 35% cases, there is an association with antiphospholipid antibodies. MRI usually reveals rather large ischemic lesions with only few thrombotic vessel occlusions or normal DSA. In young stroke patients who present with headache, multiple dissections of the craniocervical arteries should be considered. Cerebral autosomal dominant arteriopathy with subcortical infarcts and leukoencephalopathy (CADASIL) is an autosomal dominant disorder that leads to stroke and a progressive vascular encephalopathy in young adults.

Stroke may occur as a serious complication of sympathomimetic drugs including amphetamine, methamphetamine, ephedrine, cocaine, oxymetazoline, and phenoxazoline. Although intracerebral hemorrhage is the most frequent complication of the use of sympathomimetic agents, ischemic stroke may occur as well. The angiographic pattern in these patients may resemble cerebral vasculitis almost in its entirety.

Other rare conditions sometimes misdiagnosed as cerebral vasculitis include the reversible posterior leukoencephalopathy syndrome, MELAS, malignant intravascular lymphomatosis, Degos disease, amyloid angiopathy, Fabrys disease, pseudoxanthoma elasticum, lipohyalinosis, and storage diseases. Septic emboli in endocarditis may lead to a septic angiitis.

Wengenroth M, Jacobi C, Wildemann B. Cerebral vasculitis. In: Hahnel S, ed. Inflamatory Diseases of the Brain. NY: Springer; 2013:19–38

Berlit P. Diagnosis and treatment of cerebral vasculitis. Ther Adv Neurol Disorder 2010;3(1):29–42

Hajj-Ali RA, Calabrese LH. Central nervous system vasculitis. Curr Opin Rheumatol 2009;21(1):10–18

Pomper MG, Miller TJ, Stone JH, Tidmore WC, Hellmann DB. CNS vasculitis in autoimmune disease: MR imaging findings and correlation with angiography. AJNR Am J Neuroradiol 1999;20(1):75–85

8.10 Stroke

Determining whether a stroke is hemorrhagic or ischemic has important implications in the patient's prognosis and in deciding about the use of surgery or anticoagulants.

The suddenness of onset and the focal neurological signs give these syndromes the popular term stroke and help to distinguish cerebrovascular disease from other neurological disorders. Hypertension, atherosclerosis, or other evidence of vascular disease are commonly present. Disappearance of symptoms within minutes or hours allows the separation of TIA from stroke.

1. Cerebral embolism

    It is suggested by a sudden onset and a focal neurological deficit attributable to brain surface ischemia, e.g., pure aphasia, pure hemianopia.

2. Cerebral thrombosis
   A more complex and extensive neurological deficit would suggest a thrombosis, particularly when the stroke has been preceded by TIAs. When the deficits are of sudden onset, thrombus is clinically inseparable from embolus. The two mechanisms of thrombosis are difficult to separate on clinical grounds.

3. Cerebral hemorrhage
   The neurological symptoms have a characteristically smooth onset and evolution. However, if the syndrome advances within minutes or is halted at an early stage with only minor signs, the clinical picture may then become indistinguishable from that of infarction.

4. Trauma
   Sudden onset also characterizes trauma subsequent to which an epidural and subdural hematoma may occur and may mimic stroke. Although the trauma itself is sudden, the accumulation of the hematoma takes time: minutes or hours for epidural hemorrhage and as long as a week for subdural hemorrhage.

5. Seizures
   These may be a sign of lobar hemorrhage. The immediate postictal deficit mimics that caused by major stroke. A small percentage of seizures develop months or years after a stroke. A proper history may help rule out a new stroke.

6. Migraine
   It presents a major source of difficulty in the diagnosis of TIA. Migraine affects young people, has repeated attacks, experiences classic visual migraine auras at other times, and has a pounding headache contralateral to the sensory or motor symptoms in the hours after attack.

7. Cerebral neoplasia
   The focal cerebral disturbance evolves gradually in days or weeks which is longer than stroke. CT in tumors demonstrates an enhancing mass, but in contrast to ischemic stroke is often negative.

8. Cerebral abscess
   Clinical and CT findings similar to those of a brain tumor.

9. Metabolic disturbances
   In comatose patients, other diagnoses should be considered that cause focal neurological signs which often remit when the cause is reversed.
   a) Metabolic disturbances of glucose
   b) Renal failure
   c) Severe disturbances of electrolyte balance
   d) Alcohol intoxication
   e) Barbiturate intoxication

8.11 Clinical Grading Scales in Subarachnoid Hemorrhage

Botterell scale	Grade
Conscious with or without signs of bleeding in the subarachnoid space	I
Drowsy, without significant neurologic deficit	II
Drowsy, with significant neurologic deficit	III
Major neurologic deficit, deteriorating, or older with pre-existing cerebrovascular disease	IV
Moribund or near moribund, failing vital centers, extensor rigidity	V
Hunt–Hess scale	
Asymptomatic or mild headache	I
Moderate to severe headache, nuchal rigidity, can have oculomotor palsy	II
Confusion, drowsiness, or mild focal signs	III
Stupor or hemiparesis	IV
Coma, moribund appearance, and/or extensor posture	V
World Federation of Neurologic Surgeons scale	
Glasgow Coma Scale Score 15: No headache or focal signs	I
Glasgow Coma Scale Score 15: headache, nuchal rigidity, and no focal signs	II
Glasgow Coma Scale Score 13–14: may have headache, nuchal rigidity, no focal signs	III
Glasgow Coma Scale Score 13–14: may have headache, nuchal rigidity, or focal signs	IV a
Glasgow Coma Scale Score 9–12: may have headache, nuchal rigidity, or focal signs	IV b
Glasgow Coma Scale Score 8 or less: may have headaches, nuchal rigidity, or focal signs	V
Cooperative Aneurysm Study scale	
Symptom free	I
Mildly ill, alert and responsive, headache present	II
Moderately ill	III
• Lethargic, headache, no focal signs • Alert, focal signs present	
Severely ill	IV
• Stuporous, no focal signs • Drowsy, major focal signs present	

8.12 Cerebral Salt-Losing Syndrome of Inappropriate Secretion of Antidiuretic Hormone (SIADH) after a Subarachnoid Hemorrhage

Clinical parameter	Syndrome of inappropriate antidiuretic hormone release	Cerebral salt-losing syndrome
Blood pressure	Normal	Low or postural hypotension
Heart rate	Slow or normal	Resting or postural tachycardia
Blood volume	Normal or increased	Decreased
Hematocrit	Normal or low	Elevated
Hydration	Well hydrated	Dehydrated
Body weight	Normal or increased	Decreased
Glomerular filtration rate	Increased	Decreased
Blood urea nitrogen/ creatinine	Normal or low	Normal or high
Urine volume	Normal or low	Normal or low
Urine concentration	High	High
Hyponatremia	Dilutional (false)	True
Hypo-osmolality	Dilutional (false)	True
Mean day of appearance	8 (range 3–15)	4–5 (range 2–10)
Treatment	Fluid restriction (since the primary abnormality is expansion of the extracellular fluid volume with water)	Sodium and volume expansion (correction of the intravascular volume depletion and hyponatremia, replacement of ongoing urinary sodium loss with intravenous administration of isotonic/hypertonic fluids)

8.13 SIADH and Diabetes Insipidus

SIADH refers to a release of antidiuretic hormone (ADH) that is inappropriate to a low serum osmolality. On the ground of continued water ingestion, the elevated ADH results in water retention, hyponatremia, and hypo-osmolality.

SIADH results from partial damage of the supraoptic and paraventricular nuclei or neighboring areas or from production of ADH by the tumor or inflammatory tissue outside the hypothalamus.

The laboratory criteria for the diagnosis of SIADH are:
1. Low serum sodium (< 135 mEq/l)
2. Low serum osmolality (< 280 mOsm/kg)
3. Elevated urinary sodium level (25 mEq/l)
4. Urine osmolality that is inappropriately high compared to the serum osmolality
5. Absence of clinical evidence of volume depletion or diuretic use and normal thyroid, renal, and adrenal function. Symptoms of hyponatremia include confusion, muscle weakness, seizures, anorexia, nausea and vomiting, and stupor when the serum sodium falls below 110 mEq/l.

Diabetes insipidus (DI) refers to the lack of free water from a partial or complete deficiency of ADH. The clinical symptoms include polyuria (urine output greater than 300 ml/hour or 500 ml/2 hours), thirst, dehydration, hypovolemia, and polydipsia.

DI results from destruction of at least 90% of the large neurons in the supraoptic and paraventricular nuclei. The lesion often involves the supraoptic–hypophysial tract rather than the neuronal bodies themselves.

The laboratory criteria for the diagnosis of DI are:
1. Urine specific gravity of less than 1.005
2. Urine osmolality between 50 and 150 mOsm/kg
3. Serum sodium greater than 150 mEq/l unaccompanied by a corresponding fluid deficiency. Sodium levels reaching 170 mEq/l are attended by muscle cramping, tenderness and weakness, fever, anorexia, paranoia, and lethargy.

8.14 Syndromes of Cerebral Ischemia

Occluded artery	Signs and symptoms
Common carotid artery	• May be asymptomatic
	• Ipsilateral blindness
Middle cerebral artery	• Contralateral hemiplegia (face and arm greater than leg)
	• Contralateral hemisensory deficit (face and arm greater than leg)
	• Homonymous hemianopsia
	• Horizontal gaze palsy
	• Language and cognitive deficits
	◦ Left hemisphere:
	– Aphasia (i.e., motor, sensory, global)
	– Apraxia (i.e., ideomotor and ideational)
	– Gerstmann syndrome (i.e., agraphia, acalculia, left-right confusion, and finger agnosia)
	◦ Right hemisphere:
	– Constructional/spatial defects (i.e., constructional apraxia, or apractognosia, dressing apraxia)
	– Agnosias (i.e., topographagnosia, prosopagnosia, anosognosia, and asomatognosia)
	– Left-sided hemineglect
	– Amusia
Anterior cerebral artery	• Contralateral hemiparesis (distal leg more than arm)
	• Contralateral sensory loss (distal leg more than arm)
	• Urinary incontinence
	• Left-sided ideomotor apraxia or tactile anomia
	• Severe behavior disturbance (apathy or "abulia," motor inertia, "akinetic mutism," suck and grasp reflexes, and diffuse rigidity—gegenhalten)
	• Eye deviation toward side of infarction
	• Reduction in spontaneous speech, perseveration

(Continued)

▶ (Continued)

Occluded artery	Signs and symptoms
Posterior cerebral artery	• Contralateral homonymous hemianopia or quadrantanopia
	• Memory disturbance with bilateral inferior temporal lobe involvement
	• Optokinetic nystagmus, visual perseveration (palinopsia), hallucinations of the blind field
	• There may be alexia (without aphasia or agraphia), and anomia for colors, in dominant hemisphere involvement
	• Cortical blindness with patient not recognizing or admitting the loss of vision (Anton's syndrome), with or without macular sparing, poor eye–hand coordination, metamorphopsia and visual agnosia when cortical infarction is bilateral
	• Pure sensory stroke; may leave anesthesia dolorosa with "spontaneous pain" in cortical and thalamic ischemia
	• Contralateral hemiballismus and choreoathetosis in subthalamic nucleus involvement
	• Oculomotor palsy, internuclear ophthalmoplegia, loss of vertical gaze, convergence spasm, lid retraction (Collier sign), corectopia (eccentrically positioned pupils), and sometimes lethargy and coma with midbrain involvement
Anterior choroidal artery	May cause varying combinations of:
	• Contralateral hemiplegia
	• Sensory loss
	• Homonymous hemianopia (sometimes with a striking sparing of a beak-like zone horizontally)

8.15 Brainstem Vascular Syndromes

8.15.1 Midbrain

(▶ Fig. 8.3a)

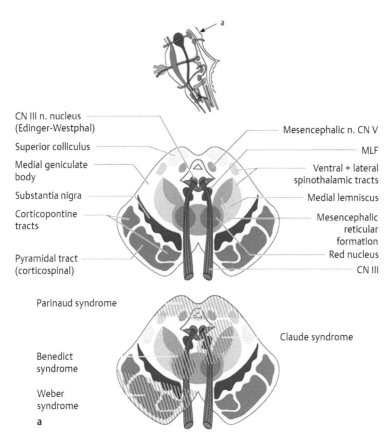

Fig. 8.3a Brainstem vascular syndromes.

Midbrain (superior colliculus): *Weber's syndrome:* (a) corticospinal and corticopontine tracts (contralateral hemiplegia including the face); (b) parasympathetic root fibers of CN III (ipsilateral oculomotor nerve paresis with fixed and dilated pupil); (c) substantia nigra (Parkinsonian akinesia). *Benedikt's syndrome:* (a) red nucleus (contralateral involuntary movements, including intention tremor, hemichorea, and hemiathetosis; (b) brachium conjunctivum (ipsilateral ataxia); (c) parasympathetic root fibers of CN III (ipsilateral oculomotor paresis with fixed and dilated pupil). *Claude's syndrome:* (a) dorsal red nucleus (contralateral involuntary movements, including intention tremor, hemichorea, and hemiathetosis; (b) brachium conjunctivum (prominent cerebellar signs and no hemiballismus); (c) dorsal midbrain tegmentum. *Parinaud's syndrome:* (a) superior colliculi (conjugated gaze paralysis upward); (b) medial longitudinal fasciculus (nystagmus and internal ophthalmoplegia); (c) eventual paresis of the CNs III and IV; (d) cerebral aqueduct stenosis/obstruction (hydrocephalus). Involvement of the inferior colliculi produces hearing loss.

389

Syndrome	Structures involved	Manifestations
Weber's syndrome	Ventral midbrain, CN III, corticospinal track	1. Ipsilateral CN III palsy including parasympathetic paresis (i.e., dilated pupil) 2. Contralateral hemiplegia
Benedikt's syndrome	Midbrain tegmentum, red nucleus, CN III, brachium conjunctivum	1. Ipsilateral CN III palsy, usually with a dilated pupil 2. Contralateral involuntary movements (intention tremor, hemichorea, or hemiathetosis)
Claude's syndrome	Dorsal mesencephalic tegmentum, dorsal red nucleus, brachium conjunctivum, CN III	1. Ipsilateral CN III palsy, usually with a dilated pupil 2. Prominent cerebellar signs 3. Contralateral involuntary movements (rubral tremor, hemiataxia, and no hemiballismus)
Parinaud's syndrome	Dorsal rostral midbrain, pretectal area, posterior commissure	1. Paralysis of conjugate upward gaze (occasionally downward gaze) 2. Pupillary abnormalities (light-near dissociation of pupil response) 3. Convergence–retraction nystagmus on upward gaze 4. Pathologic lid retraction (Collier's sign) 5. Lid lag 6. Pseudo-abducens palsy

8.15.2 Pons

(▶ Fig. 8.3b, c)

Syndrome	Structures involved	Manifestations
Millard–Gubler syndrome	Ventral paramedian pons, CN VI and VII fascicles Corticospinal tract	1. Contralateral hemiplegia (sparing the face) 2. Ipsilateral lateral rectus palsy with diplopia 3. Ipsilateral peripheral facial paresis
Dysarthria (clumsy hand syndrome)	Basis pontis (lacunar infarction) at the junction of the upper one-third and lower two-third of the pons, CN VII	1. Clumsiness and paresis of the hand, ipsilateral hyperreflexia and a Babinski sign 2. Facial weakness 3. Severe dysarthria and dysphagia

▶ (*Continued*)

Syndrome	Structures involved	Manifestations
Differential diagnosis: This syndrome has also been described with lesions in: a. The genu of the internal capsule b. Small, deep cerebellar hemorrhages		
Pure motor hemi-paresis	Lacunar infarction involving the corticospinal tracts in the basis pontis	1. Pure motor hemiplegia 2. With or without facial involvement
Ataxic hemiparesis	Lacunar infarction involving the basis pontis at the junction of the upper one-third and the lower two-third of the pons	1. Hemiparesis more severe in the lower extremity 2. Ipsilateral hemiataxia 3. Occasional dysarthria, nystagmus, and paresthesias
Differential diagnosis: This syndrome has also been described with lesions in: a. Contralateral thalamocapsular area b. Contralateral posterior limb of the internal capsule c. Contralateral red nucleus		
Locked-in syndrome (de-efferented state)	Bilateral ventral pontine lesions (infarction, tumor, hemorrhage, trauma, central pontine myelinolysis)	1. Tetraplegia due to bilateral corticospinal tract involvement 2. Aphonia due to involvement of the corticobulbar fibers destined to the lower cranial nerves 3. Occasional impairment of horizontal eye movements due to bilateral involvement of the fascicles of CN VI
Primary pontine hemorrhage syndromes	Classic type (60%): Severe pontine destruction	Tetraparesis, coma, and death
	Hemipontine type (20%)	Hemiparesis, skew deviation, dysarthria, unilateral absent corneal reflex, CN VII palsy, ipsilateral facial sensory changes, survival with functional recovery
	Dorsolateral tegmental type (20%)	Gaze paresis and/or ipsilateral CN VI palsy, unilateral CN VII palsy, contralateral extremity and ipsilateral facial sensory loss, dysarthria, preserved consciousness, motor sparing, occasional gait or limb ataxia

(*Continued*)

Cerebrovascular Disease (Stroke)

▶ (*Continued*)

Syndrome	Structures involved	Manifestations
Foville's syndrome	Dorsal pontine tegmentum in the caudal third of the pons, paramedian pontine reticular formation (PPRF)	1. Contralateral hemiplegia (with facial sparing) 2. Ipsilateral peripheral-type facial palsy (involvement of CV VII fascicles) 3. Gaze palsy to side of lesion
Raymond–Cestan syndrome	Rostral lesions of the dorsal pons	1. Cerebellar signs (ataxia) 2. Contralateral reduction of all sensory modalities (face and extremities) 3. Contralateral hemiparesis 4. Paralysis of conjugate gaze in involvement of PPRF
Marie–Foix syndrome	Lateral pontine lesions (especially brachium pontis)	1. Ipsilateral cerebellar ataxia 2. Contralateral hemiparesis 3. Variable contralateral hemihypesthesia for pain and temperature

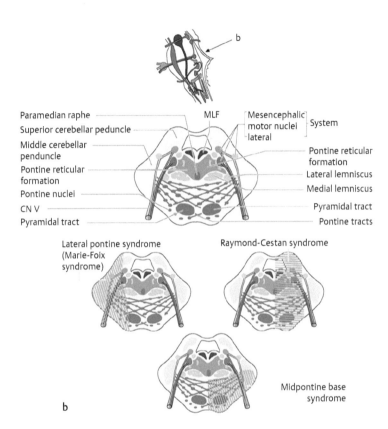

Fig. 8.3b (*Continued*) Pons (rostral): *Raymond–Cestan syndrome*: (a) superior cerebellar peduncle (cerebellar ataxia with a coarse "rubral" tremor); (b) medial lemniscus and spinothalamic tract (contralateral decrease in all sensory modalities, involving face and extremities). Ventral extension of the lesion involves additionally; (c) corticospinal tract (contralateral hemiparesis), (d) paramedian pontine reticular formation (paralysis of the conjugate gaze towards the side of the lesion). *Marie–Foix syndrome*: (a) superior and middle cerebellar peduncles (ipsilateral cerebellar ataxia); (b) corticospinal tract (contralateral hemiparesis); (c) spinothalamic tract (variable contralateral hemihypesthesia for pain and temperature). *Mid pontine base syndrome*: (a) middle cerebellar peduncle (ipsilateral ataxia and asynergy); (b) corticospinal tract (contralateral hemiparesis); (c) corticopontine fibers (ipsilateral dystaxia); (d) root fibers of CN V (ipsilateral hemianesthesia of all modalities and flaccid paralysis of chewing muscles). (*Continued*)

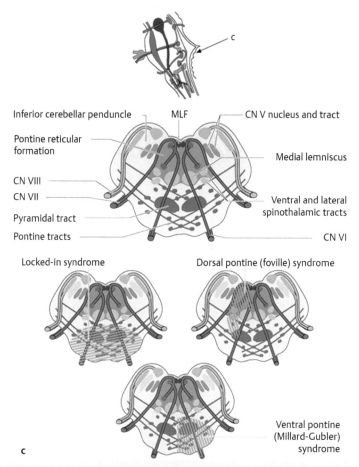

Fig. 8.3c *(Continued)* Pons (caudal): *Foville's syndrome*: (a) nucleus and fascicles of CN VII (ipsilateral peripheral type facial palsy); (b)nucleus of CN VI (gaze is "away from" the lesion); (c) corticospinal tract (contralateral hemiplegia with sparing of the face); (d) paramedian pontine reticular formation. *Millard–Gubler syndrome*: (a) pyramidal tract (contralateral hemiplegia sparing the face); (b) CN VI (diplopia accentuated when the patient "looks toward" the lesion); (c) CN VII (ipsilateral peripheral facial nerve paresis). *Locked-in syndrome*: (a) bilateral corticospinal tracts in the basis pontis (tetraplegia); (b) corticobulbar fibers of the lower CNs (aphonia); (c) occasionally bilateral fascicles of the CN VI (impairment of horizontal eye movements).

8.15.3 Medulla

(▶ Fig. 8.3d, e)

Syndrome	Structures involved	Manifestations
Dejerine anterior bulbar syndrome	Medial medulla oblongata (corticospinal tract, medial lemniscus, CN XII)	1. Ipsilateral paresis, atrophy (tongue deviates toward the lesion) 2. Contralateral hemiplegia with sparing of the face 3. Contralateral loss of position and vibratory sensation. Pain and temperature sensation are spared
Wallenberg's syndrome	Lateral medulla and inferior cerebellum (inferior cerebellar peduncle, descending sympathetic tract, spinothalamic tract, CN V nucleus)	1. Ipsilateral facial hypalgesia and thermoanesthesia 2. Contralateral trunk and extremity hypalgesia and thermoanesthesia 3. Ipsilateral palatal, pharyngeal, and vocal cord paralysis with dysphagia and dysarthria 4. Ipsilateral Horner's syndrome 5. Vertigo, nausea, and vomiting 6. Ipsilateral cerebellar signs and symptoms 7. Occasional hiccups and diplopia
Lateral ponto-medullary syndrome	Lateral medulla, inferior cerebellum, and lower pons (to the region of exit of CNs VII and VIII)	1. All clinical findings seen in the lateral medullary syndrome 2. Ipsilateral facial weakness 3. Ipsilateral tinnitus and occasional hearing disturbance

Wall M. Brainstem syndromes. In: Bradley WG, et al. eds. Neurology in Clinical Practice: Principles of diagnosis and management. 4th ed. Butterworth-Heinemann-Elsevier; 2004

Nouh A, Remke J, Ruland S. Ischemic posterior circulation stroke: a review of anatomy, clinical presentations, diagnosis, and current management. Front Neurol 2014; 5:30

Sinha KK. Brain stem infarction: Clinical clues to localize them. J Indian Acad Clin Med 2000;1(3):213–221

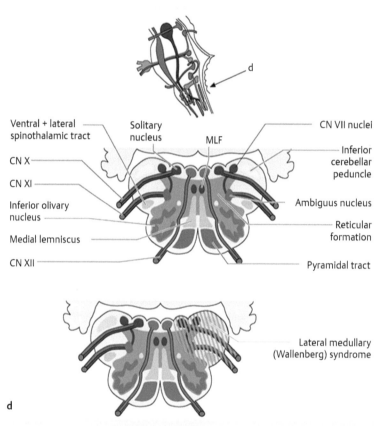

Fig. 8.3d *(Continued)* Medulla (rostral): *Lateral medullary (Wallenberg's) syndrome*: (a) nucleus and tract of CN V (ipsilateral facial pain and hypalgesia and thermoanesthesia); (b) spinothalamic tract (contralateral trunk and extremity hypalgesia and thermoanesthesia); (c) nucleus ambiguus (ipsilateral palatal, pharyngeal, and vocal cord paralysis with dysphagia and dysarthria); (d) vestibular nuclei (vertigo, nausea, and vomiting); (e) descending sympathetic fibers (ipsilateral Horner's syndrome); (f) inferior cerebellar peduncle and cerebellum (ipsilateral cerebellar signs and symptoms); (g) medullary respiratory centers (hiccups); (h) lower pons (diplopia).

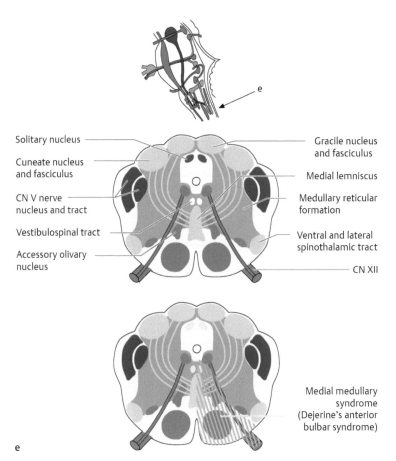

Solitary nucleus

Cuneate nucleus
and fasciculus

CN V nerve
nucleus and tract

Vestibulospinal tract

Accessory olivary
nucleus

Gracile nucleus
and fasciculus

Medial lemniscus

Medullary reticular
formation

Ventral and lateral
spinothalamic tract

CN XII

Medial medullary
syndrome
(Dejerine's anterior
bulbar syndrome)

e

Fig. 8.3e (*Continued*) Medulla (caudal): *Medial medullary (Dejerine) syndrome*: (a) CN XII (ipsilateral paresis atrophy, and fibrillation of the tongue; (b) pyramidal tract (contralateral hemiplegia with sparing of the face); (c) medial lemniscus (contralateral loss of position sense and vibration occasionally); (d) medial longitudinal nystagmus (upbeat nystagmus).

8.16 Differentiation of Various Types of Cerebral Vascular Ischemic Lesions

Ischemic vascular lesion	Clinical and radiologic characteristics			
	Risk factors	Onset/cause	Anatomic characteristics	Associated signs	Imaging characteristics CT/MRI
Systemic hypoperfusion	Heart disease, trauma, GI bleeding	Systemic disease present (cardiac arrest, bleeding hypotension)	Border zone regions between ACA, MCA, PCA and SCAs, PICA, AICA	Pallor, sweating, hypotension	Located in watershed areas CT: Low density (dark) MRI: Hypointensity (dark) in T1-WI and hyperintensity (white) in T2-WI
Embolism	Heart/coronary disease, peripheral vascular disease in white men, smoking and hyperlipidemia	Sudden onset in 80% of cases during first 24 hours; progressive in 20% of cases	MCA region most frequently, followed by the PCA or PICA distribution	Headache during and after the onset of cerebral embolism is prominent in 25% of patients	Superficial or deep wedge-shaped areas CT: Low density (dark) MRI: Hypointensity (dark) in T1-WI and hyperintensity (white) in T2-WI
Large artery thrombosis	Heart/coronary disease, peripheral vascular disease in white men, smoking hyperlipidemia	Fluctuating, progressive and remitting, manifested by a TIA in approximately 40% of patients	MCA region most frequently, followed by the PCA or PICA distribution	Headache during and after the onset of cerebral embolism is prominent in 25% of patients	Located in watershed areas or center of arterial supply CT: Low density (dark) MRI: Hypointensity (dark) in T1-WI and hyperintensity (white) in T2-WI
Small artery thrombosis	Systemic hypertension, diabetes, polycythemia	Fluctuating, progressive and remitting, manifested by a TIA in approximately 25% of patients	Small perforating arteries of deep brain structures, basal ganglia, thalamus, pons, cerebellum, cerebral white matter	Usually none	Small, deep lesions (lacunar infarcts) CT: Low density (dark) MRI: Hypointensity (dark) in T1-WI and hyperintensity (white) in T2-WI

8.17 Predisposing Factors and Associated Disorders of Cerebral Veins and Sinuses Thrombosis

1. Primary idiopathic thrombosis
2. Secondary thrombosis
   a) Pregnancy
   b) Postpartum
   c) Head injury
   d) Tumors
      i. Meningioma
      ii. Metastatic neoplasia
   e) Malnutrition and dehydration (marasmus in infancy)
   f) Infection involving sinuses, mastoids, and leptomeninges
   g) Hypercoagulable states and coagulopathies
      i. Polycythemia
      ii. Sickle cell anemia
      iii. Leukemia
      iv. Disseminated intravascular coagulation (DIC)
      v. Oral contraceptives
      vi. Inflammatory bowel disease
      vii. Nephrotic syndrome
      viii. Protein S and protein C deficiencies
      ix. Antithrombin III deficiency
   h) Paraneoplastic syndromes
      i. Cerebellar degeneration
      ii. Encephalomyelitis
      iii. Subacute necrotizing myelopathy
      iv. Peripheral polyneuropathy
      v. Cerebrovascular disease
      vi. Neuromuscular junction
   i) Chemotherapeutic agents (L-asparaginase)
   j) Cyanotic congenital heart disease

8.18 Cerebral Venous Thrombosis

Vessel involved	Structures involved	Clinical findings
Superior sagittal sinus	Venous drainage from the hemispheres and medial cerebral cortex	1. New onset headaches (simple or severe headaches that can be positionally aggravated) 2. Increased intracranial pressure with bilateral *Extension of clot into the larger cerebral veins as is common in septic thrombosis and in high percentage in the nonseptic type may cause:* 3. Convulsive seizures 4. Hemiplegia 5. Aphasia 6. Hemianopia 7. Lethargy or coma
Lateral sinus	Venous drainage from the posterior fossa, as well as drainage from the confluence of sinuses (secondary to otitis media and mastoiditis)	1. Pain, especially behind the ear (coincidental with an acute or chronic otitis or mastoiditis) 2. Increased intracranial pressure *Extension of infection into the veins draining the lateral surface of the hemisphere may cause:* 3. Jacksonian seizures 4. Hemiplegia 5. Gradenigo's syndrome 6. CNs IX, X, XI (jugular foramen distention) 7. Drowsiness and coma

Differential diagnosis: cerebral abscess

Cavernous sinus	CNs IV, V, and/or VI; internal carotid artery, possible ophthalmic artery (originates in suppurative	1. Retro-orbital pain 2. Proptosis 3. Orbital congestion with edema and chemosis of the conjunctivae and eyelids 4. Ptosis

▶ *(Continued)*

Vessel involved	Structures involved	Clinical findings
	processes of the orbit, nasal sinuses, upper half of face)	5. Facial sensory loss
		6. Signs of carotid artery occlusion
		7. Visual loss
		8. Discs are swollen with small hemorrhages

Differential diagnosis:
a. Orbital tumors in the region of the sphenoid
b. Malignant exophthalmos
c. Arteriovenous aneurysms

Bushnell C, Saposnik G. Evaluation and management of cerebral venous thrombosis. Continuum (Minneap Minn) 2014; 20(2 Cerebrovascular Disease):335–351

Bousser MG, Ferro JM. Cerebral venous thrombosis: an update. Lancet Neurol 2007;6(2):162–170

deVeber G, Andrew M, Adams C, et al; Canadian Pediatric Ischemic Stroke Study Group. Cerebral sinovenous thrombosis in children. N Engl J Med 2001;345(6):417–423

Stam J. Thrombosis of the cerebral veins and sinuses. N Engl J Med 2005;352(17):1791–1798

Ferro JM, Canhão P, Stam J, Bousser MG, Barinagarrementeria F; ISCVT Investigators. Prognosis of cerebral vein and dural sinus thrombosis: results of the International Study on Cerebral Vein and Dural Sinus Thrombosis (ISCVT). Stroke 2004;35(3):664–670

8.19 Spontaneous Intracerebral Hemorrhage (ICH)

Spontaneous intracerebral hemorrhage (ICH) accounts for approximately 10% of all strokes. The arterial hypertension is by far the most common cause of ICH; other causes being intracranial aneurysms, vascular malformation, bleeding diathesis, cerebral amyloidosis, brain tumors, vasculitis, or drug abuse.

The clinical features of ICH depend on the location, size, direction of spread, and rate of development of the hematoma. The clinical presentation of lobar hemorrhages is often misinterpreted as a thromboembolic cerebral infarction.

Posterior fossa spontaneous hemorrhages occur in 10% of patients and may affect either the cerebellum or the pons. Differentiation of cerebellar or pontine hemorrhages often is not possible on clinical grounds, since they share the sudden presenting symptoms and often signs. An accurate diagnosis is achieved quickly by CT and MR scans.

Structure involved	Clinical manifestations
Lobar hemorrhage	
• Frontal lobe	1. Abulia
	2. Contralateral hemiparesis
	3. Bifrontal headache (maximum ipsilateral)
	4. Occasionally mild gaze preference away from the hemiparesis
• Parietal lobe	1. Contralateral hemisensory loss
	2. Neglect of the contralateral visual field
	3. Headache (usually anterior temporal location)
	4. Mild hemiparesis
	5. Occasional hemianopia or anosognosia
• Temporal lobe	1. Wernicke's aphasia (dominant temporal lobe)
	2. Conduction or global aphasia (dominant temporal-parietal lobe)
	3. Variable degrees of visual field deficit
	4. Headache around or anterior to ipsilateral ear
	5. Occasional agitated delirium
• Occipital lobe	1. Ipsilateral orbital pain
	2. Contralateral homonymous hemianopia
Putaminal hemorrhage	The putamen is the most common site for hypertensive ICH
	1. Hemiparesis or hemiplegia and, to a lesser degree, hemisensory deficit
	2. Transient global aphasia with dominant hemispheric lesions
	3. Agnosia or unilateral neglect with nondominant hemispheric lesions
	4. Homonymous hemianopia
	5. Contralateral gaze palsy: the patient looks toward the hematoma and away from the hemiplegia
	6. Alloesthesia (a noxious stimulus on the side of the hemisensory disturbance is perceived at the corresponding area of the other (normal) side)
Thalamic hemorrhage	Findings:
	1. Hemisensory deficit and, to a lesser degree, hemiparesis
	2. Anomic aphasia with impaired comprehension with lesions of the dominant thalamus
	3. Convergence-retraction nystagmoid movements, impairment of vertical gaze, and pupillary light-near dissociation
	4. Downward–inward deviation of the eyes
	5. Unilateral or bilateral pseudo-VI nerve paresis
	6. Skew deviation
	7. Conjugate gaze palsy to the side of the lesion (wrong side) or conjugate horizontal gaze deviation

▶ (*Continued*)

Structure involved	Clinical manifestations
Cerebellar hemorrhage	This is most common in the area of the dentate nucleus
	Symptoms:
	1. Sudden occipital headache
	2. Nausea and repeated vomiting
	3. Dizziness, vertigo
	4. Inability to stand
	Findings:
	1. Variable degrees of alertness
	2. Small reactive pupils
	3. Skew deviation
	4. Ipsilateral gaze palsy
	5. Ocular bobbing and nystagmus toward the gaze paresis
	6. Ipsilateral peripheral facial weakness
	7. Ipsilateral absence or decrease of corneal reflex
	8. Slurred speech
	9. Gait or truncal ataxia
	10. Bilateral hyperreflexia and Babinski signs
Pontine hemorrhage	Symptoms:
	1. Headache, vomiting, vertigo, dysarthria
	2. Sudden loss of consciousness often progressing into deep coma
	Findings:
	1. Sudden-onset coma
	2. Quadriparesis/quadriplegia
	3. Respiratory abnormalities
	4. Hyperthermia
	5. Pinpoint reactive pupils
	6. Eyes fixed in a central position
	7. Loss of brainstem reflexes, including the oculocephalic (doll's head) and the oculovestibular reflexes
	8. Ocular bobbing (▶ Fig. 8.4)

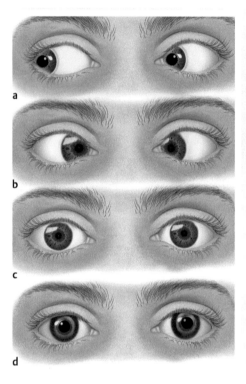

Fig. 8.4 Pupillary signs in patients with intracerebral hemorrhage. **(a)** Putaminal hemorrhage (contralateral gaze palsy; the patient looks towards the hematoma and away from the hemiplegia). **(b)** Thalamic hemorrhage (downward-inward deviation of the eyes, skew deviation, conjugate gaze palsy to the side of the lesion or horizontal gaze deviation; convergence-retraction, nystagmoid movements, impaired vertical gaze, and pupillary light-near dissociation). **(c)** Pontine hemorrhage (eyes fixed in central position; pin point reacting pupils; loss of oculocephalic reflex (doll's head) and the oculovestibular reflexes; ocular bobbing). **(d)** Cerebellar hemorrhage (skew deviation; small reacting pupils; ipsilateral gaze palsy; ocular bobbing and nystagmus towards the gaze paresis).

Tsementzis SA. Surgical management of intracerebral hematomas. Neurosurgery 1985;16(4):562–572

Silvera S, Oppenheim C, Touzé E, et al. Spontaneous intracerebral hematoma on diffusion-weighted images: influence of T2-shine-through and T2-blackout effects. AJNR Am J Neuroradiol 2005;26(2):236–241

Finelli PF. A diagnostic approach to multiple simultaneous intracerebral hemorrhages. Neurocrit Care 2006;4(3):267–271

Mauriño J, Saposnik G, Lepera S, Rey RC, Sica RE. Multiple simultaneous intracerebral hemorrhages: clinical features and outcome. Arch Neurol 2001;58(4):629–632

Lo WD, Lee J, Rusin J, Perkins E, Roach ES. Intracranial hemorrhage in children: an evolving spectrum. Arch Neurol 2008;65(12):1629–1633

Morgenstern LB, Hemphill JC, Anderson G, et al. Guidelines for the management of spontaneous intracerebral hemorrhage: A guideline for health care professionals from the American Heart Association Stroke 2010;41(9):2108–2129

9 Spinal Disorders

9.1 Failed Back Surgery Syndrome

Recurrent or residual low back pain after lumbar disc surgery; incidence ranges between 5 and 40%

1. Incorrect original diagnosis
2. Permanent nerve root injury from the original disc herniation
   Deafferentation pain which is usually constant and burning
3. Residual or recurrent disk
4. Postoperative complications
   a) Immediate
      i. Permanent injury to the nerve roots from surgery
         Deafferentation pain which is usually constant and burning and is responsible for 6–16% of persistent symptoms in postoperative patients
      ii. Epidural hematoma
      iii. Infection
      iv. Postoperative swelling
   b) Late
      i. Pseudomeningocele
         Due to a dural tear at the time of surgery; the differential includes postoperative serous fluid collections and infected collections
      ii. Epidural fibrosis
         Scar or granulation tissue formation causing compression and mechanical distortion of the nerve root
      iii. Arachnoiditis
         Once very common after contrast myelography, particularly with the combination of hemorrhage from myelography/surgery and retained contrast material. The differential includes: (a) intradural mass, (b) cerebrospinal fluid (CSF) tumor spread and (c) spinal stenosis
      iv. Discitis
         Incidence after lumbar discectomy 0.2%; intractable back pain 1–4 weeks postop after a period of symptomatic relief. The differential includes: (a) neoplasm, (b) degenerative disease, and (c) osteomyelitis
5. Insufficient root decompression by residual soft tissue or bone (i.e., stenosis of exit foramen, residual soft tissue such as a synovial cyst)
6. Surgery at wrong level
7. Disc herniation at another level
8. Mechanical segmental instability

9. Cauda equina tumor
10. Lumbar spinal stenosis
    Recurrence at operated level many years later, secondary stenosis after surgery at adjacent level or at level fused in the midline
11. Causes of back pain unrelated to the original condition (i.e., myofascial syndrome, paraspinal muscle spasm
12. Psychological factors such as secondary gains, drug addiction, poor motivation, psychological problems

9.2 Diffuse Thickening of the Nerve Root

1. Carcinomatous meningitis
2. Lymphoma
3. Leukemia
4. Arachnoiditis
5. Neurofibroma
6. Toxic neuropathy
7. Sarcoidosis
8. Histiocytosis
9. Vascular anomalies (i.e., spinal arteriovenous malformation)

9.3 Scar versus Residual Disc

MRI without intravenous contrast is at least equivalent to contrast CT in distinguishing scar tissue from disk material and yielding an accuracy of 83%. The addition of Gadolinium (Gd)-DTPA increases further the diagnostic accuracy from 89 to 96%. Overall sagittal and axial T1-weighted pre- and post-Gd-DTPA MRI remains the single most effective method of evaluating the postoperative lumbar spine patient (▶ Fig. 9.1). The important criteria for evaluating of scar tissue versus disk material in the postoperative patient based on Gd-DTPA-enhanced MRI can be summarized as follows:

1. Scar tissue enhances immediately after injection, irrespective of the time since surgery (some scars continue to enhance for more than 20 years).
2. Disk material does not enhance immediately following injection.
3. Smoothly marginated, polypoid anterior epidural mass showing continuity with the parent disc space (except for free fragments) is disk material.
4. Scar tissue can have mass effect and be contiguous to the disk space.
5. Retraction of the thecal sac toward aberrant epidural soft tissue can be a helpful sign of scar tissue when present.

Note: The presence or absence of mass effect should be a secondary consideration when compared to the presence or absence of enhancement.

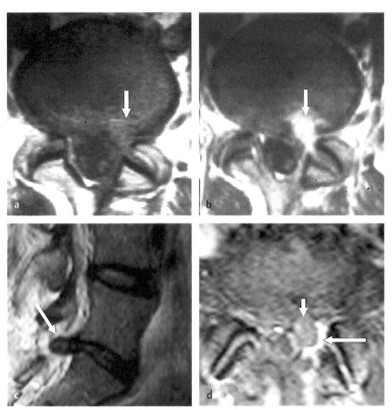

Fig. 9.1 (a-d) Radiologic characteristics between scar versus disc material. The hallmark sign distinguishing scar from recurrent or residual disc herniation is the pattern of enhancement. Scar tissue tends to enhance homogeneously, while disc herniation tends to enhance peripherally. In the early postoperative period (less than 3–6 months) it may be impossible to distinguish peripherally enhancing scar type changes from recurrent/residual disc herniation.

9.4 Multiple Lumbar Spine Surgery (Failed Back Syndromes)

A history of failed lumbar spine surgery is a diagnostic and therapeutic challenge to a physician. The first step is to differentiate those patients whose back or leg pain originates from a systemic cause (e.g., pancreatitis, diabetes, abdominal aneurysm) from those with a mechanical problem, and therefore, a thorough medical evaluation should be undertaken in this group at the same time the neurosurgical evaluation is done.

Patients with profound emotional disturbances and instability (e.g., alcoholism, drug abuse, depression) and those involved with compensation and litigation should undergo a thorough psychiatric evaluation. Even if they are found to have a genuine neurosurgical problem, their psychosocial problem should be dealt with first, because additional low back surgery would fail again. After exclusion of the psychosocial group of patients, a smaller group of patients with back and/or leg pain due to mechanical instability or scar tissue is separated; only the patients with mechanical instability will benefit from additional surgery.

9.4.1 Causes of failed back syndromes

These affect 10–40% of patients following low back surgery. Recurrent or residual back and/or leg pain after lumbar disc surgery constitutes the "failed back syndrome" (excluding secondary gain, and other nonmedical causes).

1. Residual or recurrent disc
2. Epidural fibrosis/arachnoiditis
3. Spinal stenosis
4. Mechanical instability
5. Surgery at wrong level
6. Thoracic, high lumbar disc herniation
7. Conus tumor
8. Postoperative complications (e.g., nerve root trauma, hematoma, infection)

9.4.2 Differential diagnosis

1. **Herniated intervertebral disc**
   a) Clinical assessment:
      i. Original disc not removed: This may occur if a disc fragment is left in the intervertebral disc space or if the wrong disc level was removed. Patients will continue to have the preoperative leg pain because of continued mechanical compression and inflammation of the same nerve root. Patients will wake up from surgery complaining of the same preoperative pain and will continue without ever being pain free. Patients will benefit from reoperation.
      ii. Recurrent disc at the same level: Patients will develop a sudden onset of leg pain as preoperatively, following a pain-free period of greater than months. An additional operation is indicated. In the case of a recurrent disc at different level, patients will have a pain-free interval greater than 6 months, and suffer a sudden onset of leg and/or back pain. The neurologic symptoms and the radiologic

findings, however, will be at different level than preoperatively. Reoperation will yield very good results.

b) CT scan:
   i. Without enhancement: Recurrent disc material causes a nonspecific mass effect, density greater than 90 Hounsfield units, may reveal gas or calcium collection, and nodularity, does not conform to the margins of the thecal sac, and the margins tend to be sharp. The majority of the disc material is centered at the intervertebral disc space.
   ii. With intravenous contrast enhancement: Herniated disc material does not enhance early on following contrast administration. The disc material, however, enhances on the delayed CT scan images (e.g., 40 minutes after injection of the contrast material). Discs are typically seen as areas of decreased attenuation with a peripheral rim of enhancement, whereas epidural scar enhances homogeneously.

c) MRI: Within 6 weeks following surgery at the operative site, there is a large amount of tissue disruption and edema (producing mass effect on the anterior thecal wall) that is heterogeneously isointense to muscle on T1-WI and increased on T2-WI. These disruptions will heel within 2–6 months postoperatively. MRI may be used in the immediate postoperative period for a more gross view of the thecal sac and epidural space, to exclude significant hemorrhage, pseudomeningocele, or disc space infection. Even with the use of CT-myelography, distinction between these entities on MRI is extremely difficult, as all will appear as nonspecific extradural mass effects. Herniated disks will show contiguity with the parent disc space (except for free fragments) and mass effect. Small protruded discs are low in signal intensity on T2-WI, whereas larger protruded, extruded, and free fragments can show central high-signal intensity on T2-WI. Recurrent herniations display a smooth polyploid configuration, and an hypointense rim outlining the high-signal intensity herniations, which helps to separate the herniated material from the adjacent CSF on T2-WI.

2. **Fibrosis (scar tissue)**
Six weeks to 6 months following lumbar spina surgery, there is gradual replacement of the immediate postoperative changes by posterior scar tissue. Fibrosis can be extradural (most common type) and intradural (arachnoiditis). Patients with arachnoiditis have a history of multiple lumbar spine surgeries, with pain-free intervals ranging between 1 and 6 months. They usually complain of both back and leg pain in varying degrees and the neurological evaluation is inconclusive.

The diagnosis of scar tissue versus disc is extremely important. Surgery is not indicated for scar (epidural fibrosis) but would be beneficial if disc can be diagnosed as a cause of the radiculopathy.

a) The definitive study for diagnosing arachnoiditis is:
   i. Myelographic findings of mild arachnoiditis are blunting of the caudal nerve root sleeves, segmental nerve root fusion, and small irregularities of the thecal sac margin. Multisegmental nerve root fusion with root sleeve obliteration, intradural scarring, and loculation is seen with moderate arachnoiditis. Severe adhesive arachnoiditis may cause a myelographic block.
   ii. Postmyelogram CT scan reveals nodular, or cordlike intradural masses with moderate disease. Sometimes the nerve roots are annealed against the dura and the thecal sac appears empty or featureless.
   iii. MRI findings of arachnoiditis include intradural fibrosis, nerve root clumping, loculation and sacculation, root retraction, and adhesions.
b) The best means of trying to identify epidural scar tissue are:
   i. CT scan with and without enhancement
      CT without contrast was correct 43% of the time, while CT with contrast was correct 74% of the time in differentiating scar tissue from disc material
      – Scar tissue causes retraction of the thecal sac to the surgical site and conforms to the thecal sac margin.
      – Linear strandlike densities occur within scar tissue
      – The majority of the scar tissue is seen above or below the particular disc level
      – Scar tissue shows attenuation of 75 Hounsfield units or less and shows contrast enhancement
   ii. MRI with enhancement
      Pre- and postcontrast MRI gives 96% accuracy in differentiating scar tissue from disc material
      – Scar tissue is consistently enhancing immediately following injection on T1-WI. This enhancement occurs regardless of the time since surgery; even when surgery was more than 20 years ago.
      – Scar tissue may occasionally show mass effect and should not be used as a major discriminator of epidural fibrosis versus disc material

3. **Lumbar spinal stenosis**
   Cauda equina compression from central spinal stenosis results in neurogenic claudication with bilateral leg pain that begins after walking a short distance. The pain is not well localized and often is more of a dysesthesia than true pain.

a) Plain X-rays: The interpediculate distance increases from T12 to L5. Interpediculate measurements of less than 16 mm at the L4–5 or less than 20 mm at L5–S1 and canal cross-sectional areas of less than 1.45 cm² are considered abnormal.

b) CT scanning will show bony encroachment upon the neural elements and is especially useful in evaluating the lateral recesses and foraminae. A cross-sectional area of less than 100 mm² is abnormal.

c) MRI is useful as soft tissue, such as the intervertebral disc and ligamentum flavum, contributes significantly to most cases of stenosis. Sclerotic bone will have low signal intensity on T1-WI and T2-WI, and is recognized by the encroachment upon the epidural and foraminal fat. Osteophytes containing fatty marrow are recognized by their high signal intensity on T1-WI. Sagittal images are most useful in defining bony foraminal stenosis or more generalized stenosis secondary to disc degeneration with lost disc space height and rostrocaudal subluxation of the facets.

4. **Lumbar instability**

Instability of the lumbar spine will cause pain on a mechanical basis in the multiple spine surgery patient. A coexisting spondylolisthesis, pseudoarthrosis, or an excessively wide bilateral laminectomy can cause spinal instability. These patients complain of back pain associated with activity (mechanical) and their physical examination may be negative. The diagnosis of lumbar spinal instability is based on plain X-ray features.

Radiologic elements	Point value
1. Destruction or loss of function of the anterior elements	2
2. Destruction or loss of function of the posterior elements	2
3. Radiographic criteria	4
4. Flexion–extension X-rays	
a. Sagittal plane translation > 4.5 mm or 15%	2
b. Sagittal plane rotation > 15% at L1–2, L2–3, and L3–4 > 20% at L4–5 > 25% at L5–S1	2
5. Cauda equina damage	3
6. Dangerous loading anticipated	1
Unstable = Total score of 5 or more	

Wong CB, Chen WJ, Chen LH, Niu CC, Lai PL. Clinical outcomes of revision lumbar spinal surgery: 124 patients with a minimum of two years of follow-up. Chang Gung Med J 2002;25(3):175–182

Arts MP, Kols NI, Onderwater SM, Peul WC. Clinical outcome of instrumented fusion for the treatment of failed back surgery syndrome: a case series of 100 patients. Acta Neurochir (Wien) 2012;154(7):1213–1217

Walker BF. Failed back surgery syndrome. COMSIG Rev 1992;1(1):3–6

Long DM. Failed back surgery syndrome. Neurosurg Clin N Am 1991;2(4):899–919

Guyer RD, Patterson M, Ohnmeiss DD. Failed back surgery syndrome: diagnostic evaluation. J Am Acad Orthop Surg 2006;14(9):534–543

Block AR, Gatchel RJ, Deardorff WW, Guyer RD. The Psychology of Spine Surgery. Washington DC: American Psychological Association; 2003

Louw JA. The differential diagnosis of neurogenic and referred leg pain. SA Orthop J 2014;13(2)

Mavrocordatos P, Cahana A. Minimally invasive procedures for the treatment of failed back surgery syndrome. In: Pickard JP, ed. Advances and Technical Standard in Neurosurgery. Vol. 31. Springer-Verlag; 2006:212–247

Bundschuh CV, Modic MT, Ross JS, et al. Epidural fibrosis and recurrent disk herniation in the lumbar spine: MR imaging assessment AJNR Am J Neuroradiol 2009;30:1082–1097

Small J, Schaefer W. Neuroradiology:Key differential diagnosis and clinical questions. Elsevier-Saunders; 2013

9.5 Low Back Pain

In the vast majority of patients (> 80%) no specific pathoanatomical diagnosis can be made. Low back pain is the second most common reason for people to seek medical help; its prevalence ranges from 60–90% and has an incidence rate of approximately 5%. Only 1% will develop nerve root symptoms and only 1–3% of patients have lumbar disc herniation. Low back pain is only a symptom which can result from several conditions and therefore, the term should not be equated with herniated lumbar disc.

1. **Acute and subacute low back pain**

   Acute low back pain is self-limited and the majority of patients start getting better within 6 weeks. Approximately 10% of patients will persist having symptoms for more than 6 weeks thus entering a subacute phase

   a) Trauma

      i. Musculoligamentous sprain/lumbosacral strain
      ii. Myofascial syndrome
          A localized pain complaint associated with a tense muscle containing a very tender spot, i.e. trigger point, identifiable by palpation and which may be distant to the source of pain.
      iii. Spondylolysis and spondylolisthesis
          Overuse injuries secondary to repetitive, unrepaired microtrauma are frequent particularly to athletes engaging in high-impact sports)
      iv. Posttraumatic disc herniation
      v. Postoperative

b) Infections

Immunocompromised and debilitated patients, drug abusers, diabetics, and alcoholics are at increased risk. Local spinal tenderness to percussion has 80% sensitivity with bacterial pyogenic infections, but a low specificity.

   i. Spondylitis and discitis
- Pyogenic spondylitis
  Staphylococcus aureus is the most common organism accounting for 60% of infections; *Enterobacter* for 30%; other organisms are *Escherichia coli*, *Salmonella*, *Pseudomonas aeruginosa*, and *Klebsiella pneumoniae.*
- Granulomatous and miscellaneous spondylitis
  Granulomatous spondylitis—*Mycobacterium tuberculosis* most commonly involved; *Brucella melitensis.* Fungal spondylitis—blastomycosis, aspergillosis, actinomycosis, cryptococcosis, and coccidioidomycosis. Parasitic spondylitis—*Echinococccus.*)

  ii. Epidural and subdural abscesses (*S. aureus* is by far the most common organism)

 iii. Meningitis
Spinal meningitis can be caused by bacterial, fungal, parasitic, or viral organisms, often as a manifestation of cerebral meningitis.

 iv. Myelitis
Viral infections such as herpes, coxsackie, and polio viruses are the most common organisms, and the HIV-related myelitis is increasing recently.

c) Spinal tumors

Patients aged > 50 years with an unexplained weight loss and relentless pain of > 4–5 months (range 3 days to 3.8 years) not responding to bed rest or other conservative treatment may have spinal tumors.

   i. Extradural spinal cord tumors (55%)
- Metastatic (> 70%)
  - Lung (most common in men)
  - Breast (most common in women)
  - Lymphoma
  - Prostate
- Primary spinal cord tumors (< 30%)
  - Multiple myeloma (most common bone tumor;10–15%)
  - Osteogenic sarcoma (the second most common primary bone tumor in childhood and adolescence)
  - Chordoma
  - Chondrosarcoma
  - Ewing's sarcoma

- ◦ Giant cell tumor
- ◦ Benign bone tumors (osteoid osteoma, osteoblastoma)
  ii. Intradural spinal cord tumors (40%)
  - – Meningioma
  - – Nerve sheath tumors
  - – Vascular malformations and tumors
  - – Epidermoid and dermoid cysts and teratomas
  - – Lipoma
  iii. Intramedullary spinal cord tumors (5%)
  - – Ependymoma
  - – Astrocytoma
  - – Metastases (Lung cancer, breast cancer, lymphoma, colorectal cancer)
  - – Hemangioblastoma
  - – Lipoma
  - – Schwannoma
d) Inflammatory
  i. Sacroiliitis
  An acute inflammatory disorder which may be seen early in ankylosing spondylitis. It causes morning back stiffness, hip pain and swelling, failure to get relief at rest and improvement with exercise
e) Referred pain of visceral origin
  Patients writhing in pain should be evaluated for an intra-abdominal or vascular pathology; e.g., in aortic dissection the pain is described as a "tearing" pain whereas in patients with neurogenic low back pain it tends to remain still and moving only to change positions at intervals.
  i. Abdominal aortic aneurysm eroding the vertebrae
  ii. Occlusive vascular disease causing radicular or plexus ischemia
  iii. Direct involvement of lumbosacral plexus or sciatic nerve (e.g., trauma, tumors, injections into or close to the sciatic nerve)
f) Pathologic fracture
  Patients at risk for osteoporosis or with known cancer.
  i. Lumbar compression fractures
  ii. Sacral insufficiency fractures (e.g., patients in rheumatoid arthritis on chronic treatment with steroids)

2. **Chronic low back pain**
From all patients with an acute low back pain, 5% of them will continue having persistent symptoms and fall into chronicity after 3 months. These patients account for 85% of the cost in lost work and line-up in the workman's compensation list.
a) All causes of acute and subacute low back pain listed earlier.

b) Degenerative diseases
   i. Spondylosis, spondylolysis, and spondylolisthesis
   Spondylosis refers to osteoarthritis involving the articular surfaces (joints and discs) of the spine, often with osteophyte formation and cord or root compression. Spondylolysis refers to a separation at the pars articularis which permits the vertebrae to slip. Spondylolisthesis is defined as the anterior subluxation of the suprajacent vertebra, often producing central stenosis; it is the slipping of one vertebra forward on the one below.
   ii. Lumbar spinal stenosis
   Multiple nerve roots are involved and the pain in the spine is significantly greater than that in the limb. Symptoms aggravate when standing or walking. Impairment in the bowel, bladder, or sexual function may occur.
   iii. Lateral recess syndrome
   Single or multiple nerve roots on one or both sides become compressed. Pain in the limb is usually equal to or greater than that in the spine. Symptoms are brought on by either walking or standing and are relieved with sitting. Testing by straight leg raising may be negative.
   iv. Facet arthrosis and synovial cysts
   v. Lumbar disc disease (bulge-herniation)
   Clinical features include positive straight leg raising and radicular pain in the limb disproportionate to that in the spine. Loss of strength, reflex, and sensation occurs in that root's territory.
c) Inflammatory disorders involving
   i. Vertebrae
      - Ankylosing spondylitis
      - Rheumatoid arthritis
   ii. Meninges
      - Arachnoiditis
d) Metabolic
   i. Osteoporosis (particularly in postmenopausal females)
   ii. Paget's disease (osteitis deformans)
   iii. Hyperparathyroidism
   iv. Diabetic neuropathy
   v. Gout
e) Nonorganic causes
   i. Psychiatric causes
   ii. Malingering or secondary gain (e.g., financial, emotional)
   iii. Substance abuse

Werneke M, Hart DL. Centralization phenomenon as a prognostic factor for chronic low back pain and disability. Spine 2001;26(7):758–764, discussion 765

Kinkade S. Evaluation and treatment of acute low back pain. Am Fam Physician 2007;75(8):1181–1188

Rush AJ, Polatin P, Gatchel RJ. Depression and chronic low back pain: establishing priorities in treatment. Spine 2000;25(20):2566–2571

Patrick N, Emanski E, Knaub MA. Acute and chronic low back pain. Med Clin North Am 2014;98(4):777–789, xii

Atlas SJ, Deyo RA. Evaluating and managing acute low back pain in the primary care setting. J Gen Intern Med 2001;16(2):120–131

Rives PA, Douglass AB. Evaluation and treatment of low back pain in family practice. J Am Board Fam Pract 2004;17(Suppl):S23–S31

Chou R, Qaseem A, Snow V, et al. Prognosis and treatment of low back pain: A joint clinical practice. Guideline from the American College of Physicians and the American Pain Society clinical guidelines Ann Intern Med 2007;147:478–491

9.6 Claudication Pain

Claudication pain is a cramp-like pain that is always induced by exercise at a constant distance that the patient walks; it can be either unilateral or bilateral and is relieved by rest. The most important disorder of claudication is that of peripheral arterial disease and must be distinguished from pseudoclaudication caused by lumbar spinal stenosis. Intermittent claudication must also be differentiated from lower extremity pain caused by nonvascular etiologies that may include neurologic, musculoskeletal, and venous pathologies.

9.6.1 Differential diagnosis

1. Cardiovascular
   a) Arteritis (Takayasu, giant cell)
   b) Aortic coarctation
   c) Aortic dissection
   d) Embolic disease
   e) Thromboangiitis obliterans
   f) Venous congestion (chronic venous insufficiency, postthrombotic syndrome after deep venous thrombosis)
2. Neurologic
   a) Lumbar spinal stenosis
   b) Spondylolisthesis
3. Musculoskeletal
   a) Arthritis
   b) Compartment syndrome
   c) Baker's cyst
   d) Degenerative joint disease

e) Popliteal artery entrapment syndrome
f) Popliteal vein compression
g) Fibromuscular dysplasia
h) Myopathy

9.6.2 Differentiating signs and symptoms

1. Lumbar spinal stenosis claudication
   Lumbar spinal stenosis is due to nerve root compression by herniated disks or osteophytes and the pain typically follows the dermatome of the affected root.
   a) The pain usually begins immediately upon walking and may be felt in the calf or in the lower leg and it is associated sometimes with numbness and paresthesia.
   b) The pain is not quickly relieved by rest and may even be present at rest.
   c) A sensation of pain running down the back of the leg as well as a history of back problems may be present.
   d) Symptoms are usually associated with walking; however, upright standing may produce pain, weakness, or discomfort in the hips, thighs and buttocks.
   e) Symptoms are alleviated by sitting or flexing the lumbar spine forward as opposed to standing which alleviates pain caused by intermittent claudication.
   f) In patients with cauda equina syndrome, upright positioning aggravates the narrowing of the spinal canal and therefore causes the symptoms.
2. Venous claudication
   Venous claudication occurs in patients with chronic venous insufficiency and those who develop postthrombotic syndrome after deep venous thrombosis. Baseline venous hypertension in the obstructed veins worsens with exercise.
   a) Venous claudication produces a tight bursting pressure in the limb following exercise, usually worse in the thigh and uncommonly in the calf.
   b) It is usually associated with venous edema in the leg.
   c) Leg elevation helps in relieving the symptoms.
   d) Venous claudication tends to improve with cessation of exercise but total resolution takes much longer time than the resolution of intermittent claudication.
3. Chronic compartment syndrome
   Chronic compartment syndrome is an uncommon cause of exercise-induced leg pain, which results from thickened fascia, muscular hypertrophy or when external pressure is applied to the leg. It occurs in young athletes

who develop increased pressure within a fixed compartment which compromises the perfusion and the function of the tissues within that space. The diagnosis is based on testing the intercompartmental pressure before and after exercise.

  a) Chronic compartment syndrome presents as tight bursting pressure in the calf or foot after endurance sports or other robust exercise.
  b) Pain subsides slowly with rest.
4. Hip and knee osteoarthritis
  a) Osteoarthritis in joints is typically worse in the morning or at the initiation of movement and does not cease upon stopping exercise or standing.
  b) The pain improves after sitting, lying down, or leaning against an object to alleviate weight-bearing on the joint.
  c) The pain may be affected by weather changes and may be present at rest.

Mufson I. Intermittent limping—intermittent claudication: their differential diagnosis. Ann Intern Med 1941;14(12):2240–2245

Comer CM, Redmond AC, Bird HA, Conaghan PG. Assessment and management of neurogenic claudication associated with lumbar spinal stenosis in a UK primary care musculoskeletal service: a survey of current practice among physiotherapists. BMC Musculoskelet Disord 2009;10:121

Weinberg I, Jaff MR. Nonatherosclerotic arterial disorders of the lower extremities. Circulation 2012;126(2):213–222

9.7 Differential Diagnosis of Claudicant Leg Pain

Both the backache and the leg symptoms of lumbar spinal canal stenosis are considered mechanical in nature. That is, they are aggravated by activity and often relieved significantly by rest. They are distinguished from vascular claudication in that the rest required for relief is usually of many minutes rather than a brief interruption in activities.

Clinical findings	Neurogenic claudication	Vascular claudication
Back pain	Always in the past or present history	Rare
Leg pain		
• Type	Vague and variously described as radicular, having heaviness, cramping	Sharp, cramping
• Location	Radicular distribution or extremely diffuse and almost always affects buttock, thigh and calf; in canal stenosis both legs are involved	Affects the exercised muscles (often calf, but may be buttock and thigh); often may affect one leg

▶ (Continued)

Clinical findings	Neurogenic claudication	Vascular claudication
• Radiation	Common after onset, usually proximal to distal	Rare after onset, but may be distal to proximal
• Aggravating activity	Usually walking, but can also be standing	Walking, not standing
• Walking uphill	Better (because back is flexed)	Worse (harder exercise)
• Walking downhill	Worse (because back is extended)	Better (less muscular energy needed)
• Relief	Walking in forward, flexed position is more comfortable; once pain occurs, relief comes only with lying down or sitting down	Stopping muscular activity even in the standing position
• Time to relief	Slow (many minutes)	Quick (minutes)
Neurologic symptoms	Commonly present	Not present
Straight leg raising test	Mildly positive or negative	Negative
Neurologic examination	Mildly positive or negative	Negative
Vascular examination	Pulses present	Pulses absent
Skin appearance	No change	Atrophic changes

It is important to remember that spinal stenosis has many ways of presentation, some not clearly defined until the end of complete vascular and spinal examination. Although vascular claudication is the number one differential diagnosis, other conditions that cause upset in walking also have to be included in the **differential diagnosis**. These include:

1. Bilateral hip joint disease
   a) Pain in groin along with the thigh (both aggravated by walking)
   b) Inability to rotate the hip for daily tasks (e.g., putting on socks and shoes) and an associated loss of hip range of motion
   c) X-ray changes in hips
2. Referred leg pain
   a) Although it may occur with walking, it does not limit walking distance
   b) It rarely goes below the knees
   c) It is not associated with neurologic symptoms (numbness, paresthesia)
   d) The associated backache dominates the history
3. Peripheral neuropathy
   Peripheral neuropathy (PN) is the most difficult differential diagnosis of all and missing it has to be the most common reason for a failed outcome following surgery for lumbar spinal stenosis.

a) Spinal stenosis and PN coexist in the same age group
b) PN is dominated by neurologic symptoms more than pain
c) PN produces a more uniform distal stocking pattern on neurologic deficits
d) Walking does not necessarily aggravate the pain in the patients with PN, but they do experience unsteadiness that interferes with walking
e) Electrophysiologic testing is required to differentiate among these conditions
f) Absence of stenotic lesion on MRI

9.8 Thoracic Pain

1. Neurogenic
   a) Thoracic disc herniation
   b) Thoracic spinal tumor
      i. Extradural
         – Metastatic neoplasms (66%)
         – Metastatic tumors are more common (66%) than primary spinal tumors (30%); the remaining 4% were prevertebral tumors invading the spinal canal. The frequency of skeletal metastases was much higher for some tumors: 84% for prostatic cancer and 74% of breast cancer.
         – Primary spinal tumors (30%)
            ○ Multiple myeloma
            ○ Osteogenic sarcoma
            ○ Chordoma
            ○ Chondrosarcoma
            ○ Ewing's sarcoma
            ○ Benign tumors and tumor-like conditions (e.g., exostosis, osteoid osteoma, fibrous dysplasia, aneurysmal bone cyst, hemangioma etc.)
      ii. Intradural–extramedullary
         – Meningioma
           Comprise approximately 25% of primary spinal tumors; 90% of spinal meningiomas are purely intradural and the remaining 7–10% may be extradural. Among the spinal meningiomas, 17% were in the cervical spine, 75–81% in the thoracic spine, and 2–7% in the lumbar region
         – Nerve sheath tumors (e.g., schwannoma, neurofibroma, neurinoma, and neurilemoma perineurofibroblastoma)
         – Spinal vascular malformations (e.g., dural/intradural arteriovenous malformations, cavernous angioma, capillary telangiectasia, venous malformation)

- – Spinal vascular tumors (e.g., hemangioblastomas)
- – Epidermoid and dermoid cysts and teratomas
- – Spinal lipoma
- – Leptomeningeal metastases
  - iii. Intramedullary spinal cord tumors
    - – Ependymoma
    - – Astrocytoma
    - – Intramedullary metastasis
- c) Intramedullary lesions (excluding spinal cord tumors)
  - i. Multiple sclerosis
  - ii. Amyotrophic lateral sclerosis
  - iii. Transverse myelitis
  - iv. Subacute combined degeneration
  - v. Radiation myelopathy
  - vi. Syringomyelia
  - vii. Remote effects of cancer
    - – Paraneoplastic necrotizing myelopathy
- d) Intercostal neuralgia
- e) Herpes zoster
- f) Post-thoracotomy syndrome
2. Musculoskeletal
   - a) Muscular
     - i. Strain
     - ii. Myofascial pain syndrome
     - iii. Polymyalgia rheumatica
   - b) Degenerative
     - i. Spondylosis
     - ii. Spinal stenosis
     - iii. Herniated intervertebral disk
     - iv. Facet syndrome
   - c) Traumatic
     - i. Vertebral fracture
     - ii. Postoperative
   - d) Infectious
     - i. Discitis
     - ii. Osteomyelitis
     - iii. Paraspinal and spinal abscess
     - iv. Meningitis
   - e) Neoplastic
   - f) Metabolic
     - i. Osteoporosis with vertebral collapse

        ii. Osteomalacia
        iii. Paget's disease
    g) Inflammatory
        i. Ankylosing spondylitis
        ii. Rheumatoid arthritis
        iii. Arachnoiditis
    h) Deformity
        i. Scoliosis
        ii. Kyphosis
3. Visceral referred pain
    a) Heart (T 1–5 roots; pain referred to: chest and arm)
    b) Stomach (T 5–9 root; pain referred to manubrial xiphoid)
    c) Duodenum (T 6–10 root; pain referred to xiphoid to umbilicus)
    d) Pancreas (T 7–9 root; pain referred to upper abdomen or back)
    e) Gallbladder (T 6–10; right upper abdomen)
    f) Appendix (T11–L2; right lower quadrant)
    g) Kidney, glans (T9–L2; costovertebral angle, penis)
    h) Dissecting aortic aneurysm (T8–L2 costovertebral angle)
4. Nonorganic causes
    a) Psychiatric causes
    b) Malingering
    c) Substance abuse

Fruth SJ. Differential diagnosis and treatment in a patient with posterior upper thoracic pain. Phys Ther 2006;86(2):254–268

van Kleef M, Stolker RJ, Lataster A, Geurts J, Benzon HT, Mekhail N. 10. Thoracic pain. Pain Pract 2010;10(4):327–338

Sizer PS Jr, Phelps V, Dedrick G, Matthijs O. Differential diagnosis and management of spinal nerve root-related pain. Pain Pract 2002;2(2):98–121

9.9 Thoracic Outlet Syndrome

(Scalenus anterior syndrome, cervical rib syndrome, costoclavicular syndrome, hyperabduction syndrome, upper thoracic neurovascular syndrome; ▶ Fig. 9.2)

    Neurovascular compression occurs in three possible spaces:

1. *Scalene triangle*: Most common site of brachial plexus compression
    a) Bounded by anterior/middle scalene and first rib.
    b) Cervical and anomalous rib the compression point
2. *Costoclavicular space*: Area between first rib and clavicle.
    a) Subclavian vein compression at this site.
3. *Pectoralis minor space*: Area between pectoralis minor and chest wall.
    a) Second most common site of neurovascular compression

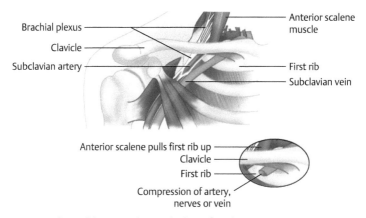

Fig. 9.2 Boundaries of thoracic outlet-spinal column, first rib, sternum.

Group of poorly categorized syndromes that include a variety of pain, motor loss (wasting and weakness of muscles in the hand) and paresthesias in the neck, shoulder, arms, and hand (4th and 5th digits). Symptoms and signs emanate from continuous or intermittent pressure on portions of the brachial plexus (C8, and T1 nerve roots, and lower trunk) and the auxiliary or subclavian vessels by anatomical structures (cervical rib, an enlarged first thoracic rib, fibrous bands, and hypertrophic scalenus muscles). Rare causes include a poor posture, head or neck trauma, repetitive occupational movements, atherosclerotic plaque formation, a Pancoast tumor. Rarely found under the age of 20 years.

1. **Neurologic type** (95% of cases): 20–60 years
   Caused by compression of the lower portion of the brachial plexus by a band of tissue that joins the transverse process at C7 to the first rib. Women are most commonly affected. Characterized by a variety of pain and paresthesias in the head, neck, arms, and hand.

2. **Venous type** (4% of cases): 20–35 years
   Results from the compression of the subclavian vein. Young men are most often affected. Characterized by arm claudication, edema, cyanosis, and venous dilatation.

3. **Arterial type** (1% of cases; atherosclerosis): older than 50 years
   Caused by the compression of the subclavian artery by a cervical rib, and it is the most serious form of the syndrome. Men and women are equally affected. Characterized by digital vasospasm, potential thrombosis or embolism, aneurysm, muscle atrophy, and gangrene.

Cooke RA. Thoracic outlet syndrome—aspects of diagnosis in the differential diagnosis of hand-arm vibration syndrome. Occup Med (Lond) 2003;53(5):331–336

Stallworth JM, Horne JB. Diagnosis and management of thoracic outlet syndrome. Arch Surg 1984;119(10):1149–1151

Dragu A, Lang W, Unglaub F, Horch RE. [Thoracic outlet syndrome: differential diagnosis and surgical therapeutic options] Chirurg 2009;80(1):65–76

Hooper TL, Denton J, McGalliard MK, Brismée JM, Sizer PS Jr. Thoracic outlet syndrome: a controversial clinical condition. Part 1: anatomy, and clinical examination/diagnosis. J Manual Manip Ther 2010;18(2): 74–83

9.10 Cervical Radiculopathy

Patients with a cervical radiculopathy usually report axial spine and upper extremity pain that often is accompanied by numbness, paresthesias, and weakness. A number of musculoskeletal disorders, however, generate pain referral and weakness patterns similar to radicular patterns and may be present in individuals with or without radiculopathy.

It is frequently difficult to differentiate whether the pain source is secondary to cervical nerve root compression or secondary to a soft-tissue disorder. Upper extremity musculoskeletal disorders and cervical radiculopathy may present with similar pain-referral patterns, in a similar patient population, and may be present concomitantly.

9.10.1 Differential diagnosis

Differential diagnosis of entities causing upper extremity pain, weakness, and sensory changes:

1. Neurologic
   a) Thoracic outlet syndrome
   b) Pancoast tumor
   c) Brachial plexopathy
   d) Herpes zoster
   e) Peripheral mononeuropathy (suprascapular, long thoracic, accessory, musculocutaneous, or ulnar neuropathy, carpal tunnel syndrome, etc.)
   f) Multiple sclerosis
   g) Syringomyelia
   h) Raised intracranial pressure
   i) Intracranial tumor
2. Shoulder abnormalities
   a) Impingement syndrome (rotator cuff tendinitis, subacromial bursitis)
   b) Rotator cuff tears
   c) Adhesive capsulitis

    d) Biceps tendinitis
    e) Glenohumeral instability
    f) Glenoid cyst
3. Elbow abnormalities
    a) Medial epicondylitis
    b) Lateral epicondylitis
4. Wrist or hand abnormalities
    a) Wrist/finger flexor and extensor tendinitis (DeQuervain's tenosynovitis)
5. Muscle or connective tissue
    a) Myofascial pain syndrome, pain referral patterns from individual muscles
    b) Fibromyalgia
    c) Polymyalgia rheumatica
6. Vascular
    a) Thoracic outlet syndrome
    b) Aortic arch syndrome
    c) Vertebral artery dissection
7. Other
    a) Dental pain (premolars)
    b) Neck-tongue syndrome (C2 root compression)

Radhakrishnan K, Litchy WJ, O'Fallon WM, Kurland LT. Epidemiology of cervical radiculopathy. A population-based study from Rochester, Minnesota, 1976 through 1990. Brain 1994;117(Pt 2):325–335

Rubinstein SM, Pool JJ, van Tulder MW, Riphagen II, de Vet HC. A systematic review of the diagnostic accuracy of provocative tests of the neck for diagnosing cervical radiculopathy. Eur Spine J 2007;16(3):307–319

Rao R. Neck pain, cervical radiculopathy, and cervical myelopathy: pathophysiology, natural history, and clinical evaluation. J Bone Joint Surg Am 2002;84-A(10):1872–1881

Jackson R. The classic: the cervical syndrome. 1949. Clin Orthop Relat Res 2010;468(7):1739–1745

9.11 Mononeuropathy of the Lower Extremity

Mononeuropathies are common clinical entities and may result from pathology located anywhere along the course of the peripheral nerve. Dysfunction can lead to weakness, pain, or sensory deficits. As individual nerves are affected, one does not see the distal and symmetric (stocking-glove type) distribution of deficits typical of a generalized polyneuropathy, at least early on.

Mononeuropathies are thought of as compressive or noncompressive. *Compressive neuropathies* produce symptoms in the distribution of the affected nerve root, plexus, or individual nerve. *Noncompressive neuropathies* may be sequelae of underlying systemic disease (e.g., diabetes, malignancy, infection, and inflammatory conditions). Viral infections such as herpes zoster, herpes simplex virus (HSV), Epstein–Barr virus (EBV), and cytomegalovirus can involve nerve roots, leading to painful radiculitis, or may trigger a Guillain–Barre syndrome 1–3 weeks after infection, usually in individuals with a reduced immune function (e.g., older people, or in HIV). Cancer can produce nerve dysfunction secondary to compression by solid tumors, infiltration by malignant cells, or paraneoplastic immune-mediated attack.

Vasculitic neuropathy usually occurs suddenly and is painful. The typical vasculitic picture is stepwise involvement of multiple individual nerves (mononeuritis multiplex) rather than an isolated mononeuropathy.

9.11.1 Differential diagnosis

1. Metabolic
   a) Diabetic amyotrophy
      Technically a radiculoplexopathy; a common clinical entity in diabetic patients with some immune-mediated microvasculitic component.
2. Compressive
   a) Lumbosacral plexopathies
      Uncommon neuropathies that may mimic a mononeuropathy. Causes include compression from a solid tumor, abscess, hematoma, or infiltrating malignancies.
   b) Lumbosacral radiculopathies
      The lower nerve roots L5/S1 followed by L4/L5 are most commonly affected. The most common causes are disk herniation, chronic degenerative changes, metastatic tumors (if known primary malignancy)
   c) Peroneal neuropathy
      The most common mononeuropathy affecting the lower extremity, manifesting as a foot drop. Most often the nerve is injured at the fibular neck due to compression (e.g., surgical positioning, crossing legs, or trauma).
   d) Meralgia paresthetica
      Due to compression of the lateral femoral cutaneous nerve. Often seen in overweight people, but patients who wear tight-fitting clothes and workers using heavy tool belts are also at risk.
   e) Morton neuroma (metatarsalgia)
      This is a relatively common source of foot pain at the base of the third and fourth toes, and is due to perineural fibrosis of an intermetatarsal nerve.
   f) Obturator neuropathy
      Seen most commonly in women who have undergone obstetric/gynecologic procedures.

g) Sciatic neuropathy
   The sciatic nerve arises from the L4–S2 nerve root and lumbosacral plexus before exiting through the greater sciatic foramen.

h) Tibial neuropathy
   The tibial nerve is rarely involved in isolation, and when involved it usually occurs distally at the level of the ankle.

i) Tarsal tunnel syndrome (distal tibial neuropathy)
   Compression of the distal tibial nerve as it passes through the tarsal tunnel (flexor retinaculum, at the medial side of the ankle), manifesting as perimalleolar pain.

j) Femoral mononeuropathy
   The femoral nerve originates from the posterior divisions of the L2, L3, and L4 nerve roots. This can result in weakness when walking and falls due to buckling of the knee.

k) Hereditary neuropathy with liability to pressure palsies (HNPP)
   Dominantly inherited condition producing relapsing and remitting episodes of painless compression neuropathy at the common sites of entrapment (e.g., peroneal neuropathy at the fibular head).

l) Peripheral nerve injury
   It is an important cause of compression lower extremity mononeuropathies, following trauma or injury.

3. Infectious
   a) HIV
      Patients with HIV can present with a mononeuritis multiplex pattern as well as a length-dependent sensorimotor polyneuropathy.

   b) Herpes zoster
      Caused by reactivation of a primary varicella zoster virus infection due to lowering of the cell-mediated immunity. Presents with burning or stabbing pain followed by a vesicular rash in the affected dermatomes.

   c) Herpes simplex
      Infection with HSV1 and HSV2 manifests with symptoms and signs ranging from tingling and burning with eruptions of vesicular lesions to painful oral, genital, and ocular ulcerations.

   d) Epstein–Barr virus
      Infectious mononucleosis is the clinical syndrome caused by EBV, and also can cause a myriad of neurologic illness. Pain and weakness may indicate the presence of EBV radiculopathy, especially in patients with AIDS.

   e) Cytomegalovirus
      Affects the immunocompromised patients and manifests with fever, bone marrow suppression, and tissue-invasive disease such as pneumonia, hepatitis, colitis, nephritis, and retinitis.

f) Lyme disease
   Patients can present with a mononeuritis multiplex or polyradicular pattern.
g) Leprosy
   In endemic areas
4. Inflammatory
   a) Sarcoidosis
      Unknown etiology, possibly multifactorial including genetic, immunologic, and infectious causes (e.g., viruses, *Borrelia burgdorferi*, *Mycobacterium tuberculosis*, and *Mycoplasma*).
   b) Sjogren's syndrome
      Chronic inflammatory and autoimmune disorder characterized by diminished lacrimal and salivary gland secretion.
   c) Rheumatoid arthritis
      The most common inflammatory arthritis characterized by symmetric arthritis of the small joints of the hands and feet.
   d) Acquired demyelinating sensory motor polyneuropathy
      Autoimmune disorder supported by pathology changes in peripheral nerve biopsies.
5. Neoplastic-related
   a) Neoplastic compressive lumbosacral radiculopathy
      Direct compression from a malignancy, usually metastatic and can occur acutely. Suspected on cases with a known primary tumor.
   b) Neoplastic compressive lumbosacral plexopathy
      Direct compression from malignancy, mostly due to intra-abdominal extension, but growth from metastases is also possible.
   c) Radiation-induced plexopathy
      Radiation may give rise to localized ischemia and fibrosis because of microvascular insufficiency.
   d) Lymphoma
      Group of malignancies of the lymphoid system linked to infectious causes with bacteria and viruses, autoimmune disorders, immunodeficiency states, and environmental factors
   e) Amyloidosis
      An amyloid protein deposition disease that may have a primary cause or be secondary to other diseases, it can be localized, systemic, inherited, senile systemic, or dialysis amyloidosis.
   f) Paraneoplastic immune-mediated attacks
      Tumor-induced autoimmunity against the nervous system can cause lumbosacral plexopathy.

g) Nerve sheath tumors
Neurofibrosarcoma is probably the most important death-causing complication of neurofibromatosis type 1.

9.12 Radiculopathy of the Lower Extremities

1. Congenital
    a) Meningeal or perineural cyst
    b) Conjoint nerve root
2. Acquired
    a) Lumbar spinal stenosis
    b) Spondylosis, spondylolysis, and spondylolisthesis
    c) Facet arthrosis and synovial cysts
    d) Lateral recess syndrome
    e) Hip joint disease and pelvic abnormalities
3. Infectious
    a) Discitis
    b) Osteomyelitis
    c) Paraspinal and spinal abscess
    d) Herpes zoster
    e) Meningitis
    f) Lyme disease
4. Primary or metastatic tumors (e.g., intra-abdominal or pelvic)
5. Vascular especially with iliofemoral occlusive vascular disease
Related to exertion and may be mimicked by intermittent claudication
Caveat: Lumbar stenosis often produces numbness and weakness, vascular disease does not.
6. Referred pain
    a) Visceral (e.g., neoplastic and inflammatory) and vascular lesions of chest, abdomen, and pelvis
    b) Retroperitoneal lesions
7. Piriform syndrome
Since a portion of the sciatic nerve is passing through or close to the piriform muscle, the nerve may become compressed and irritated when the muscle is in spasm.
8. Peripheral neuropathies—spinal mononeuropathies that may be confused with radiculopathies
Examples are diabetic neuropathy, sarcoid spinal mononeuropathy, paraneoplastic sensory neuropathy, combined system disease—B12 deficiency, pharmaceutical and industrial toxins neuropathy, ischemic neuropathy

9.13 Spinal Cord Lesions

1. Complete transection
   Most commonly the spinal cord section is incomplete and irregular, and the neurological findings reflect the extent of the damage (▶ Fig. 9.3a–o).
   Causes include:
   a) Traumatic spinal injuries
   b) Tumor
      i. Metastatic carcinoma
      ii. Lymphoma
   c) Multiple sclerosis
   d) Vascular disorders
   e) Spinal epidural hematoma (secondary to anticoagulation)
   f) Spinal abscess
   g) Intervertebral disc herniation
   h) Parainfectious or postvaccinal syndromes

   Neurologic manifestations:
   a) Sensory disturbances
      Loss of all sensory modalities below the level of the lesion, e.g., pain, temperature, light touch, position sense, and vibration. Localized vertebral pain accentuated by vertebral palpation or percussion may occur with destructive lesions (e.g., infections and tumors) and may have some lesion-localizing value. Pain that is worse when recumbent and better when sitting or standing is common with spinal malignancies.
   b) Motor disturbances
      i. Paraplegia or tetraplegia
         Initially flaccid and areflexic because of spinal shock; 3–4 weeks later become hypertonic and hyperreflexic. Complete and lower spinal cord lesions result in flexion at the hip and the knee, whereas incomplete and high spinal cord lesions result in extension at the hip and knee.
      ii. Absent superficial abdominal and cremasteric reflexes
      iii. Lower motor neuron signs at the level of lesion (paresis, atrophy, fasciculations, and areflexia)
   c) Autonomic disturbances below the level of the lesion
      i. Urinary and rectal sphincter dysfunction
      ii. Anhidrosis
      iii. Trophic skin changes
      iv. Temperature control impairment
      v. Vasomotor instability
      vi. Sexual dysfunction

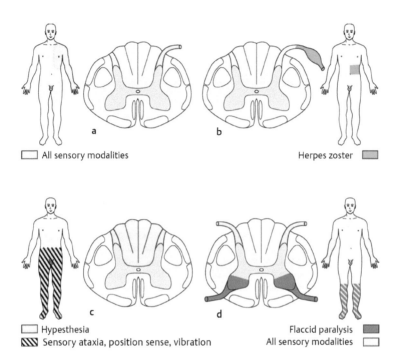

All sensory modalities

Herpes zoster

Hypesthesia
Sensory ataxia, position sense, vibration

Flaccid paralysis
All sensory modalities

Fig. 9.3 Syndromes of spinal cord and peripheral nerves lesions: **(a)** Syndrome of posterior roots (C4–T6) lesion causes lancinating pain and abolition of all sensory modalities in the corresponding dermatomes. Interruption of the peripheral reflex arc leads additionally to hypotonia and hypo- or areflexia. **(b)** Syndrome of the spinal ganglion (T6) following viral infections (herpes zoster) is causing lancinating and annoying pain and paresthesias of the involved dermatomes. **(c)** Syndrome of the posterior columns (T8) selectively damaged by tabes dorsalis (neurosyphilis) results in impaired vibration and position sense and decreased tactile localization. Also, tactile and postural hallucinations (as if walking on cotton wool), temporal and spatial disturbance of the extremities sensory gait ataxia (worse in darkness or with eyes closed), and a Roberg's sign. Patients often develop lancinating pains in the legs, urinary incontinence, and areflexia of the patellar and ankle stretch reflexes. **(d)** Syndrome of the anterior and posterior roots and peripheral nerves (neuronal muscular dystrophy) causes abolition of all sensory modalities, and flaccid paralysis in the corresponding dermotomes and myotomes. There is also areflexia, paresthesias, and occasionally pain. The peripheral nerves appear thickened and sensitive to touch. (*Continued*)

431

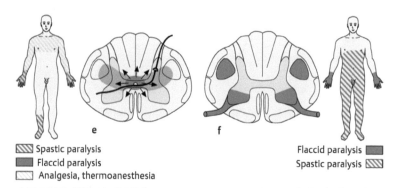

Spastic paralysis

Flaccid paralysis

Analgesia, thermoanesthesia

Flaccid paralysis

Spastic paralysis

Fig. 9.3 (*Continued*) **(e)** Syndrome of the central spinal cord (C4–T4), as in syringomyelia, hydromyelia, and intramedullary cord tumors, where the central cord damage spreads centrifugally to involve the surrounding spinal cord structures. Characteristically this results in bilateral "vest-like" thermoanesthesia and analgesia with preservation of soft touch sensation and proprioception (i.e., dissociation of sensory loss). Anterior extension with involvement of the anterior horns results in segmental neurogenic atrophy, paresis, and areflexia. Dorsal extension involves the dorsal columns causing ipsilateral position sense and vibration loss. Lateral extension causes ipsilateral Horner's syndrome (C8–T2 lesions), kyphoscoliosis, and spastic paralysis below the level of damage. Ventrolateral extension affects the spinothalamic tract resulting in thermoanesthesia and analgesia below the spinal cord lesion with sacral sparing due to its lamination (cervical sensation medial, and sacral lateral). **(f)** Syndrome of combined lesions in anterior horns and lateral pyramidal tract (amyotrophic lateral sclerosis or motor neuron disease) syndrome causes lower motor neuron signs (muscular atrophy, flaccid paresis, and fasciculation) superimposed on the symptoms and signs of upper motor neuron disease (spastic paresis and extensor plantar responses). If the nuclei of the medullary cranial nerves are involved, there will be explosive dysarthria dysphagia (bulbar or pseudobulbar paralysis).

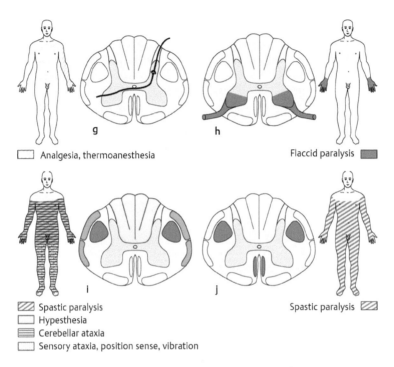

g

Analgesia, thermoanesthesia

h

Flaccid paralysis

i

j

Spastic paralysis
Hypesthesia
Cerebellar ataxia
Sensory ataxia, position sense, vibration

Spastic paralysis

Fig. 9.3 (*Continued*) **(g)** Syndrome of the posterior horns (C5–C8) causes ipsilateral segmental sensory loss, essentially of pain and temperature, but due to absence of damage to the spinothalamic tracts there is preservation of pain and temperature sensation below the level of damage. Spontaneous attacks of pain may develop in the analgesic area. **(h)** Syndrome of the anterior horns (C7–C8) where the anterior horns are selectively involved in acute poliomyelitis and in progressive spinal muscular atrophies resulting in diffuse weakness, atrophy, and fasciculations in muscles of the extremities and the trunk, reduction of muscle tone and hypo- or areflexia of muscle stretch reflexes. **(i)** Syndrome of combined lesions in posterior tracts, spinocerebellar tracts and eventually the pyramidal tracts (Friedreich's ataxia). The disease commences with loss of position sense, discrimination, and stereognosis, leading to ataxia and Romberg's sign. Pain and temperature sensations are involved to a lesser extent. Later, spastic paresis appears indicating degeneration of the pyramidal tracts. **(j)** Syndrome of the corticospinal tracts (progressive spastic spinal paralysis) presents initially with heaviness if the legs, progressing to spastic paresis, spastic gait, and hyperreflexia. Spastic paresis of the arms develops later in the course of the disease.

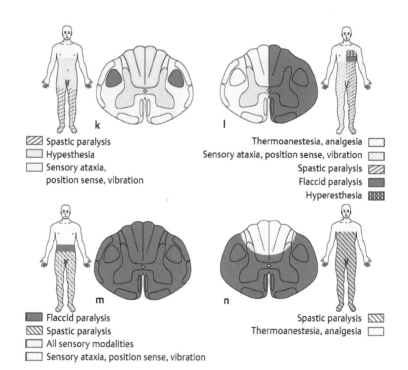

Spastic paralysis
Hypesthesia
Sensory ataxia,
position sense, vibration

Thermoanesthesia, analgesia
Sensory ataxia, position sense, vibration
Spastic paralysis
Flaccid paralysis
Hyperesthesia

Flaccid paralysis
Spastic paralysis
All sensory modalities
Sensory ataxia, position sense, vibration

Spastic paralysis
Thermoanesthesia, analgesia

Fig. 9.3 *(Continued)* **(k)** Syndrome of posterolateral column (T6) (subacute combined degeneration) due to selective damage from vitamin B12 deficiency or vacuolar myelopathy of AIDS or extrinsic cord compression, resulting in paresthesias of the feet, loss of proprioception and vibration sense and sensory ataxia. Bilateral spasticity, hyperreflexia, and bilateral extensor toe signs. Hypo- or areflexia due to peripheral neuropathy. **(l)** Syndrome of hemisection of the spinal cord (Brown–Séquard syndrome) is characteristically produced by extramedullary lesions and contralateral to the hemisection, ipsilateral loss of proprioception below the level of the lesion, ipsilateral spastic weakness and segmental lower motor neuron and sensory signs at the level of the lesion due to damage of the roots and anterior horn cells at this level. **(m)** Syndrome of complete spinal cord transection (transverse myelitis) causes impairment of all sensory modalities (light touch, position sense, vibration, temperature, and pain) below the level of the lesion. Paraplegia or tetraplegia below the level of the lesion, initially flaccid and areflexic due to spinal shock but progressively hypertonic and hyperreflexic. Segmental lower motor neuron signs (paresis, atrophy, fasciculations, and areflexia). Urinary and anal sphincter dysfunction, sexual dysfunction, anhidrosis, skin changes, and vasomotor instability. **(n)** The anterior spinal artery syndrome presents with an abrupt radicular girdle pain, loss of motor function (flaccid paraplegia), bilateral thermoanesthesia and analgesia, bladder and bowel dysfunction. Position sense, vibration, and light touch are intact.

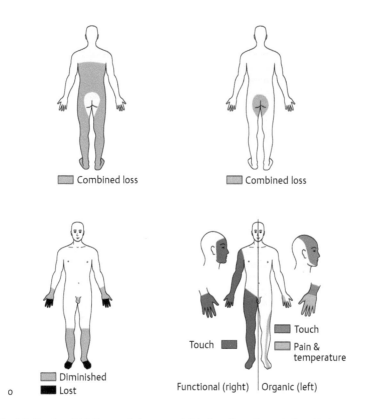

Fig. 9.3 (*Continued*) **(o)** Characteristic sensory deficits found in various spinal cord lesions in comparison to peripheral neuropathy: (1) Advanced intra-axial lesion of thoracic cord at T3–T6 (sacral sparing). (2) Cauda equina lesion. (3) Stocking-glove pattern of sensory loss of an advanced stage of peripheral neuropathy. (4) Organic sensory loss follows an anatomic distribution on the left side of the face, upper and lower extremities. Functional facial anesthesia includes the angle of the mandible and may stop at the hair line; functional loss of upper extremity sensation usually cuts off transversely at the wrist, elbow, or shoulder; functional loss of lower extremity sensation cuts off at the inguinal line ventrally, or at a joint or the gluteal fold dorsally, or it may cut off transversely at any lower level.

2. Hemisection (Brown–Sequard Syndrome)
   The Brown–Sequard syndrome is characteristically produced by extramedullary lesions (e.g., metastases, meningioma, neurofibroma, spinal vascular malformation and vascular tumors, epidermoid and dermoid cysts.
   Neurologic manifestations:
   a) Sensory disturbances
      i. Loss of pain and temperature sensation contralateral to the lesion usually one or two segments below the level of the lesion.
      ii. Ipsilateral loss of proprioception, especially vibratory and position sense, whereas tactile sensation may be normal or minimally decreased.
   b) Motor disturbances
      i. Ipsilateral spastic weakness
      ii. Segmental lower motor neuron and sensory signs
3. Central cord syndrome
   Caused by:
   a) Syringomyelia, hydromyelia
   b) Intramedullary cord lesions (e.g., tumors, hematoma)
   c) Severe hyperextension neck injuries

   Neurologic manifestations:
   a) Dissociation of sensory loss
      Thermoanesthesia and analgesia in a "vest-like" bilateral distribution with preservation of sacral sensation due to lamination of the spinothalamic tract (sacral sparing), light touch sensation and proprioception.
   b) Segmental neurogenic atrophy, paresis, and areflexia
   c) Ipsilateral Horner's syndrome (with C8–T2 lesions)
   d) Spastic paralysis and kyphoscoliosis
   e) Ipsilateral position sense and vibratory loss
4. Posterolateral column disease
   Caused by:
   a) Subacute combined degeneration of the spinal cord (due to vitamin B12 deficiency)
   b) Vacuolar myelopathy associated with AIDS
   c) Extrinsic cord compression (e.g., cervical spondylosis)

   Neurologic manifestations:
   a) Paresthesias of the feet
   b) Dorsal column dysfunction
      i. Loss of proprioception and vibration sense
      ii. Sensory ataxia
   c) Bilateral spasticity, hyperreflexia, and extensor toe signs (In a case of superimposed neuropathy, there may be hyporeflexia or areflexia.)

5. Posterior column disease

   The posterior columns are selectively damaged by tabes dorsalis neurosyphilis.

   Neurologic manifestations:
   a) Impaired vibration and position sense
   b) Decreased tactile localization
   c) Tactile and postural hallucinations
   d) Temporal and spatial disturbances
   e) Sensory ataxia (gait ataxic, or "double tapping" is characteristic)
   f) Lhermitte's sign (when the lesion is at the level of the cervical cord)

6. Anterior horn cell syndromes

   Exemplified by the spinal muscular atrophies (i.e., progressive spinal muscular atrophy in motor neuron disease, infantile spinal muscular atrophy of Werdnig–Hoffman syndrome) in which there is a selective damage of the anterior horn cells of the spinal cord.

   Neurologic manifestations:
   a) Diffuse weakness, atrophy, and fasciculations in muscles of the trunk and extremities
   b) Muscle tone is usually reduced
   c) Absent or reduced muscle stretch reflexes

7. Combined anterior horn cell and pyramidal tract disease

   Exemplified by the syndrome of amyotrophic lateral sclerosis (motor neuron disease) in which there are selective degenerative changes in the anterior horn cells of the spinal cord and the brain stem motor nuclei and in the corticospinal tracts.

   Neurologic manifestations:
   a) Mixed motor disturbances (all striated muscles may be affected except the pelvic floor sphincter and external ocular muscles)
      i. Diffuse lower motor neuron disease (progressive paresis, muscular atrophy, and fasciculations)
      ii. Upper motor neuron dysfunction (paresis, spasticity, and extensor toe signs)
      iii. The muscle stretch reflexes may be depressed, but more often exaggerated
      iv. Bulbar or pseudobulbar impairment (dysarthria, dysphagia, tongue spasticity, atrophy, or weakness)
   b) Sensory changes are absent

8. Vascular syndromes
   a) The anterior spinal artery syndrome
      It supplies the anterior funiculi, anterior horns, base of the dorsal horns, periependymal area, and anteromedial aspects of the lateral funiculi.

Spinal cord infarction often occurs in boundary zones or "watersheds" especially at the T1–T4 segments and the L1 segment.

Caused by:
  i. Aortic dissection
  ii. Atherosclerosis of the aorta and its branches
  iii. Postsurgical of the abdominal aorta
  iv. Syphilitic arteritis
  v. Following fracture-dislocation of the spine
  vi. Vasculitis
  vii. Unknown (in a substantial number of patients)

Neurologic manifestations:
  i. Sudden radicular or "girdle" pain
  ii. Thermoanesthesia and analgesia bilaterally
  iii. Loss of motor function below the level of ischemia within minutes or hours (e.g., flaccid paraplegia)
  iv. Impaired bladder and bowel control
b) The posterior spinal artery syndrome
   It supplies the dorsal columns. Infarction in this area supply is uncommon.
   Neurologic manifestations:
  i. Loss of proprioception and vibration sense below the level of lesion
  ii. Loss of segmental reflexes

Schwenkreis P, Pennekamp W, Tegenthoff M. Differential diagnosis of acute and subacute non-traumatic paraplegia. Disch Arzbebt 2006;103(44):A2948–A2954

Dickman CA, Fehling MG, Gokaslan JL. Spinal cord and spinal column tumors: Principals and Practice. New York: Thieme Medical Publishers; 2006

Schwartzman RJ. Differential Diagnosis in Neurology. IOS Press; 2006

Bradley WG, et al. Neurology in Clinical Practice. Butterworth-Heinemann-Elsevier; 2004

9.14 Cauda Equina Mass Lesions

Compression of the lumbar and sacral roots below the L3 vertebral level causes the cauda equina syndrome which is characterized by:
1. Early bilateral and asymmetrical radicular pain in the distribution of the lumbosacral roots, increased by the Valsalva maneuver (▶ Fig. 9.4).
2. The Achilles reflexes (S1–S2 roots) are absent; the patellar reflexes (L2–L4 roots) have a variable response.
3. Flaccid, hypotonic, areflexic paralysis that affects the glutei, posterior thigh muscles, and the anterolateral muscles of the leg and foot (true peripheral type paraplegia)

4. Late asymmetrical sensory loss in the saddle region, involving the anal, perineal, and genital regions extending to the dorsal aspect of the thigh, the anterolateral area of the leg, and the outer aspect of the foot.
5. Late sphincter dysfunction, autonomous neurogenic bladder, constipation, impaired erection and ejaculation.
    a) Central disc herniation
        A small central disc herniation can put tension and deform the richly innervated posterior longitudinal ligament with pain fibers and cause marked low back pain. A larger central disc herniation results in neurological compression of cauda equina.
    b) Tumors of the cauda equina
        i.   Ependymoma
             Smooth or nodular rings of ependymal cells, which are surrounding and incorporating the nerves of the cauda equina
        ii. Epidermoid and dermoid tumors
             Discrete tumor masses, which tend to occur along the cauda equina and may be bound to the surrounding nerve roots
        iii. Neurofibromas
             Well-circumscribed lesions involving initially a single nerve root until late in their courses
        iv. Meningioma
             Very rarely occurs in the lumbar canal
        v.   Lipoma
        vi. Metastatic disease of the bones
        vii. Meningeal infiltration by various tumors

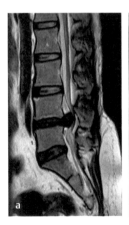
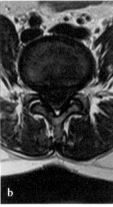

Fig. 9.4 T2-weighted **(a)** sagittal and **(b)** axial images of a 34-year-old woman who presented with an acute cauda equine syndrome and magnetic resonance imaging showing a large central L4–L5 disk prolapse with bilateral L5 nerve root compression. After an L4–L5 diskectomy, she made a complete recovery. (Reproduced from 21.7 Lumbar Spine. In: Loftus C, ed. Neurosurgical Emergencies. 3rd edition. Thieme; 2017.)

Clinical differentiation of cauda equina and conus medullaris syndromes

Clinical symptom	Conus medullaris	Cauda equina
Spontaneous pain	Uncommon	Prominent, early
	Relatively mild	Severe
	Bilateral, symmetric	Asymmetric
	Perineum and thighs	Radicular
Sensory findings	Saddle distribution	Saddle distribution
	Bilateral, symmetric	Asymmetric
	Sensory dissociation (Present)	Sensory dissociation (Absent)
	Presents early	Presents relatively late
Motor findings	Symmetric	Asymmetric
	Mild	Moderate to severe
	Atrophy absent	Atrophy more prominent
Reflex changes	Achilles reflex absent	Reflexes variably involved
	Patellar reflex normal	
Sphincter dysfunction	Early, severe	Late, less severe
	Absent anal and bulbocavernosus reflex	Reflex abnormalities less common
Sexual dysfunction	Erection and Ejaculation impaired	Less common

Source: Modified from DeJong RN: The neurologic examination, ed. 4, New York, Harper & Row Publishers Inc. 1979.

Characteristics in the differential diagnosis between extramedullary and intramedullary spinal cord tumors

Symptom	Extramedullary tumors	Intramedullary tumors
Spontaneous pain	Radicular or regional in type and distribution; an early and important symptom	Funicular; burning in type poorly localized
Sensory changes	Contralateral loss of pain and temperature; ipsilateral loss of proprioception (Brown–Sequard type)	Dissociation of sensation; spotty changes
Changes in pain and temperature sensations in the saddle area	More marked than at level of lesion. Sensory level may be located below site of lesion	Less marked than at level Sensory loss can be suspended

▶ (*Continued*)

Symptom	Extramedullary tumors	Intramedullary tumors
Lower motor neuron involvement	Segmental	Can be marked and widespread with atrophy and fasciculations
Upper motor neuron paresis and hyperreflexia	Prominent	Can be late and less prominent
Trophic changes	Usually not marked	Can be marked
Spinal subarachnoid block and changes in spinal fluid	Early and marked	Late and less marked

Source: Adapted from DeJong, RN: The neurologic examination, ed. 4, New York, Harper & Row Publishers Inc. 1979.

Ebner FH, Roser F, Acioly MA, Schoeber W, Tatagiba M. Intramedullary lesions of the conus medullaris: differential diagnosis and surgical management. Neurosurg Rev 2009;32(3):287–300, discussion 300–301

Koeller KK, Rosenblum RS, Morrison AL. Neoplasms of the spinal cord and filum terminale: radiologic-pathologic correlation. Radiographics 2000;20(6):1721–1749

9.15 Cervical Spondylotic Myelopathy

In its complete form, it is characterized by neck pain and brachialgia, with radicular motor-sensory-reflex signs in the upper extremities in association with myelopathy. Similar clinical findings may be produced by other causes of spinal cord compression such as:

1. Extradural spinal neoplasms
   Associated with a more rapid temporal clinical evolution than spondylosis and there is often a history of prior malignancy, and the radiologic studies show findings of neoplasia.
   a) Metastatic neoplasms
      i. Lung (53% in men and 12% in women)
      ii. Breast (59% in women)
      iii. Lymphoma (20% in men and 9% in women)
      iv. Prostate (8% in men)
      v. Kidney (12% in men and 6% in women)
      vi. Miscellaneous
   b) Primary spinal tumors
      i. Multiple myeloma (10–15% of cases)
      ii. Osteogenic sarcoma
      iii. Chordoma
      iv. Chondrosarcoma

v. Benign tumors and tumor-like conditions
  - Vertebral hemangiomas
  - Osteochondroma or exostosis
  - Giant cell tumors
  - Aneurysmal bone cysts
  - Fibrous dysplasia
vi. Lipoma

2. Intradural–extramedullary tumors
   a) Meningioma (25%)
   b) Nerve sheath tumors (29%)
   c) Vascular malformations and tumors
   d) Epidermoid and dermoid cysts and teratomas (1–2%)
   e) Lipoma (0.5%)

3. Intramedullary tumors
   a) Ependymoma (13% including those found in the filum terminale)
   b) Astrocytoma (10%)
      The most common among tumors arising within the spinal cord per se
   c) Metastases

4. Chronic progressive radiation myelopathy

5. Syringomyelia
   Most frequently occurs in younger age groups than is typical for cervical spondylosis

6. Noncompressive forms of myelopathy
   a) Multiple sclerosis
      There is often a history or findings on examination of disease above the foramen magnum, such as optic neuritis, nystagmus, or internuclear ophthalmoplegia.
   b) Motor neuron disease or amyotrophic lateral sclerosis Producesmotor disturbances without sensory findings and eventually signs of lower motor neuron disease are seen in muscles above the foramen magnum. The CSF and spinal imaging studies are not revealing in the ALS.
   c) Subacute combined degeneration due to vitamin 12 deficiency
      Unlike spondylosis, signs of PN are often present and loss of position sense in the lower extremities is more marked in this kind of combined disease. Lab findings of vitamin 12 deficiency are usually diagnostic.

Crandall PH, Batzdorf U. Cervical spondylotic myelopathy. J Neurosurg 1966;25(1):57–66

Baron EM, Young WF. Cervical spondylotic myelopathy: a brief review of its pathophysiology, clinical course, and diagnosis. Neurosurgery 2007;60(1, Suppl 1):S35–S41

Young WF. Cervical spondylotic myelopathy: a common cause of spinal cord dysfunction in older persons. Am Fam Physician 2000;62(5):1064–1070, 1073

9.16 Spontaneous Spinal Epidural Hematoma

Spontaneous spinal epidural hematoma is a rare case of back pain in the emergency room (0.1 in 100,000 cases per year), but one that carries a high morbidity (▸ Fig. 9.5). The classical presentation is acute onset of severe, often radiating, back pain followed by signs and symptoms of nerve root and/or spinal cord compression, which develops minutes to days later.

The true etiology remains unknown, but associations with some predisposing conditions, such as coagulopathies, blood dyscrasias, and arteriovenous malformation, have been reported.

9.16.1 Differential diagnosis

1. Herniated disc
2. Neoplasm
   a) Extradural
   b) Intradural-extramedullary
   c) Intramedullary
3. Abscess
4. Sequelae of trauma

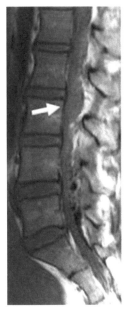 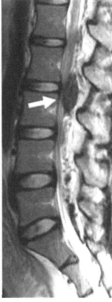

Fig. 9.5 Spontaneous spinal epidural hematoma: MRI lumbar spine: T1- and T2-weighted images demonstrate a posterior spinal epidural hematoma causing significant canal stenosis and marked compression over thecal sac and nerve roots of cauda equine.

5. Intramedullary diseases
   a) Acute and subacute transverse myelitis
   b) Demyelinating disease
6. Spinal cord infarction

Licata C, Zoppetti MC, Perini SS, Bazzan A, Gerosa M, Da Pian R. Spontaneous spinal haematomas. Acta Neurochir (Wien) 1988;95(3–4):126–130

Lee JS, Yu CY, Huang KC, Lin HW, Huang CC, Chen HH. Spontaneous spinal epidural hematoma in a 4-month-old infant. Spinal Cord 2007;45(8):586–590

9.17 Spinal Cord Compression

1. Nonneoplastic causes
   a) Spondylosis
   b) Intervertebral disc herniation
   c) Spinal stenosis and neurogenic claudication
   d) Paget's disease (osteitis deformans)
   e) Osteoporosis
   f) Syringomyelia
   g) Arachnoid cysts
   h) Pyogenic infections
   i) Other infectious and inflammatory diseases
      i. Tuberculosis
      ii. Fungal infections
      iii. Parasitic disease
      iv. Sarcoidosis
      v. Rheumatoid arthritis
      vi. Ankylosing spondylitis
   j) Spinal hemorrhage (intramedullary, subarachnoid, subdural, and epidural)
2. Neoplastic causes
   a) Epidural tumors
      i. Metastatic
         – Lung
         – Breast
         – Prostate
         – Kidney
         – Myeloma
         – Lymphoma
         – GI
         – Miscellaneous

- ii. Primary spinal neoplasms
    - – Multiple myeloma
    - – Osteogenic sarcoma
    - – Chordoma
    - – Chondrosarcoma
    - – Ewing's sarcoma
    - – Fibrous histiocytoma
    - – Giant cell tumor
    - – Benign tumors
- b) Intradural-extramedullary tumors
    - i. Meningioma
    - ii. Nerve sheath tumors
        - – Schwannomas
        - – Neurofibromas
    - iii. Vascular malformations and tumors
    - iv. Epidural and dermoid cysts and teratomas
    - v. Lipoma
- c) Intramedullary tumors
    - i. Ependymoma
    - ii. Astrocytoma
    - iii. Intramedullary metastases
- d) Leptomeningeal metastases
3. Noncompressive myelopathies simulating spinal cord compression
    - a) Transverse and Ascending myelitis
        - i. Postinfectious and postvaccination myelitis
        - ii. Multiple sclerosis
        - iii. Devic's disease (optic neuromyelitis)
        - iv. Acute necrotizing myelitis
    - b) Viral myelitis
        - i. Acute anterior poliomyelitis
        - ii. Postpoliomyelitis syndrome
        - iii. Herpes zoster
        - iv. AIDS-related myelopathies
    - c) Spirochetal disease of the spinal cord
        - i. Syphilis
        - ii. Lyme disease (*Borrelia burgdorferi*)
    - d) Toxic and deficiency myelopathies
        - i. Toxic myelopathies
            - – Myelopathy following aortography

- Myelopathy due to intrathecal agents
  - ∘ Penicillin
  - ∘ Methylene blue
  - ∘ Spinal anesthetics
  - ∘ Intrathecal chemotherapy
    (methotrexate, cytocine, arabinoside, and thiotepa)
- Spinal arachnoiditis
- Radiation myelopathy
- Electrical injuries

e) Metabolic and nutritional myelopathy
  - i. Subacute combined degeneration of the cord (multiple nutritional deficiencies)
  - ii. Nutritional myelopathy (nicotinic acid and several other vitamin deficiencies as well as caloric malnutrition)
  - iii. Myelopathy associated with liver disease
f) Spinal cord infarction
  - i. Arterial infarction
  - ii. Venous infarction
g) Autoimmune diseases
  - i. Sjogren's syndrome
  - ii. Systemic lupus erythematosus
h) Paraneoplastic myelopathy
i) Neuronal degeneration
  - i. Spinocerebellar ataxia (Friederichs's ataxia)
  - ii. Hereditary motor neuron disease
  - iii. Charcot–Marie–Tooth disease
  - iv. Warding–Hoffmann disease

Gilbert RW, Kim JH, Posner JB. Epidural spinal cord compression from metastatic tumor: diagnosis and treatment. Ann Neurol 1978;3(1):40–51

Alexiadou-Rudolf C, Ernestus RI, Nanassis K, Lanfermann H, Klug N. Acute nontraumatic spinal epidural hematomas. An important differential diagnosis in spinal emergencies. Spine 1998;23(16):1810–1813

Yamashita Y, Takahashi H, Matsuno Y, et al. Spinal cord compression due to ossification of ligaments: MR imaging Radiology 1990;175(3):211

9.18 Epidural Spinal Cord Compression

The MRI and myelographic pictures may identify most spinal epidural illnesses causing myelopathy from spinal cord compression, such as intramedullary tumors, leptomeningeal metastases, radiation myelopathy, arteriovenous malformations, and epidural lipomatosis. Some epidural diseases, however, can be confused both clinically and radiologically with epidural spinal cord compression from systemic tumor, e.g., epidural hematoma, epidural abscess, herniated disc and rarely, extradural hematopoiesis.

9.18.1 Differential diagnosis

1. Intradural-extramedullary tumors
   a) Meningioma (25% of primary spinal tumors)
   b) Nerve sheath tumors (among the most common primary spinal tumors, constituting 29% of all cases)
   c) Vascular malformations and tumors
   d) Epidermoid and dermoid tumors
   e) Teratomas
   f) Lipoma and epidural lipomatosis
   g) Drop metastasis from primary brain tumor (e.g., medulloblastoma)
2. Intramedullary tumors (▶ Fig. 9.6 and ▶ Fig. 9.7)
   a) Ependymoma (13% of primary spinal tumors)
   b) Astrocytoma (7% of primary spinal tumors)
   c) Intramedullary metastasis
3. Leptomeningeal metastases
   Clinical findings comprise early multifocal cranial or spinal nerve dysfunction, symptoms or signs of meningeal irritation, and even changes in the CSF such as mild pleocytosis and high protein (▶ Fig. 9.8). Differentiation of leptomeningeal metastases from other parenchymal or epidural metastases requires:

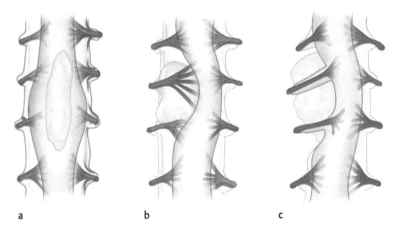

Fig. 9.6 Spinal cord tumors: (a) Intradural, intramedullary: astrocytoma, ependymoma, hemangioma, cavernoma, dermoid/epidermoid. (b) Intradural, extramedullary: nerve sheath tumors, meningioma (c) Extradural: bone neoplasms, metastases.

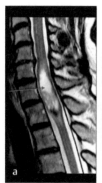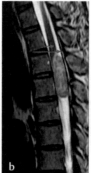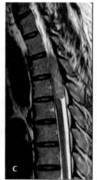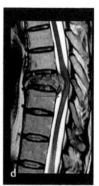

Fig. 9.7 Tumor localization in the spinal canal. **(a)** Sagittal T2-weighted image demonstrates an intramedullary tumor expanding the spinal cord. **(b, c)** Sagittal T2-weighted images in a different patient demonstrate a tubular mass between the spinal cord (**b,** *short arrow*) and dura (**b,** *long arrow*). The meniscus of CSF at the margin of the lesion (**c,** *arrow*) confirms that the lesion expands the subarachnoid space, indicating that it is in the extramedullary intradural compartment. This was a schwannoma. **(d)** Sagittal T2-weighted image in a third patient shows a mass arising from a partially collapsed vertebral body extending into the spinal canal and compressing the spinal cord. The mass narrows (*arrow*) the CSF space rather than expands it, indicating that the mass is extradural. This was a rectal carcinoma metastasis. (Reproduced from Tumor Characterization. In: Bernstein M, Berger M, ed. Neuro-Oncology: The Essentials. 3rd edition. Thieme; 2014.)

a) MRI with gadolinium enhancement of the brain and spine to reveal or exclude any mass lesions
b) CSF cytology for malignant cells. The presence of malignant cells confirms the existence of leptomeningeal tumor, despite whatever else the patient may have
4. Radiation myelopathy
Late-delayed radiation myelopathy has three forms: a progressive myelopathy, a lower motor neuron syndrome, and hemorrhage of spinal cord.
a) Progressive myelopathy (12–50 months after radiation therapy (RT))
Ascending paresthesias and weakness in one leg and a decrease in temperature and pain sensation in the other (Brown–Sequard syndrome) is the first clinical symptom in most patients. Some patients exhibit a transverse myelopathy with both legs equally affected by weakness and sensory loss that rise to the level of the radiation portal.
   i. CSF analysis is usually normal but may show an increased protein level

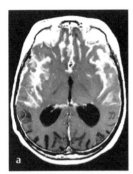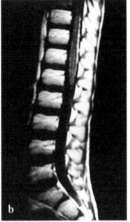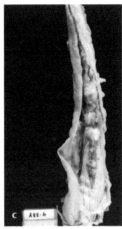

Fig. 9.8 (a) Axial T1-weighted MRI with contrast shows enhancement in the subarachnoid spaces over the hemispheres and in the sylvian fissures bilaterally. This is indicative of diffuse cerebrospinal fluid dissemination in a medulloblastoma patient. **(b)** Midsagittal T1-weighted MRI of the spine showing drop metastases from medulloblastoma as enhancement along the posterior aspect of the spinal cord and conus medullaris. **(c)** Postmortem specimen of the thecal sac, spinal cord, and cauda equina with extensive metastases from a medulloblastoma. (Reproduced from Medulloblastoma. In: Bernstein M, Berger M, ed. Neuro-Oncology: The Essentials. 3rd edition. Thieme; 2014.)

  ii. MRI
    – In the acute stage: reveals spinal cord swelling that may lead to a complete spinal block, and contrast enhancement of the area of damage
    – In late stages: the spinal cord appears to be atrophic
  iii. Motor conduction velocity in the spinal cord pathways is reduced
b) Lower motor neuron syndrome (after pelvic RT for testicular tumors)
   Subacute onset of a flaccid weakness of the legs affecting both proximal and distal muscles with atrophy, fasciculations, and areflexia. Sensory changes are absent, and sphincter function remains normal.
    i. CSF analysis may show increased protein content
    ii. The myelogram is normal
    iii. The electromyogram reveals varying degrees of denervation
    iv. Central conduction velocities are normal
c) Spinal cord hemorrhage (8–30 years after RT, and a few patients only)
   Sudden back pain and leg weakness during a few hours to a few days, in

a patient without previous neurologic symptoms. The pathogenesis is considered to be hemorrhage from telangiectasia caused by RT.

    i. MRI reveals acute or subacute hemorrhage in the spinal cord, which may be atrophic, but no other lesions are found (▶ Fig. 9.9)

5. Transverse and ascending myelopathy

Postinfectious or parainfectious myelopathy, postvaccination myelopathy, multiple sclerosis, and acute and subacute necrotizing myelopathy are the most common causes of acute transverse and ascending myelopathy. Patients commonly present with sensory cord symptoms primarily from posterior column involvement, such as painful electric-like shock sensations, elicited by neck flexion or extension (Lhermitte's sign), which involve the body below the neck.

Differential diagnosis of Lhermitte's signs include:

The pathogenesis of the Lhermitte's sign is thought to be a reversible damage to myelin in the ascending sensory tracts of the spinal cord, which allows axons to be abnormally sensitive to mechanical deformation.

a) Spinal metastasis
b) Cervical spondylosis
c) Cervical disk herniation
d) Multiple sclerosis

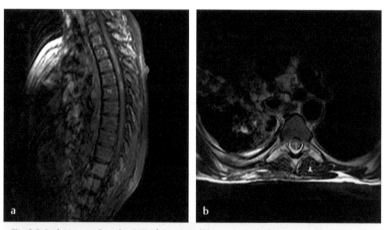

Fig. 9.9 Radiation myelopathy: MRI of spinal cord demonstrated a long segment intramedullary lesion extending from T3–T6 level. The spinal cord appeared diffusely enlarged over the involved segment and partially enhancing lesion was seen after gadolinium enhancement. **(a)** T1 contrast-enhancing sequence on sagittal plane and **(b)** T2 sequence on axial plane at level of T5 vertebra.

e) Posttraumatic syndrome
f) Subacute combined degeneration
g) Cisplatin chemotherapy
h) Cervical radiation

Patients may also present with progressive weakness, sometimes with lower motor neuron signs including fasciculations, in association with sensory loss and autonomic dysfunction such as incontinence and postural hypotension.

a) CSF analysis typically shows inflammatory changes
b) MRI usually shows normal spinal cord on T1-WI, but hyperintensity occasionally can be identified on T2-WI; contrast enhancement may be noted

6. Epidural hematoma

Epidural spinal hematomas in cancer patients usually occur spontaneously, because of concurrent severe thrombocytopenia, and less often in systemic vasculitis, as in polyarteritis nodosa.

a) Rapidly evolving symptoms and signs (acute back pain progressing to sensory and motor loss, within minutes to hours rather than days or weeks)
b) CT scan and MRI
    i. No evidence of vertebral involvement by tumor
    ii. The epidural block usually covers several segments rather than the one or two segments characteristic of epidural spinal cord compression from other causes
    iii. The density characteristics of hemorrhage on MRI are different from those of epidural tumor (except for a hemorrhagic tumor)
c) At times the diagnosis cannot be made without a biopsy
    Thrombocytopenia is a contraindication to any surgical removal of the hematoma, which would confirm the diagnosis and treat the illness

7. Epidural abscess

Differentiating leptomeningeal metastases from CNS infection, particularly in immunosuppressed patients and particularly those with lymphomas, who are susceptible to both illnesses, is very difficult and confusing. Patients with leptomeningeal metastases develop **early** signs of cranial and spinal nerve abnormalities, whereas patients with CNS infections tend to develop these signs **late**, if at all. Therefore:

a) Signs of meningeal irritation associated with fever and abnormal CSF without neurologic abnormalities suggest CNS infection.
b) Plain X-rays of the spine characteristically demonstrate two vertebral bodies across a disk space are destroyed. This is a hallmark of infection because it is rare for metastatic tumor to cross the disk space and involve two contiguous vertebral bodies.

   c) Cranial and spinal nerve dysfunction without meningeal signs and with modest CSF changes suggests tumor.

   d) To complicate the diagnosis further, and although this is rare, epidural abscess may form at the site of a metastatic epidural tumor.

   e) Needle biopsy of the involved vertebra is necessary to confirm the diagnosis. Often needle aspiration and drainage of the spinal abscess is used therapeutically (▶ Fig. 9.10).

8. Herniated disk

Cervical or lumbar, and rarely thoracic disk herniation manifests local and radicular pain, occasionally associated by dermatomal sensory and motor loss. Characteristically:

   a) The pain of a herniated disk is worse when the patient is sitting or walking but usually gets relief when lying down. Conversely, spinal cord epidural tumor is usually worse in the lying position than when sitting or standing.

   b) MRI with enhancement should establish the diagnosis of disk herniation, and also identify those cases in which disk herniation is caused by a vertebral body tumor.

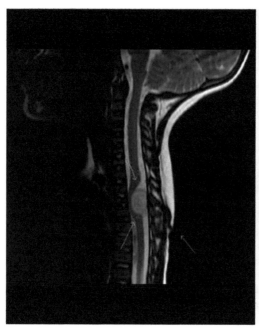

Fig. 9.10 Epidural abscess developing in association with a congenital dermal sinus tract in an infant. This T2-weighted sagittal magnetic resonance image shows significant cord compression from a well defined abscess. The arrows show both the dorsally placed globular lesion and the immediately adjacent sinus tract coursing cephalad from its origin on the skin. The abscess was surgically drained and the sinus tract excised, with normal development thereafter. (Reproduced from Unusual Bacteria Causing Epidural Abscess. In: Hall W, Kim P, ed. Neurosurgical Infectious Disease. Surgical and Nonsurgical Management. 1st edition. Thieme; 2013.)

Paterson DL. Gbranuloma Inguinale causing spinal cord compression: a case report and review of Donovanosis involving bone Clin Infect Dis 1998;26(2):379–383

Schiff D. Spinal cord compression. Neurol Clin 2003;21(1):67–86, viii

Jacob A, Weinshenker BG. An approach to the diagnosis of acute transverse myelitis. Semin Neurol 2008;28(1):105–120

Poortmans P, Vulto A, Raaijmakers E. Always on a Friday? Time pattern of referral for spinal cord compression Acta Oncol (Madr) 2009;40(1):88–91

St George E, Hillier CE, Hatfield R. Spinal cord compression: an unusual neurological complication of gout. Rheumatology (Oxford) 2001;40(6):711–712

9.19 Paediatric Intraspinal Cysts

1. Spinal intradural cysts
   a) Neurenteric cysts
      The intraspinal neurenteric cysts form a spectrum that merges with intraspinal teratomas and intraspinal dermoids and epidermoids (▶ Fig. 9.11). More than 60% of the cases are diagnosed in the first 20 years of life and 44% are located totally or partially in the cervical spinal canal, 37% are located in the thoracic spinal canal, and 19% in the lumbosacral spinal canal. The neurological signs and symptoms of a slowly progressing mass are associated by congenital anomalies, such as thickened or pigmented skin, a cutaneous dimple or dermal sinus, or a tuft of hair may occur in the midline of the back.

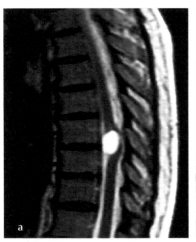
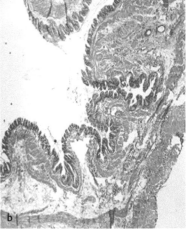

Fig. 9.11 (a, b) MRI of the spinal cord showing ventral intraspinal cyst: Radiological suspicion of a dermoid was made, but pathology examination revealed a cyst lined up by columnar epithelium of intestinal type confirming the diagnosis of a spinal intradural neurenteric cyst.

b) Epidermoid and dermoid cysts

These cysts account for 0.2–2% of the primary spinal tumors of adults; among children, however, these cysts comprise 3–13% of such spinal tumors and within the first year if life the incidence rises further to 17%. At least 62% of the dermoid cysts and 63% of the epidermoid cysts occur at or below the thoracolumbar junction. Of the intraspinal dermoids, 30% are wholly or partially intramedullary in location and of the intraspinal epidermoids 28% are wholly or partially intramedullary. In regard to associated defects, 25% have posterior spina bifida, and 34% of dermoid cysts and 20% of epidermoid cysts had a posterior dermal sinus tract. Among 11 of 12 sinus tracts in the thoracic region terminated in intradural congenital tumor. Scoliosis may develop as the cyst enlarges in a child. CT and MR are proven useful in the diagnosis workup; high signal on T1-WI and T2-WI (▶ Fig. 9.12).

c) Arachnoid cysts

These cysts are composed of arachnoid and are filled with CSF. These cysts are not associated with spinal dysraphism or any other congenital anomalies. They typically occur in the thoracic area, posterior to the spinal cord. Initially asymptomatic, but when enlarge in size they may cause back pain usually relieved when the patient lies down, radicular pain, paraparesis. Occasionally kyphoscoliosis will develop as the cyst

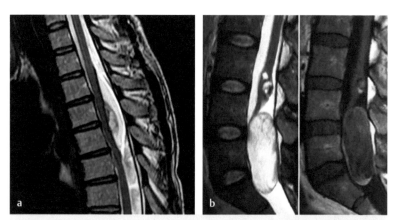

Fig. 9.12 MRI of epidermoid cysts A and B **(a)** An intradural extramedullary mass having mixed fat and solid enhancing components displacing the cord anteriorly. **(b)** An extramedullary intradural mass located behind the spinal cord. It is composed of tissue which follows fat on all sequences (bright on both T1 and T2) including fat saturated postcontrast T1.

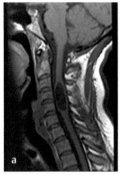 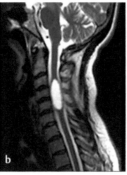

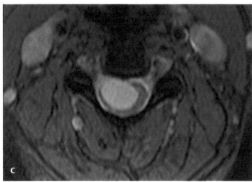

Fig. 9.13 Magnetic resonance imaging of the cervical spine is demonstrating a 36×13 mm intramedullary arachnoid cyst. (a) The lesion is hypointense in the sagittal T1-WI scan. (b) The lesion has a similar intensity of cerebrospinal fluid, but it is hyperintense on the sagittal T2-WI scan. (c) the lesion has a significant mass effect, especially at the C4-C5 level. (Reproduced from Baeesa S, Aljameely A. Intramedullary Arachnoid Cyst of the Cervical Spine: Case Report and Literature Review. Arquivos Brasileiros de Neurocirurgia: Brazilian Neurosurgery 2017;36(04): 256–259.)

grows. On MR focal impression of the cord can be seen with intensity similar to that of CSF without enhancement (▶ Fig. 9.13).

   i. Developmental
  ii. Inflammatory
 iii. Post-traumatic

d) Ependymal (neuroepithelial) cysts
A thin wall composed of connective tissue lined by a single layer of cells that resemble ependymal cells similar to a neurenteric cyst; but contrary to the latter one the epithelium of the ependymal cells do not have a basement membrane or contain mucin. These cysts are located between C2 and L5, but nearly 45% at the thoracolumbar junction and most of them have intramedullary extensions.

e) Other intramedullary cysts of the conus medullaris
A few intramedullary cysts occurring within the conus which have a thin transparent wall cyst composed of narrow bands of glial tissue lined by a layer of ependymal cells.

    f) Spinal cysticercosis

      The average incidence of intraspinal forms is about 5–6%. The parasites grow in the subarachnoid spinal space forming multiple cysts rather than within the spinal cord where the cysts are usually solitary. Myelography, CT, and MR scanning are the key diagnostic modalities. The specific diagnosis can be suspected if there is known disease elsewhere, or if in the CSF there is either eosinophilia, or a positive complement fixation test for cysticercosis.

    g) Chronic spinal subdural hematomas

2. Spinal extradural cysts

    a) Congenital extradural spinal cysts

      These cysts arise as an evagination or herniation of the arachnoid that gradually enlarges, its neck eventually closes, creating a cyst no longer communicating with the CSF space. They are located exclusively or primarily in the thoracic spine in 86% of cases and less frequently in the cervical (2.5%) and lumbosacral region (11.5%). Of the patients with congenital extradural spinal cysts, nearly 40% have Scheuermann's disease (kyphosis dorsalis juvenilis) or preoperative dorsal kyphosis without definite vertebral epiphysitis.

    b) Spontaneous spinal nerve root diverticula and cysts (Tarlov cysts)

      These cysts are extensions of the subarachnoid space along spinal nerve roots primarily located on the posterior spinal nerve roots and spinal ganglia containing fluid that is either clear and colorless or faintly yellow. Occasionally a perineural cyst can become large enough to cause a sciatic or cauda equina syndrome.

    c) Occult intrasacral meningoceles

      Results from a defect in the embryologic development of the spinal meninges in the sacral area, and become symptomatic in adult life causing pain and urinary dysfunction, suggesting that it enlarges with time probably due to hydrostatic effect of the CSF.

    d) Posttraumatic or postoperative meningeal diverticula

      Following spinal fracture-dislocation or nerve root avulsion, or after operative laminectomy, the CSF will collect and stimulate the formation of a pseudomeningocele.

    e) Spinal ganglion cysts and spinal synovial cysts

      Cysts arising from the periarticular tissue are distinguished to synovial cysts if they have synovial lining and to ganglion cysts if they have no specific lining. Most often occur in the posterolateral epidural space, attached to or adjacent to the facet joint of the L4–L5 vertebral level and are primarily unilateral.

    f) Extradural spinal hydatidosis

In about 1–2.5% of patients with hydatid disease, there are osseous lesions and half of these involve the spine. They are located in the cervical (10%), thoracic (50%), lumbar (20%), and sacral spine (20%). Epidural involvement may grow sufficiently to cause neural compression. CT imaging is good to show the initial involvement of spongy bone, and MRI seems to provide more detail about neural involvement than CT.

g) Spinal cysts associated with ankylosing spondylitis
In rare cases ankylosing spondylitis may be associated by multiple meningeal diverticula extending into the posterior bony arches of the lumbar spinal canal.

h) Ependymal cysts, neurenteric cysts, and epidermoid and dermoid cysts
These are similar but less frequent to their intradural counterparts.

i) Aneurysmal bone cyst
This benign paediatric vascular tumor occurs as a solitary lesion in a long bone or of a vertebra especially at the lumbar area. The interior of the cyst is composed of blood-filled cavernous spaces with fibrous walls that contain osteoid and giant cells and covered by a thin bony shell. Pain involving the back or neck is an early symptom, and as the tumor enlarges into the spinal canal, symptoms of cord compression or radiculopathy may develop (▶ Fig. 9.14).

j) Other spinal extradural cysts
A large midline mesothelial cyst extending from L5 to S3 with a translucent wall and filled with xanthochromic fluid, and also an intradiscal disc cyst postoperatively filled with straw-colored fluid have been reported.

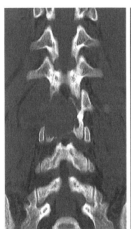 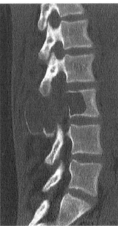

Fig. 9.14 Aneurysmal bone cyst: CT scan of the lumbar spine showing destruction of the right pedicle, a missing calcified tumor matrix and a nonsclerotic zone of transition to adjacent bone, which is not typical in benign bone lesions, but can occur in aneurysmal bone cysts.

Khosla A, Wippold FJ II. CT myelography and MR imaging of extramedullary cysts of the spinal canal in adult and pediatric patients. AJR Am J Roentgenol 2002;178(1):201–207

Kumar R, Jain R, Rao KM, Hussain N. Intraspinal neurenteric cysts–report of three paediatric cases. Childs Nerv Syst 2001;17(10):584–588

Wilson PE, Oleszek JL, Clayton GH. Pediatric spinal cord tumors and masses. J Spinal Cord Med 2007;30(Suppl 1):S15–S20

Koeller KK, Rosenblum RS, Morrison AL. Neoplasms of the spinal cord and filum terminale: radiologic-pathologic correlation. Radiographics 2000;20(6):1721–1749

Grainger & Allison's Diagnostic Radiology. Adam A, et al, eds. 6th ed. Churchill-Livingstone-Elsevier; 2015

Brooks BS, Duvall ER, el Gammal T, et al. Neuroimaging features of neurenteric cysts: analysis of nine cases and review of the literature. AJNR Am J Neuroradiol 1993;14(3):735–746

9.20 Myelopathy in Cancer Patients

Myelopathy is a devastating neurologic complication of cancer. The resultant **pain, paralysis**, and **incontinence** can turn a patient with cancer from a functioning individual to one who is confined to a chair or bed. Accurate neurologic assessment of patients is crucial for early diagnosis and correct therapy. Myelopathy in patients with cancer is not rare. Epidural spinal cord compression affects an estimated 5% of patients with cancer. Other disorders such as intramedullary spinal cord metastases, adverse effects of therapy, and paraneoplastic spinal cord syndromes, although less common, are equally devastating.

1. Metastatic cancer
   a) Epidural (in 5% of patients with cancer)
   b) Leptomeningeal
   c) Intramedullary (in fewer than 1% of patients affecting preferably the cervical cord and conus medullaris and mostly reported in small cell lung cancer)
2. Toxicity from therapy
   a) Radiation myelopathy (weeks or months after radiation to the spine)
   b) Myelopathy due to chemotherapy (after the intrathecal injection of cytarabine or methotrexate sodium high dose monotherapy; also in association with carmustine, cisplatin, and thiotepa treatment)
   c) Infectious disease
      Patients with cancer are immunocompromised due either to tumor (lymphoma) or chemotherapy and become susceptible to infections, such as varicella zoster virus, cytomegalovirus, EBV, and HSV1 or HSV2. Epidural abscess or osteomyelitis can result from the placement of epidural catheters. Also cases of syphilis, tuberculosis, aspergillosis, and toxoplasmosis cause myelitis.

   d) Vascular disease
   Surgical interventions such as aortic clamping or paravertebral surgery.
   Thrombotic states, common in cancer patients, may cause ischemia.
   Intravascular lymphomas can present with ischemic cord lesions and
   may mimic multiple sclerosis. Sudden onset of spinal cord deficits may
   signify hemorrhage into a spinal tumor.

   e) Paraneoplastic syndromes
   Pathogenesis is believed to be an autoimmune reaction to antigens
   shared by the tumor in the nervous system.

   f) Motor neuron disease
   Motor neuron disease has been described in association with multiple
   cancers (lung, breast, lymphoma, ovarian, testicular, and melanoma) and
   a variety of paraneoplastic antibodies have been found (Hu, Yo, Ma2,
   spectrin, and GM1)

Graber JJ, Nolan CP. Myelopathies in patients with cancer. Arch Neurol 2010;67(3):298–304

Reagan TJ, Thomas JE, Colby MY Jr. Chronic progressive radiation myelopathy. Its clinical aspects and differential diagnosis. JAMA 1968;203(2):106–110

Seidenwarm DJ, et al. Myelopathy AJNR 2008;29:1032–1037

Winkelman MD, Adelstein DJ, Karlins NL. Intramedullary spinal cord metastasis. Diagnostic and therapeutic considerations. Arch Neurol 1987;44(5):526–531

Mueller S, Dubal DB, Josephson SA. A case of paraneoplastic myelopathy associated with the neuromyelitis optica antibody. Nat Clin Pract Neurol 2008;4(5):284–288

Rees JH. Paraneoplastic syndromes: when to suspect, how to confirm, and how to manage. J Neurol Neurosurg Psychiatry 2004;75(Suppl 2):ii43–ii50

Lee EQ, Schiff D, Wen PY. Neurologic complications of cancer therapy. Demos Medical; 2012

9.21 Lumbar Disc Protrusion

1. Spinal stenosis
   a) Congenital: developmental acquired (hypertrophic osteoarthritis)
   b) Central lumbar canal stenosis
   c) Lateral recess syndrome
   d) "Claudication" syndrome of cauda equina
2. Spondylolisthesis
   Defects in pars interarticularis and forward slip of vertebral body in relation
   to vertebral below
3. Tumor (primary or metastatic in bone)
4. Infection
   a) Acute (e.g., *Staphylococcus aureus*)
   b) Chronic (e.g., tuberculosis)

5. Paget's disease (Osteitis deformans)
6. Ankylosing spondylitis
7. Pelvic lesions
   a) Lumbosacral plexus involved by abdominal or pelvic mass
   b) Tumor invading pelvis or sacrum
   c) Hip joint osteoarthritis
8. Leg lesion
   a) Vascular insufficiency (intermittent claudication)
   b) Peripheral nerve lesion (tumor, neuropathy)
   c) Local leg legion

9.22 Disorders of Spinal Nerve Roots

Radicular pain in nerve root distribution (e.g., brachialgia, "girdle" pain, sciatica); pain is aggravated by: cough (increased intraspinal pressure), movement of that part of spine, and stretch (e.g., straight leg raising L4, L5, S1; femoral stretch test L2, L3, L4). Impaired conduction:

- Motor: Of lower motor neuron type (e.g., weakness, tendon reflexes decreased or absent, flaccidity, fasciculations, and atrophy if existing for long enough time)
- Sensory (e.g., all modalities decreased or absent in dermatome; dermatomes often overlap so sensory loss may be subtle). Disorders may affect the spinal roots in spinal canal or intervertebral foramen.

1. Intrinsic lesions
   a) Herpes zoster
   b) Tabes dorsalis
   c) Inflammatory "radiculitis"
2. Compressive lesions
   a) Intervertebral disc protrusion
   b) Bony lesions
      i. Spinal stenosis
      ii. Osteophytes
      iii. Metastatic carcinoma
      iv. Trauma
      v. Rare (e.g., Paget's, disease)
   c) Tumors
      i. Schwannoma, neurofibroma
      ii. Meningioma
      iii. Others
   d) Infections (e.g., tuberculosis)

9.23 Foot Drop

When the dorsal extensor muscles of the foot and the toes (tibialis anterior, extensor digitorum longus, and extensor hallucis longus) innervated by the deep peroneal nerve are paralyzed, there is a foot drop. Because the tibialis anterior muscle is innervated from the L4 to S1 roots (especially L5 and to a lesser extend L4), through the sciatic and ultimately the deep peroneal nerves, a lesion of any of these can cause a foot drop. The toe extensors are primarily L5 with some S1 contribution.

Causes of foot drop:

1. Peripheral causes (more common)
   a) Peroneal nerve injury
      i. Superficial peroneal nerve: It supplies the peroneus longus and brevis muscles (L5, S1), weakness of which is causing loss of foot eversion and plantar flexion, but **NO** foot drop. The sensory changes are less helpful, in as much as there is an overlap between the dermatomes, however, commonly there is sensory loss in the lateral aspect of the lower half of leg and foot.
      ii. Deep peroneal nerve: It supplies the tibialis anterior, extensor digitorum longus, extensor hallucis longus, peronius tertius, extensor digitorum brevis and the 1st dorsal interosseous muscles, weakness of which is causing an isolated foot drop. The sensory loss is minimal affecting the great toe web space.
      iii. Common peroneal nerve: It supplies all the above muscles with sparing of tibialis posterior (foot inversion). Damage to the common peroneal nerve causes a foot drop because it supplies all foot and toe extensors. The patient cannot dorsiflex the foot, and the toes will drag when the patient walks. There is a sensory loss of the lateral aspect of lower half of leg and foot. (The superficial position of the nerve accounts for a common cause of foot drop, the so-called "crossed knee palsy." A painless foot drop is more likely to be due to a peroneal neuropathy than to radiculopathy.)
   b) L5 radiculopathy (or less commonly, L4) caused most commonly by a herniated lumbar disc (L4–5 disc space)
      i. Weakness affecting peronius, toe extensors, possibly anterior tibialis. The patient has trouble supporting weight on heel or presence of foot drop, complaining that his toes get caught on carpet.
      ii. Pain and sensory loss over the anterolateral aspect of the affected leg below the knee and extending to the dorsum of the foot and toes including the big toe.
      iii. Diminished or absent internal hamstring tendon reflex.

  c) Lumbosacral plexus neuropathy
     i. Idiopathic plexitis
     ii. Diabetic plexus neuropathy (possibly secondary to vascular injury to nerves)
     iii. Vasculitis
     iv. Trauma
     v. Following radiation treatment
     vi. Retroperitoneal or intrapelvic lesions
  d) Peripheral neuropathy: The most common inherited disorder is Carcot–Marie–Tooth syndrome or peroneal muscular atrophy. Diabetes, alcohol, and Guillain–Barre account for 90% of cases.
2. Central causes
  a) Cortical lesion located in the paracentral lobule of the motor strip (Parasagittal meningioma, metastasis). Sensation may be spared.
  b) Spinal cord injury
  c) Motor neuron disease
  d) Amyotrophic lateral sclerosis (corticospinal tracts and anterior horn cells involvement)

9.23.1 Differential diagnosis

A complete palsy of the foot dorsiflexors is strongly suggestive of peroneal nerve palsy. Most radiculopathies partially spare these muscles due to overlap of nerve root innervation. An L5 radiculopathy resembles a peroneal palsy, but is differentiated from it by: (1) weakness of foot inversion, (2) sensory loss occurring well above the midpoint of the calf, (3) more weakness of the extensor hallucis than of the anterior tibialis muscle (which receives more L4 innervation than does the extensor hallucis muscle and is, thus, less involved), and (4) back pain.

The peroneal nerve may be damaged at different levels below the knee. The deep peroneal nerve may be injured by an anterior compartment syndrome with resultant foot drop, but with sparing of the foot evertors. The distal deep peroneal nerve may be involved in an anterior tarsal tunnel syndrome. This may produce asymptomatic atrophy of the extensor digitorum brevis as well as a sensory loss in the web space between the first and second toes.

A sciatic nerve lesion may present with predominantly peroneal signs because of the more frequent and severe involvement of the peroneal nerve compared to the tibial nerve. The additional absence of the ankle reflex atrophy or weakness of the hamstring or calf muscles, or sensory loss on the sole of the foot may indicate that the sciatic nerve is affected.

Peripheral neuropathies may also cause peroneal nerve dysfunction. The common peroneal nerve is also frequent site on involvement of diabetic peripheral neuropathy.

Lumbar root syndrome versus hip pain

	Lumbar root syndrome	Hip pain
History	Sudden onset	Gradual onset
	Pain while sitting	Pain when walking and/or standing
	Improvement with standing and walking	Improvement with sitting
Physical findings	Free hip movements	Restricted hip movement
	Sciatic nerve testing positive	Sciatic nerve testing negative
	Lumbar traction test positive	Lumbar traction test negative
Diagnosis aided by	CT scan	Plain X-rays
	MRI	Intra-articular injection with a local anesthetic
	Myelography (obsolete)	

Jarvik JG, Deyo RA. Diagnostic evaluation of low back pain with emphasis on imaging. Ann Intern Med 2002;137(7):586–597

Maroon JC, Kopitnik TA, Schulhof LA, Abla A, Wilberger JE. Diagnosis and microsurgical approach to far-lateral disc herniation in the lumbar spine. J Neurosurg 1990;72(3):378–382

Jackson RP, Glah JJ. Foraminal and extraforaminal lumbar disc herniation: diagnosis and treatment. Spine 1987;12(6):577–585

Sizer PS Jr, Phelps V, Dedrick G, Matthijs O. Differential diagnosis and management of spinal nerve root-related pain. Pain Pract 2002;2(2):98–121

Westhout FD, Paré LS, Linskey ME. Central causes of foot drop: rare and underappreciated differential diagnoses. J Spinal Cord Med 2007;30(1):62–66

Bendszus M, Wessig C, Reiners K, Bartsch AJ, Solymosi L, Koltzenberg M. MR imaging in the differential diagnosis of neurogenic foot drop. AJNR Am J Neuroradiol 2003;24(7):1283–1289

Baker RA, Coles AJ, Scolding NJ, et al. The A-Z of Neurological Practice. A guide to clinical neurology. Cambridge University Press; 2005

9.24 Sacroiliac Joint Dysfunction (Syndrome)

Although many conditions refer pain to the sacroiliac (SI) joint, low back, and legs, the SI joint itself can also cause pain in those areas.

The pain is described as a dull ache or sharp, stabbing, or knifelike; pain may be aggravated by sitting or lying on the affected side and worsens with prolonged sitting, weight bearing through the affected side, Valsalva maneuver, and trunk flexion with straight legs. Patients report pain distributions in the buttocks (94%) at or near the posterior superior iliac spine (PSIS; 50%), back of the thigh (10%), and upper back in one or both sides.

Many risk factors are associated with lower back pain, and many are directly associated with lumbar disk injury. These include, but are not limited to, smoking, poor physical condition, positive family history, and occupational lifting.

Factors that specifically increase the likelihood of mechanical injury to the SI joint have not been identified. Pregnancy is one particular condition attributed to SI joint dysfunction. Was reported that 58% of patients diagnosed with SI joint pain based on clinical examination findings had some inciting traumatic injury.

9.24.1 Causes of SI joint dysfunction

There are a number of diseases that can attack, including those that cause SI dysfunction and its resulting pain in the SI joints. Most common are:
1. Sacroiliatis
2. Osteoarthritis
3. SI joint injury
4. Altered walking pattern
5. Infection
6. Prior lumbar fusion
7. Pregnancy

9.24.2 Symptoms

1. Low back pain: Usually a dull ache on one side of lower back that may extend into the thigh. It is usually below the L5 or lowest lumbar vertebra.
2. Buttock pain: Pain can range from an ache to a sharp stabbing pain that extends down one or both legs.
3. Low back pain while climbing stairs: Activities that require the pelvis to twist may produce SI joint pain.
4. Difficulty sitting or lying on one side: After experienced as an ache on one side that causes someone to shift weight to one side to relieve the pain in the other.

Provocation tests include:
1. Compression/distraction tests
2. Patrick's sign
3. Thigh thrust/sacral thrust tests
4. Drop test
5. Fortin's test
6. Gillet test

9.24.3 Differential diagnoses

1. Ankylosing spondylitis and undifferentiated spondyloarthropathy
2. Hip fracture
3. Hip overuse syndrome
4. Iliotibial band syndrome

5. Lumbosacral discogenic pain syndrome
6. Lumbosacral facet syndrome
7. Lumbosacral radiculopathy
8. Piriformis syndrome
9. Sacroiliac joint infection
10. Seronegative spondyloarthropathy
11. Superior cluneal nerve (iliac crest) syndrome
12. Trochanteric bursitis

Tibor LM, Sekiya JK. Differential diagnosis of pain around the hip joint. Arthroscopy 2008;24(12):1407–1421

Slipman CW, Sterenfeld EB, Chou LH, Herzog R, Vresilovic E. The predictive value of provocative sacroiliac joint stress maneuvers in the diagnosis of sacroiliac joint syndrome. Arch Phys Med Rehabil 1998;79(3):288–292

Maigne JY, Aivaliklis A, Pfefer F. Results of sacroiliac joint double block and value of sacroiliac pain provocation tests in 54 patients with low back pain. Spine 1996;21(16):1889–1892

9.25 Sciatica

It is the pain along the course of the sciatic nerve, originating from irritation of or trauma to its fibers above the knee.

The prevalence of true nerve-related sciatica was at 5% in men and 4% in women. It is thought that back pain affects approximately 14% of adults annually; about 1–2% also have sciatica. This amounts to 13% of 40,000,000 backpain cases per year: more than 5,000,000 cases annually.

1. Vertebral causes
   a) Intervertebral disc disease
      In most cases, sciatica is disk related and is caused by degenerative changes of the two lower lumbar motion segments.
   b) Spinal stenosis
      In many cases is caused indirectly by a disorder of the intervertebral disk.
   c) Spondylolisthesis
      Is usually bilateral and is little influenced by position changes or/and traction.
   d) Spondylitis
      Nerve root irritation is bilateral and not influenced by motion or traction. Night pain is characteristic.
   e) Vertebral tumors
      Usually metastatic and less often primary tumors. They cause severe sciatic symptoms with a bilateral Lasegue's sign and severe intractable pain with segmental radiation.
   f) Paget's disease
      Rare cause producing spinal stenosis from the new bone formation.

2. Extravertebral causes
   a) Hip disease
      Severe degenerative or inflammatory joint disease is often mistaken for a lumbar root syndrome because both diseases occur frequently and pain radiation into hip and thigh often affects the same areas. Neurologic deficits are often discrete or missing; Lasegue's sign and reverse Lasegue's sign are negative; Traction test with traction brace is negative in hip pathology whereas disk-related pain diminishes with traction, the patient is better able to bend forward. Diagnosis confirmed by intra-articular injection of local anesthetic and by X-ray.
   b) Sacroiliac disease
      Inflammatory or degenerative diseases of the sacroiliac joints can cause symptoms similar to the proximal pain area of sciatica.
   c) Extravertebral retroperitoneal tumors
      Originating from rectum, uterus or prostate may produce symptoms of displacement of the lumbosacral nerve plexus when they reach large size.
   d) Aneurysm of the common iliac artery
   e) Peripheral vascular disease
      Patients usually complain of leg pain increased by walking.
   f) Sciatic neuropathic disease
       i. Diabetic neuropathy
      ii. Alcoholic neuritis
     iii. Herpes zoster neuritis
      iv. Periarteritis nodosa
       v. Neuritis caused by leprosy
   g) Sciatic nerve damage from injection
      There is a local circumscribed tender area at the site of injection, pressure on which elicits projected pain. It also involves symptoms of autonomic nerve involvement as opposed to lumbar nerve root syndromes.

Distad BJ, Weiss MD. Clinical and electrodiagnostic features of sciatic neuropathies. Phys Med Rehabil Clin N Am 2013;24(1):107–120

Spittell PC, Spittell JA Jr, Joyce JW, et al. Clinical features and differential diagnosis of aortic dissection: experience with 236 cases (1980 through 1990). Mayo Clin Proc 1993;68(7):642–651

Magnuson PB. Differential diagnosis of causes of pain in the lower back accompanied by sciatic pain Ann Surg 1944;119(6):878–891

Kulcu DG, Naderi S. Differential diagnosis of intraspinal and extraspinal non-discogenic sciatica. J Clin Neurosci 2008;15(11):1246–1252

Millikan CH. Sciatica; differential diagnosis and treatment. J Am Med Assoc 1951;145(1):1–4

9.26 Posterior Knee Pain

Posterior knee pain is a relatively uncommon patient complaint with challenging and often elusive etiology. The differential diagnosis for posterior knee pain can be vast, so clues for distinguishing causes are important.

Soft-tissue and tendon injuries are perhaps more common causes of posterior knee pain than are vascular, neurologic, and iatrogenic injuries, but these less common origins should not be overlooked in patients who present with posterior knee pain.

Diagnosis	Clinical symptoms and signs
Support structures and tumors	
Baker's cyst	May be asymptomatic: patient may have a feeling of fullness in the popliteal fossa. Crescent sign: may simulate venous thrombosis
Soft-tissue or bone tumor	Knee locking; palpable mass; pain without weight bearing. Limited knee flexion; may mimic a meniscal scar
Meniscal scar	Increasing pain with deep knee flexion. Point joint-line tenderness; positive McMurray's test; effusion
Tendons	
Hamstring injury	Positive knee pain with sudden acceleration or deceleration. Tenderness at distal biceps femoris tendon; pain with knee flexion
Gastrocnemius tendon Calcification	Posterior knee pain with knee extension and ankle dorsiflexion. Patient may have tenderness over areas of CPPD deposition
Popliteus tendon injury	Pain with running, especially downhill. Knee flexion with internal rotation of the tibia in prone position may cause pain
Ligaments	
Posterolateral corner injury	Varus thrust in stance or with ambulation; hyperextension, external rotation; peroneal nerve may also be injured. Varus thrust; positive external recurvatum test; positive dial test
Blood vessels	
Popliteal artery entrapment	Hypertrophy of calf muscles; claudication; paresthesias below the knee. Distal pulses may disappear with hyperextension and active plantar flexion or passive dorsiflexion; trophic changes below the knee

(*Continued*)

▶ (Continued)

Diagnosis	Clinical symptoms and signs
Nerves	
Common peroneal nerve entrapment	Tenderness over area of entrapment; pain may increase with exertion. Local tenderness over area of entrapment
Tibial nerve entrapment	Tenderness over area of entrapment; pain may increase with exertion. Local tenderness over area of entrapment
Iatrogenic	
Postsurgical arthrofibrosis	Limited range of motion; stiffness. Limited knee extension
Bioabsorbable tacks	Sharp posterior knee pain exacerbated with knee extension. Focal tenderness over points of tack placement; stable knee
Other	
Degenerative joint disease	Pain increases with loading; morning stiffness
	Crepitus; limited range of motion; change in structural alignment

English S, Perret D. Posterior knee pain. Curr Rev Musculoskelet Med 2010;3(1–4):3–10

Pluche JA, Lento PH. Posterior knee pain and its causes: A Clinician's Guide to Expediting Diagnosis. Phys Sportsmed 2004;32(3):23–30

Houghton KM. Review for the generalist: evaluation of anterior knee pain. Pediatr Rheumatol Online J 2007;5:8

Calmbach WC, Hutchens M. Evaluation of patients presenting with knee pain: Part 1. Am Fam Physician 2003;68(3):907–912

9.27 Pregnancy-Related Low Back Pain

Pregnancy-related low backpain can be defined as any type of idiopathic pain arising between the 12th rib and the gluteal folds during the course of the pregnancy. As such, this does not include any situation in which the pain can be attributed to a specific pathological condition (e.g., a disk herniation) that arises either before or during the pregnancy. True sciatica has been diagnosed in 1% of the pregnant population.

Preexisting conditions may be aggravated by pregnancy and may present as low back pain. *Rheumatoid arthritis* can worsen with pregnancy with symptoms usually increasing in intensity postpartum. *Ankylosing spondylitis* can also flare up during pregnancy and present with low back pain. In cases of *idiopathic scoliosis* pregnancy does not affect the progression of scoliosis; however these patients have a slightly increased risk of back pain. Other disease pathologies (*coccidynia, osteomyelitis, osteoarthritis, spontaneous abortion, cancer, urinary tract infection*) may mimic the symptoms of "primary" low back pain associated with pregnancy.

Low back pain with radiation into the buttocks and legs is a common problem during pregnancy. However, low back pain must be carefully **differentiated** from radicular and other neurologic symptoms:

1. Posterior facet syndrome can present with pain radiation down the posterior thigh and mimic radicular pain.
2. Meralgia paraesthetica follows the distribution of the lateral femoral cutaneous nerve and may be confused with referred pain symptoms experienced with low back pain.
3. Muscle syndromes or myofascial pain syndromes: Often cause low back pain and patients may experience discomfort over the affected area and a "ropy" feeling on palpation.
4. Transient osteoporosis of the hip and osteonecrosis of the femoral head: They often potential sources of low back pain, surface in the third trimester, are commonly mistaken for pelvic instability and are of unknown etiology.

Kanakaris NK, Roberts CS, Giannoudis PV. Pregnancy-related pelvic girdle pain: an update. BMC Med 2011;9:15

Kristiansson P, Svärdsudd K, von Schoultz B. Back pain during pregnancy: a prospective study. Spine 1996;21(6):702–709

Albert H, Godskesen M, Westergaard J. Evaluation of clinical tests used in classification procedures in pregnancy-related pelvic joint pain. Eur Spine J 2000;9(2):161–166

9.28 Systemic Diseases Producing Backache

Disease	Effects
Metabolic syndromes	
Diabetes mellitus	Produces polyneuropathy, affects the vasa vasorum of nerve. Dorsal spine disease, manifested by rapid onset of pain, weakness in distribution of one or two nerves of leg (usually femoral and sciatic). Mimics herniated nucleus pulposus
Guillain–Barre syndrome	Acute idiopathic, autoimmune, demyelinating polyneuritis. Produces ascending motor weakness, and in half of the cases patients have bulbar involvement, some needing ventilatory support to sustain life. Polyneuropathy, paresthesia in glove-and-stocking distribution, elevated level of CSF with minimal cellular response
Osteoporosis	Loss of bone mineral content more than what is expected for age and sex matched controls. Causes back pain due to compression fractures of thoracic and lumbar vertebrae with secondary impingement of neural structures, as well as primary bone pain. Marked kyphosis, correction of primary spinal disorder without treating osteoporosis will result in therapeutic failure

(*Continued*)

Spinal Disorders

▶ (*Continued*)

Disease	Effects
Paget's disease	Localized alteration of bone metabolism and architecture. Low back pain without radiculopathy. Spine involved frequently, diagnosis of exclusion
Gout and pseudogout	Diagnosed by aspiration of crystals from articular joints. Rare causes of back pain. Concomitant, acute, peripheral, crystal induced articular pain and spinal pain
Porphyria	Group of inborn error s of metabolism related to heme synthesis. Pain, weakness, and paresthesia in the paraspinous musculature and extremities. Depression, deep tendon reflex suppression, cranial nerve abnormalities, extremity weakness, either single or multiple. Sensory changes include hypoesthesia and anesthesia. Neurodiagnostic studies may be altered
Malignant conditions	Usually metastatic from breast, prostate, lung or thyroid tumors. Malignant tissue replaces bony structures or occurs indirectly as a result of hormonal factors. Perineoplastic syndrome produces pure sensory and sensorimotor neuropathy, primarily in elderly patients and secondary to carcinoma of lung, ovary, breast, stomach, and colon
Infectious diseases	Rarely involve spine. Spinal epidural abscess causes symptoms localized to area of spinal involvement. Increased incidence of infections in diabetic patients. Disc space infections can result from investigative prosses, vertebral osteomyelitis, or Pott's disease. Varicella zoster remains sequestered in paraspinal ganglia after childhood infection and produces dermatomal vesicular eruptions
Inflammatory disorders	
Myofascial pain syndromes	Painful muscle groups associated with trigger points. Pain is produced distal to site of stimulation but within same muscle group
Nonarticular rheumatism	Vague collection of symptoms originating from muscles and tendons as opposed to bones and joints. Myofascial pain syndrome. Fibromyalgia involving the axial skeleton and proximal extremities
Seronegative spondyloarthropathies	Inflammatory rheumatologic disorders, including ankylosing spondylitis, psoriatic arthritis, enteropathic arthropathy, juvenile chronic arthropathy, Behcet's syndrome, and Whipple's disease. Enthesis, secondary infections, sacroiliitis. Men are more likely to have progressive spinal disease and women show peripheral joint manifestations. Low back pain with morning stiffness common, improves with exercise. Diminished mobility of spine in both AP and lateral planes
Reiter's syndrome	Occurs in patients with HLA-B27 positive, diagnosed as a triad of urethritis, conjunctivitis and arthritis. Spondyloarthropathy causing inflammatory oligoarthropathy in young male patients. Sacroiliitis, ascending spinal sacroiliitis disease. May occur with AIDS syndrome

9.29 Differential Diagnosis of Hip and Pelvis Pain in Young and Athletes

Hip joint pain may be perceived in various locations due to its multiple sensory innervations. In general, hip pain is felt in the groin or in the anterior or medial aspect of the proximal thigh, but knee pain can be a predominant feature (i.e., referred pain from the obturator nerve). Pain produced by a pathologic condition in the spine or pelvis is often referred to the hip. Hip pain referred from the lower lumbar vertebrae and sacrum is usually felt in the gluteal region, often radiating down the back or the outer side of the thigh. In contrast, lesions from the upper lumbar vertebrae often refer pain to the proximal anterior hip and thigh region. Intrapelvic or lower abdominal conditions often refer pain to the groin and proximal part of the thigh.

1. Soft-tissue injuries
   a) Contusions
      Soft tissue damage and disruption of underlying muscle fibers are common. Occasionally contusions cause significant muscular hemorrhage, producing prolonged muscle spasm, disuse atrophy, and decreased range of motion. Severe contusions can lead to myositis ossificans, wherein a hematoma develops secondary to trauma. Within 2–8 weeks the calcific flocculations mature into heterotopic bone after injury. Adjacent hip motion may be lost as a result of restricted muscle function.
   b) Muscle strains
      Muscle strains around the hip result from excessive tension/stretching of the muscles beyond their limits. If the injury is on the tendinous part, it is usually painless and involves minimal hemorrhages. If the muscle portion is involved, hemorrhage is always present. Usually there is pain and tenderness on palpation immediately at the time of injury.
   c) Musculotendinous strains
      i. Osteitis pubis: Unusual injury, most commonly seen in soccer players, race walkers and long-distance runners. There is a gradual onset of localized pain around the pubis and extending to the groin, lower abdomen, and occasionally the hip, and in severe conditions adductor spasm develops resulting in a waddling gait.
      ii. Iliac apophysitis: Affects adolescent long-distance runners and manifested by nonspecific pain along the anterior iliac crest.
   d) Sprains
      Ligamentous sprains are rare but should be suspected when there has been a violent injury to the hip.
   e) Hip snaps, clicks, and pops
      Snaps, clicks, and pops around the hip joint are noted mostly in dancers and gymnasts, but they can also be seen in various other athletes. They

are caused by the iliopsoaw snap syndrome, the proximal iliotibial band snap, and the acetabular lateral tears.

f) Bursitis

Numerous synovial lined sacs called bursae overlie bony prominences or separate tendons from muscles in the hip area. These can become inflamed and cause localized pain, tenderness and significant disability. *Bursitis of the greater trochanter* is the most common form in this area and is caused by increased stress in the iliotibial band over the bursa. *The iscial bursa* can become inflamed after a direct blow to the ischial tuberosity, as in a fall on the buttocks, or after prolonged sitting with the legs crossed or on a hard surface ("bench warmer's bursitis"). Pain may often radiate to the hamstrings and to the hip area. *The iliopectineal bursitis* appears after a sudden increase in performance requirements as in tournaments or trying new dance steps. Pain can be referred to the anterior thigh, hip, or knee as a result of adjacent irritation of the femoral nerve.

g) Neuritis

i. Sciatic neuritis occurs in athletes who have little adipose tissue, placing the sciatic nerve at risk of a direct trauma in a fall as the buttocks the floor. The athlete is complaining of pain in the posterior buttocks and hip, associated with paresthesias.

ii. Pyriformis syndrome is irritation of the sciatic nerve as it passes through a tight piriformis muscle. The pain occurs both with active external rotation with resistance and with passive stretch into internal rotation, associated with tenderness and paresthesias on palpation over the piriformis.

iii. Meralgia paressthetica is due to inflammation and trauma of the lateral cutaneous nerve of the thigh from a direct blow to the anterior hip (e.g., from a helmet or fall onto to the hard surface) causing dysesthesias or paresthesias along the lateral thigh down to the knee.

2. Skeletal injuries

a) Avulsion fractures

Avulsion injuries of the hip and pelvis occur more frequently in the competitive athletes in the course of exerting extreme effort, but they generally occur in sprinters, jumpers, and soccer and football players. Pain may be intense.

b) Nonphyseal fractures

Unstable pelvic ring and acetabular fractures, stable pelvic fractures, femoral neck fractures, and subtrochanteric femur fractures all result from violent injury to the athletes. The athlete is disabled and complains of excruciating pain in the hip region. Any attempt to move through the range of motion causes severe pain.

c) Stress fractures

There is a history of high training intensity and frequently a recent increase in the training regimen. Sharp, persistent, progressive pain or a deep, persistent, dull ache located over the bone are the most common symptoms of stress fracture. Common sites are *pubic ramus stress fractures, femoral neck stress fractures and subtrochanteric stress fractures.*

d) Growth plate injuries

Salter–Harris physeal fractures of the proximal femur and acetabulum, and slipped capital femoral epiphysis affect children and adolescents and should be considered in any young athlete who complains of pain in the hip, thigh or groin. Contributing factors include the adolescent growth spurt, a deficiency of sex hormones relative to hormones, excess weight, and sternuous physical activity or after injury such as a fall, tackle, or collision. The patient complains of pain in the region of groin, which is often referred to the anteromedial aspect of the thigh and knee, with associated muscle spasm.

e) Avascular necrosis of the femoral head

Must be considered in any *child athlete* who has a persistent limp and symptoms of intermittent hip pain, involving the groin, anterior thigh and knee, antalgic gait, spasm of the adductor muscles and iliopsoas on the affected side, atrophy of the thigh and buttocks muscles, limited hip motion and flexor contracture. The *adult athlete* has hip pain and a limp, and the mechanism is the mechanical interruption of the blood supply to the femoral head.

Causes also include:

  i. Traumatic interruption of blood supply (i.e., femoral head dislocation, femoral neck fracture)
  ii. Exogenous steroid therapy (i.e., corticosteroids, anabolic steroids)
  iii. Alcoholism
  iv. Dysbaric disorders (i.e., deep sea diving)
  v. Hemoglobinopathies (i.e., sickle cell trait, sickle cell disease, sickle cell thalassemia)
  vi. Lipid storage disease (i.e., Gaucher's disease)
  vii. Cushing's disease
  viii. Pregnancy
  ix. Radiation therapy
  x. Idiopathic (Chandler's disease)

f) Traumatic dislocation of the hip

This injury represents a severe disruption of the hip joint and is seen in such sports as skiing, football, rugby, soccer, and hockey. Acute hip dislocation is one of the few emergencies encountered in sports.

3. Structural abnormalities

Structural abnormalities of the hip can predispose to overuse problems and cause hip pain.

a) Femoral anteversion

The head of the femur is uncovered anteriorly if the patella and knee point straight forward. To bear weight adequately, the leg must be internally rotated to cover the lateral head completely. When walking the patella points medially, and the gait is noticeably intoed, which is of particular concern in ballet dancers and gymnasts.

b) Leg length discrepancy

Athletes with anatomic leg length discrepancy may have developed a compensatory scoliosis, hip abduction contracture on the affected leg, and adduction contracture on the contralateral leg. Athletes with functional leg length discrepancy must be evaluated for primary scoliosis,hip adduction and abduction contractures, and an uneven medial longitudinal arch.

4. Inflammatory disorders

a) Transient synovitis

Acute transient synovitis of the hip is a nonspecific, self-limited condition of unknown etiology although trauma, infection, and allergy may be implicated. Manifests with acute pain in the groin and anteromedial thigh, antalgic gait and painful, restricted hip motion and palpation reveals tenderness over the anterior hip.

b) Septic arthritis

Acute septic arthritis is a true emergency that primarily affects the neonate and young child, although it may occur at any age. There is a history of recent injury or infection, such as otitis media or dermatitis. Patients are unable to bear weight on the affected leg because of severe pain, are apprehensive, irritable, anorectic, and feverish (temperature reaching as high as 104–105°F.

c) Osteoarthritis

It is a common painful condition affecting the hip joint causing significant disability in senior athletes. It is characterized by progressive degenerative changes in the articular cartilage and bone, synovial inflammation leading to capsular fibrosis and restricted motion. Osteoarthritis manifests with progressive pain, more like an aching sensation exacerbated by movement and relieved by rest. Stiffness occurs after rest and then disappears with movement. Patient is easily fatigued with walking, has night pain (which may be the dominant feature), and has tenderness over the anterior and posterior aspect of the hip. Crepitations are often palpable and audible.

5. Pathologic conditions

Pathological conditions present either with an acute fracture through a lesion or with complaints of persistent, activity-related pain similar to that of an overuse injury. Often athletes with pathological fractures are initially treated at a sports facility for a sprain or strain and then later develop the pathologic fracture.

Pathologic bone lesions include: (a) Benign: *osteoid osteoma, osteochondroma, giant cell tumor, and fibrous dysplasia.* (b) Malignant: *osteogenic sarcoma, chondrosarcoma, Ewing's sarcoma, and multiple myeloma.* (c) Metastatic (more common in older people): *carcinoma of the breast, lung, kidney, thyroid, prostate, and colon.* (d) Endocrinopathies: *hyperthyroidism, Paget's disease, osteomalacia, and osteoporosis.*

6. Medical conditions

   a) Pain of urologic origin (*ureteral stone, cystitis, or urethritis*) is often referred to the respective lower abdomen quadrant, groin, hip, medial thigh and the testicle, associated with nocturia, polyuria or dysuria. Appropriate lab tests confirm the diagnosis.

   b) Gynecologic problems (*pelvic inflammatory disease = vaginitis, endometriosis, salpingitis, and ovarian cyst disease, as well as an ectopic pregnancy*) should also be considered. A pap smear and appropriate cultures should be used.

   c) In male patients (*prostatitis, epididymitis, and orchitis*) often present with pain in the groin and medial thigh. Appropriate labs and a physical exam will help with the diagnosis.

   d) Other diseases (*proctitis, perirectal abscess*) cannot be overlooked.

9.29.1 Differential diagnosis of common radiculopathies

Root level	Features		Differential diagnosis
	Clinical	Electrodiagnostic	
C5	Paresthesia/dysesthesia over the deltoid, weak deltoid; ± biceps weakness; decreased biceps muscle strength reflex	Romboids (C5 only), supraspinatus, biceps, infraspinatus, deltoid	Rotator cuff abnormality, acromioclavicular joint, suprascapular nerve, axillary nerve, "stinger", brachial neuritis
C6	Paresthesia/dysesthesia over shoulder to lateral forearm and thumb; weak biceps, wrist decreased biceps and pronator muscle strength reflex	Pronator teres, extensor carpi radialis, brachioradialis biceps; normal extensors; deltoids, supraspinatus, infraspinatus	Carpal tunnel syndrome, "stinger", brachial neuritis, musculocutaneous nerve entrapment

(Continued)

▶ *(Continued)*

Root level	Features		Differential diagnosis
	Clinical	Electrodiagnostic	
C7	Paresthesia/dysesthesia in index and long fingers; decreased triceps muscle strength reflex; weak elbow extension, wrist flexion	Triceps, pronator teres, flexor carpi radialis, extensor digitorum communis, extensor carpi radialis, extensor carpi ulnaris; median flexor carpi radialis H-reflex may be abnormal	Carpal tunnel syndrome, proximal median nerve entrapment
C8	Paresthesia/dysesthesia radiating to ulnar aspect of arm into 4th and 5th digits; weak intrinsics of hand	Extensor digitorum communis, 1st digit, abductor pollicis brevis; prolonged median and ulnar F waves	Ulnar entrapments at elbow or Guyon's canal; thoracic outlet syndrome
T8–10	Paresthesia/dysesthesia in bandlike distribution	Local paraspinals, possibly intercostal muscles	Herpes zoster
L3	Paresthesia/dysesthesia in groin, medial thigh, weak hip flexion	Adductors, iliopsoas	Psoas and adductor strain
L4	Paresthesia/dysesthesia in hip to groin and anterior thigh to medial leg and foot; decreased knee muscle strength reflex; weak knee extensors, ankle dorsiflexors	Anterior tibialis quadriceps	Saphenous nerve entrapment, anterior compartment syndrome
L5	Paresthesia/dysesthesia in back of thigh and anterior tibial region to 1st web space on dorsum of foot; weak ankle dorsiflexion, great toe extension; diminished medial hamstring muscle strength reflex; straight leg raising (SLR) positive	Anterior tibialis hamstrings, hip abductors, tensor fascia lata, medial gastrocnemius; peroneal F wave may be abnormal	Peroneal neuropathy at the fibular head or anterior compartment syndrome
S1	Paresthesia/dysesthesia from hip to posterior thigh and calf to lateral aspect of foot; weak plantar flexors and ankle eversion; diminished ankle muscle strength reflex; straight leg raising (SLR) positive	Gluteus maximus, medial hamstrings, lateral gastrocnemius; ± sural sensory nerve action potential	Deep posterior compartment syndrome, anterior cruciate ligament injury with posterior tibial translation, plantar fasciitis; "chronic" hamstring strain; persistent "tennis leg"

9.30 Juvenile Idiopathic Scoliosis

Juvenile idiopathic scoliosis is essentially a diagnosis of exclusion; to that a detailed medical history, and physical examination, and a careful review of the radiographs will help yield the correct diagnosis.

9.30.1 Differential diagnosis

1. Neurofibromatosis
2. Benign bone tumors (e.g., osteoid osteoma)
3. Malignant or benign intraspinal tumors
4. Spinal infection
5. Connective tissue disease (e.g., Marfan's syndrome, Ehlers–Danlos syndrome)
6. Chromosomal abnormalities (e.g., Down's syndrome)
7. Congenital scoliosis
8. Syringomyelia
9. Tethered cord syndrome
10. Metabolic bone disease (e.g., rickets)
11. Degenerative neurologic conditions (e.g., Fredrich's ataxia, primary muscle disease)
12. Paediatric disc pathology

Ramirez N, Johnston CE, Browne RH. The prevalence of back pain in children who have idiopathic scoliosis. J Bone Joint Surg Am 1997;79(3):364–368

Robinson CM, McMaster MJ. Juvenile idiopathic scoliosis. Curve patterns and prognosis in one hundred and nine patients. J Bone Joint Surg Am 1996;78(8):1140–1148

Herring JA. In Tachdjian's Pediatric Orthopedics from the Texas Scotish Rite Hospitan for Children. 5th ed. Elsevier/Saunders; 2005

9.31 Cervicocephalic Syndrome versus Migraine versus Meniere's Disease

Cervicocephalic syndrome	Migraine	Meniere's disease
Headaches		
Triggered by certain positions of the head	Spontaneous	Spontaneous
Influenced by changes in head position	Cannot be influenced by changes in head position	Cannot be influenced by changes in head position
Short duration (position-dependent)	Persists for hours	Pain persists for hours
Nausea/vomiting		
None	Nausea and vomiting	Vomiting
Spine movements	Spine movements	Spine movements
Limitation of cervical spine motion	Free motion	Not limited
Cervical muscle spasm		
Treatment		
Improvement with cervical traction, cervical collar	Improvement with ergotamine alkaloids	Improvement with 20% glucose infusion and dehydration with loop diuretics (Lasix)

9.32 Differentiation of Spasticity and Rigidity

Spasticity is a component of the pyramidal syndromes. Rigidity is a component of the extrapyramidal syndromes. Brain lesions may affect both pyramidal and extrapyramidal neural pathways resulting in mixtures of spasticity and rigidity, as in cerebral palsy.

Spasticity	Rigidity
Clinical findings	
• Characteristics of hypertonicity	• Characteristics of hypertonicity
Clasp-knife phenomenon (A catch and yield sensation, elicited by a quick jerk of the resting extremity)	Lead-pipe phenomenon (Lead-pipe resistance, elicited by a slow movement of the patient's resting extremity)
Clonus	No clonus
Muscle stretch reflexes: Hyperactive	Muscle stretch reflexes: Not necessarily altered
Extensor toe sign	Normal plantar reflexes
• Distribution of hypertonicity	• Distribution of hypertonicity
Monoplegic, hemiplegic, paraplegic, tetraplegic	Usually in all four extremities, but may have a "hemi" distribution
Predominates in one set of muscles such as flexors of the upper extremity and the extensors of the knee and plantar flexors of the ankle.	Affects antagonistic pairs of muscles about equally
• Associated neurological signs	• Associated neurological signs
None specific	Cogwheeling and tremor at rest
Electrophysiological findings	
EMG	EMG
No muscle activity at complete rest	Electrical activity with the muscle as relaxed as the patient can make it

10 Peripheral Nerve Disorders

10.1 Carpal Tunnel Syndrome

Carpal tunnel syndrome (CTS) is a common clinical condition, occurring in 1 out of 50 people at any one time; over 50% present with bilateral disease. CTS is caused by compression of median nerve in the carpal tunnel. The ulnar nerve is *not* affected, as it lies above the carpal tunnel (▶ Fig. 10.1).

Clinically, CTS presents with numbness, tingling, burning, and dull ache. Symptoms are predominantly in the thumb, index, middle finger, and parts of the ring finger and sometimes the palm as well. Symptoms are most common at night and often relieved by shaking the hands on waking. These symptoms may recur during the day with activities such as driving, carrying objects, or typing. In some people, pain radiates up the forearm, sometimes even up to the neck. Rarely, people get weakness or clumsiness, skin changes (dryness, altered color).

10.1.1 Tests which aid in the diagnosis of CTS

1. Physical tests
   a) Median nerve percussion test (Tinel's sign): The test is positive when tapping the area over the median nerve at the wrist can produce paresthesia in the median nerve distribution. Sensitivity: 28–73%, specificity: 44–95%.

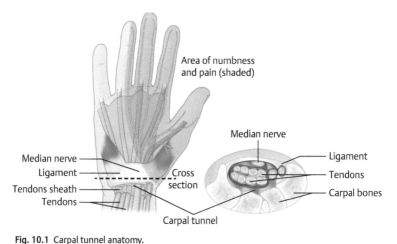

Fig. 10.1 Carpal tunnel anatomy.

b) Carpal tunnel compression test: The test is considered positive when after applying pressure over the carpal tunnel for 30 seconds the patient's sensory symptoms are duplicated. Sensitivity: 87%, specificity: 90%.

c) Phalen wrist flexion test (Prayer sign): It is positive when full flexion of the wrist for 60 seconds produces the patient's symptoms. Sensitivity: 46–80%, specificity: 51–91%.

2. Electrodiagnostic tests
   a) Nerve conduction studies
      These are considered the gold standard in the diagnosis of CTS. This works by comparing the latency and amplitude of a median nerve segment across the carpal tunnel to another nerve segment that does not go through the carpal tunnel, such as the radial or ulnar nerve. A lot of factors, such as age, gender, finger diameter, concurrent systemic disease, obesity and temperature, may influence the amplitude and latency of an individual nerve. This is the most sensitive and accurate technique, with a sensitivity of 80–92% and specificity of 80–99%. However, false negative and false positives result in 16–34% of clinically defined CTS being mixed with NCS.

   b) Electromyogram
      This test is normal (false negative cases) in up to 31% of CTS. Abnormal electromyography (EMG) with increased polyphasicity, positive waves, fibrillation potentials, and decreased motor unit numbers of maximal thenar muscle contraction is considered severe in degree and is an indication for surgery.

3. Ultrasound (US)
   The use of US has been implicated in the diagnosis of CTS because thickening of the median nerve, flattening of the nerve within the tunnel, and bowing of the flexor retinaculum are features diagnostic of CTS. Comparison of the diagnostic utility of US with that of electrodiagnostic studies (EDS) found that the two techniques had almost equal sensitivities (i.e., 67.1 and 64.7% respectively). When these techniques were used together the sensitivity increased to 76.5%. However, a significant flaw is that 23.5% of patients with CTS remained undetected.

4. Magnetic resonance imaging (MRI)
   MRI is excellent for picking up rare pathological causes of CTS (i.e., ganglion, hemangioma, or bony deformity). Furthermore, sagittal images may show accurately and allow the determination of the severity of nerve compression with a sensitivity of 96%, although specificity is extremely low at 33–38%. MRI is able to predict those patients who would benefit from surgical interventions, although the results do not correlate well with

patient's perceived severity of symptoms because MRI provides anatomical information as opposed to information on nerve impairment and function.

10.1.2 Contributing risk factors

CTS remains an idiopathic syndrome, but there are certain risk factors that have been associated with this condition. The most significant of these are:

1. Environmental factors
   a) Prolonged postures in extremes of wrist flexion or extension
   b) Repetitive use of flexor muscles
   c) Exposure to vibration
2. Medical risk factors
   a) Extrinsic factors that increase the volume within the tunnel (outside or inside the nerve)
      i. Pregnancy
      ii. Menopause
      iii. Obesity
      iv. Renal failure
      v. Hypothyroidism
      vi. The use of oral contraceptives
      vii. Congestive heart failure
      viii. Advancing age
      ix. Female gender
      x. Autoimmune diseases (scleroderma, lupus)
   b) Extrinsic factors that alter the contour of the tunnel
      i. Fracture of the distal radius (Colle's fracture)
         – Directly
         – Posttraumatic arthritis
         – Ligamentous or synovial thickening
         – Acromegaly
         – Paget's disease
   c) Intrinsic factors within the nerve that increase the volume within the tunnel
      i. Tumors (neurofibroma, lipoma, xanthoma)
      ii. Tumor-like lesions (aneurysm, hemangioma, gouty tophi)
   d) Neuropathic factors
      i. Diabetes
      ii. Alcoholism
      iii. Vitamin toxicity or deficiency
      iv. Exposure to toxins
      v. Amyloidosis (infiltration of flexor retinaculum)

10.1.3 Differential diagnosis

1. Cervical radiculopathy (C6, C7)
   a) Sensory symptoms (numbness and paresthesia)
      May involve the thumb, index and middle fingers like in CTS although they may often radiate along the lateral forearm and occasionally the radial dorsum of the hand. In cervical radiculopathy, the pins and needles come and go, day and night, in an irregular way, never lasting more than an hour at a time whereas in CTS the pins and needles appear on using the hand. There are no paresthesias at rest, nor are they felt above the wrist.
   b) Pain
      Unlike the CTS, pain in cervical radiculopathy frequently involves the neck and may be precipitated by neck movements. Nocturnal exacerbation of pain is more prominent with CTS. Patients with radicular pain tend to keep their arms and neck still, whereas in CTS patients shake their arms and rub their hands to relieve the pain. Symptoms aggravated by coughing and sneezing are much more likely to be due to cervical radiculopathy than CTS.
   c) Weakness and atrophy
      It involves C6, C7-innervated muscles, not median-innervated C8 muscles. Brachioredialis and triceps tendon reflexes may be decreased or absent in radiculopathy.
   d) In CTS, the symptoms are reproduced by provocative tests:
      i. By tapping over the carpal tunnel (Tinel's signs)
      ii. By flexion of the wrist (Phalen's sign)
      iii. By a blood pressure cuff with compression above systolic pressure; median paresthesias and pain may be aggravated (cuff compression test of Gilliatt and Wilson)
   e) EDS
      They are usually diagnostic although both C6, C7 root compression and distal median nerve entrapment may coexist (double crush injury). Somatosensory evoked response EMG, orthodromic/antidromic etc.
2. Brachial plexopathy
   It is usually incomplete and characterized by the involvement of more than one spinal or peripheral nerve producing clinical deficits such as muscle paresis and atrophy, loss of muscle stretch reflexes, patchy sensory changes, and often shoulder and arm pain which is usually accentuated by arm movement.
   a) CTS versus C6 radiculopathy
      i. The two conditions can coexist

    ii. C6 radiculopathy:
- Neck and shoulder pain
- Weakness in C6-innervated muscles, reflex changes
- Sensory loss restricted to the thumb
- The absence of nocturnal paresthesias and reproduction of the paresthesias with root compression maneuvers

b) Upper plexus paralysis (Erb–Duchenne type)
The muscles supplied by the C5 and C6 roots are paretic and atrophic (i.e., deltoid, biceps, brachioradialis, radialis, and occasionally the supraspinatus, infraspinatus, and subscapularis) producing a characteristic position of the limb: *Porter's tip* position (i.e., internal rotation and adduction of the arm, extension and pronation of the forearm and the palm is facing out and backward). The biceps and brachioradialis reflexes are depressed or absent. There may be some sensory loss over the deltoid muscle area.

c) Lower plexus paralysis (Dejerine–Klumpke type)
The muscles supplied by the C8 and T1 roots are paretic and eventually atrophic (i.e., weakness of wrist and finger flexion and weakness of the small hand muscles) producing a *"claw hand"* deformity. The finger flexor reflex is depressed or absent. Sensation may be intact or lost over the medial arm, forearm, and ulnar aspect of the hand. Ipsilateral Horner's syndrome with injury of the T1 root.

d) Neuralgic amyotrophy (Parsonage–Turner syndrome)
Otherwise known as idiopathic brachial plexitis. It begins typically with a prodrome of severe proximal limb pain followed in 7–10 days by marked weakness in one or more peripheral nerves with little numbness. Typically the distribution is not specifically in the distal median nerve distribution, although more proximal branches of the median nerve, such as the anterior interosseous nerve, may be affected. Such findings, out of the distribution of the median nerve in the carpal tunnel, argue strongly against the diagnosis of CTS. In doubtful cases, EDS can help sort out the pathology. The pain usually disappears within few days. The condition is idiopathic, but it is thought to be a plexitis and may follow viral illness or immunizations.

e) Thoracic outlet syndrome (cervicobrachial neurovascular compression syndrome)
The thoracic outlet syndrome may be purely vascular, purely neuropathic, or rarely, mixed. The true neurogenic thoracic outlet syndrome is rare that occurs more frequently in young women and affects the lower trunk of the brachial plexus. Initially the pins and needles are strictly nocturnal. There is mutational numbness, but hardly any symptoms during the day. This is the release phenomenon, i.e., the paresthesia appears

only after cessation of the compression; the interval is related to the duration of the compression. Intermittent pain in the medial arm and forearm and the ulnar border of the hand is the most common symptom. Paresthesias and sensory loss involve the same distribution. The motor and reflex findings are essentially those of lower brachial plexus palsy, with particular involvement of the C8 root causing weakness and wasting of the thenar muscles similar to CTS. However, in contrast to the latter one, in the thoracic outlet syndrome wasting and paresis also tend to involve the hypothenar muscles which derive innervation from the C8 and T1 roots, and the sensory symptoms involve the medial arm and forearm where the arm discomfort is made worse with movement. EDS reveal evidence of lower trunk brachial plexus dysfunction.

f) Pancoast tumor
   This tumor can be confused with CTS in that the symptoms may be present in the hand, but the neurological distribution will be rather different depending on the specific location of the Pancoast tumor. It would be extremely unlikely for a tumor at the lung apex to specifically affect only the fibers pointing to the median nerve, particularly as some of these come from the medial cord and some from the lateral cord of the brachial plexus.

g) Postradiation neuritis
   Similarly, postradiation neuritis of the brachial plexus can cause extreme pain, hand numbness, and hand weakness, but the pattern will not be limited to the median nerve distribution, and EDS will localize to the plexus and not to the wrist.

3. Proximal medial nerve neuropathy
   a) The pronator teres syndrome
      It results due to the compression of the median nerve as it passes between the two heads of the pronator teres. It is characterized by:
      i. Diffuse aching of the forearm
      ii. Paresthesias in the median nerve distribution over the hand.
      iii. Weakness of the thenar and forearm musculature (ranging from mild involvement to none)
      iv. Pain in the proximal forearm upon forced wrist supination and wrist extension
   b) The lacertus fibrosus syndrome
      Pain in the proximal forearm is caused upon resisting forced forearm pronation of the fully supinated and flexed forearm.
   c) The flexor superficialis arch syndrome
      Pain in the proximal forearm is caused upon forced flexion of the proximal interphalangeal (IP) joint of the middle finger.

d) The anterior interosseous syndrome (purely a motor branch)
   i. Weakness of the flexor pollicis longus (FPL), pronator quadratus, and the median-innervated profundus muscles. Impaired flexion of the terminal phalanx of the thumb and the index finger is characteristic.
   ii. There is no associated sensory loss.
   iii. Excessive supination/pronation seems to aggravate the pain.
e) Entrapment at the elbow (ligament of Struthers)
   i. Weakness of median-innervated muscles, including the pronator teres
   ii. Associated loss of the radial pulse when the arm is extended. Electrodiagnosis:
      – Nerve conduction studies in proximal median nerve compression syndromes are frequently normal.
      – Needle EMG will consistently show neurogenic changes in median innervated forearm and hand median muscles.

4. Intracranial neoplasms
   These can sometimes present with history of numbness or tingling in the hand, weakness in the hand, or loss of coordination in the hand. Often, these findings will be associated with hyperreflexia indicating that the diagnosis is more central. In addition, the pattern of weakness or hypoesthesia will typically not be in a distribution limited to that of the median nerve. Thus, a careful neurological examination, combined with appropriate imaging studies such as MRI, is the key factor in sorting out CNS neoplasia from CTS.

5. Multiple sclerosis
   Multiple sclerosis can be superficially confused with CTS but can be readily distinguished by a careful neurological evaluation, since the diagnosis of multiple sclerosis requires, as its name suggests, multiple events and multiple sites of pathology, none of which would be typical for CTS. Other CNS disorders, such as amyotrophic lateral sclerosis or Charcot–Marie–Tooth (CMT) disease, are pure motor neuropathies that affect distal muscles diffusely, so that all the intrinsic muscles show weakness, and not just those of the thenar eminence.

6. Cervical syringomyelia
   This condition can also be confused with CTS. The characteristic patterns of numbness and weakness, however, are quite different reflecting the cervical spine origin of the symptoms.

7. Tumors within the peripheral nerves
   Peripheral nerve tumors can simulate CTS. This can be particularly difficult if the tumor is within the carpal tunnel as is often the case with lipofibroma-

tous hamartoma of nerve. The key distinction here will be a relatively long history of a mass. Unlike the swelling of the flexor synovium that one can see in CTS, the nerve tumor enlargement will not move with active finger motion. MRI is oftentimes useful in sorting out the diagnosis more specifically.

Amadio PC. Differential diagnosis of carpal tunnel syndrome. Springer-Verlag Berlin; 2007:89–94

Ibrahim I, Khan WS, Goddard N. Carpal tunnel syndrome: A review of the recent literature Open Orthop J 2012;6:69–76

Atroshi I, Gummesson C, Johnsson R, Ornstein E, Ranstam J, Rosén I. Prevalence of carpal tunnel syndrome in a general population. JAMA 1999;282(2):153–158

Burns TM. Mechanism of acute and chronic conversion neuropathy. In: Dyck PJ, Thomas PK, eds. Peripheral Neuropathy. 4th ed. Amsterdam Elsevier; 2005:1391–1402

Werner RA, Andary M. Carpal tunnel syndrome: pathophysiology and clinical neurophysiology. (Review) Clin Neurophysiol 2002;113(9):1373–1381

10.2 Ulnar Neuropathy

Ulnar nerve entrapment is the second most frequent entrapment neuropathy in the upper extremity. The elbow is the most common area of entrapment. Less common sites of entrapment include the arcade of Struthers, the medial intermuscular septum, the medial epicondyle, and the deep flexor pronator aponeurosis (▶ Fig. 10.2).

10.2.1 Ulnar entrapment at the elbow (cubital tunnel syndrome)

The most common location (62–69%) is the nerve entrapment at the epicondylar groove from repeated subluxation of the nerve with elbow flexion over the medial epicondyle. Entrapment of the ulnar nerve as it enters the cubital tunnel is the next most common site (23–28%), and results as it enters the forearm via a narrow opening (cubital tunnel) formed by the medial humeral epicondyle, the medial collateral ligament of the joint, and the firm aponeurotic band to which the flexor carpi ulnaris is attached. Elbow flexion reduces the size of the opening under the aponeurotic band, while extension widens it. The frequency of ulnar nerve compression is increasing, partly due to the use of mobile phones, as the elbow is held flexed for long periods of time. "Tardy ulnar palsy" results from narrowing of the cubital tunnel secondary to an elbow fracture or in osteoarthritis, ganglion cysts, lipomas, or neuropathic (Charcot) joints.

- Total paralysis of the nerve, including branches of the nerve serving the flexor digitorum profundus and flexor carpi ulnaris muscles, causes wasting along the medial side of the forearm.

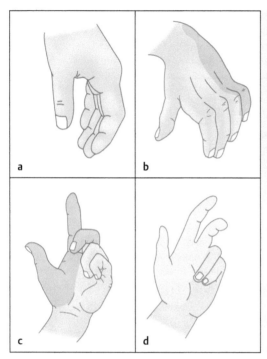

Fig. 10.2 (Clockwise from top left) **(a)** Radial nerve palsy. **(b)** Ulnar nerve palsy. **(c)** Median nerve palsy ("Lover's paresis or Blessing hand"). **(d)** Median and ulnar nerve palsies ("monkey hand").

- Paralysis of the nerve also leads to weakness of flexion of the fourth and fifth fingers; if proximal portions of these fingers are held steady, the patient is unable to flex the terminal phalanges.
- With paralysis of the hypothenar muscles, abduction of the fifth finger is impossible.
- Paralysis of interossei and the medial two lumbricals causes "claw hand" deformity, mainly seen in the ulnar fingers.
- There may be wasting of the hypothenar muscles, interossei, and the medial part of the thenar eminence. Further, there may be weakness in movement of fingers and abduction of the extended thumb against the palm.
- There is sensory loss of the dorsal and palmar aspects of the medial side of the hand together with the medial one and a half fingers.
- With compression of the ulnar nerve, the ulnar nerve is often palpably enlarged in the ulnar groove and for a short distance proximal to the elbow.
- Tinel's sign may be present and finger crossing usually abnormal.

10.2.2 Differential diagnosis

1. Cervical radiculopathy (C8/T1)
    a) May cause sensory symptoms in the fourth and fifth fingers, and also along the medial forearm. Although the elbow is a common C8 referral site, pain is more proximal centering in the shoulder and neck.
    b) Electrodiagnosis
        i. Ulnar sensory potentials in C8 are intact in radiculopathies and no focal conduction abnormalities across the elbow segment.
        ii. Needle EMG demonstrates denervation in C8/T1 median-innervated thenar muscles as well as ulnar-innervated muscles.
2. Thoracic outlet syndrome/lower brachial plexopathy
    a) Sensory symptoms involve not only the fourth and fifth fingers, but also medial forearm.
    b) Weakness involves both the hypothenar and more severely the thenar muscles. If index finger extension is spared, you would tend to think lower trunk, not medial cord.
    c) EDS show normal conduction and a lesion in the lower trunk of brachial plexus.
3. Syringomyelia
    a) Dissociated sensory loss is characteristic with sparing of large-fiber sensation.
    b) Median-innervated C8 motor function is impaired as well as ulnar function. There are often associated long track findings in the legs.
    c) Electrodiagnosis shows normal ulnar sensory potentials due to the preganglionic nature of the lesion.
    d) MRI is diagnostic.
4. Motor neuron disease
    a) Sensory disturbances are not found.
    b) Weakness and wasting of intrinsic hand muscles. Thenar muscles as well as the hypothenar muscles are often affected. Fasciculations may be present indicating the widespread nature of the disease.
5. Ulnar neuropathy at the wrist (Guyon's canal)
    Also known as *handlebar palsy* (seen in cyclists). The wrist is the second most common area of entrapment. It is caused by direct compression of the ulnar nerve in Guyon's canal due to any of the following reasons:
    a) Ganglion cyst (80% of nontraumatic causes)
    b) Lipoma
    c) Repetitive trauma
    d) Ulnar artery thrombosis
    e) Hook of hamate fracture or nonunion/pisiform dislocation

f) Inflammatory arthritis
g) Fibrous band, muscle, or bony anomaly
h) Palmaris brevis hypertrophy

10.2.3 Clinical presentation

- Cutaneous sensation of the hand and fingers is often spared.
- If the lesion is just proximal to the wrist, it causes impaired sensation of the palmar aspects of the hand and the fourth and fifth fingers, and muscle weakness, especially in the hypothenar eminence.
- Clawing of ring and little fingers from loss of intrinsic muscles (adductor pollicis, deep head flexor pollicis brevis, interossei, and lumbricals 4 and 5).
- Weakened grasp from loss of MCP joint flexion power.
- Weak pinch from loss of thumb adduction (as much as 70% of pinch strength is lost).
- Positive Tinel's signs on percussion over the ulnar nerve at the wrist (light percussion over the nerve causes a sensation of "pins and needles" in the distribution of the nerve, i.e., the ulnar side of the hand and the fourth and fifth fingers).
- Positive Phalen's test with paraesthesias in the fourth and fifth fingers (the patient holds their wrist in maximum flexion for 30–60 seconds)
- Froment's sign:
  - IP flexion compensating for loss of thumb adduction when attempting to hold a piece of paper.
  - Loss of MCP flexion and adduction by adductor pollicis (ulnar nerve)
  - Compensatory IP hyperflexion by FPL (anterior interosseous nerve)
- Jeane's sign:
  - A compensatory thumb MCP hyperextension and thumb adduction by extensor pollicis longus (radial nerve)
  - Compensates for loss of IP extension and thumb adduction by adductor pollicis (ulnar nerve)
- Wartenberg's sign: abduction posturing of the little finger
- Electrodiagnosis
  - The most specific study is a prolonged distal motor latency to the first dorsal interosseus compared to the abductor digiti minimi.
  - Needle EMG may demonstrate active or chronic denervation in either thenar or hypothenar muscles with sparing or ulnar-innervated forearm muscles.

Difference between *ulnar tunnel syndrome* and *cubital tunnel syndrome*:
  Cubital tunnel demonstrates:
- Less clawing
- Sensory deficit to dorsum of the hand

- Motor deficit to ulnar-innervated extrinsic muscles
- Tinel's sign at the elbow
- Positive elbow flexion test

Kimura J. Mononeuropathies and entrapment syndromes: In: Kimura J, ed. Electrodiagnosis in Diseases of Nerve and Muscle: Principles and Practice. 3rd ed. Oxford-New York; 2001:711–750

Tagliafico A, Resmini E, Nizzo R, et al. The pathology of the ulnar nerve in acromegaly. Eur J Endocrinol 2008;159(4):369–373

Andreisek G, Crook DW, Burg D, Marincek B, Weishaupt D. Peripheral neuropathies of the median, radial, and ulnar nerves: MR imaging features. Radiographics 2006;26(5):1267–1287

Murata K, Shih JT, Tsai TM. Causes of ulnar tunnel syndrome: a retrospective be study of 31 subjects J Hand Surg Am 2003;28A:647–651

Posner MA. Compressive ulnar neuropathies at the elbow: I. Etiology and diagnosis. J Am Acad Orthop Surg 1998;6(5):282–288

10.3 Claw Hand

(Also known as Spinster's claw or ulnar claw)

It is a common clinical deformity, also known as the "intrinsic minus" hand. This is characterized by hyperextension of the metacarpophalangeal (MCP) joints and flexion of the proximal and distal IP joints (▶ Fig. 10.2).

The ulnar nerve paralysis results in ulnar claw, where the clawing is confined to the little and ring fingers. The high ulnar palsy has less obvious clawing than the low ulnar palsy. There is loss of abduction/adduction of the fingers and wasting of the interosseous muscles, most obvious in the first web space and the hypothenar eminence. There will be numbness in the distribution of the involved nerve or nerves. Frequently in ulnar paralysis, the little finger remains permanently abducted from the ring finger (Wartenberg's sign).

10.3.1 Causes

1. Ulnar nerve palsy
   In this condition, all interossei as well as the ulnar-sided lumbricals are paralyzed, but the median nerve-innervated lumbricals to the index and middle fingers are preserved. As a consequence, the clawing is confined to the ring and little fingers and the thumb. The most common cause of ulnar nerve palsy is wrist laceration. Ulnar nerve compression at the elbow will cause ulnar claw and ulnar sensory loss. Spontaneous ulnar clawing with no sensory loss is most likely due to compression of the motor branch by a ganglion in the region of the pisohamate joint.

2. Paralysis of the ulna and median nerves
   This produces a full claw hand. This deformity will also result from C8 and T1 nerve root lesions.

3. Nerve palsy due to leprosy
   On a worldwide basis, leprosy still remains the most common cause of the claw hand.

10.3.2 Differential diagnosis

Certain conditions mimic the claw hand.

1. **Volkmann's contracture**
   This deep flexor compartment compression syndrome results in ischemic necrosis of the profundus tendons in the forearm causing flexion contracture of the fingers. The superficialis tendons are usually spared, but intrinsic tendons may also be contracted. This produces flexion of all joints of the fingers rather than hyperextension of the MCP joints. The flexor tendons are tight.

2. **Intrinsic muscle contracture**
   This can be of ischemic origin, due to crash injuries and produces the opposite deformity in the claw hand, namely tight intrinsics, or intrinsic plus hand, rather the loose intrinsic minus claw hand. This condition spontaneously occurs in rheumatoid arthritis and may lead to Swan-neck deformity.

3. **Dupuytren's contracture**
   This typically involves the little and ring fingers and can mimic a claw hand, but the MCP joint is flexed and the contracted fingers cannot passively be extended. Palpation of the Dupuytren's tissue in the palm confirms the diagnosis.

4. **Congenital flexion contracture (camptodactyly)**
   This condition usually involves only the little finger, it is often bilateral and is hereditary. It is present at birth. The finger is flexed at the proximal IP joint and often cannot be passively fully straightened.

   a) Spastic hand
      This condition results from an upper motor neuron palsy and usually involves a clasping deformity of the thumb in the palm and tightening of the flexor tendons that cannot be easily passively extended. The wrist is also characteristically flexed.

   b) Neuropathies
      Various muscular dystrophies present as bizarre hand deformities of an atypical type.

Preston DC, Shapiro BE. Proximal, distal, and generalzed weakness. In: Daroff RB, Fenickel GM, Jankovic J, Mazziott JC, eds. Bradley's Neurology in Clinical Practice. 6th ed. Philadelphia PA: Elsevier; 2012:chap 25
Sapienza A, Green S. Correction of the claw hand. Hand Clin 2012;28(1):53–66

10.4 Dupuytren's Contracture

Dupuytren's disease must be distinguished from several other conditions that affect the hand, including trigger finger, stenosing tenosynovitis, a ganglion cyst, or a soft-tissue mass. Unlike Dupuytren's contracture, trigger finger typically involves pain with flexion followed by the inability to extend the affected digit (▶ Fig. 10.3).

Stenosing tenosynovitis may be distinguished from Dupuytren's disease by pain and a history of overuse or trauma. A small, movable nodule that is tender to palpation at the MCP joint is likely a ganglion cyst. A soft-tissue mass must also be excluded from the diagnosis, especially if the patient is significantly younger than the typical patient with Dupuytren's disease and if he or she has no other risk factors.

A patient younger than age 40 years without involvement of the dorsal hand or foot is unlikely to have Dupuytren's disease; however, then possibility of a sarcoma must be ruled out. Although the pathologic findings of a biopsy will most likely reveal a benign etiology (e.g., lipoma, inclusion cyst).

10.4.1 Differential diagnosis

- Epitheliod sarcoma
- Fibroma /neurofibroma
- Lipoma
- Giant cell tumor
- Tendon nodule of stenosing tenosynovitis
- Palmar tendinitis
- Traumatic scar
- Ganglion cyst

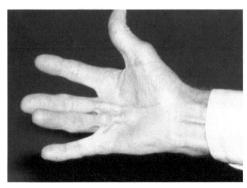

Fig. 10.3 Dupuytren's contracture demonstrating lumps on palm, fascial shortening, puckering, dimpling, and thickening in the palm, with variable flexion deformity of two fingers.

- Callus formation
- Palmar ganglion
- Changes secondary to rheumatoid arthritis
- Hyperkeratosis
- Non-Dupuytren's disease

Rayan GM. Dupuytren disease: Anatomy, pathology, presentation, and treatment. J Bone Joint Surg Am 2007;89(1):189–198

Young DM, Hansen SL. Current diagnosis and treatment: Surgery 13e; In: Doherty GM, ed. Chap 42 Hand Surgery. New York: The Mcgraw Hill Company; 2010

10.5 Radial Nerve Palsy

The radial nerve is a continuation of the posterior cord of the brachial plexus and is composed of fibers from spinal levels C5–C8. It descends beyond the posterior wall of the axilla entering in the triangular space. It then continues distally in the spiral groove of the humerus on bare bone. Within the proximal forearm it gives off the posterior interosseous branch, while it continues in the dorsal forearm giving off branches to the remaining extensor muscles of the wrist and fingers (▶ Fig. 10.2).

1. Compression in the axilla

   Lesions in the axilla affecting the posterior cord of the radial nerve are uncommon. These lesions can result from compression of the nerve by crutches against the humerus or muscles of the axilla ("crutch paralysis"), improper arm positioning during drunken sleep, a pacemaker catheter, missile injuries, shoulder dislocation, or proximal humeral fracture.

   High axillary lesions would result in:

   a) Weakness of triceps and more distal muscles innervated by the radial nerve

   b) Abnormal appearance of the hand (wrist drop)

   c) Hyporeflexia or areflexia of the triceps (C6–C8) and brachioradialis (C5–C6) reflexes

   d) Sensory loss of the extensor area of the arm and forearm and the back of the hand and dorsum of the first four fingers

2. Compression within the spiral groove of the humerus

   Lesions of the radial nerve occur most commonly in this region. The midshaft segment of the radial nerve directly behind humerus is susceptible to direct compression lesions. Lesions are usually due to displaced fractures of the humeral shaft. The most classical radial nerve injuries occur following a drunken sleep during which the arm is left to hang off the bed or bench ("Saturday night" palsy), arm misposition during general anesthesia, or from callus formation due to old humeral fracture. There may be a familial history or underlying diseases such as alcoholism, lead and arsenic poisoning, diabetes mellitus, polyarteritis nodosa, serum sickness, or advanced Parkinsonism.

The clinical findings should be similar to an axillary lesion except that:

a) The triceps muscle and the triceps reflex are normal.
b) Sensibility on the extensor aspect of the arm is normal whereas that of the forearm may or may not be spared depending on the site of origin of this nerve from the radial nerve proper. Lesions distal to the spiral groove and above the elbow just prior to the bifurcation of the radial nerve and distal to the origin of the brachioradialis and extensor carpi radialis longus, produce symptoms similar to those seen with a spiral groove lesion with the following exceptions:
    i. The triceps reflex is normal.
    ii. The brachioradialis and extensor carpi radialis longus muscles are spared.

3. Compression at the elbow

The radial nerve just above the elbow and before its entering to the anterior compartment of the arm, gives off branches to the brachialis, the coracobrachialis and extensor carpi radialis longus before dividing into the posterior interosseous nerve and the superficial radial nerve. The posterior interosseous nerve is the deep motor branch of the radial nerve passing through a fibrous band (the arcade of Frohse) of the supinator muscle in the upper forearm. Entrapment is thought to be due to:

a) A fibrotendinous arch where the nerve enters the supinator muscle (arcade of Frohse)
b) Within the substance of the supinator muscle (supinator tunnel syndrome)
c) The sharp edge of the extensor carpi radialis brevis
d) A constricting band at the radiohumeral joint capsule

There are two recognizable clinical syndromes for this disorder which are discussed in subsequent text.

Radial tunnel syndrome (RTS)

The radial tunnel contains the radial nerve and its two main branches, the posterior interosseous and superficial radial nerves. Forced repeated pronation, supination, or inflammation of supinator muscle attachments (as in tennis elbow) may traumatize the nerve, sometimes by the sharp tendinous margins of the extensor carpi radialis brevis muscle.

Although it is the same posterior interosseous nerve that is being compressed in both RTS and posterior interosseous neuropathy (PIN) syndrome, patients present with altogether different symptoms. Rather than weakness or paralysis as their chief report, patients with RTS typically present with lateral proximal forearm pain which must be distinguished from lateral epicondylitis. It is a pain-only phenomenon with no significant findings on imaging or EDS. The latter are almost always unrevealing in the absence of a PIN syndrome.

The diagnosis is mainly clinical. It is characterized by lateral dull ache deep in the extensor muscle mass of the upper forearm. There is tenderness over the extensor radialis longus muscle just where the posterior interosseous nerve enters the supinator muscle mass. Pain increases with forced supination or with resisted extension of the middle finger (the middle finger test) while the patient's elbow and wrist are extended. Even though the site of entrapment is similar to posterior interosseous neuropathy, unlike it, there is usually no muscle weakness. Operative decompression relieves the symptoms in most patients.

Posterior interosseous neuropathy

Structural pathologies, such as lipomas, ganglia, rheumatoid synovial over-growths, fibromas, and dislocations of the elbow, may all account for compression of the radial and the posterior interossseous nerves at this site resulting in PIN. The latter may also be the result of entrapment. Entrapment is thought to be due to:

a) A fibrotendinous arch where the nerve enters the supinator muscle (arcade of Frohse)
b) Within the substance of the supinator muscle (supinator tunnel syndrome)
c) The sharp edge of the extensor carpi radialis brevis
d) A constricting band at the radiohumeral joint capsule

Clinically, there is marked extensor weakness of thumb and fingers (finger drop). Distinguished from radial nerve palsy by less wrist extensor weakness (no wrist drop) due to sparing of extensor carpi radialis longus and brevis, and while the extensor carpi ulnaris is paretic the wrist will deviate radially. The brachioradialis and supinator muscles are also spared. Sensory loss is not present. Pain may be present at the onset, but is usually not a prominent feature of the syndrome.

Although clinical examination is the key in making diagnosis of PIN syndrome, EDS should be used for additional information. As loss of motor function is the hallmark of PIN syndrome, EMG evaluation is usually positive (in contrast to RTS). EDS may demonstrate slowing of motor conduction across the elbow segment in severe cases or slightly reduced distal motor potential amplitudes. Needle EMG may demonstrate neurogenic change.

Once PIN palsy has been diagnosed, lipomas should be considered as a causative factor, because they are the most commonly reported tumor to cause PIN syndrome. Other sources of compression include ganglia from the anterior capsule, rheumatoid pannus, septic arthritis of the elbow, synovial chondromatosis, and vasculitis. Other more proximal etiologies should be ruled out, such as lesions of the cervical spine (C7 radiculopathy will not produce weakness of the triceps and wrist flexors, unlike a PIN lesion), brachial plexus, and radial nerve proper at the level of humeral shaft. Finally, extensor tendon rupture or extensor digitorum communis tendon subluxation may mimic PIN palsy.

Operative release of the posterior interosseous nerve and lysis of any constrictions including the arcade of Frohse should be employed in cases that do not respond to a 4–8 weeks of expectant management.

4. Radial nerve injury at the wrist

   Wrist injuries frequently involve the superficial radial sensory branch as a consequence of its exposed position (cross the extensor pollicis longus tendon; can often be palpated at this point with the thumb in extension). Tight casts, watch bands, athletic bands, and handcuffs may cause transient compression of the superficial radial sensory branch resulting in anesthesia, hypoesthesia, or hyperesthesia over the dorsum of the radial side of the hand. It is often not the loss of sensation that is troublesome, but the development of painful paresthesias or dysesthesias that is a much more difficult problem and may be resistant to all forms of treatment. Nonsurgical therapy involves the removal of precipitating or exacerbating causes and this often suffices to a spontaneous recovery of radial nerve dysfunction within weeks. Neither steroid injection nor release of the nerve from adhering scar tissue is usually indicated.

5. Differential diagnosis of radial palsies
   a) Cerebral lesion
      i. Dorsal extension is possible during firm grasping of an object as an involuntary synesthesia mechanism.
      ii. Hyperreflexia, pathological reflexes (triceps reflex, finger flexion reflex—Tromner's test, Hoffman's test)
   b) Radiculopathy of C7 root
      i. There is extensor as well as flexor muscle weakness
      ii. Neck pain
      iii. Sensory disturbances
      iv. Associated with weakness of the thenar muscles sometimes
   c) Spinal muscular atrophy
   d) Myotonic dystrophy of Steinert (distal atrophy of the forearm)
   e) Rupture of the thumb and finger extensors that can occur in rheumatoid arthritis
   f) Ischemic muscle necrosis at the forearm
   g) Rheumatologic diseases may mimic neuromuscular weakness of the forearm extensor compartment. For instance, De Quervain tenosynovitis can cause pain in the distribution of the superficial branch of the radial nerve.

Böhringer E, Weber P. Isolated radial nerve palsy in newborns-case report of a bilateral manifestation and literature review. Eur J Pediatr 2014;173(4):537–539

Green's Operative Hand Surgery. 6th ed. In: Wolfe-Hotchkiss et al –Churchill-Livingstone; 2010

Andreisek G, Crook DW, Burg D, Marincek B, Weishaupt D. Peripheral neuropathies of the median, radial, and ulnar nerves: MR imaging features. Radiographics 2006;26(5):1267–1287

Wang LH, Weiss MD. Anatomical, clinical, and electrodiagnostic features of radial neuropathies. Phys Med Rehabil Clin N Am 2013;24(1):33–47

Jou IM, Wang HN, Wang PH, Yong IS, Su WR. Compression of the radial nerve at the elbow by a ganglion: two case reports. J Med Case Reports 2009;3:7258

10.6 Meralgia Paresthetica

(The Bernhardt–Roth syndrome)

The lateral cutaneous nerve is a purely sensory branch arising from the lumbar plexus (L2–L3). It passes obliquely across the iliac muscle and enters the thigh under the lateral part of the inguinal ligament. It supplies the skin over the anterolateral aspect of the thigh.

Meralgia paresthetica is a condition caused by entrapment of this nerve as it passes through the opening between the inguinal ligament and its attachment 1–2 cm medial to the anterior superior iliac spine. Numbness is the earliest and most common symptom. Patients also complain of pain, paresthesias (tingling and burning), and often touch-pain-temperature hypoesthesia over anterolateral aspect of the thigh. It occurs especially in obese individuals who wear constricting garments (e.g., belts, tight jeans, corsets, and camping gear). Intra-abdominal or intrapelvic processes may directly impinge on the nerve during its long course, abdominal distention (as a result of ascites, pregnancy, tumor, or systemic sclerosis), after an intertrachaderic osteotomy and following removal of iliac crest bone graft crest if taken too far close (< 2 cm) to the anterior superior iliac spine.

10.6.1 Differential diagnosis

1. Femoral neuropathy
   Sensory changes tend to be more anteromedial than in meralgia paresthetica, at time extending to the medial malleolus and the great toe.
2. L2 and L3 radiculopathy
   There is usually an associated weakness of knee extension due to quadriceps paresis and also impairment of hip flexion due to iliopsoas weakness.
3. Nerve compression by an abdominal or pelvic tumor
   There are concomitant gastrointestinal or genitourinary symptoms.

Cheatham SW, Kolber MJ, Salamh PA. Meralgia paresthetica: a review of the literature. Int J Sports Phys Ther 2013;8(6):883–893

Erbay H. Meralgia paresthetica in differential diagnosis of low-back pain. Clin J Pain 2002;18(2):132–135

10.7 Femoral Neuropathy

The femoral nerve arises in the lumbar plexus from branches of the posterior division of the L2, 3, 4 roots. The nerve passes between and innervates the iliac and psoas muscles. It then descends beneath the inguinal ligament, just lateral to the femoral artery, to enter the femoral triangle in the thigh, where it divides into the anterior and posterior divisions. The nerve may be damaged by penetrating lacerations or missile wounds, complications of femoral angiography, retroperitoneal tumors or abscesses, irradiation, fractures of the pelvis or femur, surgical table malpositioning, hip arthroplasty, and renal transplantation.

Femoral nerve injury produces weakness of knee extension due to quadriceps paresis. Proximal lesions may also impair hip flexion due to iliopsoas weakness. Sensory loss over the anterior and medial aspect of the thigh, at times extending to the medial malleolus and the great toe. EMG demonstrates neurogenic changes and electrophysiologic studies show reduced motor potential amplitude.

10.7.1 Differential diagnosis

1. High lumbar herniated disc
   a) In pure femoral nerve palsy, the function of the adductors and their reflexes remain intact, whereas in a L2–3 root lesion the adductors are weak.
   b) In an L4 root lesion, the tibialis anterior is also involved.
   c) The distribution of sensory loss is characteristic for each type of lesion.
2. Diabetic neuropathy
3. Lumbar plexus palsies
4. Multiple sclerosis
5. Arthritic muscle atrophy
6. Sarcoma of the proximal femur
7. Sarcoidosis, polyarteritis nodosa, systemic Lupus erythematosus
8. HIV-1 associated multiple mononeuropathies
9. Arthritic muscle atrophy
10. Ischemic infarction of the knee extensors
11. Muscular dystrophy of the quadriceps
12. A lipodystrophy after insulin injection in diabetics

Al-Ajmi A, Rousseff RT, Khuraibet AJ. Iatrogenic femoral neuropathy: two cases and literature update. J Clin Neuromuscul Dis 2010;12(2):66–75

Barr K. Electrodiagnosis of lumbar radiculopathy. Phys Med Rehabil Clin N Am 2013;24(1):79–91

Pendergrass TL, Moore JH. Saphenous neuropathy following medial knee trauma. J Orthop Sports Phys Ther 2004;34(6):328–334

10.8 Peroneal Neuropathy

See section "Foot Drop" in Chapter 9.

10.9 Coccydynia

(Coccyx pain or tailbone pain)

Causes of coccyx pain include trauma, dislocations, and primary or metastatic malignancies. Most of the tumors of the sacrum or coccyx are more likely to be malignant. Sources of acute, abrupt trauma include internal trauma (e.g., giving birth) and external trauma (e.g., falling onto the coccyx). Nonabrupt trauma may include prolonged sitting. Tailbone pain may begin after certain medical procedures, such as colonoscopy. Some cases of coccydynia are idiopathic.

10.9.1 Differential diagnosis

1. Coccygeal fracture
2. Complex regional pain syndrome
3. Endometriosis
4. Fibroid uterus
5. Intracoccygeal dislocation
6. Sacrococcygeal dislocation
7. Intrapelvic malignancy
8. Ischial bursitis
9. Hemorrhoids
10. Lumbar degenerative disc disease
11. Ovarian cyst
12. Pain referred from the sacroiliac joint, lumbosacral area, uterus, or ovaries
13. Perirectal abscess
14. Pilonidal cyst
15. Lumbar facet arthropathy
16. Lumbar spondylosis and spondylolisthesis
17. Mechanical low backpain
18. Piriformis syndrome
19. Proctalgia fugax

Blocker O, Hill S, Woodacre T. Persistent coccydynia–the importance of a differential diagnosis. BMJ Case Rep 2011;2011

Patijin J, Janssen M, Hayek S, et al. Coccygodynia Pain Pract 2010;10(6):554–559

Johnson A, Rochester AP. Coccydynia. J Woman's Health Phys Ther 2006;30(2):40

10.10 Tarsal Tunnel Syndrome

A syndrome resulting from the entrapment and compression of the tibial nerve. Signs and symptoms include burning sensation, tingling, and pain in the sole of the foot.

10.10.1 Anterior tarsal tunnel syndrome

Compression of the deep peroneal nerve as it passes under the extensor retinaculum on the dorsum of the ankle. It is usually related to edema, fractures, ankle sprains, or external pressure from tight boots. This compression results in paresis and atrophy of the extensor digitorum brevis muscle. The terminal sensory branch to the first dorsal web space may be affected, occasionally with Tinel's sign at the ankle (▶ Fig. 10.4).

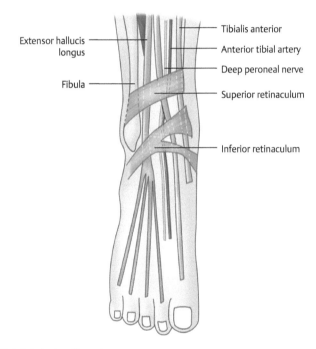

Fig. 10.4 Anterior tarsal tunnel.

10.10.2 Posterior tarsal tunnel syndrome

Compression of the tibial nerve at the ankle behind the medial malleolus where it is covered by the laciniate ligament connecting the distal tibia to the calcaneus. It is usually related to local trauma (17–43%), such as fractures near the ankle, sprains in ankle; arthrosis, tenosynovitis, and rheumatoid arthritis cause (10%) of all cases; tumors (tibial nerve schwannoma) are rare as are ganglia (up to 8%); convoluted vessels are somewhat more frequent (17%). Hypertrophic or accessory muscles and tendons may impinge on the tarsal tunnel and compress the nerve. Diabetes mellitus, hypothyroidism, gout, mucopolysaccharidosis may be precipitating causes. The entrapment results in hypoesthesia in the distribution of the medial and lateral plantar nerves, a positive Tinel's sign with percussion or pressure over the flexor retinaculum below the medial malleolus. EMG and nerve conduction velocities aid in the diagnosis (▸ Fig. 10.5).

10.10.3 Differential diagnosis

1. Polyneuropathy (diabetes)
   Paresthesia of the forefoot is a very common symptom that usually appears bilaterally.
2. L5 and S1 nerve root syndromes (radiculopathy or plexopathy)
   Weakness of dorsal flexion of the toes and atrophy of the extensor digitorum brevis could lead—especially in connection with severe pain—to the assumption of a radicular syndrome L5–S1. The nonradicular pattern of sensory deficit, which, on the contrary, corresponds exactly to the sensory area of the deep peroneal nerve, the absence of Lasegue's sign on clinical examination as well as normal function of the remaining muscles, especially the extensor hallucis longus, should establish the diagnosis.
3. Ischemia
   This possibility due to peripheral vascular diseases that must also be considered.
4. Compartment syndrome of the deep flexor compartment
   This can produce the clinical manifestations of a distal tibial nerve lesion. The pain that arises after walking a certain distance in lumbar spinal stenosis ("neurogenic claudication") is usually bilateral, unlike the pain of tarsal tunnel syndrome.
5. Morton's metatarsalgia
   The typical lancinating, shock-like pain of Morton's metatarsalgia between the third and fourth toes arises on mechanical stress and compression of

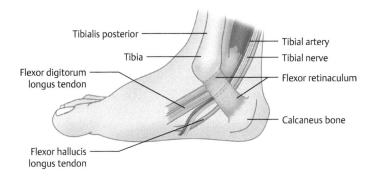

Tibialis posterior

Tibia

Flexor digitorum
longus tendon

Tibial artery

Tibial nerve

Flexor retinaculum

Calcaneus bone

Flexor hallucis
longus tendon

a

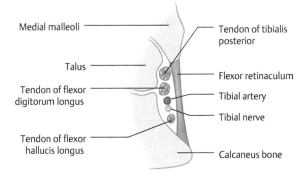

Medial malleoli

Talus

Tendon of flexor
digitorum longus

Tendon of flexor
hallucis longus

Tendon of tibialis
posterior

Flexor retinaculum

Tibial artery

Tibial nerve

Calcaneus bone

b

Fig. 10.5 (a, b) Posterior tarsal tunnel.

the vault of the foot and is thus distinct from the continual burning
dysesthesia of the sole that is found in tarsal tunnel syndrome.

6. Calcaneal spur, arthrosis, inflammatory changes of the fasciae and ligaments
   These problems do not produce pain of a characteristically neuropathic type.

Mumenthaler M. [Tarsal tunnel syndrome. Diagnosis and differential diagnosis] Wien Klin Wochenschr
   1993;105(16):459–461

Krause KH, Witt T, Ross A. The anterior tarsal tunnel syndrome. J Neurol 1977;217(1):67–74

Mahan KT, Rock JJ, Hillstrom HJ. Tarsal tunnel syndrome. A retrospective study. J Am Podiatr Med Assoc
   1996;86(2):81–91

Kushner S, Reid DC. Medial tarsal tunnel syndrome: a review. J Orthop Sports Phys Ther 1984;6(1):39–45

10.11 Morton's Neuroma (Interdigital Neuroma)

The most common presentation of an interdigital (Morton's) neuroma is pain located between the third and the fourth metatarsal heads (in the third interspace) that radiates into the third and fourth toes. Patients often describe this as a burning pain that intermittently "moves around." Usually, the pain is exacerbated by tight-fitting and/or high-heeled shoes or increased activity on the foot. The pain is often relieved by removing the shoe and rubbing the forefoot. Occasionally, these symptoms occur in the second interspace with radiation into the second and third toes. The incidence of interdigital neuromas is 8–10 times more common in females. The mechanism is probably chronic hyperextension of the metatarsophalangeal (MTP) joints (in high heels) with tethering and irritation of the nerve across the transverse metatarsal ligament. This results in an entrapment neuropathy.

10.11.1 Differential diagnosis

1. Neurogenic pain, tingling, or numbness
2. Peripheral neuropathy typically has more global numbness (entire foot or glove and stocking, rather than in the interspace and its two toes, is numb (not painful) unless early in the onset of neuropathy)
   a) Degenerative disk disease often has accompanying motor, sensory, and reflex changes rather than numbness in a single interspace and its corresponding two toes.
   b) Tarsal tunnel syndrome has a positive Tinel's sign over the tarsal tunnel (medial ankle) and numbness limited to the plantar aspect of the foot (no dorsal foot numbness)
   c) Lesions of the medial or lateral plantar nerves
3. MTP joint pathology
   a) Synovitis of the lesser MTP joint(s) from rheumatoid arthritis or non-specific synovitis has tenderness over the metatarsal head or MTP joint rather than interspace.
   b) Fat pad atrophy or degeneration of the plantar fat pad or capsule has tenderness over the metatarsal head or MTP joint rather than the interspace.
   c) Subluxation or dislocation of the lesser PTP joints has tenderness over the metatarsal head or MTP joint rather than the interspace.
   d) Arthritis of the MTP joint has tenderness over the metatarsal head or MTP joint rather than the interspace.
4. Plantar foot lesions (▶ Fig. 10.6 and ▶ Fig. 10.7)
   a) Synovial cysts are usually a tender mass but no numbness or tingling.
   b) Soft-tissue tumors of the interspace: ganglion, synovial cyst, lipoma, soft-tissue neoplasm; usually a tender mass but no numbness or tingling.
   c) Abscess; plantar abscess foot; usually a tender mass but no numbness or tingling

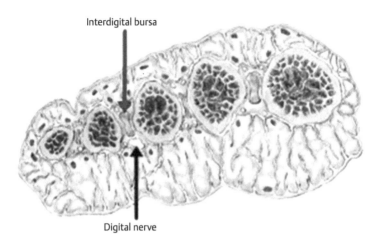

Interdigital bursa

Digital nerve

Fig. 10.6 Coronal section of the right foot across the metatarsal heads.

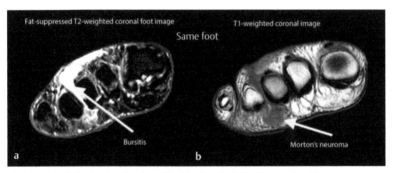

Fat-suppressed T2-weighted coronal foot image

T1-weighted coronal image

Same foot

Bursitis

Morton's neuroma

a

b

Fig. 10.7 MRI of coronal right foot section. **(a)** T2-weighted MRI image: Bursitis appears brighter and has signs of rim enhancement from fluid accumulation due to inflammation. **(b)** T1-weighted MRI image: Morton neuroma appears as a patchy enhancement due to perineural fibrosis usually along the plantar aspect of metatarsal heads.

Zanetti M, Weishaupt D. MR imaging of the forefoot: Morton neuroma and differential diagnoses. Semin Musculoskelet Radiol 2005;9(3):175–186

Sharp RJ, Wade CM, Hennessy MS, Saxby TS. The role of MRI and ultrasound imaging in Morton's neuroma and the effect of size of lesion on symptoms. J Bone Joint Surg Br 2003;85(7):999–1005

Bignotti B, Signori A, Sormani MP, Molfetta L, Martinoli C, Tagliafico A. Ultrasound versus magnetic resonance imaging for Morton neuroma: systematic review and meta-analysis. Eur Radiol 2015;25(8):2254–2262

Bencardino J, Rosenberg ZS, Beltran J, Liu X, Marty-Delfaut E; Morton's Neuroma. Morton's neuroma: is it always symptomatic? AJR Am J Roentgenol 2000;175(3):649–653

10.12 Tingling in Hands and Feet

Tingling in hands, feet, or both is a common and bothersome symptom. Such tingling can sometimes be benign (after pressure on nerves when the arm is crooked under the head as one falls asleep, or when one crosses his legs too long), is usually painless and is soon relieved by removing the pressure that caused it. In many cases, however, tingling in the hands and feet can be severe, episodic, or chronic. It also can accompany other symptoms such as pain, itching, numbness, and muscle wasting. In such cases, tingling may be a sign of nerve damage as a result of trauma, bacterial or viral infections, toxic exposure, and systemic disease.

Such nerve damage is known as peripheral neuropathy, because it affects nerves distant from the brain and spinal cord, often in the hands and feet. Over time, peripheral neuropathy can worsen, resulting in decreased mobility and even disability.

10.12.1 Causes and differential diagnosis

1. Diabetes
   It is one of the most common causes of peripheral neuropathy (30%).
   Tingling and other symptoms often first develop in both feet and go up the legs, followed by tingling and other symptoms that affect both hands and go up the arms. In another 30%, peripheral neuropathy is idiopathic, and the remaining 40% it occurs due to a variety of other causes.
2. Nerve entrapment syndromes
   a) Carpal tunnel syndrome
   b) Ulnar nerve palsy
   c) Peroneal nerve palsy
   d) Radial nerve palsy
3. Systemic diseases
   a) Kidney disorders
   b) Liver disease
   c) Vascular damage and blood diseases
   d) Amyloidosis
   e) Connective tissue disorders and chronic inflammation
   f) Amyloidosis
   g) Connective tissue disorders and chronic inflammation
   h) Hormonal imbalances (including hypothyroidism)
   i) Cancers and benign tumors that impinge on nerves
4. Vitamin deficiencies
   Vitamins E, B1, B6, B12, and niacin are essential for healthy nerve function.
   a) Thiamine: in malnourished, alcoholics, after gastric surgery
   b) Pyridoxine: overdose also causes neuropathy

c) Vitamin E: may be associated with cerebellar syndrome
d) Vitamin B12: predominantly sensory neuropathy, with spinal cord involvement
e) Strachan's syndrome: painful sensory neuropathy, optic neuropathy, and deafness, in association with orogenital dermatitis: reported from tropical countries.
f) Coeliac disease: controversial whether coeliac disease causes neuropathy in the absence of vitamin deficiency.

5. Alcoholism
   Alcoholics are more likely to have a thiamine or other important vitamin deficiencies because of poor dietary habits that commonly causes peripheral neuropathy. It is also possible that alcoholism itself can cause nerve damage, a condition that some researchers call alcoholic neuropathy.

6. Toxins
   a) Heavy metals (lead, arsenic, mercury, and thallium)
   b) Industrial and environmental chemicals (acrylamide, organophosphates, carbon disulfide, organic solvents such as n-hexane and methyl-n-butyl ketone)
   c) Medications
      i. Especially chemotherapy drugs used for lung cancer (Adriamycin, amiodarone, chloroquine, dapsone, disulfiram, ethambutol, gold, isoniazid, metronidazole, platinum: cisplatin and carboplatin, vincristine)
      ii. Some antiviral and antibiotic drugs (nitrofurantoin, nitrous oxide, nucleoside analogue reserve inhibitors, phenytoin, podophyllin, pyridoxine, suramin, thalidomide)

7. Infections
   a) Lyme disease
   b) Shingles (varicella zoster)
   c) Cytomegalovirus infection
   d) Epstein–Barr virus infection
   e) Herpes simplex virus infection
   f) Chronic active hepatitis
   g) HIV /AIDS

8. Autoimmune diseases
   a) Guillain–Barre syndrome
   b) Systemic lupus erythematosus or other connective tissue diseases
   c) Rheumatoid arthritis
   d) Monoclonal gammopathy of undetermined significance

9. Inherited disorders
   These include a group of disorders collectively known as CMT disease.

10. Injury
    Often related to trauma, nerves can be compressed, crushed, or damaged, resulting in nerve pain. Examples include nerve compression caused by a herniated disc or dislocated bone.

10.13 Peripheral Neuropathy

Peripheral nerve diseases are surprisingly common, with a prevalence of symmetrical polyneuropathy of about 2.4%; more in the elderly. While many patients are not severely disabled, pain is common and some forms of neuropathy are progressive, disabling, and ultimately fatal.

Typical symptoms of peripheral neuropathy are numbness and tingling in the feet and hands that may progress proximally with varying degrees of muscle weakness, atrophy, ataxia, painful paresthesias, and autonomic dysfunction. There are different types of peripheral neuropathies that can affect primarily sensory, motor, autonomic, or mixed fibers.

The possibility of peripheral nerve disease comes into the differential diagnosis of sensory, motor, or autonomic symptoms, and of loss of the tendon reflexes. If there are cognitive or visual symptoms, peripheral nerve disease cannot be the only diagnosis, although it may be present as well.

Other conditions that can simulate peripheral neuropathy are disorders of the spinal cord (such as syringomyelia, cervical stenosis, low-grade compressive tumors, as well as multiple sclerosis, tabes dorsalis, and lumbar stenosis producing polyradiculopathy). In the case of a possible motor neuropathy, consideration must be given to amyotrophic lateral sclerosis, myasthenia gravis, or polymyopathy. There may be a history of localized pain, trauma, or associated central neurologic symptoms that may be helpful in suggesting one of these etiologies. Careful clinical examination usually points toward one of these etiologies, particularly the sensory and reflex examinations. Nerve conduction and EMG studies are used to confirm the diagnosis of a peripheral neuropathy, though X-rays and MRIs may also be needed to exclude the presence of any of these other disorders.

10.13.1 Etiology

1. Ischemic neuropathies
   a) Peripheral nerve vasculitis
      In nondiabetics, there has been shown evidence of vasculitis with secondary nerve ischemia.
   b) Diabetes mellitus
      i. Diabetic amyotrophy (proximal diabetic neuropathy or lumbosacral radiculoplexopathy), has been associated with an inflammatory

angiitis, with nerve and muscle biopsy showing inflammatory infiltrates and sometimes necrotizing vasculitis.
  ii. Mononeuropathy multiplex (cranial nerves, thoracic, limb)
  c) Bland microvasculopathy of scleroderma
  d) Temporal arteritis
2. Inflammatory/immune mediated neuropathies
  a) Rapid onset polyneuropathy causes progressive weakness and areflexia within 4 weeks of onset and self-limiting course is acute inflammatory demyelinating polyneuropathy (AIDP); the most common form of Guillain–Barre syndrome. There are a number of autoimmune peripheral neuropathies that are associated with specific antibodies and produce characteristic clinical syndromes.
  b) Sarcoid neuropathy
  c) Multifocal demyelinating neuropathy with persistent conduction block
  d) Multifocal motor neuropathy
  e) Multifocal variants of Guillain–Barre syndrome
  f) Idiopathic brachial or lumbosacral plexopathy
  g) Primary or secondary eosinophilia (eosinophilic fasciitis, myalgia, trichinosis)
  h) Systemic lupus erythematosus
3. Infection-related neuropathies
  a) Leprosy
  b) Lyme disease
  c) Retroviral infection (HIV, HTLV-1)
  d) Herpes virus infection (herpes zoster (HZ), cytomegalovirus)
  e) Infective endocarditis
  f) Others (leptospirosis, hepatitis A, B, and C, *Mycobacterium pneumoniae, Ascaris, Plasmodium falciparum*)
4. Drug-induced neuropathies
  a) Antibiotics (penicillin, sulphonamides)
  b) Cromolyn
  c) Thiouracil
  d) Allopurinol
  e) Interferon-alpha
  f) Drugs of abuse (amphetamines, cocaine, heroin)
5. Hereditary neuropathies
  a) The largest category falls under CMT or also known as hereditary motor and sensory neuropathy (HMSN); CMT 1 is the most commonly seen (1/2,500)
  b) Hereditary neuropathy with liability to pressure palsies (HNPP)
  c) Familial amyloid polyneuropathy (FAP)
  d) CMT 3 (Dejerine–Sottas disease)

e) CMT 2 (axonal HMSN)
f) Hereditary neuralgic amyotrophy (HNA)
g) HNA with relapsing multifocal sensory neuropathy
h) Porphyria
i) Tangier's disease
6. Traumatic neuropathies
   a) Multiple peripheral nerve injuries
   b) Burns
   c) Multifocal entrapments
      i. Diabetes mellitus
      ii. HNPP
7. Neoplasia-related neuropathies
   Paraneoplastic peripheral neuropathies usually produce sensorimotor, axonal, or mononeuritis multiplex neuropathies. Small-cell carcinoma of the lung has been the neoplasm most commonly associated with peripheral neuropathy, but neuropathies have been seen with a variety of other tumors, and polyneuropathy occurring secondary to cancer chemotherapy may sometimes be mistakenly considered to be paraneoplastic. Three groups of neuropathies are associated with solid tumors: a progressive, often painful peripheral neuropathy associated with lung and other neoplasms; a predominantly axonal neuropathy; and a mononeuritis multiplex which represents a vasculitis of nerve, usually seen in small-cell lung carcinoma. A second group of paraneoplastic sensory and motor neuropathies are associated with plasma cell dyscrasias. From all the paraneoplastic antibodies associated with CNS clinical syndromes, the anti-Hu and anti-amphiphysin (motor neuron syndrome) remain the only testable antibodies. The anti-Hu, known as antineuronal nuclear antibodies type I (ANNA-1), are most closely associated with small-cell lung carcinomas, and also prostate cancer, small-cell adrenal cancer, lung adenocarcinoma, neuroblastoma, and chondrosarcoma.
   a) Infiltrative processes
      i. Non-Hodgkin's lymphoma (B cells >T cells)
      ii. Leukemia (T, B, NK cell)
      iii. Angiocentropin lymphoma (B>>T cell)
      iv. Hodgkin's lymphoma (rare)
      v. Multiple myeloma (rare)
      vi. Carcinoma (with leptomeningeal metastases)
   b) Mass lesions
      i. Schwannomas (neurofibromatosis-1, 2)
      ii. Extranodal lymphoma
      iii. Chloroma (granulocytic sarcoma)

8. Other conditions
   a) Warternberg's migrant sensory neuritis
   b) Sensory perineuritis
   c) Cholesterol emboli syndrome
   d) Idiopathic thrombocytopenic purpura
   e) Gastrointestinal conditions (Chron's, ulcerative colitis, celiac sprue)
   f) Radiation plexopathy

10.13.2 Differential diagnosis

1. Distal numbness and paresthesia are commonly caused by peripheral neuropathy but may also be caused by spinal cord disease (e.g., multiple sclerosis), and have to be distinguished from symptoms of hyperventilation.
2. Foot pain in small-fiber neuropathy has to be distinguished from arthritis and ischemic pain.
3. Bilateral weakness of toes and feet is usually due to peripheral neuropathy but can be caused by bilateral L5 root lesions or distal myopathy.
4. The proximal weakness of polyradiculoneuropathy has to be distinguished from muscle disease and from myelopathy.
5. Involvement of the sphincters brings to mind spinal cord disease but can occur with peripheral neuropathy; for example, inability to pass urine and ileus are features of severe Guillain–Barre syndrome.
6. Loss of tendon reflexes is usually due to peripheral neuropathy but also occurs in root lesions, Holmes–Adie syndrome, tabes dorsalis, and spinal shock.
7. In an acute, painful diabetic third-nerve palsy, compression of the nerve from an intracranial aneurysm is the most important condition to enter into the differential diagnosis. Diabetic third-nerve lesions characteristically spare pupillary function, whereas this is not true of compression neuropathy.
8. Diabetic amyotrophy has to be distinguished from cauda equina and other lumbosacral plexus lesions such as malignant invasion. The evolution of diabetic amyotrophy often provides the solution, with a rapid onset and subsequent improvement.

Azhary H, Farooq MU, Bhanushali M, Majid A, Kassab MY. Peripheral neuropathy: differential diagnosis and management. Am Fam Physician 2010;81(7):887–892

Willison HJ, Winer JB. Clinical evaluation and investigation of neuropathy. J Neurol Neurosurg Psychiatry 2003;74(2, Suppl 2):ii3–ii8

Thomas PK. Classification, differential diagnosis, and staging of diabetic peripheral neuropathy. Diabetes 1997;46(Suppl 2):S54–S57

Devigili G, Tugnoli V, Penza P, et al. The diagnostic criteria for small fibre neuropathy: from symptoms to neuropathology. Brain 2008;131(Pt 7):1912–1925

Dyck PJ, Dyck PJ, Grant IA, Fealey RD. Ten steps in characterizing and diagnosing patients with peripheral neuropathy. Neurology 1996;47(1):10–17

10.14 Lumbosacral Radiculopathy

Lumbosacral radiculopathy (LSR) is one of the most common disorders with approximately 3–5% prevalence affecting men and women equally. Degenerative spondyloarthropathies are the principal underlying cause of these syndromes and are increased with age.

In the majority of cases, LSR is caused by compression of nerve roots from pathology in the intervertebral disk or associated structures. The differential diagnosis, however, is broad and includes neoplastic, infectious, and inflammatory disorders.

Sciatica, the classic presenting symptom of LSR, is characterized by a sharp, dull, aching, burning, or throbbing pain in the back, radiating into the leg. Pain related to disk herniation is exacerbated by bending forward, sitting, coughing, or straining and relieved by lying down or sometimes walking. Conversely, pain related to lumbar spinal stenosis characteristically is worsened by walking and improved by forward bending. Pain that is exacerbated by or fails to respond to the recumbent position is a distinctive feature of radiculopathy produced by inflammatory or neoplastic lesions and other nonmechanical causes of backpain. The distribution of pain radiation along a dermatome may be helpful in localizing the level of involvement; when present, the dermatomal distribution of paresthesias is more specific.

10.14.1 Lumbosacral monoradiculopathy

Differential diagnosis
1. L1 radiculopathy
   Extremely rare; disk herniation at this level is uncommon. Features are pain, paresthesias, and sensory loss in the inguinal area without significant weakness.
   Differential diagnoses: include inguinal and genitofemoral neuropathies.
2. L2 radiculopathy
   Disk herniation rare; L2 radiculopathy produces pain, paresthesias, and sensory loss in the anterolateral thigh. Weakness of hip flexion may occur.
   Differential diagnoses: Lateral femoral cutaneous neuropathy (meralgia paresthetica) may mimic L2 radiculopathy; the presence of hip flexor weakness suggests radiculopathy rather than meralgia. Femoral neuropathy and upper lumbar plexopathy may present similarly.
3. L3 radiculopathy
   Disk herniation is an uncommon cause. Pain and paresthesias involve the medial thigh and knee, with weakness of hip flexors, hip adductors, and knee extensors; knee jerk may be depressed or absent.

Differential diagnoses: L3 radiculopathy may be confused with femoral neuropathy, obturator neuropathy, diabetic amyotrophy, or upper lumbar plexopathy. Combined weakness of hip adduction and hip flexion differentiates L3 radiculopathy from femoral and obturator mononeuropathies.

4. L4 radiculopathy

    Produced most commonly by disk herniation. Spinal stenosis frequently involves this nerve root in conjunction with adjacent spinal roots. Sensory symptoms involve the medial lower leg in the distribution of the saphenous nerve. Knee extension and hip adduction may be weak; additionally, foot dorsiflexion weakness uncommonly may be observed. When present, ankle dorsiflexion weakness generally is less prominent than in L5 radiculopathy. The knee jerk may be depressed or absent.

    Differential diagnoses: Lumbosacral plexopathy is the main differential diagnostic consideration; saphenous neuropathy also is pure sensory syndromes.

5. L5 radiculopathy

    The most common cause is disk herniation. Foot drop is the salient clinical feature, with associated sensory symptoms involving the anterolateral leg and dorsum of the foot. In addition to weakness of ankle dorsiflexion, L5 radiculopathy commonly produces weakness of toe extension and flexion, foot inversion and eversion, and hip abduction.

    Differential diagnoses: Common peroneal neuropathy closely mimics L5 radiculopathy. Physical examination may help in localization as weakness of foot eversion (mediated by the L5/peroneal-innervated peroneus muscle) in conjunction with inversion (mediated by the L5/tibial-innervated tibialis posterior) places the lesion proximal to the peroneal nerve. Lumbosacral plexopathy and sciatic neuropathy are important differential diagnostic considerations. The involvement of the hip abductors (gluteus medius and minimus) indicates a lesion proximal to the sciatic nerve but does not differentiate L5 radiculopathy from lumbosacral plexopathy. An asymmetric internal hamstring reflex can support its presence.

6. S1 radiculopathy

    Caused commonly by disk herniation, with associated weakness of foot plantar flexion, knee flexion, and hip extension. Subtle weakness of foot plantar flexion may be demonstrated by having the patients stand or walk on their toes. Sensory symptoms typically involve the lateral foot and sole. The ankle jerk is depressed or absent.

    Differential diagnoses: Sciatic neuropathy and lower lumbosacral plexopathy may mimic S1 radiculopathy. Both of these conditions, however, also are expected to affect L5-innervated muscles.

10.14.2 Lumbosacral polyradiculopathy

The majority of lesions causing lumbosacral polyradiculopathy are compressive in nature and result from disk herniation or spondylosis with entrapment of nerve roots. It is important, however, to recognize a variety of other lesions that may produce LSR including several neoplastic, infectious, and inflammatory disorders. Differential diagnosis

1. Degenerative
   a) Intervertebral disk herniation
   b) Degenerative lumbar spondylosis
2. Neoplastic
   Radiculopathy may result from tumors in various locations within the spinal canal; usually, these lesions are extramedullary. Primary tumors tend to be intradural, whereas metastatic lesions are extradural. Furthermore, primary lesions tend to be solitary (neurofibromatosis 1 being a notable exception), whereas metastatic lesions frequently are multiple.
   a) Primary tumors
   Most are benign and slow growing characterized by back pain, the nature of which is distinctive, as compared to that of disk herniation, as it becomes increasingly severe over time and is worse when lying down, often interacting with sleep. Most frequent tumors are:
   i. Neurofibromas (often associated with neurofibromatosis type 1)
   ii. Ependymomas
   iii. Schwannomas (less common, associated with neurofibromatosis type 2)
   iv. Meningiomas
   v. Lipomas
   vi. Dermoids
   vii. Lipomas
   Ependymomas and neurofibromas typically affect the filum terminale, producing a cauda equina syndrome.
   b) Epidural and vertebral metastases
   The three most common cancers involving the LS spine are breast, lung, and prostate cancers, each accounting approximately for 10–20% of cases, and may produce metastatic spinal cord compression. Tumors in pelvic region, including colon and prostate, preferably metastasize to the LS region. Back pain is the most common complaint and is unremitting and characteristically worse with recumbency. Percussion tenderness at the site of the lesion is noteworthy. Bowel and bladder disturbances occur at onset and become more common with the disease progress. Cancer cells may infiltrate the leptomeninges producing most commonly radiculop-

athy, from involvement of the cauda equine. The most likely primary tumors to do so are leukemia, lymphoma, and breast carcinoma. Other tumors include melanoma, lung cancer, gastrointestinal cancers, and sarcomas.

3. Infectious
   a) Herpes zoster or shingles
      A common disorder prevalent in immunocompromised and elderly populations. Ophthalmic and thoracic dermatomes are affected most commonly, whereas lumbosacral zoster accounts for approximately 20% of cases. The pain of acute HZ, frequently overwhelming at the onset, gradually subsides as the vesicles crust over in most patients.
   b) Spinal epidural abscess (SEA)
      Risk factors include diabetes mellitus, IV drug abuse, spinal surgery, epidural catheter placement, and immunocompromised status. Classical clinical triad of fever, back pain, and neurological deficits is seen in 20% of patients.
   c) Polyradiculopathy in HIV and AIDS
      Polyradiculopathy in AIDS tend to involve the lumbosacral nerve roots, producing a rapidly progressive cauda equina syndrome with severe lower back pain. Other causes of HIV radiculopathy include herpes simplex virus, lymphomatous meningitis, mycobacteria, *Cryptococci*, and treponemal infections.
   d) Lyme radiculopathy
      Seen most commonly in the first 2 months of infection (classic rash of erythema migrans and a flu-like illness) and mimics structural disk herniation.

4. Inflammatory—metabolic
   a) Diabetic amyotrophy
      Type 2 diabetes may cause a syndrome of severe lower extremity (groin, anterior thigh, and lower legs) pain followed shortly after by weakness and weight loss in middle-aged or older patients. Nerve ischemia, inflammation, and metabolic causes are implicated.
   b) Ankylosing spondylitis
   c) Paget's disease
   d) Arachnoiditis
      Classically caused by a reaction to intrathecal oil-based contrast dye for myelography; other causes include neurocysticercosis and other infections, blood in the intrathecal space, surgical interventions in the spine, intrathecal corticosteroids, and trauma.
   e) Sarcoidosis
      Can affect any level of the neuraxis; cauda equina syndrome and lumbosacral polyradiculopathy are manifestations of sarcoid.

5. Developmental
   a) Tethered cord syndrome

      Characterized by an abnormally low-lying conus medullaris tethered to an intradural abnormality. Uncommonly presents in adulthood most often as pain centered around the anorectal or inguinal regions, but sometimes diffusely in the legs or in a radicular distribution.

6. Other
   a) Spinal hematomas

      Uncommon; usually occur in patients who have coagulopathies, who take anticoagulants, who have recently undergone epidural injections or instrumentation of the lumbosacral spine.

   b) Lumbar spinal cysts (incidence 4.6–17%)

      Most sacral meningeal cysts are dural diverticula (Tarlov cysts) may produce radicular pain often relieved when patients are recumbent and aggravated by Valsalva's maneuver.

Van Boxem K, Cheng J, Patijn J, et al. 11. Lumbosacral radicular pain. Pain Pract 2010;10(4):339–358

Barr K. Electrodiagnosis of lumbar radiculopathy. Phys Med Rehabil Clin N Am 2013;24(1):79–91

Lee-Robinson A, Lee AT. Clinical and diagnostic findings in patients with lumbar radiculopathy and polyneuropathy. Am J Clin Med 2010;7(2):80–85

Lin JT, Lutz GE. Postpartum sacral fracture presenting as lumbar radiculopathy: a case report. Arch Phys Med Rehabil 2004;85(8):1358–1361

Pascual AM, Coret F, Casanova B, Láinez MJ. Anterior lumbosacral polyradiculopathy after intrathecal administration of methotrexate. J Neurol Sci 2008;267(1–2):158–161

10.15 Electrophysiologic Abnormalities of the Neuraxis

The electrophysiological findings vary among the diseases that diffusely affect the neuraxis. These include the following:

10.15.1 The anterior horn cell disease

Anterior horn cell diseases include poliomyelitis, motor neuron disease or amyotrophic lateral sclerosis, infantile spinal muscular atrophy (SMA) type I and juvenile SAM types II and III, Werdnig–Hoffman disease; rarely it can occur secondary to Hodgkin's disease or macroglobulinemia.

Motor conduction velocities are normal and as more axons degenerate, the evoked compound muscle action potentials decrease until there is no response at all. Proximal slowing of conduction may be documented by a collision technique or by F wave studies. Typically, the sensory nerve action potentials are normal. The EMG shows diffuse abnormalities in the extremities and occasionally in the bulbar muscles, such as fibrillation potentials, positive sharp waves, complex repetitive discharges; in addition, voluntary effort may produce recruitment patterns, long duration polyphasic, "giant" motor unit potentials and synchronization of motor units. The H reflex is usually evoked easier than in normal individuals and may occur in peroneal and ulnar muscles. Fasciculation potentials at a rate of 5–15 / second triggered by voluntary movement and lasting for hours even during sleep.

10.15.2 Radiculopathy

Most radicular problems are caused by isolated compression of an individual root. Many diffuse polyradiculopathies, however, extend to the proximal aspect of the neuron and technically should be termed a polyradiculoneuropathy. Examples of the latter include Guillain–Barre syndrome, diphtheria, hereditary hypertrophic neuropathy, and diabetes mellitus. Meningeal infiltration by organisms, neoplastic cells, or inflammatory cells after intrathecal injections can also involve multiple roots.

The clinical differentiation of patients with polyradiculoneuropathies from those with polyneuropathy may be difficult. Root involvement may be demonstrated by EMG sampling of paraspinal muscles. In addition, conduction of the proximal segments can be measured using F responses and H reflexes. If the lesion is restricted to the roots, the sensory nerve action potentials are relatively preserved, even in the presence of sensory findings.

10.15.3 Polyneuropathy

Peripheral neuropathies are manifested by motor, sensory, and autonomic symptoms and signs, frequently in a distal or "stocking-glove" distribution. The etiology remains undiagnosed in 24–43% of the patients, even after extensive work-up. In some diseases, there is predominantly myelin dysfunction, i.e., diphtheria, Dejerine–Sottas disease, metachromatic leukodystrophy, Krabbe's globoid leukodystrophy, Guillain–Barre syndrome. Other diseases show primary axonal involvement, i.e., alcoholic polyneuropathy, drug toxicities, amyloidosis, Friedreich's ataxia, metabolic neuropathies such as porphyria. Many diseases, however, have mixed features.
The EDS can:
1. Establish the presence of polyneuropathy
2. Delineate the pattern (i.e., proximal–distal, arms–legs, motor–sensory, symmetric–asymmetric)
3. Distinguish between myelin and/or axonal involvement. The distribution between proximal–distal may be shown by EMG sampling, whereas proximal conduction can be compared with distal conduction by using F responses.

10.15.4 Neuromuscular junction disease

A change in the amplitude of the evoked compound muscle action potential on repetitive supramaximal stimulation is the hallmark of these conditions.

Myasthenia gravis is the most common of the neuromuscular junction diseases. It is clinically characterized by muscular exhaustion after exercise with rapid recovery after rest and after Tensilon (edrophonium) injection. The EDS using repetitive supramaximal stimulation at a rate of 3 per second show a decrement of greater than 10% by the fifth evoked response, which then reach a plateau or increase. After a period of exertion (tetanic or voluntary), the response is increased at first (postactivation facilitation) and subsequently the decrement is exaggerated (postactivation exhaustion). Postactivation exhaustion with a response to rest or anticholinesterase agents has been reported in *multiple sclerosis, amyotrophic lateral sclerosis, hypothyroidism, and McArdle's disease.*

Decrement on repetitive supramaximal stimulation can also occur in many other conditions, such as *hemiplegia, parkinsonism, poliomyelitis, cervical radiculopathy, polyneuropathy, dermatomyositis, polymyositis, and systemic lupus erythematosus.* It also occurs with the use of *Dilantin, antibiotics, carnitine treatment, and other drugs.* With the use of single-fiber EMG, it is possible to record action potentials of individual muscle fibers. The interval between action potentials from two muscle fibers of the same motor unit varies somewhat in normal subjects (*jitter phenomenon*), whereas in myasthenic patients the jitter increases in magnitude, and the second action potential may even be blocked. These single-fiber EMG findings may be the most sensitive, but they are not specific to myasthenia gravis, since they occur in polyneuropathy as well.

Increments on repetitive supramaximal stimulation at rapid rates (20–50/sec) are reported in *Lambert–Eaton myasthenic syndrome* and *botulism.* After a period of exertion (voluntary or tetanic) there is a pronounced facilitation that may be prolonged, but is not followed by exhaustion. Other electrical features are less specific. The initial evoked response is low and may decrease at slow rates of repetitive supramaximal stimulation. On needle EMG, there is a tendency for a decrease in amplitude and duration of the motor unit potentials and an increase in polyphasic characteristics.

10.15.5 Myopathy

Myopathic conditions may be primary or secondary, genetic or acquired, and most frequently affect the proximal musculature and sometimes distal musculature also. Myopathies are associated with EMG changes that include:

1. Motor unit potentials (MUPs) of decreased duration and amplitude, with polyphasic qualities, occurring in abundance even on minimal exertion.

MUPs can occur in nonmyopathic conditions, as in reinnervation, giant axonal neuropathy, botulism, motor neuron disease, and hypokalemic periodic paralysis.

2. A decrease in the total amplitude on maximal effort
3. A decrease in territory of the motor units (using multilead recording). There are many reports of "neuropathic" characteristics, including fibrillation potentials, positive sharp waves, and complex repetitive discharges in conditions considered myopathies. Such findings occur in polymyositis and dermatomyositis, muscular dystrophy, type II glycogenosis, carnitine deficiency, cytochrome-related myopathy, myotubular myopathy, centronuclear myopathy, and other myopathic conditions.

Summary of the electrodiagnostic findings in various diffuse abnormalities

	Anterior Horn cell disease	Radiculopathy	Neuropathy	Neuromuscular junction disorder	Myopathy
Motor unit potentials					
Amplitude/ duration	Markedly increased	Increased	Increased	Occasionally increased	Decreased
(All can have polyphasic potentials)					
Recruitment Pattern	Decreased	Decreased	Decreased	Normal	Increased
At rest					
Fasciculations	Present	Rare	Rare	Absent	Rare
(All can have fibrillation potentials, positive sharp waves, and complex repetitive discharges)					
Conduction studies	Normal or slightly slowed	Normal	Normal, slightly or markedly slowed	Usually normal	Normal
Repetitive Supramaximal stimulation	Usually normal	Normal	Usually normal	Abnormal	Usually normal

It is important to remember that many electrodiagnostic abnormalities to patients with diffuse processes are nonspecific. That is a lesion anywhere in the lower motor neuron—muscle apparatus may be associated with fibrillation potentials, positive sharp waves (during the acute phase), and complex repetitive discharges, plus a tendency to polyphasic qualities in the motor unit potentials.

11 Movement Disorders

11.1 Hyperkinetic Movement Disorders

Disorder	Movement characteristics
Athetosis	Slow, distal, writhing, and involuntary with a propensity to affect the arms and hands
Chorea	Rapid, semipurposeful, graceful, dancelike, nonpatterned moving involving distal or proximal muscle groups
Dystonia	Involuntary, patterned, sustained or repeated muscle contractions, often leading to twisting movements and abnormal posture
Myoclonus	Sudden, brief (< 100 millisecond), shock-like, arrhythmic muscle twitches
Ticks	Brief, repeated, stereotyped muscle contractions that are often suppressible. Can be simple and involve a single muscle group or complex and affect a range of motor activities
Tremor	Rhythmic oscillation of the body part due to intermittent muscle contractions

11.2 Chorea

Chorea has been defined as "a state of excessive, spontaneous, irregular, nonrepetitive, brief, rapid, and randomly distributed movements. These movements may vary in severity from restlessness with mild intermittent exaggeration of gesture and expression, fidgeting movements of the hands, unstable dance-like gait to a continuous flow of disabling, violent movements."

Patients with chorea cannot maintain a sustained posture; when attempting to grip an object, they alternately squeeze and release ("milkmaid's grip"); when attempting to protrude the tongue, the tongue often pops in and out ("harlequin's tongue"); patients involuntarily drop objects frequently and voluntarily augment the choreiform movements with semipurposeful movements in order to mask the chorea. Hypotonia is very common in many conditions causing chorea, but strength is unaffected.

Related terms to chorea are: athetosis, choreoathetosis, and ballismus.

Athetosis (Greek athetos = not fixed) is a slow form of chorea, where the movements have a writhing (i.e., twisting, snakelike) appearance. *Choreoathetosis* is essentially an intermittent form (i.e., moderately slow or moderately rapid chorea). Athetosis without chorea is almost always due to perinatal brain injury (i.e., asphyxia, kernicterus). *Ballismus* (Greek ballismos = jumping about or dancing) is considered a very severe form of chorea presenting with "continuous, violent, coordinated involuntary activity involving the axial and proximal appendicular musculature such that the limbs are flung about." The movement disorders most often involve only one side of the body (i.e., hemiballismus). More typically occur in the elderly hypertensive and/or diabetic patients as a result of stroke involving mainly the subthalamic nucleus. Hemiballismus due to stroke usually remits spontaneously over 3–6 months.

Chorea may commence at any age. (1) Early infancy, (2) at approximately 1 year (the most common age of onset), and (3) during late childhood or adolescence. The pathophysiology causing chorea is attributed to a degeneration or fixed injuries to the striatum (caudate nucleus, globus pallidus, and putamen), or to a biochemical imbalance affecting these parts of the brain.

11.2.1 Differential diagnosis of chorea

1. Genetic disorders
   a) *Huntington's disease (HD)*
      Rare, autosomal dominant, caused by a trinucleotide (CAG) repeat expansion in the gene encoding Huntington on chromosome 4 (*4p16.3*). The cardinal pathologic findings in HD are neuronal loss and gliosis in the cortex and striatum, especially the caudate nucleus. Onset between 20 and 50 years of age, characterized by chorea, personality disorders, cognitive decline leading to dementia, and psychiatric disorders (▶ Fig. 11.1). In 10% cases of HD, the onset is before age 20 (*Westphal variant*); the disease is then characterized by the combination of progressive parkinsonism, dementia, ataxia, and seizures. As the disease progresses, patients develop increasing rigidity and akinesia. Finally, patient becomes bed ridden with marked weight loss and death occurs 15–20 years from onset. Despite the wide spectrum of clinical manifestations of HD, the diagnosis is now straightforward with genetic testing.
   b) *HD-like 2 and other HD-like syndromes*
      Up to 7% of patients bearing striking resemblance to HD do not have the Huntington gene mutation. Dystonia and parkinsonism appear to be more prominent than in HD. HD-L2 is caused by mutations in the gene encoding juctophilin-3, autosomal dominant, and shows increased prevalence among individuals of African ancestry.
   c) *Ataxia telangiectasia*
      It is an autosomal recessive disorder. The responsible gene, called ATM, is on chromosome 11q. Affected individuals develop telangiectasias by 2–4 years of age on exposed areas of skin (frequent infections, vitiligo, café-au-lait spots, premature aging and scleroderma-like lesions) and conjunctiva; progressive cerebellar ataxia, diminished muscle bulk, atonia, choreoathetosis; decreased or absent IgA, IgE, IgG3, IgG4, and lymphoid tissue; and defective cellular DNA repair leading to induced

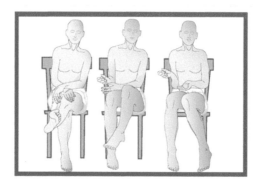

Cardinal Features

- Characterized by involuntary arrhythmic movements of a forcible, rapid, jerky type
- Typically involves distal parts of extremities early, proximal parts later
- Tongue movements and facial grimacing are manifest in advanced cases
- Often incorporated into normal voluntary movements to make less noticeable
- Huntington's chorea, a genetically determined progressive degenerative condition associated with eventual cognitive decline, is classic example

Fig. 11.1 Huntington's chorea. (Reproduced from Chorea. In: Alberstone C, Benzel E, Najm I, et al., ed. Anatomic Basis of Neurologic Diagnosis. 1st edition. Thieme; 2009)

chromosomal aberrations with increased risk of malignancy, particularly leukemia and lymphoma and infection.

d) *Neuroacanthocytosis (choreoacanthocytosis) syndromes*
Neuroacanthocytosis (NA) syndromes present in young/mid adulthood with orofacial tics, behavioral changes, psychiatric disease, subtle cognitive dysfunction, chorea, parkinsonism, and lingual-buccal-facial dystonia with lip and tongue biting develop subsequently. A total of 40% of patients have seizures, peripheral motor neuropathy with areflexia, and muscle atrophy. Typical dystonic tongue protrusion on eating strongly suggests this diagnosis. The autosomal recessive type is most common and is due to mutations of VOS13A localized to chromosome 9. Degeneration of the basal ganglia is a consistent feature.

McLoed syndrome: McLeod NA syndrome is similar in presentation to autosomal recessive NA syndromes, with the additional involvement of other organs. Cardiac involvement develops in two-thirds of these patients, elevation of liver enzymes and frank myopathy. It is diagnosed by decreased expression of Kell and Kx antigens on erythrocytes, caused by mutation of the XK gene.

All the NA syndromes are *differentiated* from:

  i. *Bassen–Kornzweig syndrome*: An autosomal recessive disorder of childhood in which abetalipoproteinemia and acanthocytosis occur along with steatorrhea, retinitis pigmentosa, and cerebellar ataxia

 ii. *Pallidal degeneration syndrome*: Hypobetalipoproteinemia, acanthocytosis, and retinitis pigmentosa, a disease of childhood akin to *Hallervorden–Spatz disease* and a defect in the gene for pantothenate kinase

iii. *HD and HD-L2*

 iv. *Wilson's disease*

e) *Benign familial (hereditary) chorea*

Benign hereditary chorea may develop in childhood, and is not associated with cognitive impairment or other significant neurologic abnormalities apart from mild hypotonia and ataxia. It is transmitted by autosomal dominant inheritance; mutations may be found in the gene for thyroid transcription factor 1 (TITF-1, also NKX2.1) or other genes.

f) *Spinocerebellar ataxia (types 2, 3, or 17)*

Movement disorders can be seen in several of the spinocerebellar ataxias (SCAs) due to trinucleotide repeat expansions/mutations of a variety of genes. Cerebellar findings are typically present, including eye movement abnormalities and gait ataxia. SCA3 (*Machado–Joseph disease*), the *most* common SCA can present with parkinsonism, dystonia, and chorea. Patients with SCA1 and SCA2 may occasionally present with or develop chorea. Parkinsonism, dystonia, and chorea may be seen in SCA17, in addition to the typical phenotype of ataxia, dementia, and hyperreflexia.

g) *Fahr's disease (idiopathic basal ganglia calcification)*

Fahr's disease refers to a heterogeneous group of disorders defined by the radiologic findings of calcium deposition in the basal ganglia and other regions often including the deep cerebellar nuclei. Dystonia, parkinsonism, chorea, ataxia, cognitive impairment, and behavioral changes may be seen. It is likely that several different genes may be implicated, including those for mitochondrial functions.

h) *Wilson's disease*

Chorea may occasionally be seen in Wilson's disease but is not common as a presenting symptom. However, it is essential to exclude this treatable disorder by ophthalmological slit-lamp examination, serum ceruloplasmin, and 24-hour copper excretion.

Differential diagnosis: If work-up for this is negative, then McLeod syndrome, tardive dyskinesia or NA syndrome should be considered.

i) *Neurodegeneration with brain iron accumulation*
Abnormal brain iron accumulation in the basal ganglia is seen in an increasing number of disorders including, *neuroferritinopathy, pantothenate-kinase-associated neurodegeneration, infantile neuroaxonal dystrophy, FA2H-associated neurodegeneration, and aceruloplasminemia.* The diagnostic MRI shows the "eye of the tiger." Clinically, dystonia, parkinsonism, and chorea are characteristic. Retinal degeneration and diabetes mellitus precede these symptoms by about 10 years. Cognitive impairment may be present initially.

j) *Inborn errors of metabolism*
There is a number of metabolic disorders in which movement disorders may be seen, typically in combination with other neurologic features. The presentation may vary with age of onset, dystonia, chorea, and encephalopathy being more prominent at younger ages, often precipitated by febrile illness or medication. The associated neurologic and non-neurologic features help guide the evaluation, which may involve assaying blood and urine for amino acids, lymphocytic enzymes, and/or genetic testing.
    i. Glutamic acidemia
    ii. Propionic acidemia
    iii. Homocystinuria
    iv. Phenylketonuria
    v. Pyruvate dehydrogenase deficiency
    vi. Niemann–Pick C
    vii. Late onset GM1 gangliosidoses and chronic GM2
    viii. Neuronal intranuclear inclusion disease
    ix. Metachromatic leukodystrophy

k) *Lesch–Nyhan syndrome*
Occurs due to mutation of hypoxanthine phosphoribosyltransferase resulting in the accumulation of uric acid. It presents at 3–6 months with psychomotor retardation and hypotonia, with subsequent development of spasticity, dystonia, and choreoathetosis. Self-mutilation with biting of the hands and lips is a classical feature.

l) *Mitochondrial causes of chorea (Leigh's syndrome)*
Leigh's syndrome may be seen with various mutations of mitochondrial DNA. Onset is in early childhood and occasionally adulthood. Presents with acute encephalopathy, psychomotor retardation, hypotonia, spasticity, myopathy, dysarthria, seizures, and dystonia. MRI shows lesions in the thalamus or caudate/putamen.

2. Infectious and postinfectious
   a) *Sydenham's chorea (rheumatic chorea)*
      This condition is seen as a consequence of streptococcal infection (group A β-hemolytic streptococcus) of immune mechanisms—antibodies mistakenly attack cells in the basal ganglia and cause inflammation. Chorea occurs in 26% of children with rheumatic fever between the ages of 7 and 15 years of age. Chorea, hypotonia, dysarthria, and emotional lability are cardinal features. The chorea and psychological disturbances slowly recover over 1–3 months, but may recur. Those who have suffered one or more attacks of Sydenham's chorea are at particular risk of developing it again in adult life during pregnancy (*chorea gravidarum*) or when exposed to drugs such as oral contraceptives, digoxin, or phenytoin. The *diagnosis* is established by the clinical features and cannot be confirmed by laboratory tests. In clinical practice, Sydenham's chorea is the most common form of childhood chorea, whereas HD and drug-induced chorea account for the majority of adult onset cases. *The differential diagnosis* is mainly between Sydenham's chorea, lupus-associated chorea, and drug-induced chorea.
   b) *HIV infection*
      HIV and its complications are the most commonly reported infectious cause of chorea, either as a result of a secondary mass lesion, such as lymphoma or abscess from opportunistic infections (e.g., toxoplasmosis, syphilis, tuberculous meningitis and others) or directly from HIV encephalopathy, or the HIV drug therapy.
   c) *Creutzfeldt–Jakob disease*
      New variant Creutzfeldt–Jakob disease should be considered in an adult with a time course of subacute cognitive and motor deterioration over months.
   d) *Viral meningoencephalitis*
      In children, striatal necrosis may occur as a complication of encephalitis from various infectious agents, including *measles, mumps, parvovirus, mycoplasma pneumoniae, and herpes simplex.*
3. Autoimmune choreas
   The basal ganglia may be vulnerable in systemic autoimmune disorders:
   a) *Systemic lupus erythematosus (SLE)*
      Lupus-associated chorea is the initial feature and appears 7 years before the steady and for 3 consecutive years after the appearance of systemic features of lupus (ataxia, psychosis, and seizures). When chorea is the initial feature of lupus, it must be differentiated from Sydenham's chorea.

b) *Antiphospholipid antibody syndrome (AAS)*
   Chorea may occur in patients with AAS and no other evidence of SLE.
c) *Vasculitis*
d) *Paraneoplastic syndromes*
   As new autoantibodies are being identified, it becomes critical to exclude cancer in a patient with a subacute or acute presentation of chorea, in whom other etiologies have been excluded. *Renal, small cell lung, breast, Hodgkin's, and non-Hodgkin's lymphoma* have been reported as causative. Antibodies detected include anti-CRMP-5/CV2, anti-Hu or anti-Yo.

4. Drug-induced chorea (as a toxic or an idiosyncratic reaction)
   Chorea might result from the use of various drugs, and drug-induced chorea is probably the most commonly encountered type of chorea in neurological practice and in the community.
   a) *Dopamine receptor blocking agents* (phenothiazines, benzamides, butyrophenones)
      Patients with chronic use of these agents develop tardive dyskinesia and generalized chorea as well and 50% or more are irreversible.
   b) *Antiparkinsonian drugs* (L-dopa, dopamine agonists, anticholinergics)
   c) *Anticonvulsants* (phenytoin, carbamazepine, valproic acid, phenobarbital, gabapentin, lamotrigine)
   d) *Central nervous system (CNS) stimulants* (amphetamines, cocaine, phenylphenidate, pemoline, and specifically crack—"crack dancing"—after binging)
   e) *Calcium channel blockers* (verapamil, flunarizine, cinnarizine)
   f) *Typical neuroleptics* (haloperidol, chlorpromazine, and fluphenazine)
   g) *Antiemetics* (prochlorperazine and metoclopramide)
   h) *Estrogen*
      Induces reversible chorea when administered in the contraceptive pill or as hormone replacement therapy, with the same mechanism as in chorea gravidarum.
   i) *Others* (lithium, tricyclic antidepressants, cyclosporin, intrathecal baclofen, intrathecal methotrexate, digoxin)

5. Vascular choreas
   Cerebrovascular disease is regarded as the most common cause of non-genetic chorea, accounting for 50% of cases. Conversely, chorea is a rare complication of acute vascular lesions (> 1% of cases).
   a) *Ischemic or hemorrhagic lesions of the basal ganglia*
   b) *Arteriovenous malformation (AVM)*
      Acquired paroxysmal choreoathetosis precipitated by sound and light was attributed to an AVM of the parietal lobe)

c) *Polycythemia*
d) *Vasculopathies/vasculitis*
   i. Moyamoya disease
   ii. Churg–Strauss syndrome
   iii. Cardiopulmonary bypass—"post-pump chorea" (reversible, usually complication of extracorporeal circulation)
6. Metabolic or toxic encephalopathies
   a) Hyperthyroidism
   b) Hypoparathyroidism
   c) Acute intermittent porphyria
   d) Hypo/hypernatremia and central pontine myelinolysis
   e) Hypocalcaemia
   f) Hypoglycemia and hyperglycemia
   g) Hepatic/renal failure
   h) Carbon monoxide poisoning
   i) Manganese poisoning
   j) Mercury poisoning
   k) Organophosphate poisoning
   l) Vitamin B12 deficiency in infants
   m) Wernicke encephalopathy

Walker RH. Differential diagnosis of Chorea. Curr Neurol Neurosci Rep 2011;11(4):385–395

Cardoso F, Seppi K, Mair KJ, Wenning GK, Poewe W. Seminar on choreas. Lancet Neurol 2006;5(7):589–602

Wild EJ, Tabrizi SJ. The differential diagnosis of chorea. Pract Neurol 2007;7(6):360–373

Beal ME. In: Danel A, ed. Neuroacanthocytosis Syndromes. Springer; 2005

11.3 Dystonia

Dystonia is a disorder characterized by involuntary muscle contractions that cause slow repetitive movements or abnormal postures. The movements may be painful, and some individuals with dystonia may have tremors or other neurologic features. There are several different forms of dystonia that may affect only one muscle, groups of muscles, or muscles throughout the body.

Dystonia can affect many different parts of the body and the symptoms are different depending on the form of dystonia. Early symptoms may include a foot cramp or a tendency for one foot to turn or drag after walking some distance or running, or a worsening in handwriting after writing several lines. Sometimes, both eyes might blink rapidly and uncontrollably; other times, spasms will cause the eyes to close. Symptoms may also include tremor (71%) or difficulties in speaking (12%). The initial symptoms can be very mild and may be noticeable only after prolonged exertion, stress, or fatigue. Over a period of time, the symptoms may become more noticeable or widespread.

The cause of dystonia is not known, but is believed to result from an abnormality in or damage to the basal ganglia or other brain regions that control movement.

One way to classify the dystonia is on the basis of the parts of the body which they affect:

1. Focal dystonia (is localized to a specific part of the body)
   a) *Cervical dystonia* (also called spasmodic torticollis or torticollis)
   b) *Blepharospasm*
   c) *Craniofacial dystonia*

   When dystonia affects the muscles of the head, face, and neck (such as blepharospasm) it is called craniofacial dystonia. The term *Meige's syndrome* is sometimes applied to craniofacial dystonia accompanied by blepharospasm. *Oromandibular dystonia* affects the muscles of the jaw, lips, and tongue. This dystonia may cause difficulties in opening the jaw, and speech and swallowing can be affected. *Spasmodic dystonia* involves the muscles that control the vocal cords, resulting in strained or breathy speech.

   d) *Task-specific dystonias*

   Focal dystonias that tend to occur only when undertaking a particular repetitive activity. Examples include *writer's cramp* that affect the muscles of the hand and sometimes the forearm, and only occurs during handwriting. Similar focal dystonias have also been called *typist's cramp, pianist's cramp, and musician's cramp. Musician's dystonia* is a term used to classify focal dystonias affecting musicians, specifically their ability to play an instrument or to perform. It can involve the hand in keyboard or string players, the mouth and lips in wind players, or the voice in singers.

2. Generalized dystonias (affect most or all of the body)
   a) *Genetic disorders*

   There are several genetic causes of dystonia. Some forms appear to be inherited in a dominant manner. Each child of a parent having the abnormal gene will have a 50% chance of carrying the defective gene, sufficient to cause the chemical imbalance that may lead to dystonia. It is important to note the symptoms may vary widely in type and severity even among members of the same family. Different forms of dystonia that may have a genetic cause are as follows:

   i. *DYT1* dystonia (aka dystonia musculorum deformans or idiopathic torsion dystonia)

   A rare form of dominantly inherited with reduced penetrance (30–40%) and variable expression, caused by mutation in the *DYT1* gene. This form of dystonia typically begins in childhood, affects the limbs first, and progresses, often causing significant disability.

      ii. Dopa-responsive dystonia (DRD) (aka Segawa's disease)
          Individuals typically experience onset during childhood and have progressive difficulty with walking. Some forms of DRD are due to mutations in the *DYT5* gene. Patients have dramatic improvement in symptoms after treatment with levodopa.

      iii. *DYT6* dystonia is caused by *DYT6* mutations and is often presents as craniofacial dystonia, cervical dystonia, or arm dystonia. Rarely a leg is affected at the onset.

      iv. *DYT3* mutation causes dystonia associated with parkinsonism.

      v. *DYT5* (GTP cyclohydrolase 1), which is associated with DRD

      vi. DYT6 (THAP1) associated with several clinical presentations of dystonia

      vii. DYT11, which causes dystonia associated with myoclonus

      viii. DYT12, which causes rapid onset dystonia associated with parkinsonism

  b) *Acquired dystonia* (also called secondary dystonia)
     Result from environmental or other damage to the brain, or from exposure to certain types of medications. Dystonia can be a symptom of other diseases, some of which may be hereditary. Acquired dystonia often plateaus and does not spread to other parts of the body. Drug-induced dystonia often ceases if the medications are stopped quickly. Some causes of acquired dystonia include:

      i. Birth injury (including hypoxia, and neonatal brain hemorrhage.

      ii. Certain infections

      iii. Reactions to certain drugs, heavy metal, or carbon monoxide poisoning

      iv. Trauma (posttraumatic encephalopathy)

      v. Stroke (postischemic encephalopathy)

      vi. Basal ganglia tumors

3. Cervical dystonia (spasmodic torticollis, wryneck, nuchal dystonia)
It is the most common of the focal dystonias, and most often occurs in middle-aged women more than men. The muscles in the neck that control the position of the head are affected, causing laterocollis 42%, retrocollis in 29%, and anterocollis in 25% of the cases; however, the majority of cases (66%) had a combination of these abnormal postures. The neck muscles produce repetitive, patterned, clonic (spasmodic) head movements or tonic (sustained) abnormal postures of the head. It is commonly called spasmodic torticollis, but since it is not always spasmodic and does not always consist of torticollis (neck turning, wryneck), the term cervical dystonia is preferred. Cervical dystonia often begins slowly and usually reaches a plateau over a few months or years. The most common types of dystonia which affects the neck muscles are:

a) *Idiopathic cervical dystonia (ICD)*
   It is the most common form of adult-onset (age group of 31–40 years of age) focal dystonia. Although the pathogenesis is idiopathic, following causes have been hypothesized to play a role:
   i. Genetics
      Observations that support the hypothesis of an abnormal gene include: (i) the presence of individuals with adult-onset dystonia in families with childhood-onset dystonia, (ii) adult-onset dystonia may affect multiple generations, and (iii) the prevalence of focal dystonia is very high in families of patients with idiopathic dystonia.
   ii. Trauma
      The prevalence of patients with cervical dystonia related to trauma is 5–21%. Posttraumatic onset of cervical dystonia occurred within a few days, never relieved for 4 years and there was absence of family history of focal dystonia. Distinguishing acute cervical trauma from traumatic torticollis may be difficult. Postconcussive syndromes self-limited contrary to acute posttraumatic torticollis is usually a chronic syndrome.
   iii. Abnormalities in the lentiform nuclei
      Another possible cause of ICD is bilateral abnormalities in the lentiform nuclei, seen as increased echogenity on transcranial sonography, whereas the MRI is normal.
4. Dystonia secondary to structural causes
   a) *Structural (mechanical)*
      i. Atlantoaxial dislocation
      ii. Cervical spine fracture
      iii. Disc herniation
      iv. Cervical spine abscess (osteomyelitis)
      v. Klippel–Feil syndrome (Congenital—when a child is born, the bones in a child's neck do not form correctly, causing his neck to twist)
   b) *Fibromuscular*
      i. Fibrosis from local trauma or hemorrhage
      ii. Post-radiation fibrosis
      iii. Acute stiff neck
      iv. Congenital torticollis associated with absence or fibrosis of cervical muscles
   c) *Infectious*
      i. Pharyngitis
      ii. Local painful lymphadenopathy
   d) *Neurologic*
      i. Vestibulo-ocular dysfunction (CN IV paresis, hemianopia, nystagmus, or labyrinthine disease)

    ii. Posterior fossa tumor
- Cerebellar astrocytoma
- Cerebellar hemangioblastoma (von Hippel–Lindau disease)
- Ependymoma
- Medulloblastoma

   iii. Cervicomedullary malformations
- Chiari malformation
- Cerebellar malformations (hemisphere hypoplasia, vermal aplasia)
- Atlantoaxial dislocation
- Basilar impression

   iv. Bobble-head doll syndrome (third ventricular cyst)

    v. Spinal cord tumor
- Astrocytomas
- Ependymomas
- Neuroblastomas
- Sarcomas
- Other (neurofibroma, teratoma, dermoid, chondroma)

   vi. Syringomyelia/syringobulbia

  vii. Extraocular muscle palsies, strabismus

 viii. Focal seizures

   ix. Myasthenia gravis

e) *Psychogenic*

Suggestive symptoms include previous somatization, abrupt onset, secondary gain, and absence of sensory trick. Psychogenic dystonia is rare and should be diagnosed with caution.

Albanese A, Barnes MP, Bhatia KP, et al. A systematic review on the diagnosis and treatment of primary (idiopathic) dystonia and dystonia plus syndromes: report of an EFNS/MDS-ES Task Force. Eur J Neurol 2006;13(5):433–444

Jankovic J, Tsui J, Bergeron C. Prevalence of cervical dystonia and spasmodic torticollis in the United States general population. Parkinsonism Relat Disord 2007;13(7):411–416

11.4 Torticollis in Children (Head Tilt)

Torticollis is a clinical symptom and sign characterized by a lateral head tilt and chin rotation toward the side opposite to the tilt (▶ Fig. 11.2). Torticollis can appear temporarily and go away again. It can also be present at birth (congenital). Both boys and girls get all types of torticollis. The differential diagnosis is different for infants than for children and adolescents. Children, infants, and newborns may acquire torticollis from congenital causes or trauma due to childbirth.

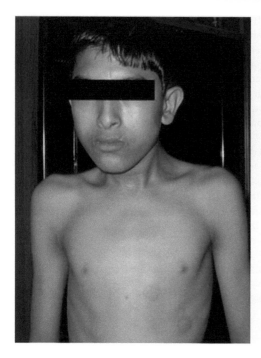

Fig. 11.2 Photo showing a torticollis, short neck, and neck muscles in spasm. (Reproduced from Diagnosis. In: Goel A, Cacciola F, ed. The Craniovertebral Junction. Diagnosis–Pathology–Surgical Techniques. 1st edition. Thieme; 2011.)

11.4.1 Neonates and infants

1. Infant torticollis or congenital muscular torticollis
   Congenital muscular torticollis is the most common cause of torticollis in infants. Boys and girls are equally likely to develop the head tilt. It can be present at birth or take up to 3 months to develop. No one knows why some babies get torticollis and others do not. Most doctors believe it could be related to the cramping of a fetus inside the uterus or abnormal positioning (such as being in the breech position, where the baby's buttocks face the birth canal). The use of forceps or vacuum devices to deliver a baby during childbirth also makes a baby more likely to develop torticollis. These factors put extra pressure on a baby's sternomastoid muscle, causing it to tighten and making it difficult for a bay to turn the neck.
   Differential diagnosis:
   a) Congenital anomalies of the occipital condyles
   b) Congenital anomalies of upper cervical spine (C1 and C2)
   c) Eye muscle imbalance problems

2. Benign paroxysmal torticollis
   It occurs in infants and toddlers with a family history of migraine and is
   remitting spontaneously. The cause is not fully understood. It is believed to
   be a variant closely related to benign paroxysmal vertigo in some infants
   but not in others.
3. Sandifer's syndrome
   Abnormal truncal posturing associated with gastroesophageal reflux,
   neural axis abnormalities, and benign paroxysmal torticollis. Hyperextension or extreme lateral flexion of the trunk occurs during any activity
   including walking, giving bizarre forms of gait. Effective management of
   hiatus hernia and reflux leads to complete resolution of the problem.
4. Klippel–Feil syndrome or hemivertebrae
   Klippel–Feil syndrome is present when *a child is born* (congenital). It
   presents with a head tilt and may have associated cervicothoracic scoliosis,
   and troubled hearing since the bones in their ears may not form correctly.
5. Craniosynostosis
   Craniofacial asymmetry resulting from craniosynostosis, so that the faces of
   some infants with fixed torticollis may look unbalanced or flattened (plagiocephaly). For example, posterior plagiocephaly produces a parallelo-
   gram-shaped head while unilateral lambdoid synostosis produces a
   trapezium-shaped head.

11.4.2 Toddlers and schoolchildren

1. Grisel's syndrome
   Torticollis in the older child is most frequently a manifestation of atlantoaxial rotatory displacement resulting from trauma or oropharyngeal
   inflammation.
2. Intermittent torticollis
   Intermittent torticollis associated with headaches, vomiting, or neurologic
   symptoms may be caused by tumors of the posterior fossa. Benign and
   malignant neoplasms of the upper cervical spine are rare causes of
   torticollis in children, and are associated with corticospianl tract signs.
3. Ocular torticollis
   Children with congenital superior oblique palsy tend to tilt their head away
   from the side of the weak superior oblique muscle to correct diplopia and
   to restore binocular vision.
4. Temporary torticollis
   Retropharyngeal abscesses and pyogenic cervical spondylitis are unusual
   infectious causes of torticollis. For most children, torticollis goes away after
   successful treatment.

5. Torticollis without associated symptoms/signs
   a) Cervical dystonia: It is rare in children but may be seen in older adolescents.
   b) Juvenile rheumatoid arthritis
   c) Sternomastoid injuries
6. Tic and Tourette syndrome (motor tics, attention deficits, obsessive compulsive behavior)

Karmel-Ross K, ed. Torticollis: Differential Diagnosis, Assesment and Treatment, Surgical Management and Bracing. The Haworth Press New York-London; 1997

Huang MH, Gruss JS, Clarren SK, et al. The differential diagnosis of posterior plagiocephaly: true lambdoid synostosis versus positional molding. Plast Reconstr Surg 1996;98(5):765–774, discussion 775–776

Golden KA, Beals SP, Littlefield TR, Pomatto JK. Sternocleidomastoid imbalance versus congenital muscular torticollis: their relationship to positional plagiocephaly. Cleft Palate Craniofac J 1999;36(3):256–261

11.5 Blepharospasm

The most frequent feature of cranial dystonia is blepharospasm. If the dystonia is limited to the eyelids it is termed *essential blepharospasm*. Blepharospasm associated with dystonic movements of other muscle groups of the face, neck or limbs, is known as *Meige's syndrome*. It affects middle or older age women and it never begins in childhood. Blepharospasm in children is almost always drug induced. In most patients, early symptoms include an increase in the frequency of blinking, dry eye symptoms (foreign-body sensations, grittiness and eye irritation) and photophobia. In 25% of patients, the symptoms begin in one eye, but they become bilateral in almost all cases.

1. Occiliar diseases
   a) External
      i. Foreign bodies
      ii. Inflammation (of eyelids, cornea, conjunctiva)
   b) Internal
      i. Uveitis
      ii. Cataract
      iii. Retinal disease
2. Neurologic diseases
   a) Common disorders
      i. Parkinson's disease (PD)
      ii. Postencephalitic PD
   b) Uncommon disorders
      i. HD
      ii. Wilson's disease (hepatolenticular degeneration)

      iii. Hallervorden–Spatz disease

      iv. Multiple sclerosis (MS): A disorder which may cause "writhing" muscle movements anywhere on the face, often called *myotonia* or *myotonic contractions.* These muscle contractions appear "like a worm crawling under the skin" and do not resemble the tonic or clonic facial muscle spasms.

3. Brainstem and diencephalic disease
   a) Ischemia
   b) Demyelination
4. Hemifacial spasm: Characterized by spastic contractions of muscles involving an entire half of the face. Often progresses to show some weakness of the face muscles on the same side, which always follows spasms. Most often due to vascular compression and irritation of the root entry zone facial nerve near the brain stem.
5. Bell's palsy/facial nerve injury with aberrant regeneration: After injury, as this nerve recovers, it may grow back in strange ways (so called *aberrant regeneration*), and cause spasms, something like hemifacial spasm. Repeated episodes of facial weakness on one side of the face or episodes on both sides of the face may indicate a disorder called *Melkersson–Rosenthal syndrome.* Here facial weakness precedes facial spasm.
6. Benign eyelid twitch (eyelid myokymia): Tiny muscle contractions generally affecting one eyelid (more often the lower). Twitching is episodic, lasting seconds to hours over minutes to months, but always eventually resolves on its own. Affected with stress, fatigue, and caffeine use.
7. Gilles de la Tourette's syndrome, other tic disorders
8. Miscellaneous rare associations
   a) Seizure disorders (absence status, partial complex)
   b) Encephalitis
   c) Tetany
   d) Tetanus
   e) Progressive external ophthalmoplegia
   f) Schwartz–Jampel syndrome (osteochondromuscular dystrophy): Infants have a characteristic triad, e.g., blepharophimosis, pursing of the mouth, and puckering of the chin.
9. Drug induced
   a) Neuroleptics (tardive dyskinesia, tardive dystonia)
   b) Dopamine agonists (levodopa)
   c) Nasal decongestants (long-term use)
   d) Sympathomimetics

10. Psychogenic disorder: Hysterical spasms (blepharospasm is only rarely due to psychogenic factors. The diagnosis is difficult, in view of the response to organic blepharospasm stress its common association with depression and the unusual response of the movements to various stimuli)

Jankovic J, Havins WE, Wilkins RB. Blinking and blepharospasm. Mechanism, diagnosis, and management. JAMA 1982;248(23):3160–3164

Pina-Garza JE. Blepharospasm in Felichel's Clinical Pediatric Neurology. 7th ed. Elsevier-Saunders; 2013

11.6 Parkinsonian Syndromes (Hypokinetic Movement Disorders)

11.6.1 Classification of parkinsonism

1. Primary (idiopathic) parkinsonism (▶ Fig. 11.3)
   a) PD
   b) Juvenile parkinsonism
2. Secondary (acquired, symptomatic) parkinsonism
   a) Vascular (multi-infarct)
   b) Infectious (e.g., postencephalitic, slow virus)
   c) Drugs (e.g., antipsychotic, reserpine, α-methyldopa, lithium)
   d) Toxins (e.g., CO poisoning, methanol, ethanol, Hg)
   e) Trauma
   f) Miscellaneous (e.g., brain tumor, normotensive hydrocephalus, syringobulbia, hypothyroidism, parathyroidism)

11.6.2 Multiple system degenerations (parkinsonism-plus syndromes)

1. Progressive supranuclear palsy (PSP) (Steele–Richardson–Olszewski syndrome)
2. Multiple system atrophy
   a) Shy–Drager syndrome (SDS)
   b) Striatonigral degeneration (SND)
   c) Olivopontocerebellar atrophy (OPCA)
3. Corticobasal ganglionic degeneration (CBGD)
4. Autosomal dominant Lewy body disease

11.6.3 Heredodegenerative parkinsonism

1. HD
2. Wilson's disease

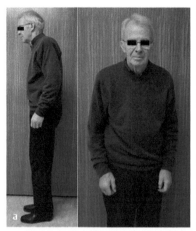
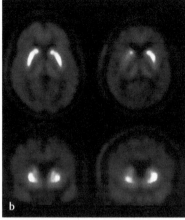

Fig. 11.3 (a) Parkinson disease. Typical posture with stooped head and upper body and lightly flexed elbows, hips, and knees. (b) Hypomimia (paucity of facial expression) and the asymmetry of manifestations that is typical in idiopathic Parkinson disease (the right elbow is somewhat more strongly flexed than the left). (c) An 18F-DOPA-PET scan in a normal person (left, top and bottom) and in a patient with incipient Parkinson disease, worse on the left side of the body (right, top and bottom). The basal ganglia are seen in axial and coronal section (upper and lower rows of images, respectively). The patient with Parkinson disease has a more than 20% reduction in the activity of dopamine decarboxylase in the right putamen (particularly in its dorsal aspect), with relatively normal activity in the caudate nucleus. (Image provided courtesy of Dr. F. Jüngling, PET/CT-Zentrum NW-Schweiz, St. Claraspital, Basel, Switzerland.) (Reproduced from 6.9 Parkinson Disease and Other Hypertonic–Hypokinetic Syndromes. In: Mattle H, Mumenthaler M, Taub E, ed. Fundamentals of Neurology: An Illustrated Guide. 2nd edition. Thieme; 2017.)

3. Hallervorden–Spatz disease
4. Familial basal ganglia calcification
5. Familial parkinsonism with peripheral neuropathy
6. Neuroacanthocytosis

11.6.4 Dementia syndromes

1. Parkinsonism–dementia– amyotrophic lateral sclerosis (ALS) complex of Guam
2. Alzheimer's disease (AD)
3. Creutzfeldt–Jakob disease
4. Normal pressure hydrocephalus

11.6.5 Differential diagnosis of parkinsonism

Parkinson's disease

PD is a progressive neurological disease with the following clinical characteristics:

Manifestations (+)	Possible other features (±)
Bradykinesia	Dystonia
Rigidity	Dysautonomia
Gait disturbance	Dementia
Tremor	Dysarthria/dysphagia
Asymmetric findings	Myoclonus
Levodopa response/dyskinesia	Sleep impairment
Lewy bodies	Family history

The clinical heterogeneity of PD makes it difficult to differentiate it from other parkinsonian disorders based on the clinical criteria alone. The pathological examination may prove the diagnosis of PD wrong in 10–15% of patients. Pathologically, Lewy bodies are present in pigmented neurons of the substantia nigra and other CNS areas. There is a therapeutic response to levodopa, which tends to support the diagnosis of PD (in over 77% of patients the response was "good" or "excellent"), but the drug cannot be used to reliably differentiate PD from other parkinsonian disorders.

Progressive supranuclear palsy

The diagnosis of PSP should be considered in any patient with progressive parkinsonism and disturbance of ocular motility.

The earliest and most disabling clinical symptom relates to gait and balance impairment. Supranuclear downgaze palsy is the most important distinguishing feature of PSP, but it may also occur in diffuse Lewy body disease (DLBD), CBGD, and other atypical parkinsonian disorders.

Manifestations (+)	Possible other features (±)
Bradykinesia	Dystonia
Rigidity	Dysautonomia
Gait disturbance	Sleep impairment
Dementia	Levodopa response
Dysarthria/dysphagia	Putaminal T2 hypointensity
Eyelid apraxia	
Supranuclear downgaze palsy	

The pathological findings reflect neuronal degeneration in the basal nucleus of Meynert, globus pallidus, subthalamic nucleus, superior colliculi, mesencephalic tegmentum, substantia nigra, locus coeruleus, red nucleus, reticular formation, vestibular nuclei, cerebellum, and spinal cord. Neurodiagnostic studies are not helpful in confirming the diagnosis of PSP. Neurochemically the most striking abnormality is a marked depletion of striatal dopamine, reduction in dopamine receptor density, choline acetyltransferase activity, and loss of nicotine (but nor muscarinic) cholinergic receptors in the basal forebrain.

Multiple system atrophy

Multiple system atrophy (MSA) is characterized clinically by the combination of parkinsonian, pyramidal, cerebellar, and autonomic symptoms. Contrary to PD, rest tremor is usually absent and the findings are relatively symmetric. The autonomic symptoms are disabling and help differentiate MSA from other parkinsonian disorders.

The pathological features include cell loss and gliosis in the striatum, substantia nigra, locus coeruleus, inferior olives, pontine nuclei, dorsal vagal nuclei, Purkinje cells of the cerebellum, and Onuf's nucleus of the caudal spinal cord.

Neurochemically low levels of dopamine in the substantia nigra and striatum have been shown in postmortem studies.

Neuroimaging using MRI often reveals areas of bilateral decrease in signal density in the posterolateral putamen on T2WI. Positron emission tomography (PET) studies showed reduced striatal and frontal lobe metabolism.

Shy–Drager syndrome

Dysautonomia is the most characteristic clinical feature of SDS. Patients showed reduced 18F 6-fluodopa uptake, indicating nigrostriatal dysfunction.

Manifestations (+)	Possible other features (±)
Bradykinesia	Ataxia
Rigidity	Dementia
Gait disturbance	Dysarthria/dysphagia
Dysautonomia	Motor neuron disease
Sleep impairment	Neuropathy
Putaminal T2 hypointensity	Oculomotor deficit
Levodopa response	
Lewy bodies	

Striatonigral degenerations

Respiratory dysregulation with laryngeal stridor and sleep apnea are often prominent clinical features in SND. Decreased D2-receptor density was found in patients with SND. Vasomotor impairment in SND has been attributed to selective loss of tyrosine hydroxylase-immunoreactive neurons in the A1 and A2 regions of the medulla oblongata.

Manifestations (+)	Possible other features (±)
Bradykinesia	Dysautonomia
Rigidity	Dystonia
Gait disturbance	Eyelid apraxia
Dysarthria/dysphagia	Motor neuron disease
Putaminal T2 hypointensity	Sleep impairment
Levodopa dyskinesia	
Lewy bodies	

Olivopontocerebellar atrophy

Cerebellar ataxia is the most frequent presenting symptom in patients with OPCA. MRI on T2-WI shows pancerebellar and brainstem atrophy, enlarged fourth ventricle and cerebellopontine angle (CPA) cisterns, and demyelination of transverse pontine fibers. A reduction in dopamine has been found accounting to 53% in putamen, 35% in caudate, and 31% in nucleus accumbens. Mitochondrial deoxyribonucleic acid abnormalities may be important in the pathogenesis of OPCA.

Manifestations (+)	Possible other features (±)
Rigidity	Bradykinesia
Gait disturbance	Tremor
Ataxia	Dysautonomia
Dysarthria/dysphagia	Neuropathy
Oculomotor deficit	Sleep impairment
Putaminal T2 hypointesity	Lewy bodies

Corticobasal ganglionic degeneration

The most striking features of CBGD include marked asymmetry of involvement, movement disorders, cortical sensory loss, apraxias and the "alien limb" phenomenon. Dementia is a late feature.

Manifestations (+)	Possible other features (±)
Bradykinesia	Tremor
Rigidity	Dementia
Gait disturbance	Eyelid apraxia
Dysarthria/dysphagia	Lewy bodies
Dystonia	
Limp apraxia	
Myoclonus	
Oculomotor deficit	
Asymmetric findings	

Neuroimaging with CT scans showed asymmetrical parietal lobe atrophy corresponding to the most affected side in 54% of patients and bilateral parietal atrophy in 40% of them. PET scanning reveals reduced fluorodopa uptake in the caudate and putamen, and markedly asymmetrical cortical hypometabolism, especially in the superior temporal and inferior parietal lobe.

Pathological features of CBGD include neuronal degeneration in the pre- and post-central cortical areas, the basal ganglia, and the presence of achromatic neural inclusions in the cortex, thalamus, subthalamic nucleus, red nucleus, and substantia nigra. There is a clinical and pathological overlap with "parietal Pick's disease."

The dopamine concentration in the striatum and substantia nigra was reduced, when compared with age-matched controls.

Diffuse lewy body disease

DLBD is considered a variant or overlap between AD and PD. Clinical differentiation therefore may be difficult. In most cases with DLBD, however, psychosis and dementia were often found to precede parkinsonism (gait disturbance, rigidity, and resting tremor). The differentiation between DLBD and other parkinsonian syndrome, especially PSP, is particularly difficult when a patient with parkinsonism and dementia is also found to have oculomotor deficit.

Manifestations (+)	Possible other features (±)
Dementia	Bradykinesia
Lewy bodies	Rigidity
	Gait disturbance
	Dysautonomia
	Dysarthria/dysphagia
	Limb apraxia
	Myoclonus
	Oculomotor deficit
	Sleep impairment

Neuroimaging studies, including MRI and PET scan, cannot reliably differentiate among PD, AD, and DLBD. Immunocytochemical staining techniques using antibodies against ubiquitin have improved the identification of Lewy bodies. More than 30% of patients with AD have Lewy bodies in the cortex and substantia nigra, whereas all PD patients have cortical Lewy bodies. In addition to the diffuse distribution of Lewy bodies throughout the basal forebrain, brainstem, and hypothalamus, the lack of neurofibrillary tangles in DLBD helps differentiate it from AD.

Parkinsonism–dementia–amyotrophic lateral sclerosis complex of Guam

Dementia coupled with motor neuron disease are the most frequent presenting features besides the Parkinsonian findings.

Manifestations (+)	Possible other features (±)
Bradykinesia	Ataxia
Rigidity	Dysautonomia
Gait disturbance	Oculomotor deficit
Tremor	
Dementia	
Dysarthria/dysphagia	
Motor neuron disease	

Quinn N. Parkinsonism—recognition and differential diagnosis. BMJ 1995;310(6977):447–452

Braune S. The role of cardiac metaiodobenzylguanidine uptake in the differential diagnosis of parkinsonian syndromes. Clin Auton Res 2001;11(6):351–355

Hughes AJ, Daniel SE, Ben-Shlomo Y, Lees AJ. The accuracy of diagnosis of parkinsonian syndromes in a specialist movement disorder service. Brain 2002;125(Pt 4):861–870

Eckert T, Barnes A, Dhawan V, et al. FDG PET in the differential diagnosis of parkinsonian disorders. Neuroimage 2005;26(3):912–921

11.7 Myoclonus

Myoclonus is a sudden, brief (most often < 100 millisecond), jerky, shock-like involuntary movement. It may be positive or negative. When positive, the cause is the contraction of a single (or a group) agonist and antagonist muscles. When negative, there is transient (< 500 millisecond) interruption of tonic muscle tone, with momentary weakness or loss of postural tone, for example, *asterixix*. Over 27% of myoclonus is transient, mostly from drug adverse effects or metabolic abnormalities. Myoclonus must be *differentiated* from other involuntary movements such as:

1. Ticks: Involuntary repetitive and complex movements of skeletal or oropharyngeal muscles; brief or prolonged and voluntarily suppressible.
2. Chorea: Movements are quick jerk-like always simple in a continuous flow which tend to affect proximal limbs, trunk and facial muscles, and are exacerbated by mental concentration or stress.
3. Tremor: Rhythmic oscillations usually of a limb; can be worse with action (cerebellar dysfunction) or be present at rest.
4. Dystonia: Consists of often painful twisting and turning movements that cause abnormal postures.
5. Exaggerated startle (hyperekplexia): Unexpected stimuli provoke proximal tonic stiffening, often with falls and associated vocalization.

Myoclonus may occur as an epileptic or nonepileptic event. It can be an isolated finding or occur as a symptom of many diseases. Although the majority of cases of myoclonus originate in the CNS, occasional cases of brief shock-like movements clinically indistinguishable from CNS myoclonus occur with spinal cord or peripheral nerve or root disorders.

An **etiologic classification** is summarized as follows:

1. *Benign essential myoclonus*: Has its onset in childhood and adolescence and is inherent autosomal dominant. Dystonia can be part of the clinical picture. The electroencephalogram (EEG) is normal. The jerks are alcohol sensitive and the disease is nonprogressive.
2. *Epileptic myoclonus*: Adolescents presenting with myoclonus may have one of a number of epileptic syndromes or neurological conditions with poor prognosis. They fall into two categories:
   a) Idiopathic generalized epilepsies
      i. Juvenile myoclonic epilepsy (JME)
      ii. Juvenile absence epilepsy (JAE)
         Myoclonic (cortical) seizures are just one of the many seizure types seen. In JME, myoclonic jerks may occur in variable frequency with minimal absences, unlike JAE where absences are the predominant seizure type. Generalized tonic–clonic seizures can occur in both JME and JAE.

b) Progressive myoclonic epilepsies

Rare genetic disorders, usually autosomal recessive, characterized by myoclonic jerks, tonic–clonic seizures and progressive neurological deterioration, especially cerebellar signs and dementia. The five principal causes are:

    i. Unverricht–Lundborg disease
    ii. Lafora disease
    iii. Myoclonic epilepsy with ragged red fibers (MERRF)
    iv. Neuronal ceroid lipofuscinosis (NCL)
    v. Sialidosis

3. *Secondary (symptomatic) myoclonus*: It occurs as a result of an underlying medical problem.

    a) Cortical, brain stem, or spinal cord lesions such as tumors, AVMs, encephalitis, ischemia, or inflammation.

    b) Basal ganglia degenerations such as multiple system atrophy, CBGD, HD, Hallervorden–Spatz disease, and PD.

    c) Spinocerebellar degenerations

    d) Dementias such as AD, Creutzfeldt–Jakob disease, and Gerstmann–Straussler–Schenker disease.

    e) Toxic encephalopathies such as a bismuth, heavy metal, methyl bromide poisoning, or drug induced such as levodopa, carbamazepine, tricyclic antidepressants, or serotonin reuptake inhibitors.

    f) Metabolic derangements such as a hepatic and renal disease, hyponatremia, hypoglycemia, dialysis syndrome from aluminum toxicity, multiple carboxylase deficiency, biotin deficiency, and mitochondrial encephalopathies.

    g) Encephalitides such as subacute sclerosing panencephalitis, herpes simplex encephalitis, subacute necrotizing encephalopathy or Leigh disease, Arbor virus encephalitis, encephalitis lethargica and others

    h) Posthypoxic encephalopathy (Lance–Adams syndrome)

4. *Physiological myoclonus*: Refers to muscle jerks occurring in normal subjects. Examples include hiccups, sneezes, or sleep starts (hypnic jerks) or during sleep (nocturnal myoclonus) and during times of anxiety.

5. *Psychogenic myoclonus*: It represents a voluntary muscle jerk. About 8% of myoclonus is psychogenic.

Krishnakumar D. Diagnostic approach to an adolescent with myoclonus. ACNR 2010;10(4):39–41

11.8 Tourette Syndrome and Other Tic Disorders

Tourette syndrome (TS) is a familial neuropsychiatric disorder that is characterized by motor and phonic tics (involuntary, rapid, repetitive, and stereotyped movements of individual muscle groups) that begin in childhood. Evidence points toward a spectrum of TS symptomatology that extends beyond the tics disorder to probably include obsessive compulsive disorder (OCD), attention deficit hyperactivity disorder (ADHD), and mood disorders.

Tic disorders are classified on a spectrum based on severity:

1. *Transient tic disorders*: Common motor tics (eye blinking, nose puckering, facial grimacing) and/or vocalizations (throat sounds, sniffing, grunting, and coughing) that last only a few weeks or months and certainly do not persist for more than 1 year. They are especially noticeable during times of excitement or fatigue. Boys are affected 3–4 times more often than girls.

2. *Chronic tic disorders*: These are differentiated from transient tic disorders not only by their duration over many years, but by their relatively unchanging character. While transient tic come and go (sniffing may be replaced by forehead furrowing), chronic tics such as facial contortions or blinking may persist unchanged for years.

3. *Tourette syndrome (TS):* It can be the most debilitating tic disorder and is characterized by multiform, frequency changing motor and phonic tics. The most distressing and most well-known complex vocal symptom in TS is coprolalia which is involuntary swearing. Some patients with TS imitate what they have just seen (echopraxia), heard (echolalia), or said (palilalia).

TS is a genetic disorder with an autosomal dominant pattern of inheritance. According to the DSM IV-TR the diagnostic criteria are:

Both multiple motor and one or more vocal tics have been present at sometimes during the illness, although not necessarily concurrently.

1. The tics occur many times a day (usually in bouts) nearly every day or intermittently throughout a period of more than 1 year, and during this period there is never a tic-free period of more than 3 consecutive months.

2. The disturbances cause marked distress or significant impairment in social, occupational, or other important areas of functioning.

3. The onset is before 18 years of age.

4. The disturbance is not due to the direct physiological effects of a substance (e.g., stimulants), or a general medical condition (e.g., HD or postviral encephalitis). Among patients with TS, 50% have ADHD. Also, 50% of patients with TS have OCD. There is a higher incidence of learning disabilities in children with TS. Approximately 65% of children and

adolescents with chronic motor or phonic tic disorder have a comorbid condition. Around 90% of those with TS develop one or more psychiatric disorders.

11.8.1 Differential diagnosis

The differentiation of TS from other tic syndromes may be no more than semantic, especially since recent genetic evidence link TS with multiple and transient tics of childhood and can only be defined in retrospect.

1. *ADHD/OCD*
   Many ADHD children have a few phonic or motor tics, grimace, or produce noises similar to those with TS, and 50% of them with TS have had ADHD and OCD. Compulsions are associated with feelings of inner anxiety and are characterized by ritualistic behavior (checking, touching, arranging, etc.) and the need to repeat them in the same manner.

2. *Other tic disorders*
   Chronic non-TS tic disorders have either motor or phonic tics, but not both. They may be just as disturbing or disabling as TS. Transient tic disorders of children resolve completely within 1 year of onset. TS may remit for weeks to months but generally returns.

3. *Seizures*
   Some partial seizures could be mistaken for tics, but these are generally not suppressible and are not preceded by a premonitory urge. Eyelid flickering (myoclonus) seen with absence seizures could resemble tics, but in absence seizures there is loss of consciousness, no suppressible, and no premonitory urge. Patients with TS, however, retain a clear consciousness during such paroxysms. If in doubt an EEG may be useful.

4. *Developmental and other neurological disorders*
   CNS injury from trauma or disease may cause a child to be vulnerable to the expression of the disorder (TS), particularly if this is a genetic predisposition. Autistic children and children with intellectual disabilities may display the entire gamut of TS symptoms.

5. *Spasms*
   Muscle spasms, such as blepharospasms or spasmodic torticollis, may be confused with TS, but the characteristics of tics in TS should allow differentiation.

6. *Myoclonus*
   Involuntary brief, jerk-like movements. Can be irregular and is not preceded by the urge to perform the movement

7. *Akathisia, dystonias*
   An abnormal state of excessive restlessness accompanied by feeling the need to move about, with brief gained after moving. Often seen in the context of dopamine receptor-blocking agent exposure.

8. *Stereotypies*
   Repetitive movements, postures, or utterances can be seen in normal children but often in children with pervasive developmental disorders or Rett syndrome. Common ones include head banging, body rocking, and repetitive finger movements.

9. *Paediatric autoimmune neuropsychiatric disorders associated with strepto-coccal infections (PANDAS)*
   It is postulated as either: (a) a dramatic increase in symptoms in children already known to have tics or OCD. or (b) as an appearance of such symptoms in children without prior history, following a Group A beta-hemolytic streptococcal infection.

10. *Paediatric acute neuropsychiatric syndrome (PANS)*
    A recently described syndrome suggests primary diagnostic criteria of acute-onset OCD with secondary features of abnormal movements, separation anxiety, frequent urination, behavioral regression, and loss of handwriting skills.
    a) Allergic rhinitis: may present with sniffing, eye blinking, and throat clearing.
    b) Conjunctivitis: may represent with eye blinking.
    c) Cough-variant asthma: chronic cough following exposure to allergens or upper respiratory infection.

11. *Genetic conditions (e.g., Huntington's chorea)*
    Involuntary choric movements not associated with an urge to move. By definition, these movements should be random and not stereotyped.

12. *Postinfectious autoimmune diseases (e.g., Sydenham's chorea)*
    Develop weeks to months after streptococcus infection, and involve choreiform and truncal movements.

13. *Metabolic diseases (e.g., Wilson's disease)*
    Findings include tremor and tic-like movements, incoordination of speech, swallowing, and gait and behavioral changes. Kayser–Fleischer rings due to copper accumulation in the eyes. Lab findings show decreased copper and ceruloplasmin levels in the blood, increased urinary excretion of copper, and copper accumulation in the liver.

14. *Postviral encephalitis*
    Differentiated by history.

15. *Substance exposure*
    a) Psychiatric medication: These are likely to cause tics but they can be associated with other movement problems, such as restlessness.
    b) Stimulant medications: These do not cause tics, although in a minority of patients they may exacerbate them.
    c) Carbamazepine: It may produce tics.
    d) Neuroleptics: Prolonged use of some of them may result in tardive dyskinesia, a neurologic syndrome which manifests as many kinds of repetitive purposeless movements, some of which may appear tic-like. These may include lip smacking, grimacing, and rapid eye blinking, and may occur in the extremities as well as the face.

Cath DC, Hedderly T, Ludolph AG, et al; ESSTS Guidelines Group. European clinical guidelines for Tourette syndrome and other tic disorders. Part I: assessment. Eur Child Adolesc Psychiatry 2011;20(4):155–171

Freeman RD; Tourette Syndrome International Database Consortium. Tic disorders and ADHD: answers from a world-wide clinical dataset on Tourette syndrome. Eur Child Adolesc Psychiatry 2007; 16(Suppl 1):15–23

11.9 Tremor

Tremor is one of the most common involuntary movement disorders seen in clinical practice. It is defined as a rhythmic, involuntary, oscillating movement of one or more body parts produced by reciprocally innervated antagonist muscles. Tremors vary in frequency and amplitude and are influenced by physiologic and psychological factors, pathologic processes, and drugs or toxins.

11.9.1 Differential diagnosis

There are a number of syndromes that may be misinterpreted as tremor. These may include:
1. *Clonus*
   There are rhythmic, uniphasic contractions and relaxations of muscle groups around joints that is stimulated through stretch reflex. Passive stretching increases the clonus but not tremor, helps to differentiate clonus from tremor on the basis of irregular movements.
2. *Rhythmic myoclonus*
   It is characterized by irregular or rhythmic, shock-like contractions of a muscle group due to CNS disease. Electrophysiologic analysis by electromyography (EMG) or EEG as well as back-averaging help to make the diagnosis.
3. *Epilepsia partialis continua*
   it is a focal motor epilepsy associated with recurrent, rhythmic clonic movements of a specific muscle group. A clinical history that is positive for epilepsy and EEG readings that show abnormal spikes help point to the correct diagnosis.

4. *Asterixis*

It is a condition in which sudden, periodic interruptions in muscle contraction lead to arrhythmic lapses of sustained posture associated with EMG pauses ranging from about 35 to 200 milliseconds or greater. This condition is sometimes referred to as "negative myoclonus."

Tremor can be classified on a clinical and etiologic basis. The first classification system is based on whether tremor occurs at rest (*resting tremor*) or with action (*action tremor*). Tremors with movement (action) are subdivided into *postural tremor* that occurs with maintained posture, *kinetic or intention tremor* that which occurs with movement from point to point, and *task-specific tremor*, occurring only when doing highly skilled activity. The second tremor classification is by cause. Tremor can be due to a variety of conditions, both physiologic and pathologic.

Disorder	Diagnosis
Physiologic tremor	Rhythmic oscillations of 8–12 Hz with posture and movement but without neurological findings; enhanced by:
	• Stress (anxiety, fatigue, emotion, exercise)
	• Endocrine (adrenocorticosteroids, hypoglycemia, thyrotoxicosis, pheochromocytoma)
	• Toxins (As, Bi, Br, Hg, ethanol withdrawal)
	• Drugs (beta-agonists, cycloserine, dopaminergic drugs, methylxanthines, valproic acid, psychiatric drugs: lithium-tricyclics-neuroleptic, stimulants: amphetamines, cocaine)
Essential tremor	Essential tremor (ET) is the most common movement disorder. It often occurs in families as an autosomal dominant trait. The frequency is between 4 and 10 Hz. Most noticeable in extremities that maintain an antigravity posture (postural tremor). No associated neurological findings. Ethanol suppresses the tremor. The tremor is most prominent in the hands, although the cranial musculature is frequently affected (titubation). Speech involvement (voice tremor) can result from tremor. ET may be associated with other movement disorders, including cervical dystonia, writer's cramp and spasmodic dysphonia. Patients with ET have increased hearing disability compared with controls or patients with PD. Tremor is bilateral and affects all age groups
Parkinsonian tremor	A pill-rolling type of tremor of 3–6 Hz most prominent in the rest and postural positions. The parkinsonian resting tremor is characteristically inhibited by voluntary movements, i.e., there is no kinetic tremor. The tremor affects the hands, chin, lips, legs, and trunk; a head tremor is unusual. Associated with other signs of parkinsonism, including bradykinesia, rigidity, positive glabellar reflexes, "mask-like" face and impaired postural reflexes. There is no history of Parkinson's tremor, and alcohol consumption does not decrease movement. Tremor onset is unilateral

(*Continued*)

▶ (*Continued*)

Disorder	Diagnosis
Tremor with other basal ganglia diseases	Tremor can be a component of the symptom complex in patients with dystonic disorders, such as spasmodic torticollis. In Wilson's disease tremor can be the presenting symptom. It can occur with postural and kinetic movements and is prominent in the proximal muscles. In the shoulder it is described as "wing-beating" tremor
Cerebellar tremor	Patients with cerebellar disease have both postural and kinetic tremors, but not resting tremor. Various types of postural tremors have been described, most common consists of oscillations of the arms or of the legs. It is referred to as titubation when it affects the trunk and head. There is also a mild postural tremor that is more rapid (frequency 10 Hz) with distal predominance. The characteristic cerebellar kinetic tremor has a frequency of 3–5 Hz. It is evident on finger-to-nose and heel-to-shin tests. Common cause of cerebellar tremor is MS, but brainstem tumors or strokes and degenerative and paraneoplastic diseases can also be responsible
Rubral (midbrain) tremor (Holmes tremor)	A combination of resting, postural, and severe kinetic tremor of 2–5 Hz. This tremor is uncommon but highly distinctive and resistant to symptomatic pharmacotherapy. Signs of ataxia and weakness may be present. Common causes include cerebrovascular accident and MS, with a possible delay of 2 weeks to 2 years in tremor onset and occurrence of lesions
Posttraumatic tremor	Tremor of 2–8 Hz that can occur days to months after a head injury, long after consciousness has been regained. It is typically proximal and made worse with movement
Alcohol withdrawal tremor	It may occur after a period of relative or absolute abstinence. Initially has the characteristic of an enhanced physiologic tremor. A more permanent postural tremor can occur in persons with chronic alcoholism even with alcohol abstinence
Drug-induced and toxic tremor	Pharmacologic agents used to treat other medical conditions may induce tremors. Types of tremors induced by drugs include enhanced physiologic tremor, rest tremor, and action tremor. Such medications may include theophylline, valproate, lithium, tricyclic antidepressants, neuroleptics, sympathomimetics, amphetamines, steroids, certain agents used to treat endocrine and metabolic disorders. Toxin-induced tremor, such as seen in manganese, arsenic, or mercury intoxication or poisoning, occurs in association with other neurologic symptoms, such as gait disturbances, rigidity, dystonia, ataxia, dysarthria, confusion etc.
Tremor due to systemic disease	Tremor occurs when the patient is moving or assumes a specific position. Associated symptoms include asterixis, mental status changes, and other signs of systemic illness. Diseases such as thyrotoxicosis and hepatic failure, delirium tremens, drug withdrawal, and peripheral neuropathies (particularly dysgammaglobulinemic neuropathies)

▶ (*Continued*)

Disorder	Diagnosis
Orthostatic tremor	Orthostatic tremor is considered to be a variant of essential tremor. This type of tremor occurs in the legs immediately on standing and is relieved by sitting down. Orthostatic tremor is usually high frequency (14–18Hz) and no other clinical signs or symptoms are present
Psychogenic tremor	Tremors are very common in hysteria. Tremors are complex and unclassifiable, have changing characteristics, and are clinically inconsistent. Tremor increases with attention and lessens with distractibility. Tremor is unresponsive to antitremor drugs and responsive to placebo. Remission of tremor with psychotherapy.

Shahani BT, Young RR. Physiological and pharmacological aids in the differential diagnosis of tremor. J Neurol Neurosurg Psychiatry 1976;39(8):772–783

Elble RJ. Diagnostic criteria for essential tremor and differential diagnosis. Neurology 2000;54(11, Suppl 4):S2–S6

Pahwa R, Lyons KE. Essential tremor: differential diagnosis and current therapy. Am J Med 2003;115(2): 134–142

11.10 Medical Conditions Associated with Gait Disorders

1. Idiopathic gait disorder
2. Affective disorders and psychiatric conditions
    a) Depression
    b) Fear of falling
    c) Sleep disorders
    d) Substance abuse
3. Neurologic disorders
    a) Cerebellar dysfunction or degeneration
    b) Delirium tremens
    c) Dementia
    d) MS myelopathy
    e) PD
    f) Stroke
    g) Vertebrobasilar insufficiency
    h) Normal pressure hydrocephalus
4. Sensory abnormalities
    a) Peripheral polyneuropathy
        i. Alcoholism

       b) Multiple sensory deficit syndrome
       c) Visual impairment
          i. Presbyopia
          ii. Cataracts
       d) Hearing impairment
          i. Benign positional vertigo
          ii. Meniere's disease
          iii. Oscillopsia (unsteadiness of the visual image)

5. Cardiovascular
    a) Arrhythmias
    b) Congestive heart failure
    c) Coronary artery disease
    d) Orthostatic hypotension
    e) Peripheral arterial disease
    f) Thromboembolic disease

6. Infectious and metabolic diseases
    a) Diabetes mellitus
    b) Hepatic encephalopathy
    c) HIV-associated neuropathy
    d) Hyper- and hypothyroidism
    e) Obesity
    f) Uremia
    g) Tertiary syphilis
    h) Vitamin B12 deficiency

7. Musculoskeletal disorders
    a) Cervical spondylosis
    b) Gout
    c) Lumbar stenosis
    d) Disc disease
    e) Muscle weakness or atrophy
    f) Osteoporosis
    g) Osteoarthritis
    h) Rheumatoid arthritis
    i) Paget's disease
    j) Congenital or acquired deformity
    k) Polymyalgia

8. Other
    a) Other acute medical illnesses
    b) Recent surgery

c) Use of certain medications (i.e., antiarrhythmics, diuretics, digoxin, narcotic psychotropics, and antidepressants), especially four or more.

Jahn K, Zwergal A, Schniepp R. Gait disturbances in old age: classification, diagnosis, and treatment from a neurological perspective. Dtsch Arztebl Int 2010;107(17):306–315, quiz 316

11.11 Neurological Disorders of Stance and Gait

1. Supratentorial lesions
   a) *White matter disease*
      - White matter disease in the elderly
        Normal histology but vascular or ischemic disease has been present in cases with pronounced changes on MR or CT
      - Leukoencephalopathies
        Familial disorder of white matter disease may manifest itself as impaired gait; e.g., MS, progressive multifocal encephalopathy, AIDS encephalopathy, radiation leukoencephalopathy
   b) *Acute vascular disease*
      i. Thalamic astasia
         Thalamic infarction and hemorrhage cause inability to stand or walk despite minimal weakness. Patients usually fall backward or toward the site contralateral to the lesion. The lesions cluster in the superior portion of the ventrolateral nucleus of the thalamus and the suprathalamic white matter.
      ii. Capsular and basal ganglia lesions
         Small capsular lesions involving the most lateral portion of the ventrolateral nucleus of the thalamus, and multiple bilateral lacunae in the basal ganglia can be attended by gait impairment.
   c) *Normotensive hydrocephalus*
      Significant dilatation of the lateral, third, and fourth ventricles and blunting of the calloso caudal angle causing spastic gait ataxia and urinary disturbances. Fibers destined for the leg region course in the posterior limb of the internal capsule and then ascend in the more medial portion of the corona radiata, near the wall of the lateral ventricle.
   d) *Bilateral subdural hematomas*
      Unilateral chronic subdural hematomas cause a mild hemiparesis, speech and language disorders, and apraxia. Bilateral lesions present with gait failure, particularly in elderly individuals.

2. Infratentorial lesions
   a) *Pontomesencephalic gait failure*
      The pedunculopontine region plays an important role in motor be-havior. Loss of neurons in the area causes an acute onset of inability to walk, without hemiparesis or sensory loss and lack of cadence or gait rhythmicity to the patient. This gait deficit resembles the gait failure experienced by many elderly individuals without a clear anatomic correlate.
   b) *Vestibular lesions*
      Unilateral lesions of the vestibular area, e.g., Wallenberg syndrome, MS, and CPA neoplasms, make patients to fall to the side of the lesion; bilat-eral findings are present in Wernicke's encephalopathy of B1 deficiency.
   c) *Cerebellar lesions*
      Acute or progressive balance impairment occurs in cerebellar lesions affecting the flocculonodular lobe, or vestibulocerebellum. Most often patients with cerebellar lesions tend to fall to the side of the lesion.
3. Myelopathy
   The initial manifestation of a myelopathy is often gait or balance impairment.
   a) *Cervical spondylosis*
      Advanced disease may lead to tetraparesis with a spastic-ataxic gait and be associated by radicular findings, such as pain and reflex changes.
   b) *MS*
      Gait or balance impairment and sensory changes may be the only man-ifestations of MS involving the spinal cord or rarely some of the higher levels of neuraxis.

11.12 Types of Stance and Gait

Watching the patient stand and walk is the single most important part of the entire neurological assessment and examination.
1. Developmental gaits
   a) *Neonatal automatic or reflex stepping*
      When the infant is held upright and its feet touch the bed surface it lifts its legs alternately and steps as reflex.
   b) *Infantile cruising*
      The infant makes steps when steadied by a parent or when holding on to a couch.
   c) *Toddler's gait*
      Broad base, short, jerky, irregular steps, a semi-flexed posture of the arms, and frequent falls comprise toddler's gait.

d) *Child's mature gait*
  A narrow-based, heel-toe stride with reciprocal swinging of the arms.
e) *Limping (walking with an unsteady gait, favoring one leg)*
  It is most likely due to pain caused by minor injury. Splinters, blisters, or tired muscles are common causes. More serious problems include:
    i. Developmental (e.g., hip dysplasia, cerebral palsy)
    ii. Trauma (e.g., fracture, puncture wound, slipped femoral epiphyses)
    iii. Infections (e.g., osteomyelitis, septic arthritis, synovitis, Lyme disease)
    iv. Osteochondroses (e.g., Calve–Legg–Perthes disease)
    v. Neoplasia (e.g., leukemia)
    vi. Inflammatory (e.g., juvenile rheumatoid arthritis)
  Nonpainful chronic limping is indicative of developmental problem, such as dysplasia of the hip or neuromuscular problem (cerebral palsy)

2. Neuromuscular gaits
  a) *Club foot gait*
    The gait depends on what type of valgus–varus deformities exists.
  b) *In-toed or pigeon-toed gait*
    It is due to tibial torsion.
  c) *Lordotic waddling gait*
    In muscular dystrophies and the polymyositis there is weakening of the proximal muscles of the shoulders, back, and hips, so the patients develop a characteristic sway-backed, waddle gait. Furthermore, these patients find it difficult of getting up on, or down from, the examining table, or when standing up from a sitting or a reclining position.
  d) *Toe-drop or foot-drop gait*
    Due to paralysis of foot dorsiflexion, the patient is unable to clear the floor, so he jerks the knee high, flipping the foot up into dorsiflexion, and characteristically slaps the foot down.
      i. Unilateral foot-drop
        Suggests a mechanical or compressive neuropathy of the common peroneal nerve or L5 root.
      ii. Bilateral foot-drop or steppage gait
        Due to a symmetrical distal neuropathy of toxic, metabolic, or familial type, as in alcoholic neuropathy or Charcot–Marie–Tooth's progressive peroneal atrophy.
  e) *Heel-drop gait*
    Due to paralysis of the tibial nerve the patient is unable to plantarflex his foot, although he can dorsiflex it.
  f) *Flail-foot gait*
    Due to a complete sciatic palsy the patient is unable to either dorsiflex or plantarflex his foot.

g) *Toe-walking gait*

Due to tight heel cords the child has a limited dorsiflexion of the foot to about 90 degrees so the child stands on the balls of his feet without a definite heel strike. Such a gait is observed in Duchenne's muscular dystrophy, in spastic diplegia, and in autistic or other retarded children.

3. Sensory gaits

   a) *Painful sole or hyperesthetic gait*

   When the patient sets the foot down, he bears as little weight on it as possible, and limbs off the foot as soon as possible, hunching the shoulders.

   i. Unilateral

   In Morton's metatarsalgia, a painful neuroma of an interdigital nerve, or gout.

   ii. Bilateral

   In painful distal neuropathies of toxic, metabolic, or alcoholic in origin.

   b) *Radicular pain gait or antalgic gait*

   Compression of the L5 root from a herniated disk causes extreme pain radiating into the big toe, aggravated by coughing, sneezing, or straight leg raising. The patient's back is lordotic, and when he walks he does not bear weight on the painful leg and takes stiff, slow, short strides with no heel strike and his trunk tilts slightly to the side opposite the pain.

   c) *Nocturnal flipping-hand gait*

   In patients with carpal tunnel syndrome, there is an excruciating nocturnal pain in the hand often awaking him. The patient paces the room flipping or shaking the hand in an effort to get some pain relief. A pathognomonic gait seen often in autistic and other retarded children who develop repetitive, self-stimulating mannerisms resembling a variety of flipping-hand gaits.

   d) *Tabetic or dorsal column or sensory ataxic gait*

   Resembles a double foot drop and it is seen in patients with tabes dorsalis, in whom a syphilitic infection causes degeneration of the dorsal columns of the spinal cords. The patients lift the knees high and slaps the feet down, placing them irregularly due to sensory ataxia. When standing the patient must use visual cues, otherwise he sways and falls over.

   e) *Blind person's gait*

   The slow, deliberate, and searching steps of a blind person are characteristic and should not confuse an experienced examiner.

4. Cerebellar gaits

   a) *Unilateral cerebellar gait*

   A unilateral cerebellar lesion, most likely from neoplasm, infarct, or demyelinating disease causes ipsilateral cerebellar signs with the patient presenting dystaxia of volitional movements (veers or falls in one direction) and of volitionally maintained postures, hence a reeling gait.

b) *Bilateral cerebellar gait*

Bilateral cerebellar signs imply a toxic, metabolic, or familiar disorder. Dystaxia of the legs and gait with little or no dystaxia of the arms, and no dysarthria or nystagmus suggests a rostral vermis syndrome, most commonly secondary to alcoholism. Truncal ataxia alone implies a flocculonodular lobe or caudal vermian lesion, often a fourth ventricular tumor.

5. Spastic gait

a) *Hemiplegic gait*

The patient circumducts the affected leg, dragging the toe, placing the ball down without a heel strike with the ipsilateral arm held in partial flexion or, less often, flaccidly at the side.

b) *Spastic gait*

The patient walks with stiff legs, not clearing the floor with either foot, giving the appearance of wading through water because he must work against the spastic opposition of his own muscles, as if walking in thick, sticky mud; the knees tend to rub together in a scissoring action.

  i. Pure spastic or paraplegic gait

  A pure spastic paraplegic gait without sensory deficits, coming on after birth, implies a corticospinal tract disorder, such as in familial spastic paraplegia.

  ii. Spastic diplegic gait

  Patients affected from diplegic cerebral palsy have small and short legs in contrast to normally developed chest, shoulders, and arms. In spastic diplegia there is severe spasticity in the legs, minimal spasticity in the arms, and little or no deficit in speaking or swallowing, whereas in double hemiplegia there is pseudobulbar palsy and more arm weakness than leg.

  iii. Spastic-ataxic gait

  If in addition to spasticity, the disease impairs the dorsal columns or cerebellum as in spinocerebellar degeneration or MS, the patient will have a wider-based unsteady gait taking irregular steps.

6. Basal ganglia gaits

a) *The marche a petits pas (the march of small steps)*

Elderly patients with small vessel disease from arteriosclerosis, shown as multiple lacunar infarcts in the basal ganglia, develop a characteristic gait with shuffling, short steps, unable to lift the feet from the ground the progress of which ceases if the patient tries to speak (unable to walk and talk or chew gum at the same time).

b) *Parkinsonian gait*
   The patient with degeneration of the substantia nigra or neuroleptic medication toxicity arises and walks slowly with short steps, lacks any arm swing, turns en bloc like a statue rotating on a pedestal, and has a tremor at rest which disappears during intentional movement.

c) *Festinating gait*
   When the patient is shoved after forewarning, he will move forward or backward on tiny steps of increasing speed and decreasing length, as if chasing the center of gravity, and may fall over.

d) *Choreiform gait*
   The patient with Huntington's or Sydenham's chorea walks and the play of finger and arm movements increases along with walking, or may even appear clearly for the first time. Random missteps mar the evenness of the strides, as the choreiform twitches supervene.

e) *Spastic-athetoid gait*
   A combination of athetosis and moderate spastic diplegia or double hemiplegia secondary to perinatal hypoxic damage of the basal ganglia and thalamus has the characteristics of spastic gait associated with slow writhing movements of fingers and arms which tend to increase during walking.

f) *Equinovarus dystonic gait*
   Dystonia may initially manifest in a child by an intermittent intoeing of the foot that impedes walking, while in later stages dystonic truncal contortions and tortipelvis may cause the trunk to incline strongly forward.

g) *Dromedary gait*
   The patient with dystonia musculorum deformans may take giant uneven strides, exhibiting flexions or rise and fall of the trunk, like the ungainly gait of a dromedary camel.

7. Cerebral gaits
   Elderly patients with severe bilateral cerebral disease secondary to AD, multi-infarct dementia, or senility have difficulty initiating the sequence of movements to rise, stand, or walk. When starting to walk, the patient makes several efforts to move the feet appearing somewhat puzzled, as if searching for lost motor engrams, or the right buttons to press to start progressing.

   a) *The dancing bear gait*
      The effort to progress may only result in stepping on the same spot as if trying to free the feet from thick, sticky mud.

b) *Apraxic gait*

When the patient does progress, his feet cling to the floor as if magnetized.

8. Psychiatric gaits

a) *Astasia-abasia*

The patient tilts, gyrates, and undulates all over the place, unwittingly proving by not falling during the marvelous demonstration of agility, that strength, balance, coordination, and sensation have to be intact.

9. Sexual behavior and biologic orientation gait

The gait is characteristic of and diagnostic of the biologic and behavioral state of a person's brain.

a) *Heterosexual male-female gait*

Alexander NB, Goldberg A. Gait disorders: search for multiple causes. Cleve Clin J Med 2005;72(7): 586–, 589–590, 592–594 passim.

12 Neurotrauma

Echoencephalogram is an obsolete examination nowadays (▶ Fig. 12.1). It was the initial and basic test of severe head injuries in the pre-CT scan era.

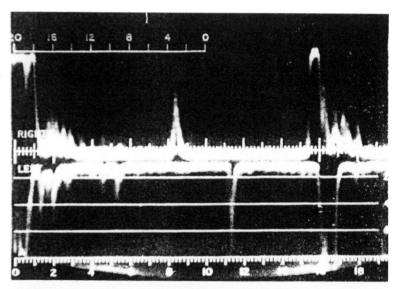

Fig. 12.1 Echoencephalogram. This ECHO demonstrates a right-to-left 1.5 cm shift of the midline (as midline was considered the calcified pineal gland) due to a right subdural hematoma.

States of altered consciousness

Confusion	Disturbed consciousness and impairment of higher cerebral functions
Delirium	Confusion with motor restlessness, transient hallucinations, and delusions
Stupor	Conscious but rousable only with intense stimulation
Coma	Unarousable unresponsiveness (GCS </= 8/15)
Vegetative state	Loss of consciousness with preservation of brainstem function
Death	Loss of consciousness and the capacity to breath spontaneously: irreversible

Abbreviation: GCS, Glasgow Coma Scale.

12.1 The Unconscious Patient

The state of arousal is determined by the function of the central reticular formation that extends from the brain stem to the thalamus. Coma occurs when this center is damaged by a metabolic abnormality or by an invasive lesion which compresses this center. Coma is also caused by damage to the cerebral cortex.

The various levels of consciousness vary from *consciousness*, which means awareness of oneself and the surroundings in a state of wakefulness, to *coma*, which is a state of unarousable unresponsiveness. Rather than using these broad terms in clinical practice it is preferable to describe the actual state of the patient in a sentence. For more details please refer to the following table.

State	Clinical features	Simplified classification
Consciousness	Aware and wakeful	Awake
Clouded consciousness	Reduced awareness and wakefulness "Alcohol effect" Confusion Drowsiness	Confused
Stupor	Unconscious Deep sleep-like state Arousal with vigorous stimuli	Responds to shake and shout
Semicomatose	Unconscious (deeper) Responds only to painful stimuli (sternal rubbing with knuckles) without arousing	Responds to pain
Coma	Deeply unconscious Unarousable and unresponsive	Unresponsive coma

Kumar PJ, Clark ML. Clinical Medicine. 5th ed. London: Bailliere Tindall; 2003

12.2 Hysterical "Unconscious" Patient

One of the most puzzling problems in emergency medicine is how to diagnose the unconscious patient caused by the conversion reaction (hysteria). These patients really experience their symptoms (as opposed to the pretending patient) and resist most normal stimuli, including painful stimuli.

- Hold the patient's eye or eyes open with your fingers and note the reaction to light.
- Now hold a mirror over the eye and watch closely for pupillary reaction. The pupil should constrict with accommodation from the patient looking at his or her own image.

12.3 Blackouts: Episodic Loss of Consciousness

Episodic or transient loss of consciousness is a common problem. The history is important to determine whether the patient is describing a true blackout or episodes of dizziness, weakness or some other sensation. Various causes of blackouts are discussed below.

1. Epilepsy

    It is the most common cause of blackouts. There are various types, the most dramatic being the tonic–clonic seizure where patients have sudden loss of consciousness without warning. Associated features are:

    a) *Cyanosis*, then heavy "snoring" breathing

    b) *Eyes rolling* "back into head"

    c) *Tongue biting* may or may not be there

    d) *Incontinence* of urine or feces may or may not be there

    With partial complex seizures there is *aura* (sensory or psychological feelings) and *automatisms* (e.g., fidgeting, lip smacking).

2. Syncope

    In syncope, there is a transient loss of consciousness, but with warning symptoms and rapid return of alertness following a brief period of unconsciousness (seconds to 3 minutes). There are several forms of syncope:

    a) Vasovagal "attack" or common faint

    The patient invariably remembers the onset of fainting. Most common syncope of the benign vasomotor type and tends to occur in young people, especially when standing still (e.g., choir boys). It is the main cause of repeated fainting attacks. The differential diagnosis includes all the other causes of transient loss of consciousness and, in particular, a seizure disorder. Its associated features are:

        i. Occurs while standing, or rarely sitting

        ii. Warning feelings of dizziness, faintness, or true vertigo

        iii. Nausea, hot and cold skin sensations

        iv. Fading hearing or blurred vision

        v. Sliding to ground (rather than heavy full-length fall)

        vi. Rapid return of consciousness

        vii. Pallor and sweating and bradycardia

        viii. Often trigger factors (e.g., emotional, upset, pain)

    b) Micturition syncope

    This uncommon event may occur after micturition in older men, especially during the night when they leave a warm bed and stand void. The cause appears to be peripheral vasodilatation associated with reduction of venous return from standing.

c) Cough syncope

Severe coughing can result in obstruction of venous return with subsequent blackout. This is also the mechanism of blackouts with breath-holding attacks.

d) Carotid sinus syncope

Caused by pressure on a hypersensitive carotid sinus (e.g., in some elderly patients who lose consciousness when their neck is touched).

e) Effort syncope

Exertion or effort syncope is due to obstructive cardiac disorders, such as aortic stenosis and hypertrophic obstructive cardiomyopathy.

f) Hyperventilation syncope

Hyperventilation is a common cause of dizziness and faintness but rarely causes syncope. It is a benign disorder which is caused by overbreathing in response to anxiety. It occurs most commonly but not exclusively in teenage or young women.

3. Choking

Sudden collapse can follow choking. Also known as "café coronary" or "barbecue coronary" when patient suddenly becomes cyanosed, is speechless, and grasps the throat while eating. This is caused by inhaling a large bolus of meat which obstructs the larynx.

4. Drop attacks

These are episodes of "blackouts" in which the patient falls to the ground and then immediately gets up again. They involve sudden attacks of weakness in the legs. Drop attacks occur in middle-aged women and are considered to be brainstem disturbances producing sudden changes in tone in the lower limbs. Other causes of drop attacks include vertebrobasilar insufficiency, Parkinson's disease, and epilepsy.

5. Cardiac arrhythmias

Stokes–Adams attacks and cardiac syncope are manifestations of recurrent episodes of loss of consciousness, especially in the elderly, caused by cardiac arrhythmias. *The blackout is sudden with the patient falling to the ground without warning and without convulsive movements,* and then by an equally rapid recovery of consciousness, the entire episode usually lasting a matter of seconds. The diagnosis can be confirmed by 24-hour ambulatory monitoring.

6. Vertebrobasilar insufficiency

Loss of consciousness can occur with vertebrobasilar insufficiency (VBI) transient ischemic attack. Typical preceding symptoms of VBI include dyspnea, vertigo, vomiting, hemisensory loss, ataxia, and transient global amnesia.

7. Hypoglycemia

   The diagnosis should be suspected if there are *feelings of hunger, sweating, nervousness and palpitations* coupled with episodes of *confusion, abnormal speech, or unusual behavior* in a patient not at risk for seizures or syncope, and most frequently in diabetics taking oral hypoglycemic agents or insulin. A blood glucose level < 2.5 mmols/l is considered to be hypoglycemia.

8. Head injuries and unconsciousness

   Some non-life-threatening head injuries are serious enough to cause significant loss of consciousness and retrograde amnesia.

9. Psychogenic factors

   Hysterical blackouts or fits are not uncommon and have to be differentiated from hyperventilation. It is unusual for hyperventilation to cause unconsciousness but it is possible that consciousness gets clouded, especially if the patient is administered oxygen.

   Other features that suggest psychogenic rather than organic factors are:

   a) Labile effect
   b) Rapidly changing levels of consciousness
   c) Well-articulated speech
   d) Bizarre thought control.

   Clinical differences between a seizure and a vasovagal attack are listed in the following table.

Clinical features	Vasovagal attack	Epileptic seizure
Posture	Upright	Any posture
Onset	Gradual	Sudden
Incontinence/tongue biting	Rare	Common
Period/unconsciousness	Seconds	Minutes
Recovery	Rapid (within seconds)	Slow
Precipitating factor	Stereotyped	Nonstereotyped
Recurring pattern	No	Yes

12.4 Glasgow Coma Scale (GCS)

12.4.1 Advantages

The advantages of the GCS are that it has face validity, wide acceptance, and established statistical associations with adverse neurological outcomes, including brain injury, neurological intervention, and mortality. However, these are offset by several important limitations.

12.4.2 Limitations

The GCS predicts mortality well at its extremes and poorly in its midrange, and thus most of its predictive capacity is anchored by the endpoints. The GCS is not reliable. A clinical scale must be reproducible to be accurate and useful. Unfortunately, the GCS contains multiple subjective elements and has repeatedly demonstrated surprisingly low interrater reliability in a variety of settings. The GCS was accurately used by experienced users, while inexperienced ones made consistent errors (up to 4- or 5-point scales) mainly in the intermediate levels of consciousness. The GCS is criticized for failure to incorporate brainstem reflexes which are considered good indicators of brainstem arousal systems' activity. In addition, the GCS does not incorporate the size and reactivity of patient's pupils to light. The reliability of the GCS is further compromised in patients with tracheal intubation because verbal response can no longer be evaluated. The GCS is only grossly predictive. The prognostic value of the GCS is weak enough that it cannot accurately predict outcomes for individual patients. Data from the German Rescue System showed that GCS scores of 3–6 during the first two posttraumatic days did not correspond to the outcome after 1 year. Several clinical conditions have great impact on GCS rating, such as sedation, high blood alcohol concentrations

	Response	Score
Eye opening	Spontaneous	4
	To command	3
	To pain	2
	No response	1
Best motor response	Obeys	6
	Localizes	5
	Withdrawal	4
	Flexor	3
	Extensor	2
	No response	1
Best verbal response	Oriented and conversed	5
	Confused conversation	4
	Inappropriate words	3
	Incomprehensible sounds	2
	No response	1

(> 240 mg/100 ml) are associated with a 2–3 point reduction in GCS. Similarly, the GCS use in the assessment of the acutely poisoned patient should not be recommended. Mechanism of injury (penetrating versus blunt) and age (> 55 years) were also found to have a major effect in the predictive value of GCS. The stimulation techniques are of utmost importance. The pressure of the finger nail bed with a pencil as was proposed in the GCS falsely lowers the level of responsiveness. The GCS is an ordinal scale. The difference between unit values is not consistent and compares only better with worse. Yet, minimal differences of GCS scores are important in terms of prognosis.

12.5 The Full Outline of Unresponsiveness (FOUR) Score Coma Scale

The FOUR score provides greater neurological detail than the GCS, recognizes a locked-in syndrome, and is superior to the GCS due to the availability of brainstem reflexes, breathing patterns, and the ability to recognize different stages of herniation. The probability of in-hospital mortality was higher for the lowest total FOUR score, when compared with the lowest total GCS score. However, it is even more complicated than the GCS (4 component scales), requires more time to calculate, and has similarly limited interrater reliability.

Eye response

- 4 = eyelids open or opened, tracking, or blinking to command
- 3 = eyelids open but not tracking
- 2 = eyelids closed but open to loud voice
- 1 = eyelids closed but open to pain
- 0 = eyelids remain closed with pain

Motor response

- 4 = thumbs-up, fist, or peace sign
- 3 = localizing to pain
- 2 = flexion response to pain
- 1 = extension response to pain
- 0 = no response to pain or generalized myoclonus status

Brainstem reflexes

- 4 = pupil and corneal reflexes present
- 3 = one pupil wide and fixed
- 2 = pupil or corneal reflexes absent

▶ (*Continued*)

- 1 = pupil and corneal reflexes absent
- 0 = absent pupil, corneal, and cough reflex

Respiration

- 4 = not intubated, regular breathing pattern
- 3 = not intubated, Cheyne–Stokes breathing pattern
- 2 = not intubated, irregular breathing
- 1 = breaths above ventilator rate
- 0 = breaths at ventilator rate or apnea

Wijdicks EF, Bamlet WR, Maramattom BV, Manno EM, McClelland RL. Validation of a new coma scale: The FOUR score. Ann Neurol 2005;58(4):585–593

12.6 Neurotrauma Paediatric Scales

Cranial traumas have different particularities in infants, toddlers, preschool children, school children, and teenagers. The assessment of these cases must be individualized according to age. It is completely different in children than in adults. Trauma scales are very useful in grading the severity and predicting outcome in traumatic brain injury (TBI), but trauma scales used in adults must be adapted for the use in children. Children have age-related specificity and anatomic particularities for each of the period of development.

12.6.1 Paediatric coma scale

	Response	Score
Eye opening	Spontaneous	4
	To voice	3
	To pain	2
	No response	1
Best motor response	Flexes/extends	4
	Withdraws	3
	Hypertonic	2
	Flaccid	1
Best verbal response	Cries	3
	Spontaneous respiration	2
	Apneic	1

12.6.2 Paediatric coma scale/children's coma scale

	Response	Score
Eye opening	Spontaneous	4
	To speech	3
	To pain	2
	None	1
Best motor response	Obeys commands	5
	Localizes pain	4
	Flexion to pain	3
	Extension to pain	2
	None	1
Verbal response	Orientated	5
	Words	4
	Vocal sounds	3
	Cries	2
	None	1

Note: The PCS is used in evaluation of brain injury severity in preverbal children. Scores must be adjusted according to child's age:
(0–6 months = 9, 6–12 months = 11, 1–2 years = 12, 2–5 years = 13, > 5 years = 14)

Simpson D, Reilly P. Pediatric coma scale. Lancet 1982;2(8295):450

12.6.3 Children's coma score (CCS)

This scale also evaluates eye-opening response and motor response to stimuli, but it is limited only for infants and toddlers. Maximum CCS assignable is 11, and minimal 3. CCS is very useful for all paediatric TBIs in infants and toddlers.

	Response	Score
Ocular response	Pursuit	4
	EOM intact, reactive pupils	3
	Fixed pupils or EOM impaired	2
	Fixed pupils or EOM paralyzed	1

(*Continued*)

▶ (*Continued*)

	Response	Score
Verbal response	Cries	3
	Spontaneous respiration	2
	Apnea	1
Motor response	Flexes and extends	4
	Withdraws from painful stimuli	3
	Hypertonic	2
	Flaccid	1

Abbreviation: EOM, extraocular muscles.
Source: Raimondi AJ, Hirschauer J. Head injury in the infant and toddler. Coma scoring and outcome scale. Childs Brain 1984;11:12–35

12.6.4 Trauma infant neurological score (TINS)

TINS is used for evaluation of TBI severity in infants and children under 3 years of age. It combines clinical and history elements: mechanism of trauma, orotracheal intubation on arrival, neurological exam, presence of subgaleal hematoma. Total score ranges from 1 to 10 points. TINS score over 2 indicates the need for a CT scan. In conclusion, TINS is very useful in TBI in 0–3-year-old children. TINS also reflects outcome of these patients (at 10 points the outcome is critical status).

	Min/max	0	1	2
Mechanism of trauma	1/2	–	Fall < 1 m or mild blow	Fall > 1 m or penetrating injury
Intubated on arrival	0/2	No	Yes	–
Alertness	0/2	Fully alert, but arousable	Decreased	Unconscious
Motor deficit	0/2	None	Localizing signs	No movement
Pupils	0/2	Reactive bilaterally	Anisocoria or nonreactive	Dilated and nonreactive
Scalp injury	0/1	None	Subgaleal hematoma	–

Source: Beni-Adani L, Flores I, Spektor S, Umansky F, Constantini S. Epidural hematoma in infants: a different entity? J Trauma 1999;46(2):306–311.

12.6.5 Liege scale

Adding information on brainstem reflexes improves the prognostic precision of the GCS for patients with severe head injury. The Glasgow-Liege scale improves the precision of prognosis especially in head trauma patients with initial and complete loss of consciousness.

Brainstem reflexes	Scores
Fronto-orbicular reflex	5
Vertical oculocephalic or oculovestibular reflex	4
Papillary light reflex	3
Horizontal oculocephalic or oculovestibular reflex	2
Oculocardiac reflex	1

Laureys S, Majerus S, Moonen G. Assessing consciousness in critically ill patients. Yearbook of Intensive Care and Emergency Medicine. JL Vincent, Heidelberg, Springer-Verlag; 2002:715–727

12.7 Comatose Patients in the Emergency Room

The problem of patients presenting in coma is common. Regardless of the cause, the approach to these patients requires rapid assessment while instituting therapeutic and diagnostic measures, which identify and correct or amend any processes that might lead to progressive and irreversible damage.

The preliminary differential diagnosis addresses the question: "Is the coma due to a primary CNS disease or secondary to a systemic illness?" Focal findings strongly suggest the presence of a structural lesion. Systemic problems, such as a lack of nutrients (glucose, oxygen) or metabolic problems (sodium, calcium) or an accumulation of toxins (carbon dioxide, carbon monoxide, alcohol) cause diffuse CNS dysfunction. Occasionally, hyponatremia, hepatic coma, or nonketotic hyperosmolar coma can present with focal neurological signs.

12.7.1 Differential diagnosis

The first 10 items in the differential diagnosis list below are the most life- and function-threatening:
1. Shock or hypertensive encephalopathy (decreased cardiac output, myocardial infarction, congestive heart failure, and pulmonary embolus)
2. CO narcosis or hypoxia (pulmonary disease, hypoventilation)
3. Hyperthermia or hypothermia
4. Hypoglycemia (insulin overdose)

5. Wernicke's encephalopathy (thiamine deficiency)
6. Exogenous toxins (opiates, carbon monoxide, cyanide, barbiturates, benzodiazepines, antidepressants, antihistamines, atropine, organic phosphates, bromides, anticholinergics, ethanol, methanol, ethylene glycol, hallucinogens, ammonium chloride, heavy metals, over-the-counter drugs including salicylates)
7. Stroke (ischemic)
8. Intracranial hemorrhage (with or without trauma)
9. Meningitis (bacterial, syphilis, fungal, carcinomatous)
10. Reye's syndrome (paediatric)
11. Trauma (diffuse axonal injury to the brain)
12. Tumors (CNS meningioma, glioma, and remote effects, e.g., lung cancer)
13. Toxins (mercury, arsenic, lead, and magnesium)
14. Infections (sepsis, any infection outside the CNS especially in elderly, AIDS, subacute bacterial endocarditis)
15. CNS infections (progressive multifocal leukoencephalopathy, Creutzfeldt–Jakob disease)
16. Seizures (status epilepticus, prolonged postictal state)
17. Blood (anemia, sickle cell disease)
18. Vascular (systemic lupus erythematosus)
19. Metabolic (hypercalcemia, uremic encephalopathy, hepatic encephalopathy, hyperosmolar state, thyrotoxicosis or myxedema coma, Cushing's disease, pituitary apoplexy, porphyria)
20. Psychiatric (especially depression, hysterical conversion reaction)
21. Other (migraine, basilar especially in children)

The mnemonics **TIPPS** on the vowels **AEIOU** list the frequent causes of coma:

A = alcohol/anoxia
E = epilepsy
I = insulin
O = opiates
U = uremia
T = trauma
I = infection
P = poisoning
P = psychogenic
S = shock, stroke

12.8 Coma in Children

- Head injuries
  Children in traumatic coma usually do not have a surgically correctable lesion. A relatively minor injury can have an apparent initial recovery, followed by

several hours or decreased level of consciousness with waxing and waning signs, then complete recovery (Posttraumatic stupor and delayed nonhemorrhagic encephalopathy).

- Seizures
  The postictal state in children can occasionally be prolonged and last two to three days.
- Reye's syndrome
  This postviral illness tends to be associated with salicylate ingestion and presents with decreased level of consciousness and elevated ammonia levels. Due to a decrease in use of aspirin for fever in children, it is now less common.

12.9 Coma in the Elderly

- Ischemic stroke
  It is more common in the elderly. Basilar artery thrombosis impairs brainstem perfusion causing onset of coma. Large hemispheric ischemic strokes may develop massive cerebral edema and result in compression of the brain stem over days from onset. Cerebellar hemisphere strokes (ischemic or hemorrhagic) can result in coma for hours to days.
- Chronic subdural hematomas
  It presents much more commonly in the elderly and about half the time a history of head trauma, which may be very minor, is obtained.
- Hypothyroidism
  Must always be considered in the elderly
- Sedatives
  The elderly patient can be very sensitive to medication including sedative hypnotic medications.
- Drug overdose
  The elderly may accidentally or intentionally take on overdose of drugs.
- Postictal
  The postictal state following seizures may be prolonged in the elderly patient

12.10 Unresponsive Patient

1. Intracranial lesions
   a) Cerebrovascular disease
      i. Hemorrhage
         - Intracerebral
         - Subarachnoid
         - Epidural hematoma
         - Subdural hematoma

    ii. Ischemia
- Watershed
- Cardioembolism
- Vasculitis
- Hypercoagulable disorder
- Hypoxic-ischemic encephalopathy
- Cerebral venous thrombosis

    iii. TBI
- Contusions
- Diffuse axonal injury

    iv. Epilepsy
- Generalized or partial complex seizures
- Status epilepticus (convulsive, nonconvulsive)
- postictal states

    v. Neoplasm
- Primary
- Metastatic

    vi. Brain edema

    vii. Infection
- Meningitis
- Encephalitis
- Abscess

    viii. Primary neuronal or glial disorders
- Progressive multifocal leukoencephalopathy (PML)
- Creutzfeldt–Jakob disease
- Adrenoleukodystrophy
- Gliomatosis cerebri

2. Toxic and metabolic encephalopathy

  a) Exogenous

    i. Sedatives or psychotropic drugs
- Ethanol
- Barbiturates
- Opiates
- Cocaine
- Tricyclic antidepressants and anticholinergic drugs
- Phenothiazines
- Heroin
- Amphetamines
- Lysergic acid diethylamide, mescaline
- Anticonvulsants
- Selective serotonin reuptake inhibitors

        ii. Acid poisons
- Methyl alcohol
- Paraldehyde

       iii. Other
- Organic phosphates
- Cyanide
- Heavy metals
- Cardiac glycosides
- Steroids (Insulin)
- Carbon monoxide exposure

b) Endogenous

      i. Hyperglycemia
- Ketotic coma
- Nonketotic coma

      ii. Hypoglycemia (endogenous insulin, liver disease, etc.)

     iii. Uremic coma (kidney failure)

     iv. Hepatic coma (liver failure)

      v. Wernicke's encephalopathy (thiamine deficiency)

     vi. CO_2 narcosis (pulmonary failure)

    vii. Electrolyte disturbance
- Dehydration
- Drug-induced
- Heat stroke
- Fever

   viii. Endocrine
- Pituitary apoplexy and necrosis
- Adrenal (Addison's disease, Cushing's disease, pheochromocytoma)
- Thyroid (myxedema "coma," thyrotoxicosis)
- Pancreas (diabetes, hypoglycemia)

     ix. Systemic illness
- Cancer
- Sepsis
- Porphyria

3. Anoxia

a) Hypoxic (decreased blood pO and O content)

      i. Pulmonary disease

     ii. Decreased atmospheric oxygen tension

b) Anemic (decreased blood O content, pO normal)

      i. CO poisoning

     ii. Anemia

     iii. Methemoglobinemia

4. Ischemia
   a) Decreased cardiac output
      i. Congestive heart failure
      ii. Cardiac arrest
      iii. Severe cardiac arrhythmias
      iv. Aortic stenosis
   b) Decreased systemic peripheral resistance
      i. Blood loss and hypovolemic shock
      ii. Syncopal attack
      iii. Anaphylactic shock
   c) Intracranial vessel disease
      i. Increased vascular resistance
         – Subarachnoid hemorrhage
         – Bacterial meningitis
         – Hyperviscosity (polycythemia, sickle cell anemia)
      ii. Widespread small-vessel occlusions
         – Subacute bacterial endocarditis
         – Disseminated intravascular coagulation (DIC)
         – CNS arteritis (systemic lupus erythematosus)
         – Fat embolism
5. Mental illness
   a) Conversion hysteria
   b) Catatonic stupor (often a manifestation of schizophrenia)
   c) Dissociative or "fugue" state
   d) Severe psychotic depression
   e) Malingering

12.11 Metabolic and Psychogenic Coma

In unresponsive patients, differences between the mental state, motor signs, breathing patterns, electroencephalogram (EEG), and oculovestibular or caloric reflexes distinguish metabolic from psychiatric disease.

12.11.1 Comatose patients with metabolic disease

Metabolic encephalopathy is, by far, the most common cause of unconsciousness in general hospitals. The striking and diagnostic finding with most metabolic agents is that they selectively depress certain susceptible functions at several different levels of the brain, but at the same time spare other functions which equally depend on structures at those selfsame levels. Obviously, no mechanical lesion could possess this combination of launching both diffuse and selective attack at the same time.

There are other helpful clues:
1. Metabolic encephalopathies cause confusion and delirium in advance of stupor and coma.
2. Many cases are accompanied by various forms of tremor or myoclonus in their pre-coma stage.
3. The motor signs are usually symmetrical.
4. The EEG is generally very slow.
5. Caloric stimulation elicits either tonic deviation of the eyes or, if the patient is deeply comatose, there is no response.
6. Seizures are common.
7. All metabolic comas spare the papillary light reflex.
8. They usually do not and they never impair central sensory pathways, except as a part of the overall depression of unconsciousness.
9. Respiratory changes are common, often because the disease itself produces acid-base changes.

12.11.2 Psychologically unresponsive patients

The diagnostic key is that patients with psychogenic responsiveness are behaviorally abnormal but physiologically normal. Not surprising, therefore, shouting, pinching, and various other traumatic assaults have an unpredictable effect or none at all. This stands in contrast to the normal results of physical examination, that is:
1. The EEG is normal
2. Caloric stimulation
   Normal response to caloric irrigation, with nystagmus having a quick phase away from the side of ice-water irrigation; there is little or no tonic deviation of the eyes. Nystagmus is present.
3. Lids close actively, whereas the lids shut more gently in true coma.
4. No pathologic reflexes are present.
5. Pupils reactive or dilated (cycloplegics).
6. Muscle tone is normal or inconsistent.

Plum and Posner's. Diagnosis of Stupor and Coma. 4th ed. Oxford University Press; 2007

12.12 Metabolic and Structural Coma

When a physician meets patients with impaired consciousness, the first and most compelling question about the cause is concerned, as to whether the condition is structural or metabolic. Often answers are found in close attention to history taking and the physical examination. A careful clinical thinking yields more important information than a scattershot of hurried laboratory tests.

Structural lesions are almost always supratentorial or infratentorial in locus, rarely both, while the metabolic disorders tend to affect the brain at several different levels at the same time.

The metabolic and structural diseases are distinguished from each other by combinations of motor signs and their evolution, and EEG changes.

12.12.1 Comatose patients with metabolic disease (60%)

Patients usually suffer from partial dysfunction affecting many levels of neuraxis simultaneously, while at the same time retain the integrity of other functions originating at the same level. In general, patients should be suspected of suffering from metabolic disease if below given findings are present.

1. Cognitive and behavioral changes (if they represent the earliest or the only signs)
    a) Cognition
        i. Poor memory
        ii. Disoriented
        iii. Language impaired
        iv. Inattentive
        v. Dyscalculia
    b) Behavior
        i. Agitated
        ii. Delusions and/or hallucinations
2. Diffusely abnormal motor signs which are bilateral and symmetric
    a) Tremor
    b) Myoclonus
    c) Bilateral asterixis
3. The EEG is diffusely, but not focally, slow
4. Acid-base abnormalities with hyper- and hypoventilation are frequent
5. Pupillary reactions are usually preserved even if the patient is comatose

12.12.2 Comatose patients with gross structural disease (40%)

Patients generally have a rostrocaudal deterioration that is characteristic of supratentorial mass lesions. This condition does not occur in metabolic brain disease, nor is the anatomic defect regionally restricted as it is the case with subtentorial damage. Light reflex loss and anisocoria suggest a structural etiology. The clinical signs are certainly helpful, but there is too much overlap to verify the diagnosis on clinical findings alone. It is not uncommon, in patients with hepatic encephalopathy or hypoglycemia, to develop focal motor signs such as hemiparesis or visual field defects that are characteristic of a structural lesion, whereas patients with multiple brain metastases may develop nothing other than a global alteration of cognitive function. Thus, laboratory screening tests are essential to exclude structural disease. Following are the screening tests:

1. CT/MR imaging with enhancement (e.g., metastases, infection)
2. Lumbar puncture (e.g., infection, meningeal carcinomatosis)
3. EEG
4. Hematological work-up
   a) Blood cultures (e.g., sepsis, septic emboli)
   b) Full blood count
   c) Coagulation tests (e.g., prothrombin time, partial thromboplastin time, fibrin degeneration product)
   d) Blood gases
5. Biochemical work-up
   a) Electrolytes (e.g., Na, K, Ca, Mg, PO_2)
   b) Blood urea nitrogen, creatinine, glucose, lactate
   c) Endocrine tests (e.g., follicle-stimulating hormone, T3, T4, cortisol)
   d) Thiamine, folic acid, Vitamin B12
6. Drug levels (e.g., digoxin, anticonvulsants, theophylline etc.)

The patient should be suspected of suffering from structural brain disease, either alone or in combination with metabolic brain disease if:

1. Abnormal focal motor signs (including focal seizures) occur, which progress rostral to caudal and are asymmetrical.
2. Neurological signs point to one anatomic area (mesencephalon, pons, medulla).
3. Specific cognitive function disorders, such as aphasia, acalculia, or agnosia, appear out of proportion to a general overall decrease in mental state.
4. The EEG may be slow, but in addition there is a focal abnormality.
5. The patient is at particular risk of developing one of the complications of cancer that may mimic metabolic brain disease, particularly disseminated intravascular coagulation (DIC) or meningitis.

Plum and Posner's. Diagnosis of Stupor and Coma. 4th ed. Oxford University Press; 2007

12.13 Coma-Like States

The basic brain structure that is responsible for arousal is the ascending reticular activating system (ARAS). This system originates in the brain stem reticular formation and extends to the cortex via the diffuse or nonspecific thalamo-frontal projection system. Reticular activation, by means of an external stimulus, alerts widespread areas of the cortex and subcortex, thus enabling the patient to be alert, think clearly, learn effectively, and relate meaningfully.

If there is damage to the extension of the brainstem reticular system in the thalamus or hypothalamus, the full picture of coma will not occur. Since the brainstem portion of the ARAS is intact, reticular activity innervates the nuclei of the extraocular nerves, and the patients can open their eyes and look about. The cortex, however, is not sufficiently stimulated to produce voluntary movement or speech. These patients are in a coma-like state.

12.13.1 Pharmacologically induced coma

The treatment of neurologic emergencies, such as refractory status epilepticus or intractable intracranial hypertension, can involve the deliberate induction of a coma-like state with sedatives or anesthetic agents (e.g., barbiturates, propofol, and midazolam). These agents are responsible for a dramatic decrease in neuronal activity with concomitant reduction in cerebral metabolism and cerebral blood flow. Pharmacologically induced coma can abolish virtually all clinical evidence of brain or brainstem activity, and confounds the clinician's ability to diagnose coma or even brain death.

12.13.2 Brain death

Represents a complete and irreversible loss of brain and brainstem function. It is recognized clinically by the abolition of consciousness, cranial nerve activity, motor reflexes, and spontaneous breathing. Before a diagnosis of brain death can be made, conditions that can confound neurologic assessment must be ruled out. In particular physiologic or metabolic derangements, severe hypothermia (temperature < 32°C), and recent exposure to toxic or pharmacologic agents might impair consciousness or neuromuscular transmission. Although not necessary for the clinical diagnosis, the EEG in brain death is silent, and cerebral metabolism is absent.

Diagnosis	Level of consciousness	Voluntary movements	Eye responses
Akinetic mutism (differentiation)	Patient seemingly awake, but silent and motionless	Lack of movement; more often patients move one side or one arm in a stereotyped fashion in response to noxious stimuli	Eyes dart in the direction of moving objects

(*Continued*)

579

▶ (*Continued*)

Diagnosis	Level of consciousness	Voluntary movements	Eye responses
Persistent vegetative state	Wakefulness accompanied by an apparent total lack of cognitive function. Sleep–wake cycles exist	Usually little or none, depending upon the brain areas damaged. Mostly primitive postural reflexes	Eyes open spontaneously in response to verbal stimuli
Apallic state	Awake; no meaningful interaction with environment	Little or no purposeful movement; mostly reflexes or mass movements	Open, searching, but no real eye contact
Locked-in syndrome (differentiation)	Awake, alert, aware of self, and capable of perceiving sensory stimuli	None; motionless	Open, with normal following and good eye contact. Vertical eye or eyelid movements (blinking) are retained. In some cases, lateral gaze is also paralyzed

Diagnosis	Speech	Muscle tone	Reflexes
Akinetic mutism (differentiation)	Vocalizing little or not at all. Can produce normal, short phrases on stimulation	Usually normal; sometimes slight increase in legs	"Frontal release signs," such as grasp or sucking may be present. Often display signs of corticospinal track involvement, such as hyperreflexia, and a Babinski sign
Persistent vegetative state	None or occasional grunts or groans. Some patients produce a few words	Variable, often increased. Extremities often in flexion	Variable, usually increased with pathologic reflexes
Apallic state	None or occasional grunting	Increased in all limbs. Extremities often in bilateral decortication and double hemiplegia	Increased in all extremities with primitive reflexes. Brainstem reflexes intact
Locked-in syndrome (differentiation)	Aphonia from interruption of corticobulbar fibers to the lower cranial nerves	Acute spastic tetraplegia	Increased in all extremities

Diagnosis	Clinical-pathological studies	EEG findings
Akinetic mutism (differentiation)	Lesions affect: (1) bilaterally the frontal region (anterior cingulate gyri), (2) the diencephalomesencephalic reticular formation and globus pallidus, (3) the hypothalamus, or (4) septal area. The most common cause is occlusion of the small vessels entering the brain stem from the tip of the basilar artery. Less commonly due to severe acute hydrocephalus, and direct compression by tumors	It shows slow wave abnormalities
Persistent vegetative state	Damage to forebrain structures causing severe mental loss but preservation of the patient's autonomic or vegetative functions	EEG in several instances were essentially isoelectric but in others regained various patterns of rhythm and amplitude, not consistent from one case to the other
Apallic state	Diffuse bilateral degeneration of the cerebral cortex and absent neocortical function but with relatively intact brainstem function. That sometimes follows anoxia, hypoglycemia, circulatory or metabolic embarrassment, or encephalitis	EEG shows severe diffuse slowing with no response to auditory or noxious stimuli
Locked-in syndrome (Differentiation)	Damage of the descending motor pathways bilaterally in the upper pontine tegmentum that interrupts all corticospinal and corticobulbar fibers at the level of the abducens and facial nuclei, but spares the more dorsal reticular formation. It is usually due to basilar artery thrombosis with ventral pontine infarction, pontine hemorrhage or tumor, or central pontine myelinolysis. In rare cases, tentorial herniation, severe polyneuropathies, or myasthenia gravis may also cause this syndrome	The EEG reflects the patient's state of wakefulness

Plum and Posner's. Diagnosis of Stupor and Coma. 4th ed. Oxford University Press; 2007

12.14 Trauma Score

The trauma score is a numerical grading system for estimating the severity of injury. The score is composed of the GCS (reduced to approximately one-third total value) and measurements of cardiopulmonary function. Each parameter is given a number (high for normal and low for impaired function). Severity of injury is estimated by summing the numbers. The lowest score is 1, and the highest score is 16.

Parameter	Range	Score
Respiratory rate	10–24/min	4
	25–35/min	3
	36/min or greater	2
	1–9/min	1
	None	0
Respiratory expansion	Normal	1
	Retractive/none	0
Systolic blood pressure	90 mmHg or greater	4
	70–80 mmHg	3
	50–69 mmHg	2
	0–49 mmHg	1
	No pulse	0
Capillary refill	Normal	2
	Delayed	1
	None	0

The following table shows the projected estimate of survival for each value in the trauma score, based on results from 1,509 patients with blunt or penetrating injury.

Trauma score	Percentage survival (%)
16	99
15	98
14	96
13	93
12	87
11	76
10	60
9	42
8	26
7	15
6	8
5	4
4	2
3	1
2	0
1	0

12.15 Respiratory Patterns in Comatose Patients

Anatomic level of pathologic lesion	Respiratory patterns (Fig. 12.2)
Forebrain damage	
Bilateral widespread cortical lesions	
Bilateral thalamic dysfunction	Eupneic, with sighs or yawns
Lesions in the descending pathways anywhere from the cerebral hemispheres to the level of the upper pons.	Cheyne–Stokes breathing
Hypothalamic-midbrain damage	
Patients with dysfunction involving the rostral brainstem tegmentum. Lesions have been found between the low midbrain and the middle third of the pons, destroying the paramedian reticular formation just ventral to the aqueduct and fourth ventricle	Sustained regular hyperventilation (despite the prolonged and rapid hyperpnea, patients are hypocapnic and relatively hypoxic and have pulmonary congestion leading rapidly to pulmonary edema. This type of breathing, therefore, cannot be called "primary hyperventilation")
Lower pontine damage	
Patients have lesion or dysfunction of the lateral tegmentum of the lower half of the pons adjacent to the trigeminal motor nucleus. More prolonged apneusis has developed when the lesions extend caudally to involve the dorsolateral pontine nuclei	Apneustic breathing
Pontomedullary junction damage	
Patients have lesions at the lower pontine or high medullary level	Cluster breathing
Medullary damage or dysfunction	
Follows lesions of the respiratory centers located in reticular formation of the dorsomedial part of the medulla and extend down to or just below the obex	Ataxic breathing (Biot) or "atrial fibrillation of respiration" (inspiratory gaps of diverse amplitude and length intermingle with periods of apnea)

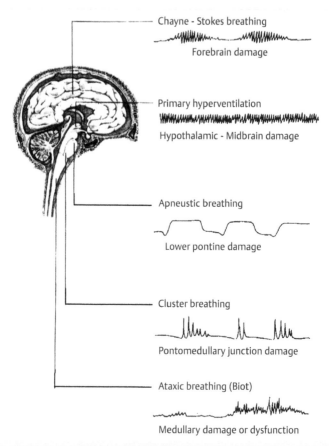

Chayne - Stokes breathing

Forebrain damage

Primary hyperventilation

Hypothalamic - Midbrain damage

Apneustic breathing

Lower pontine damage

Cluster breathing

Pontomedullary junction damage

Ataxic breathing (Biot)

Medullary damage or dysfunction

Fig. 12.2 Abnormal types of breathing in severe head injuries.

Wijdicks EFM, Bamlet WR, Maramattom BV, Manno EM, McClelland RL. Validation of a new coma scale: The FOUR score. Ann Neurol 2005;58(4):585–593

Bassetti C, Aldrich MS, Quint D. Sleep-disordered breathing in patients with acute supra- and infratentorial strokes. A prospective study of 39 patients. Stroke 1997;28(9):1765–1772

12.16 Pupillary Changes in Comatose Patients

Brain stem areas controlling consciousness are anatomically adjacent to those controlling the pupils. Pupillary changes, therefore, are a valuable guide to the presence and location of brainstem diseases producing coma.

Pupillary shape, size, symmetry, and response to light reflect patency or not of the brain stem and third nerve function. The pupillary light reflex is very sensitive to mechanical distortion, but very resistant to metabolic dysfunction. Abnormalities of this reflex, particularly when unilateral, is the single most important physical sign potentially distinguishing structural from metabolic coma.

Location of the coma-producing structural lesions	Pupils
Sleep or diencephalic dysfunction (metabolic coma)	Small, react well to light ("diencephalic pupils")
Unilateral hypothalamic damage or dysfunction	Miosis and anhidrosis (ipsilateral to the lesion)
Midbrain tectal or pretectal damage	Midsized (5–6 mm) or slightly large, "fixed" hippus (spontaneous oscillations in size) that becomes larger when neck is pinched (ciliospinal reflex)
Midbrain tegmental damage (CN III nucleus involvement)	Midsized (4–5 mm), often unequal, usually slightly irregular (irregular constriction of the sphincter of the iris results in a pear-shaped pupil), midbrain corectopia (displacement of the pupil to one side), fixed to light and lack of ciliospinal response
Pontine tegmental damage	Pinpoint, constricting to light (due to a combination of sympathetic damage and parasympathetic irritation)
Pontine lateral, lateral medullary, and ventrolateral cervical cord damage or dysfunction	Ipsilateral Horner's syndrome
Peripheral lesions	The light reflex is sluggish or absent, the pupils become widely dilated (7–8 mm) due to sparing of the sympathetic pathways (Hutchinson's pupil). Oval-shaped pupils due to nonuniform paresis of the pupil sphincter, causing an eccentric antagonistic effect of pupil dilators

Ritter AM, Muizelaar JP, Barnes T, et al. Brain stem blood flow, pupillary response, and outcome in patients with severe head injuries. Neurosurgery 1999;44(5):941–948

Cruz J, Minoja G, Okuchi K. Major clinical and physiological benefits of early high doses of mannitol for intraparenchymal temporal lobe hemorrhages with abnormal pupillary widening: a randomized trial. Neurosurgery 2002;51(3):628–637, discussion 637–638

Shlugman D, Parulekar M, Elston JS, Farmery A. Abnormal pupillary activity in a brainstem-dead patient. Br J Anaesth 2001;86(5):717–720

Tokuda Y, Nakazato N, Stein GH. Pupillary evaluation for differential diagnosis of coma. Postgrad Med J 2003;79(927):49–51

12.17 Spontaneous Eye Movements in Comatose Patients

Location of the coma-producing structural damage	Spontaneous eye movements
Bilateral cerebral damage (bilateral cerebral ischemia) with an intact brain stem. Rarely in posterior fossa hemorrhage	Periodic alternating gaze (Ping-Pong gaze). Roving of the eyes in full swing of the horizontal plane in oscillating cycles of 2–5 seconds
Mid or lower pontine damage	Nystagmoid jerking of a single eye in a horizontal, vertical, or rotatory fashion and occasional bilateral disconjugate vertical and rotatory eye movements (one eye may rise and intort as the other falls and extorts)
Intrinsic pontine lesions (hemorrhage, tumor, infarction etc.), extra-axial posterior fossa masses (hemorrhage or infarction), diffuse encephalitis, and toxic metabolic encephalopathies	Ocular bobbing (intermittent, often conjugate, brisk, bilateral downward movement of the eyes with slow return to mid-position). When associated with preservation of horizontal eye movements, it becomes a specific finding but not pathognomonic of acute pontine injury
Diffuse brain dysfunction and encephalopathy (anoxic coma or after prolonged status epilepticus). No definite brain stem lesion	Ocular dipping (slow downward eye movement with fast return to mid-position). Brain stem horizontal gaze reflexes are usually intact
Pontine hemorrhage, viral encephalitis, and metabolic encephalopathy	Reverse ocular bobbing (fast upward eye movement with a slow return to mid-position)
Pretectal area (acute hydrocephalus)	Pretectal pseudobobbing (arrhythmic, repetitive downward and inward, "V-pattern," eye movements at a rate ranging from 1 per 3 seconds to 2 per second and an amplitude of one-fifth to half of the full voluntary range). Often associated with abnormal pupillary light reactions, intact horizontal eye movements, open and often retracted eyelids, a blink frequently preceding each eye movement, and a mute or stuporous patient. This situation requires immediate surgical decompression of hydrocephalus
Severe pontine damage (locked-in patients)	Vertical ocular myoclonus (pendular, vertical isolated movements of the eyes with a frequency of 2 Hz, and other rhythmic body movements after a 6-week to 9-month delay)

Levy DE, Caronna JJ, Singer BH, Lapinski RH, Frydman H, Plum F. Predicting outcome from hypoxic-ischemic coma. JAMA 1985;253(10):1420–1426

Bateman DE. Neurological assessment of coma. J Neurol Neurosurg Psychiatry 2001;71(Suppl 1):i13–i17

12.18 Abnormal Motor Responses in Comatose Patients

Location of the coma producing structural lesion	Abnormal motor responses
Cerebral hemispheres, diencephalon, precollicular level of midbrain	Decorticate rigidity (adduction of the shoulder and arm, flexion at the elbow, and pronation and flexion at the wrist; the leg remains extended at the hip and knee)
Intercollicular level of midbrain, down to the middle of pontine tegmentum	Decerebrate rigidity (extension and pronation of the upper extremities and forcible plantar flexion of the foot. Produced by noxious stimuli; opisthotonos develops periodically with hyperextension of the trunk, hyperpronation of the arms, and clenched teeth)
Pontine tegmentum	Abnormal extension of the arms with weak flexion of the legs
Below the junction between the lower and middle third of pons, medulla	Flaccid or absent motor response (skeletal muscle flaccidity marks the initial motor phase of acute functional spinal cord transection—"spinal shock")

Jennett B, Teasdale G, Galbraith S, et al. Prognosis in patients with severe head injury. Acta Neurochir Suppl (Wien) 1979;28(1):149–152

Born JD, Albert A, Hans P, Bonnal J. Relative prognostic value of best motor response and brain stem reflexes in patients with severe head injury. Neurosurgery 1985;16(5):595–601

13 Infections of the Central Nervous System

13.1 Pathogens Responsible for Bacterial Infections

The epidemiology of bacterial meningitis has changed significantly, primarily because of widespread immunization with the conjugated *Haemophilus influenzae* vaccine (HIB) in 1990 and the *Streptococcus pneumoniae* vaccine in 2000. Before the introduction of these vaccines, *H. influenzae* accounted for nearly half of all bacterial meningitis cases (45%), followed by *S. pneumoniae* (18%) and then *Neisseria meningitides* (14%). After the introduction of the HIB vaccine, the most common pathogens were *S. pneumoniae* (47%), *N. meningitides* (25%), group B streptococcus (12%), and *Listeria monocytogenes* (8%) (refer to the following tables). It is likely that the most recent addition of the *S. pneumoniae* vaccine will change the specific epidemiology of bacterial meningitis again. Indeed, the widespread use of the pneumococcal vaccine beginning in infancy has decreased the incidence of invasive disease by *S. pneumoniae* by more than 90%.

Before introduction of *Haemophilus influenzae* type B vaccines		After introduction of *H. influenzae* type B vaccines	
H. influenzae	45%	*Streptococcus pneumoniae*	47%
S. pneumoniae	18%	*Neisseria meningitidis*	25%
N. meningitidis	14%	Streptococcus group B (*S. agalactiae*)	12%
Streptococcus group B (*S. agalactiae*)	6%	*Listeria monocytogenes*	8%
Listeria monocytogenes	3%	*H. influenzae*	7%
Others[a]	14%	Others	1%
Children < 5 years old (> 70% *H. influenzae*)			

[a]*Staphylococcus aureus*, *S. epidermidis*, Streptococcus group B, *Escherichia coli*, *Proteus mirabilis*, *Pseudomonas aeruginosa*, *Mycobacterium tuberculosis*, *Acinetobacter* species.

Predisposing factor	Common bacterial pathogens
Paediatric	
Neonate (< 30 days)	*Group B streptococci Gram negatives: (Escherichia coli, Klebsiella), Listeria monocytogenes*
Children 1–23 months	*S. pneumoniae, N. meningitidis, Group B streptococcus, H. Influenzae, E. coli*
Children 2–18 years	*S. pneumoniae, N. meningitidis*
Adult	
Young and middle aged (18–50 years)	*S. pneumoniae, N. meningitidis*
>50 years + elderly	*S. pneumoniae, N. meningitidis, L. monocytogenes*
Impaired immunity (such as HIV)	*S. pneumoniae, N. meningitidis, L. monocytogenes, aerobic Gram-negative bacilli (including Pseudomonas aeruginosa)*
Basilar skull fracture	*S. pneumoniae, H. influenzae, group A β-hemolytic streptococci*
Penetrating head trauma, post neurosurgery	*S. aureus, S. epidermidis, aerobic Gram-negative bacilli (including P. aeruginosa)*
Cerebrospinal fluid shunt (e.g., VP shunt)	*S. epidermidis, S. aureus, aerobic Gram-negative bacilli (including P. aeruginosa), Propionibacterium acnes*
Splenectomy	*S. pneumoniae, H. influenzae, N. meningitidis*
Petechial rash	*N. meningitidis, S. pneumoniae (post splenectomy), H. influenzae (post splenectomy)*
Brain stem encephalitis/abscess/early seizures	*L. monocytogenes*

Source: Wenger JD, Hightower AW, Facklam RR, et al. Bacterial meningitis in the USA in 1985. The Bacterial Meningitis Study Group. J Infect Dis 1990;162:1316–1322.
Tunkel AR, Sheid WM. Acute meningitis. In: Mandell JE, Bennett JE, Dolin R, eds. Principles and practices of infectious diseases. 5th ed. Philadelphia: Churchill Livingstone; 2000:962

The **incidence** of bacterial meningitis is 4–10 cases per 100,000 persons per year in the United States. The causative agents vary with the age of the patients. Mortality rates for all causes of meningitis were approximately 20%, except *H. influenzae* meningitis in which it is less than 3%.

13.1.1 Signs and symptoms of meningitis

In adults the symptoms include fever, headaches, stiff neck, confusion or altered mental status, lethargy, photophobia, seizures, vomiting, profuse sweating, myalgia, and generalized malaise. The classic triad is fever, neck stiffness, and altered mental status. Only 44% of adults in the community had the classic triad. Ninety-five percent of the patients had at least two of the three symptoms. Positive signs of Kerning and Brudzinski are hallmarks of meningitis yet present in only about 50% of adults. Confusion and fever suggest possible meningitis, particularly associated with a seizure. Seizures occur in 5–28% of adults with meningitis. Seizures are the presenting symptom in one-third of children, and occur more frequently with *S. pneumoniae* and *H. influenzae*, than with meningococcal meningitis. Cranial nerve palsies (CNs III, IV, VI, and VII) occur in 10–20% of patients. Focal neurologic deficits (i.e., dysphasia, hemiparesis) due to ischemia and infarction adjacent to the subarachnoid space are less frequent. A petechial rash is common with meningococcemia (up to 50% of cases) and less frequently with *Staphylococcus aureus*, *Acinetobacter* species, and *Rickettsia* species. Patients may develop signs of raised intracranial pressure with papilledema, temporal lobe herniation, and coma.

In very young infants with meningitis, the chief complaint is often nonspecific and include: irritability, lethargy, poor feeding, fever, seizures, apnea, a rash, or a bulging fontanelle.

In geriatric patients, frequently the presenting sign of meningitis is confusion or an altered mental status.

The onset of presentation differs depending on many variables including age, underlying comorbidity, immunocompetence, mental competence, ability to communicate, prior antibiotic therapy, and the specific bacterial pathogens.

The differential diagnosis of viral meningitis includes the other causes of aseptic meningitis, such as partially treated bacterial meningitis, nonpolio enteroviruses, mumps (the most common cause of aseptic meningitis) tuberculous meningitis, spirochetal infections (leptospirosis, borreliosis, Lyme disease, and syphilis), and fungal, amoebic, neoplastic, sarcoidosis, chemical meningitis/drugs (azathioprine, NSAIDs, antimicrobial trimethoprim/sulfamethoxazole [TMP/SMX], ranitidine, carbamazepine), cranial hypotension, postsurgical state, granulomatous, and idiopathic meningitides.

Mace SE. Acute bacterial meningitis. Emerg Med Clin North Am 2008;26(2):281–317, viii

Bareja R, Pottathi S, Shah RK, et al. Trends in Bacterial etiology amongst cases of Meningitis. J Acad Indus Res 2013;1(12):761–765

Bacterial Meningitis in Canada. Bacterial meningitis in Canada: hospitalizations (1994–2001). Can Commun Dis Rep 2005;31(23):241–247

Katz JT, Ellerin TB, Tunkel AR. Acute bacterial meningitis. Hospital Physician Board Review Manual. Infect Dis 2004;9(4):1–12 van de Beek D, de Gans J, Spanjaard L, Weisfelt M, Reitsma JB, Vermeulen M. Clinical features and prognostic factors in adults with bacterial meningitis. N Engl J Med 2004;351(18):1849–1859

Durand ML, Calderwood SB, Weber DJ, et al. Acute bacterial meningitis in adults. A review of 493 episodes. N Engl J Med 1993;328(1):21–28

Kim KS, Harwood-Nass A. Acute bacterial meningitis in infants and children. Lancet Infect Dis 2010;10(1): 32–42

Riordan FA, Thomson AP, Sills JA, Hart CA. Bacterial meningitis in the first three months of life. Postgrad Med J 1995;71(831):36–38

Chávez-Bueno S, McCracken GH, Jr. Bacterial meningitis in children. Pediatr Clin North Am 2005;52(3): 795–810, vii

13.2 Viral Infections

In the central nervous system (CNS), *demyelination, degenerative disorders, and neoplastic disease* are all more common than *infections,* yet the prompt and accurate diagnosis of CNS infections is perhaps more important than any of these diseases because of the profound effect accurate diagnosis of infection has on patient treatment and outcome. Prompt institution of appropriate antibacterial and/or antiviral therapy is critical.

Viruses can cause meningitis or encephalitis, and the clinical presentation may overlap, with the latter having more significant alterations in the level of consciousness and possibly new psychiatric symptoms, cognitive defects, seizures, or focal neurologic deficits. The presentation of viral CNS infections is usually of a sudden onset of illness with fever, headache, nuchal rigidity, focal neurological signs, cerebrospinal fluid (CSF) pleocytosis, and focal abnormalities may be seen on EEG, CT, and/or MRI. The diagnosis of meningitis or encephalitis is based upon which feature predominates in the illness although meningoencephalitis is also a common term that recognizes the overlap. Distinguishing between encephalitis and meningitis is important because the likely etiology and subsequent management of each is different.

A **detailed history** can provide clues for an etiologic diagnosis. Occurrence during summer suggests *arbovirus* (e.g., West Nile virus) or *enterovirus* infection, while winter disease suggests other infections (e.g., *influenza*). The travel history can reveal clues to geographically restricted viruses, such as those predominantly found in Asia (Japanese encephalitis). Other points include taking a history of sexual contacts (e.g., HIV), insect contact (e.g., mosquitos harboring Western and Eastern equine viruses, West Nile virus), animal contact (e.g., rabies virus, lymphocytic choriomeningitis virus [LCMV]), recent vaccination or viral illness (e.g., acute demyelinating meningoencephalitis); and immunosuppression (e.g., human herpes virus 6, varicella zoster virus [VZV], cytomegalovirus [CMV], or JC virus).

Mortality and **morbidity** vary according to cause, but are high, e.g., mortality 10–40% in Japanese encephalitis, with neurological sequelae in 5–75% of survivors.

On **physical examination**, patients often have fever and may have signs of meningeal irritation but clear sensorium (i.e., meningitis), or altered mental status (i.e., encephalitis). The skin examination provides additional information, such as a petechial rash suggests meningococcal meningitis; a maculopapular rash can occur with West Nile virus meningoencephalitis; and a group of vesicles in a dermatomal pattern suggests VZV. Some manifestations suggest temporal lobe features in herpes simplex encephalitis; hydrophobia in rabies; parkinsonian and extrapyramidal features in Japanese encephalitis.

A **lumbar puncture** is important. Interpreting the results can be difficult, as there is overlap between the CSF findings in bacterial and viral infections; however, broad general differences can be stated. In *acute bacterial meningitis*, CSF white cell counts are usually high (hundreds or thousands per mL), with neutrophilic predominance, accompanied by elevated proteins and hypoglycorrhachia; while in *viral meningitis*, CSF shows a mild pleocytosis and lymphocytic predominance (though in early phase it can be neutrophilic), slightly elevated protein, and normal glucose (except LCMV when glucose is low). CSF analysis remains the best test for the diagnosis of meningeal diseases.

Knowledge of the possibilities and limitations of diagnostic methods for specific viral CNS infections is vital. A positive CSF polymerase chain reaction (PCR) finding is usually reliable for etiological diagnosis. The demonstration of intrathecal antibody synthesis is useful for confirming the etiology in a later stage of disease, hitherto sufficiently evaluated in herpes simplex encephalitis and tick-borne encephalitis.

Nucleic acid amplification methods have improved the detection of common (*herpes simplex virus [HSV], enterovirus,* and *VZV*) and uncommon viral pathogens. The results of these tests are available more quickly and are more sensitive than viral cultures. Other viral causes of meningoencephalitis, such as arboviruses (including West Nile virus), can be identified by detection of IgM and IgG antibodies in CSF. Despite improved virological and differential diagnostic methods, etiology remains unknown in about half (50%) of the cases with suspected viral encephalitis.

Imaging with **CT scans** alone can be done in uncomplicated cases of meningitis, but **MRI** is the single most important diagnostic test for parenchymal infections. The MRI signal intensity, and spatial distribution patterns in the CNS help differentiate important infections from other diseases. This shall include *bacterial cerebritis* and *abscess, tuberculoma,* and *tuberculous meningitis;* various forms of *viral encephalitis,* such as herpes simplex, herpes zoster, CMV and West Nile; *viral leukoencephalopathies,* such as progressive multifocal leukoencephalopathy (PML); and the *transmissible spongiform encephalopathies,* especially Creutzfeldt–Jakob disease (CJD). Differential include comparisons to the most common *parasitic diseases,* especially cysticercosis and toxoplasmosis, and to unusual manifestations of *neoplastic, demyelinating,* and *metabolic diseases.*

The differential diagnosis of viral encephalitis includes meningitis, Behcet's disease, systemic lupus erythematosus, multiple sclerosis, secondary syphilis, leukemia, lymphoma, other infective encephalopathies (bacterial, fungal, protozoal, and parasitic), intracranial abscesses and neoplasms, toxic and metabolic encephalopathies, and heat stroke. The diagnosis of "viral encephalitis" should not be made too hastily, because it may condemn the patient with concealed cerebral malaria or some other curable encephalopathy to delayed treatment or even death.

Kenedy PGE. Viral encephalitis: causes, differential diagnosis, and management. J Neurol Neurosurg Psychiatry 2004;75:110–115

Whitley RJ, Gnann JW. Viral encephalitis: familiar infections and emerging pathogens. Lancet 2002;359(9305):507–513

Baringer JR. Herpes simplex virus encephalitis. In: Davis LE, Kennedy PGE, eds. Infectious diseases of the nervous system 1st ed. Butterworth-Heinemann; 2002:135–164

Johnson RT. Viral infections of the nervous system. 2nd ed. Philadelphia: Lippincott-Raven; 1998

Ziai WC, Lewin JJ, III. Update in the diagnosis and management of central nervous system infections. Neurol Clin 2008;26(2):427–468, viii

Tunkel AR, Glasser CA, Bloch KC, et al. Infectious Society of America. The management of encephalitis: clinical practice guidelines by the infectious Disease Society of America. Clin Infect Dis 2008;47:303–327

13.2.1 RNA Viruses

1. Enteroviruses (*polioviruses, coxsackie viruses A, B, echoviruses, and enteroviruses*)

   The CNS is the most commonly involved organ system during the spread of human enteroviruses from the alimentary tract. A number of neurologic syndromes are recognized, and each can be caused by a number of different types of enteroviruses, i.e., aseptic meningitis, encephalitis, lower motor neuron paralysis, acute cerebellar ataxia, cranial nerve palsies, chronic persistent infections. Enteroviruses are responsible for 80–90% and mumps for 10–20% of diagnosed cases of viral meningitis, with many other viruses sometimes incriminated with considerable geographical and seasonal variation.

   Differential diagnosis of paralytic poliomyelitis: postinfectious and other immunopathic polyneuroradiculopathies, such as Guillain–Bare syndrome and Landry's ascending paralysis; metabolic neuropathies such as acute porphyria; paralytic rabies; neoplastic polyradiculopathies; and rarities, such as tick paralysis and herpesvirus simiae (B virus) infection. The lack of objective sensory loss in poliomyelitis usually distinguishes it from these other entities.

2. Arboviruses

Out of the 450 RNA viruses transmitted by arthropods, the two most common families causing encephalitis are: (a) the *Togaviridae* (i.e., *Western equine encephalitis, Eastern equine encephalitis, St. Louis encephalitis*) and (b) the *Bunyaviridae* (i.e., *California encephalitis viruses*). Japanese encephalitis is the most common encephalitis in Asia. Encephalitides caused by arthropod-borne viruses accounts for about 10% of all reported cases annually. An arbovirus may produce a fulminating encephalitis or an aseptic meningitis. Neither the clinical picture not the laboratory abnormalities distinguish one arbovirus infection from another. In fact, the arboviral encephalitis cannot be differentiated from any of the other causes of encephalitis clinically. Similarly, the pathological findings in the brains are also nonspecific for arboviral infection. The diagnosis of arboviral infections is made serologically (i.e., hemagglutinating inhibition, neutralizing antibodies, and late in disease the complement fixation)

3. Measles

Encephalitis occurs in about 0.5–1 of every 1,000 measles cases. The clinical picture is characterized by a recurrence of the fever and the development of headache, lethargy, irritability, confusion, and seizures in up to 56% cases. The majority of patients return to normal within 48–72 hours, but about 30% of them progress to a persisting coma. Approximately 15% of patients with measles encephalitis will die, and in addition, 25% will develop severe brain damage and neurologic deficits such as mental retardation, seizures, deafness, hemiplegia, severe behavioral disorders. *Subacute sclerosing panencephalitis*, caused by measles virus, typically presents with very gradual onset of altered behavior, mild intellectual deterioration, and loss of energy. After that periodic involuntary movements appear; further progression is marked by intellectual deterioration, rigidity, spasticity, and increasing helplessness; 40% of patients die within a year.

4. Mumps

The CNS involvement as a complication of mumps is approximately in 15% of the patients. Meningitis is far more common than is encephalitis. The neurological features are the same as in other encephalitides and gradually resolve within 1–2 weeks. Death occurs in less than 2% of reported cases.

5. Rabies

The symptomatology of the neurologic phase presents in two different types—"furious" or "paralytic" presentation. The furious type is characterized by agitation, hyperactivity, bizarre behavior, aggressiveness with attempts to bite other persons, disorientation and hydrophobia, fever, hypersalivation, and seizures which may cause death in one-fourth of patients. The paralytic type affects approximately 10–15% of patients and presents with a progressive, ascending flaccid, symmetric paralysis or as an asymmetric paralysis involving the exposed extremity. Patient's death may occur during the acute stage from cardiac and respiratory abnormalities. The diagnosis can be made by histopathology, virus cultivation, serology, or detection of viral antigen.

Steihauer DA, Holland JJ. Rapid evolution of RNA Viruses. Ann Rev Microbiol 1987;41:409–431
Holmes EC. The evolution and Emergence of RNA Viruses. Oxford University Press; 2009

13.2.2 DNA Viruses

1. Herpes viruses
   a) *Herpes simplex virus Type 1 (HSV-1)*
      The reactivation and replication of the HSV leads to inflammation and extensive necrosis and edema of the medial temporal lobe and orbital surface of the frontal lobe of immunocompetent patients producing the characteristic clinical picture. Patients develop fever, headache, irritability, lethargy, confusion and focal neurologic signs, such as aphasia, motor and sensory deficits, and seizures (major motor, complex partial, focal, and absence attacks). CSF examination, electroencephalography (widespread, periodic, stereotyped complexes of sharp and slow waves at regular intervals of 2–3 seconds), brain imaging, and biopsy make the HSV encephalitis (HSE) most amenable to diagnosis from all other viral encephalitides.
   b) *Herpes simplex virus Type 2 (HSV-2)*
      Usually two neurologic conditions may develop:
      i. Aseptic meningitis for about 5% of all cases of aseptic meningitis in the United States are caused by the genital HSV-2. The typical clinical picture of headache, fever, stiff neck, and marked CSF lymphocytic pleocytosis often is preceded by pain in the genital or pelvic region.
      ii. Encephalitis identical to that caused by the HSV-1 encephalitis occurring most often in the newborn and rarely in the immunocompromised adult.

Differential diagnosis: Clinically, infectious diseases of the CNS can present with unspecific symptoms including headaches, nausea, and fever. Thus, *bacterial* and *fungal infections* should be considered in the differential diagnosis of *acute viral encephalitis.* Patients are often empirically treated for a potential infection with bacterial and viral pathogens with both antibiotics and antiviral agents until the diagnosis of HSE has been established. Predominantly lymphocytic or monocytic pleocytosis in the CSF can be present in *tuberculous* or *fungal CNS infection* as well as in *HSE*; however, the former infections are associated with a dramatic elevation in protein levels and with hypoglycorrhachia, which are not typical for HSE. Many other viruses, including *CMV, influenza A,* and *echovirus,* have been shown to affect the temporal lobe and mimic HSE, and HSE has no particular clinical characteristics to distinguish it from other CNS infections. In addition, *HSV-2* is a putative cause of HSE, and a 2008 study reported that 12% of all CNS infections with HSV-2 are encephalitic and often have neurological sequelae. Tumors, brain abscesses, and hematomas can also mimic HSE. In addition, vascular disorders and toxic encephalopathies can be mistaken for HSE.

   c) *Varicella zoster virus (VZV)*

      Two neurologic conditions usually develop:

         i. Causes chickenpox (varicella) in childhood, becomes latent in dorsal root ganglia, and reactivates decades later to produce shingles (zoster) in adults. Subacute encephalitis develops on a background of cancer, immunosuppression, and acquired immune deficiency syndrome (AIDS), and death is common.

        ii. Granulomatous arteritis characterized by an acute focal deficit with transient ischemic attack (TIA) or stroke and mental symptoms may develop. In immunocompetent individuals, VZV causes large-vessel vasculitis manifested as ischemic or hemorrhagic stroke, generally weeks to months after herpes zoster ophthalmicus. In immunosuppressed patients, VZV causes a multifocal small-vessel vasculopathy. On MRI it presents as ovoid, round lesions in the gray–white matter junction. PCR can detect VZV DNA in CSF; however, a negative test does not exclude the diagnosis of VZV encephalitis. Mortality is 25% of patients.

2. Cytomegalovirus (CMV)

   Most congenital CMV infections are asymptomatic, although many carriers develop sensorineural hearing loss and intellectual handicaps, and less often seizures, hypotonia, and spasticity and in severe meningoencephalitis lethargy and coma occur. The hallmark is periventricular calcifications detected by CT. CMV has a special affinity for the neuroblasts of the subependymal matrix and regional vasculature with a result of subependymal degeneration and calcification. The acquired CMV infections in the immunocompromised adults, particularly AIDS patients, are very common. CMV is an important cause of encephalitis (progressive dementia, headache, focal or diffuse weakness, and seizures, attributed to CMV vasculitis or foci of demyelination), myelitis, and polyradiculitis (beginning insidiously as a cauda equina syndrome with distal weakness, paresthesias, incontinence, and sacral sensory loss).

3. Epstein–Barr virus (EBV)

   EBV causes infectious mononucleosis and is being associated with the nasopharyngeal carcinoma and Burkitt's lymphoma. EBV meningoencephalitis affects both immunocompetent and immunocompromised individuals causing acute cerebellar ataxia, athetosis and chorea, chiasmal neuritis, or in more serious cases meningoencephalopathy stupor and coma. EBV DNA has been detected in CNS lymphoma tissue.

4. Adenovirus

Van Etten JL, Lane LC, Dunigan DD. DNA viruses: the really big ones (giruses). Annu Rev Microbiol 2010;64:83–99

Weller SK, Sawitzke JA. Recombination promoted by DNA viruses: phage ? to herpes simplex virus. Annu Rev Microbiol 2014;68:237–258

13.2.3 Slow viruses

1. Subacute sclerosing panencephalitis (SSPE)
   SSPE is a chronic measles infection of children between 5 and 15 years and young adults. The brain shows a diffuse and wide spread inflammation and necrosis in both gray and white matter. The disease leads to severe neurologic dysfunction (i.e., Stage 1: decline in school performance and behavioral changes, Stage 2: myoclonic jerks, Stage 3: decerebrate rigidity and coma, Stage 4: loss of cortical functions) and on the average patients survive about 3 years.

2. Progressive multifocal leukoencephalopathy (PML)
   PML is a subacute demyelinating disease caused by the human papovavirus JCV and the simian virus SV40 and usually affects immunocompromised individuals. Patients develop progressive multifocal neurologic symptoms and signs (i.e., mental deficits: 36.1%, visual deficits: 34.7%, motor weakness: 33.3%, speech deficits: 17.3%, incoordination: 13.0%, tone alterations: 2.8%, miscellaneous: 17.3%) that typically result in death in 6–12 months and occasionally up to 3–5 years.

3. Spongiform encephalopathies (SEs) or prion diseases
   Of the four human diseases CJD, Gerstmann–Sträussler–Scheinker syndrome (GSS), Kuru, fatal familial insomnia), CJD is by far the most common, whereas the Kuru was the first to be described. Patients with CJD have behavioral disturbances which progress to frank dementia characterized by memory loss, sleep disorders, and intellectual decline, myoclonic spasms, seizures, visual disturbances, cerebellar signs, and lower motor neuron disturbances. Most patients live 6–12 months, and few up to 5 years.

Brooks BR, Jubelt B, Swarz JR, Johnson RT. Slow viral infections. Annu Rev Neurosci 1979;2:310–340

ter Meulen V, Hall WW. Slow virus infections of the nervous system: virological, immunological and pathogenetic considerations. J Gen Virol 1978;41(1):1–25

Thomson RA, Green JR. Infectious Diseases of the centralnervous system MTP Press Ltd. International Medical Publication; 2012

13.2.4 Human Immunodeficiency Virus (HIV)

Among AIDS patients, 40–60% develop significant neurologic symptoms or signs in their life time and approximately 10–20% present with symptoms of neurologic illness. Most opportunistic CNS infections and neoplasms are associated with headache, fever, meningismus, altered level of consciousness, or focal neurological deficit. The presence of one or more of these symptoms should alert the medical care provider to the possibility of CNS infection. In people with AIDS, a normal ("nonfocal") neurologic examination can be present with PML, cryptococcal meningitis, HIV-associated dementia, or CMV encephalitis (CMVE). Bacterial or viral meningitis can occur at any stage of HIV infection and is typically accompanied by fever.

Two forms of meningitis have been described with HIV-1 infection. At the time of seroconversion to HIV-1 most patients will develop CSF abnormalities and a few of them will develop symptoms of headache, meningitis, encephalitis, myelopathy, and plexitis. This acute meningitis is clinically indistinguishable from other forms of aseptic meningitis.

Chronic recurring meningitis can also occur, characterized by headaches and CSF abnormalities without signs of meningeal irritation. Late in the course of the HIV-1 infection, particularly when immunosuppression is prominent, the patients may develop HIV-1 associated encephalopathy (AIDS–dementia complex), HIV-1 associated myelopathy (spinal vacuolar myelopathy), and neurologic problems secondary to opportunistic processes.

Infection of the CNS may occur during any stage of HIV infection, but opportunistic infection occurs only during late-stage infection, when the CD4 count falls below 200 cells/dl. Opportunistic infections may affect the brain or spinal cord, and onset may be acute, subacute, or chronic. The most common opportunistic CNS infections and neoplasms are: Toxoplasma encephalitis (TE), cryptococcal meningitis, primary CNS lymphoma (PCNSL), PML, AIDS–dementia complex (ADC, also known as HIV-associated dementia), and CMVE. Focal brain lesions occur in up to 17% of people with AIDS and are most often caused by TE, PML, or PCNSL. Since the introduction of potent antiretroviral therapy (previously called highly active antiretroviral therapy or HAART), the incidence of TE and PCNSL has decreased, whereas the incidence of PML has increased.

Evaluation of potential CNS infection should include neuroimaging with CT scanning or MRI with and without administration of an intravenous contrast agent. The most common causes of focal CNS lesions in people with AIDS are TE and PCNSL. Evaluation of a solitary ring-enhancing CNS mass lesion in a patient with AIDS should be guided by: (1) CD4 count; (2) serologic status to *Toxoplasma gondii* and *Cryptococcus neoformans*; (3) findings on neurologic examination, and (4) presence or absence of headache or fever. Lumbar puncture may be useful for differentiating between TE and PCNSL. The CSF testing should include cell count with differential, glucose, protein, bacterial culture, and VDRL. Other tests include fungal cultures, cryptococcal polysaccharide capsular antigen (CrAg), and PCR assays. If symptoms of brain imaging are consistent with herpes virus infection or PML < PCR assays are high. In people with AIDS, an elevated level of b2 microglobulin in the CSF (greater than 3.8 mg/l) is specific, but not sensitive for the diagnosis of HIV-associated dementia. If the CD4 count is greater than 200 cells/dl, opportunistic CNS infection or neoplasm is unlikely, and the **differential diagnosis** should include atypical bacterial abscess, fungal, or mycobacterial abscesses, cryptococcoma, syphilitic gumma, tuberculoma, cerebrovascular disease, and neoplasms other than PCNSL.

Stereotactic brain biopsy (SBB) of a CNS lesion may be necessary for certain clinical scenarios, such as if a solitary CNS lesion is accompanied by negative serology, if a contrast-enhancing lesion is atypical for TE or does not respond to anti-toxoplasma treatment; if a new lesion develops during anti-toxoplasma maintenance treatment protocol. SBB provides a diagnosis for 88–98% of contrast-enhancing lesions, and 67% of nonenhancing lesions.

13.3 Central Nervous System Infections in the Compromised Host: Differential Diagnosis

The differential diagnostic approach depends on the patient's clinical manifestations of CNS disease, the acuteness of the clinical presentation and the type of immune defect. Most patients with CNS infections may be grouped into those with meningeal signs, or those with mass lesions. Other common manifestations include encephalopathy, seizures, or a stroke-like presentation.

Most pathogens have a predictable clinical presentation that differs from that of the normal host. CNS *Aspergillus* infections present either as mass lesions (e.g., brain abscess) or as a meningitis. *Cryptococcus neoformans*, in contrast, usually presents as a meningitis, but not as a cerebral mass lesion even when cryptococcal elements are present. *Aspergillus* and *Cryptococcus* CNS infections are manifestations of impaired host defenses, and rarely occur in immunocompetent hosts. In contrast, the clinical presentation of *Nocardia* infections in the CNS is the same in normal and compromised hosts, although more frequently in compromised hosts.

The acuteness of the clinical presentation coupled with the CNS symptomatology further adds to limit differential diagnosis possibilities. Excluding stroke-like presentations, CNS mass lesions tend to present subacutely or chronically. Meningitis and encephalitis tend to present more acutely.

The type of immune defect predicts the range of possible pathogens likely to be responsible. Patients with diseases that decrease B-lymphocyte function are particularly susceptible to meningitis caused by encapsulated bacterial pathogens. The presentation of bacterial meningitis is essentially the same in normal and compromised hosts with impaired B-lymphocytic immunity. Compromised hosts with impaired T-lymphocyte or macrophage function are prone to develop CNS infections caused by intracellular pathogens. The most common intracellular pathogens are the fungi, particularly *Aspergillus*, other bacteria (e.g., *Nocardia*), viruses (i.e., HSV, JC, CMV, HHV-6), and parasites (e.g., *T. gondii*).

The presence of extra-CNS sites of involvement also may be helpful in the diagnosis. A patient with impaired cellular immunity with mass lesions in the lungs and brain that have appeared subacutely or chronically should suggest *Nocardia* or *Aspergillus* rather than cryptococcus or toxoplasmosis. Patients with T-lymphocyte defects presenting with meningitis generally have meningitis caused by *Listeria* or *Cryptococcus* rather than toxoplasmosis or CMV infection.

A clinician must be ever vigilant to rule out the mimics of CNS infections caused by noninfectious etiologies. Bacterial meningitis, cryptococcal meningitis, and tuberculosis easily are diagnosed accurately from stain, culture, or serology of the CSF. In contrast, patients with CNS mass lesions usually require a tissue biopsy to arrive at a specific etiologic diagnosis. In a compromised host with impaired cellular immunity in which the differential diagnosis of a CNS mass lesion is between TB, lymphoma, and toxoplasmosis, atrial of empiric therapy is warranted. Anti-toxoplasmosis therapy may be initiated empirically and usually results in clinical improvement after 2–3 weeks of therapy. The nonresponse to anti-toxoplasmosis therapy in such a patient would warrant an empiric trial of anti-tuberculous therapy. Lack of response to anti-toxoplasma and anti-tuberculous therapy should suggest a noninfectious etiology (e.g., CNS lymphoma).

Fortunately, most infections in compromised hosts are similar in their clinical presentation to those in the normal host, particularly in the case of meningitis. The compromised host is different than the normal host in the distribution of pathogens, which is determined by the nature of the host defense defect. In compromised hosts, differential diagnosis possibilities are more extensive and the likelihood of noninfectious explanations for CNS symptomatology is greater.

Nelson M, Manji H, Wilkins E. 2 Central nervous system opportunistic infections HIV Med 2011;12(Suppl 2):8–24

Zunt JR. CNS infection during immunosuppression. Neurol Clin 2002;20(1):1–v

Dougan C, Ormerod I. A neurologist's approach to the immunosuppressed patient. J Neurol Neurosurg Psychiatry 2004;75(Suppl 1):i43–i49

Porter SB, Sante MA. Toxoplasmosis of the CNS in the acquired immunodeficiency syndrome N Engl J Med 1992;327:1643–1648

Lusso P, Gallo RC. Human herpesvirus 6 in AIDS. Immunol Today 1995;16(2):67–71

13.4 Fungal Infections

Fungal infections of the CNS are becoming more frequent because of the expansion of at-risk populations and the use of treatment modalities that permit longer survival of these patients. These are patients who have received transplants, those prescribed with immunosuppressive and chemotherapeutic agents, HIV-infected patients, premature infants, the elderly, and patients undergoing major surgery. Prior to the 21st century, blood stream infections were more frequently caused by *Candida albicans, C. neoformans,* and agents of invasive pulmonary infections included primarily endemic mycoses and *Aspergillus fumigatus.* Nowadays fungi that were previously considered nonpathogenic, such as mucoraceous genera (formerly called *Zygomycetes*) and a variety of both hyaline and dematiaceous molds (*Acremonium, Scedosporium, Paecilomyces,* and *Trichoderma* species), are commonly seen in immunocompromised patients.

13.4.1 Differential diagnosis

1. *Infectious*: viral meningitis; encephalitis; brain abscess; mycobacterial meningitis; toxoplasmosis; primary HIV infection; syphilis; PML.
2. *Noninfectious*: carcinomatous meningitis; lymphomatous meningitis; cerebrovascular accident; CNS vasculitis; sarcoidosis; drugs.

Histopathology continues to be a rapid and cost-effective means of providing a presumptive or definitive diagnosis of an invasive fungal infection. However, the use of fungal silver impregnation stains cannot alone solve these challenges, and newer diagnostic techniques may be required. Recent advances in fungal genomics is helping in this regard as PCR-based identification of clinical isolates is proving to be far superior as compared to conventional biochemical identification panels (e.g., API-20C-AUX, VITEK ID-YST, etc.). Pyrosequencing (+) is a relatively inexpensive and very productive rapid DNA-sequencing method for the identification of medically important yeasts. Advanced imaging techniques, such as diffusion-weighted imaging, MR perfusion, and MR spectroscopy, when combined with clinical findings, may help in differentiating fungal disease from other mimickers such as pyogenic infection or cystic metastases.

1. *Candida albicans*

   Candida CNS infection is a manifestation of disseminated disease (candidemia) and is associated with intravenous drug use, indwelling venous catheters, abdominal surgery, and corticosteroid therapy. CNS infection with candida species often results in scattered intraparenchymal granulomatous microabscesses secondary to arteriolar occlusion. Meningitis is a common feature of CNS candidiasis, resulting from invasion of meningeal microvasculature by small group of yeast cells.

2. *Cryptococcus neoformans*

   The portal of entry of cryptococcus in the body is the lungs. The pulmonary infection is not demonstrable in healthy individuals. But it becomes invasive in immunocompromised patients. *C. neoformans* is neurotropic and most patients with cryptococcal meningitis suffer from defective cellular immunity. Cryptococcal meningitis is the most common CNS infection (50%) in chronically immunosuppressed but non-AIDS patients. It is the second most common cause of opportunistic fungal infections in AIDS patients. Cryptococcal meningitis presents as a chronic febrile syndrome with headache. The ensuing aseptic meningoencephalitis reflects cognitive changes or dementia, irritability, personality changes, mass lesions with focal neurologic deficits, and less often ocular abnormalities (papilledema, with or without loss of visual acuity, and cranial nerve palsies) in 40% of patients. Cryptococcal antigen (CrAg) is detected in 99% of serum and 91% of CSF samples; therefore, a negative serum CrAg virtually excludes the diagnosis of cryptococcal meningitis.

3. Mucormycosis (formerly zygomycosis)

   Mucormycosis describes a group of frequently lethal mold infections that have a predilection for diabetic patients, patients on steroid therapy, and severely immunocompromised hosts, such as hematopoietic stem cell transplantation (HSCT) recipients. The majority of human infections are due to fungi that mostly belong to the genera *Rhizopus, Mucor, Rhizomucor, Cunninghamella,* and *Absidia.* Despite the emergence of mucormycosis as a significant cause of mycosis, it remains much less frequent than other more common forms like invasive aspergillosis. Mucormycosis are generally acute and rapidly progressive with mortality rates of 70–100%. Rhinocerebral mucormycosis typically occurs in a patient with diabetic ketoacidosis or with leukemia, whereas pulmonary infection occurs more often in those with malignancy. The infection often begins as ulcerations in the paranasal sinuses or in the palate and may spread along perivascular and perineural channels through the cribriform plate into the frontal lobe or through the orbital apex into the cavernous sinus. *The Mucorales* characteristically invade blood vessels, causing thrombosis and hemorrhagic infarctions as well as cerebritis.

4. *Aspergillus* species

   Out of approximately 175 species of genus *Aspergillus*, only *Aspergillus fumigatus, A. flavus, A. terreus, and A. niger,* are associated with human disease. *A. fumigatus* has become the most prevalent airborne fungal pathogen accounting for > 90% of human fungal infections. Risk factors for *Aspergillus* infection (IA) include prolonged and profound neutropenia, high-grade graft-versus-host diseases (GvHD), use of corticosteroids, age > 40 years, in HSCT recipients and patients with advanced AIDS.

Aspergillosis involving the CNS has similar findings with mucormycosis. CNS aspergillosis may result either from direct extension of nasal cavity/paranasal sinus infection or more commonly from hematogenous dissemination. By a direct extension *Aspergillus* invades the cavernous sinus and circle of Willis, resulting in angiitis, thrombosis, and infarction. In hematogenous spread septic infarction occurs with associated cerebritis and abscess formation. Aspergillus infection is associated with high rates of mortality, i.e., more than 50%. Higher rates were noted in HSCT recipients (68%) and in neutropenic patients the rates were even higher (89%). Aspergillosis is also emerging as a serious form of mycosis in the ICU with a mortality rate of 75–95%. Infections by *non-fumigatus Aspergillus spp.* are becoming increasingly common, especially infections caused by *A. terreus* and *A. flavus*, which have recently been recognized as a cause of frequent lethal infections. These tend to be resistant to amphotericin B. In addition, *A. flavus* produces aflatoxin which is extremely toxic and potent hepatocarcinogen.

5. *Coccidioides immitis*
    Infection with *Coccidioides* can cause numerous problems, ranging from the usually benign *Valley fever* to a lethal meningitis. Without treatment approximately 95% of patients with coccidioidal meningitis will die within 2 years. Hematogenous spread of the endospores into the intracranial space results in meningeal inflammation with infectious purulent and caseous granulomas, particularly at the base of the brain. Multiple coccidioidal microabscesses may be found in cerebellum, periventricular area causing secondary hydrocephalus. The diagnosis is best done by examination of the CSF, where antibodies for the organism can be tested. Rarely, a biopsy of the tissues surrounding the brain (meninges) may be needed for an accurate diagnosis. Imaging is not specific, but may show hydrocephalus in up to 30–50% of patients.

6. *Blastomyces dermatitidis*
    Blastomycosis is caused by *Blastomyces dermatitidis* that is a dimorphic (mycelia/yeast) fungus found in eastern North America and parts of India and Africa. Annual incidence of the disease ranges from < 1 to 100 per 100,000 in endemic areas. Except for rare inoculation cutaneous disease, the organisms enter the body via inhalation of conidia from the environment (wind or excavation dust, digging, direct contact) into the lungs. Pulmonary blastomycosis has a wide *differential diagnosis* and may be asymptomatic or present as mild, moderate, or severe acute pneumonia. The latter may be complicated by acute respiratory distress syndrome (ARDS). Subacute to chronic infiltrates, cavitary lung disease, or both may occur instead. In addition, acute or chronic dissemination of *B. dermatitidis* to the skin, brain, genitourinary system, bone or any other organ system may

result. Hematogenous dissemination results in blastomycosis meningitis with an acute/fulminant onset of headache, stiff neck, and focal signs.

7. *Scedosporium* spp.

    Scedosporium apiospermum and *S. prolificans* represent two medically important antifungal-resistant opportunistic pathogens. *S. apiospermum* causes mycetoma and deep-seated infections (e.g., brain abscesses) and could disseminate in neutropenic bone marrow transplant (BMT) recipients and immunosuppressed individuals; crude mortality rate is about 55%. *S. prolificans* causes bone and soft-tissue infections in immunocompetent individuals and deeply invasive and disseminated infections in immuno-compromised patients with crude mortality rate of 90%.

8. *Fusarium* spp.

    These are the fungi with hyaline-branched septate hyphae. Of all filamentous fungi, *Fusarium* spp. remain the second most common cause of invasive disease in immunosuppressed patients (neutropenia, GvHD, hematological malignancies and in the HSCT recipients). Clinical manifestations of fusariosis are more often characterized by cutaneous involvement and fungemia than those of *Aspergillus* spp. Typical presentation of disseminated fusariosis includes positive blood culture (up to 75%) and the appearance of multiple purpuric cutaneous nodules with central necrosis. High mortality is due in part to high rates of resistant to available antifungals.

9. *Acremonium* spp.

    These are becoming increasingly recognized as opportunistic fungal pathogens in patients (children and adults) with prolonged corticosteroid therapy, splenectomy, neutropenia, and BMT. Following entry through penetrating injuries, they can cause foot mycetomas and corneal infections even in immunocompetent hosts.

10. *Paecilomyces* spp.

    These are cosmopolitan filamentous fungi that inhabit the soil, decaying plants, and food products. The genus *Paecilomyces* contains several species including the emerging pathogens *P. lilacinus* and *P. variotii*. *P. lilacinus* infections include oculomycosis (51.3%) and cutaneous and subcutaneous infections (35.3%); the rest (13.4%) were miscellaneous infections. Peritonitis and sinusitis are the most common infections caused by *P. variotii*. *Differential diagnoses* are usually associated with varying sets of predisposing factors. In that, while oculomycosis, subcutaneous infections occur in solid organ transplants (SOT) and neutropenic BMT recipients, neutropenic and immunodeficient hosts, and patients undergoing surgery.

11. *Trichoderma* spp.

    These have traditionally been employed in the biotechnology industry as sources of enzymes and antibiotics, as well as in agriculture as plant growth promoters and biofungicides. It is now recognized that fatal disseminated disease due to *Trichoderma longibrachiatum* occurs in patients undergoing peritoneal dialysis, in patients with hematologic malignancies and in BMT or SOT transplant recipients.

12. *Dematiaceous molds (phaeohyphomycosis)*

The long and taxonomically diverse list of infections caused by dematiaceous (pigmented thick-walled) fungi are grouped under phaeohyphomycosis. Dematiaceous molds are characterized by the presence of a pale brown-dark melanin-like pigment in the cell wall. They may cause a variety of cutaneous and subcutaneous infections in immunocompetent hosts and invasive or disseminated infections in immunocompromised hosts. The number of dematiaceous molds being reported as etiologic agents of phaeohyphomycosis is growing, several of which target the nervous system (neurotropic fungi). Common neurotropic fungi include *Cladophialophora bantiana, Bipolaris spicifera, Exophiala spp., Wangiella dermatitidis, Ramichloridium obovoideum,* and *Chaetomium atrobrunneum.* Brain abscess is the most common CNS presentation. However, *Bipolaris* ssp. and *Exserohilum rostratum* infections may initially present as sinusitis and then extend into the CNS.

13. *Histoplasmosis*

Histoplasmosis or Darling's disease is pulmonary mycosis caused by the soil-inhabiting dimorphic fungus *Histoplasma capsulatum.* There are two varieties *H. capsulatum* and *H. duboisii* that are pathogenic to humans. *H. capsulatum* is most commonly encountered in North and Central America and in Europe; *H. duboisii* occurs in Africa. In the United States, *H. capsulatum* is endemic in the Mississippi and the Ohio river valleys. It also exists in localized foci in many Middle Eastern countries. Humans acquire *H. capsulatum* infections during occupational or recreational activities in areas where the pathogen is highly endemic (disrupted soil, accumulated dirt, and guano in old buildings and bridges, or in caves where bats roost). Most individuals with histoplasmosis are asymptomatic; symptomatic episodes manifest within 3–17 days after exposure. The acute phase is characterized by nonspecific respiratory (cough or flu-like) symptoms. Chest X-ray findings are unremarkable in 40–70% of cases. In some cases, chronic histoplasmosis may resemble tuberculosis; disseminated histoplasmosis affects multiple organ systems and is often fatal unless treated. Severe infections can cause hepatosplenomegaly, lymphadenopathy, and adrenal enlargement. Leakage from scar tissues left on the retina following ocular histoplasmosis damages the retina and could result in loss of vision. Immunosuppressed patients and those who do not have effective cell-mediated immunity against the organism are likely to manifest symptomatic disease during acute/disseminated episodes.

Guarner J, Brandt ME. Histopathologic diagnosis of fungal infections in the 21st century. Clin Microbiol Rev 2011;24(2):247–280

Mathur M, Johnson CE, Sze G. Fungal infections of the central nervous system. Neuroimaging Clin N Am 2012;22(4):609–632

Abu-Elteen KH, Hamad MA. Changing epidemiology of Classical and Emerging Human Fungal Infections: A Review. Jordan J Biol Sci 2012;5(4):215–230

Richardson M, Lass-Flörl C. Changing epidemiology of systemic fungal infections. Clin Microbiol Infect 2008;14(Suppl 4):5–24

Phaller MA, Pappas PG, Wingard JR. Invasive fungal pathogens: current epidemiological trends. Clin Infect Dis 2006;43(Suppl 1):S3–S14

Miceli MH, Díaz JA, Lee SA. Emerging opportunistic yeast infections. Lancet Infect Dis 2011;11(2):142–151

Disease	Differentiating symptoms/signs	Differentiating tests
Tuberculous meningitis	History of contact or resident in endemic area	CSF smear and culture; sensitivity of smear > 50%; culture requires large CSF volume for maximum sensitivity
		Skin testing or IFN-gamma-based blood tests supportive; but negative results do not exclude diagnosis of tuberculosis
Bacterial meningitis	Relevant exposure history	Specific serology (*Borrelia, Brucella, Leptospira, Treponema pallidum*)
	With symptoms and signs (meningismus, headache, myalgias, and pharyngitis)	Culture (*Actinomyces, Nocardia, and Brucella*)
		Partially treated disease confirmed with nonculture diagnostic methods: PCR, antigen tests for meningococcal and pneumococcal infections
Viral meningitis	Relevant exposure history	Serology for herpes simplex virus, varicella zoster virus, and other viruses; CSF viral culture; PCR for enteroviruses and herpes viruses
	Difficult to distinguish clinically with symptoms and signs (meningismus, headache, myalgias, and pharyngitis)	
Noninfectious lymphocytic meningitis	History, symptoms, signs suggestive of autoimmune disease, sarcoidosis, systemic lupus, Behcet's disease, and carcinomatous meningitis. Recurrent chemical meningitis may be associated with epidermoid cysts or craniopharyngioma	Head CT/MRI may demonstrate epidermoid cysts or craniopharyngioma
		CSF cytology may demonstrate malignant cells; CSF ACE elevated in sarcoidosis
		Autoantibodies to investigate systemic manifestation

Abbreviation: ACE, angiotensin-converting enzyme; CSF, cerebrospinal fluid; IFN, interferon; PCR, polymerase chain reaction

Source: British Medical Journal, Publishing Group Ltd 2015.

13.5 Parasitic and Rickettsial Infections

13.5.1 Protozoa

Protozoal infections, though endemic to certain regions, can be seen all around the world, because of the increase in travel and migration. In addition, immunosuppression associated with various conditions, particularly with HIV infection, favors the occurrence of more severe manifestations and failure to respond to treatments. The CNS may be the only affected system; when not, it is often the most severely affected. Despite information obtained from clinical, laboratory, and imaging procedures that help to narrow the differential diagnosis of intracranial infections, there are cases that need confirmation with biopsy or autopsy. Predominant presentations are meningoencephalitis (*trypanosomiasis*), encephalopathy (*cerebral malaria*), or as single or multiple pseudotumoral-enhancing lesions (*toxoplasmosis, reactivated Chagas disease*).

1. *Toxoplasma gondii*
   a) Congenital infection
      Acute toxoplasma infection occurs in a pregnant woman in 30—45% or the entire gestation period, with the rate of transmission highest (it approaches 100%) during the third trimester. A fetal *Toxoplasma* infection early in pregnancy is likely to cause major disruption of CNS organogenesis in fetus resulting in fetal death or hydrops and severe abnormalities. The severity of complications declines with advancing pregnancy, although premature delivery, chorioretinitis, microcephaly, minor brain calcifications, and even fetal death may still result from late infection.
      The differential diagnosis consists of other congenital (intrauterine) infections grouped as the TORCH syndrome:
         i. Toxoplasmosis
         ii. Other (syphilis)
         iii. Rubella
         iv. CMV
         v. Herpes simplex viruses
   b) Acquired infection
      Most people become infected after childhood and the primary infection is usually silent and latent. Significant disease occurs if the latent infection reactivates when the immune system is compromised. Cerebral toxoplasmosis is one of the most frequent opportunistic infections associated with HIV-related immunodeficiency. Children and adults at risk for serious toxoplasmosis include those with malignancies, individuals undergoing immunosuppressive therapy for organ transplantation or connective tissue disorders, and most recently, AIDS patients. Presentation as mass lesion (begins with headache, lethargy, seizures, focal

neurologic abnormalities, and signs of increased intracranial pressure) is the most common pattern. This requires differentiation from other AIDS-associated mass lesions occurring in the CNS; mainly AIDS-related lymphoma, although PML, cerebral tuberculoma, and other CNS tumors should also be considered, since cerebral toxoplasmosis can also occur in combination with these other conditions.

2. Amoebae
   a) *Entamoeba histolytica*
      Cerebral amoebic abscess caused by *Entamoeba histolytica* infection is a rare global disease not related to immunodeficiency that causes proctocolitis with bloody dysentery, and liver abscesses and rarely cerebral abscess through hematogenous spread from liver. The cerebral lesion is usually single, located in the cortical gray matter, basal ganglia, or at the junction of cortex and white matter. Transmission is by ingestion of cysts in infected feces. Signs indicating CNS involvement include headache, altered sensorium, fever, convulsions, and focal neurologic deficits. Diagnosis is by CT scans which may reveal lesions in brain, liver, and lungs and is confirmed with serology tests.

   b) *Naegleria* and *Acanthamoeba*
      Naegleria spp. produce primary amebic meningoencephalitis in young and healthy individuals with a history of severe persistent frontal headache after swimming in a fresh-water lake during the summer months. The course of the disease is fulminating progressing from signs of meningismus to coma, which ends with death within 2–7 days in virtually all cases, and is not related to immunodeficiency. In addition, there is ageusia or parosmia due to the fact that the organism invades the nasal mucosa and enters the brain by travelling along the olfactory nerves. The ingestion of the trophozoite is harmless. Primary amoebic meningoencephalitis occurs worldwide and major epidemics have occurred in United States, Europe, Australia, West and Central Africa, India, South America. *Acanthamoeba castellanii, A. polyphaga, and Balamuthia mandrillaris*, ubiquitous within the environment in both soil and water, are the most frequent free-living amoebae that cause this pattern of disease. They produce a subacute CNS disorder consisting of altered mental status, convulsions, fever, and focal neurologic deficits. Mortality due to neurological complications is high. The main risk factors are HIV infection, lymphoma, malnutrition, cirrhosis, diabetes, broad-spectrum antibiotics or immunosuppressive therapy, radiation therapy, or pregnancy. Amoebae enter into the lungs via the nasal route, followed by hematogenous spread from where they cross the blood–brain barrier and enter into the CNS. The olfactory neuroepithelium may provide an

alternative route of entry into the CNS. CSF is not diagnostic; brain CT scan may reveal abscess and serology tests may be helpful in diagnosis.

3. Malaria

Cerebral malaria (CM), the most common complication of malaria due to *Plasmodium falciparum,* usually begins abruptly with disturbances of consciousness, acute organic brain syndromes, generalized convulsions, meningismus, cranial nerve palsies, abnormal posturing, and, in rare cases, focal neurologic signs.

Most neurological manifestations persist for 24–72 hours and then proceed either to death or to complete recovery. The latter would argue against widespread permanent hypoxic damage, or reperfusion injury as a pathological mediator. However, focal necrosis of brain white matter is known to occur (Durck's granuloma). CM is not related to immunodeficiency. It is associated with widespread morbidity and mortality, especially in infants and children, as well as during pregnancy. CM is a clinical rather than a pathological diagnosis and should be considered in the differential diagnosis of any patient who has a febrile illness with impaired consciousness who lives in or has recently travelled to malaria endemic areas (Africa, South East Asia, India, Central and South America). The differential diagnosis of cerebral malaria includes:

a) Metabolic encephalopathy secondary to uremia
b) Drugs or toxins
c) Meningitis (bacterial or viral)
d) Encephalitis (bacterial or viral)
e) Traumatic encephalopathy
f) Brain tumor

4. Trypanosomiasis

There are three species of *Trypanosoma,* i.e., *Trypanosoma brucei gambiense, T. b. rhodesiense, and T. cruzi* that affect man, all transmitted by blood-feeding insects. Though morphologically similar, they give rise to quite different diseases in Africa and South America.

Neurologic complications can occur directly from meningoencephalitis consisting of:

a) African trypanosomiasis (sleeping sickness): Caused by *T. b. rhodesiense* (East and South Africa) and *T. b.* gambiense (West Africa). Both infections cause a systemic and meningoencephalitis syndrome usually 3–4 weeks after infection by *T. b. rhodesiense*, and many months or years in case of *T. b. gambiense.* The early acute infection, usually more severe in case of *T. rhodesiense,* has little or no impact on the CNS, while infection by *T. gambiense* is responsible for subacute or chronic meningoencephalitis. CNS involvement produces insomnia, headache, loss of concentration, personality changes, hallucinations, and altered sensation.

b) American trypanosomiasis (Chagas disease): Caused by *T. Cruzi* and is widespread in South America. Acute infection tends to be a mild self-limiting febrile illness. Approximately 30% of infected individuals develop chronic Chagas disease that most commonly affects the heart (cardiomyopathy and dysrhythmias) or the digestive system (megaesophagus or megacolon). Immunosuppression from any cause may result in reactivation of latent infection causing extensive necrotizing encephalitis. Convulsions or altered level of consciousness and rarely CNS granulomas develop and induce focal neurologic deficits.

Haque R, Huston CD, Hughes M, Houpt E, Petri WA, Jr. Amebiasis. N Engl J Med 2003;348(16):1565–1573

Stanley SL, Jr. Amoebiasis. Lancet 2003;361(9362):1025–1034

Ralston KS, Petri WA, Jr. Tissue destruction and invasion be Entameoba histolytica 2011;27:254–263

Beier JC, Keating J, Githure JI, Macdonald MB, Impoinvil DE, Novak RJ. Integrated vector management for malaria control. Malar J 2008;7(Suppl 1):S4

WHO. Handbook for integrated Vector management. Feneva: WHO Press; 2012:68–978 92 4 150280 1

Sundaram C. A morphological approach to the diagnosis of protozoan infections of the central nervous system. Pathol Res Int 2011;2011:1–15 (ID 290853)

Chacko G. Parasitic diseases of the central nervous system. Semin Diagn Pathol 2010;27(3):167–185

Field MC, Lumb JH, Adung'a VO, Jones NG, Engstler M. Macromolecular trafficking and immune evasion in african trypanosomes. Int Rev Cell Mol Biol 2009;278:1–67

Murray HW, Berman JD, Davies CR, Saravia NG. Advances in leishmaniasis. Lancet 2005;366(9496):1561–1577

Malvy D, Chappuis F. Sleeping sickness. Clin Microbiol Infect 2011;17(7):986–995

Brun R, Blum J, Chappuis F, Burri C. Human African trypanosomiasis. Lancet 2010;375(9709):148–159

Stevens L, Dorn PL, Schmidt JO, Klotz JH, Lucero D, Klotz SA. Kissing bugs. The vectors of Chagas. Adv Parasitol 2011;75:169–192

Lindsay DS, Dubey JP. Toxoplasma gondii: the changing paradigm of congenital toxoplasmosis. Parasitology 2011;138(14):1829–1831

Montoya JG, Liesenfeld O. Toxoplasmosis. Lancet 2004;363(9425):1965–1976

13.5.2 Cestodes

1. Neurocysticercosis
   This disease is caused by infestation with larva forms of *Taenia solium* (pork tapeworms), *T. saginata* (bovine tapeworms), or *T. multiceps* (dog tapeworms). It is pandemic, but the most affected region of the world is Latin America (incidence of 3.6%). It is rare in Jewish and Islamic countries because of the prohibition of pork meat. The features of CNS cysticercosis depend on the number, location, and size of the cysts and the intensity of the evoked inflammatory response. Cysts can invade cerebral parenchyma and induce seizures (50% of patients), obstruct the CSF flow and produce hydrocephalus (30% of cases), involve the meninges and produce meningitis, occlude vascular structures and cause stroke, or less frequently, involve the spinal cord and cause myelitis, cord compression, and paraparesis. *T. multiceps* cysts can also involve the posterior fossa, leading to signs of

increased intracranial pressure or obstructive hydrocephalus. Among the disorders that neurocysticercosis can mimic are:

a) Tumors
b) Strokes
c) Hemorrhage
d) Abscess
e) Meningitis
f) Pseudotumor cerebri
g) Pheochromocytoma
h) Neuropsychiatric diseases

The diagnosis of neurocysticercosis (NCC) is made on histopathologic evidence of NCC, CT or MRI showing a scolex within a cystic lesion, or a clinical response to initial therapy of NCC combined with serological evidence of infection with *T. solium* using CSF ELISA in up to 90% cases. The history of exposure in an endemic area is significant.

Diagnostic criteria for NCC:

a) Absolute
   i. Histological demonstration of the parasite from biopsy of brain or spinal cord lesion
   ii. Cystic lesions with scolex on CT or MRI
   iii. Direct visualization of subretinal parasite by fundoscopy
b) Major
   i. Lesions highly suggestive of NCC on neuroimaging
   ii. Positive serum electroimmunotransfer blot (EITB) for detection of anticysticercal antibodies
   iii. Resolution of cysts after antiparasitic therapy
   iv. Spontaneous resolution of small single enhancing lesions
c) Minor
   i. Lesions compatible with NCC on neuroimaging
   ii. Clinical manifestations suggestive of NCC
   iii. Positive CSF-ELISA for detection of anticysticercal antibodies
   iv. Cysticercal antigens
   v. Cysticercosis outside the CNS

Epidemiology

a) Evidence of household contact with *T. solium* infection
b) Individual coming from living in an endemic area
c) History of travel to an endemic area

2. *Echinococcus granulosus* (hydatid disease)

It is of worldwide distribution and is endemic in sheep- and cattle-breeding countries, such as tropical countries, Middle East, England and Wales. Eating offal from sheep and other herbivores with hydatid cysts infects the dog. The adult worms develop in the intestine of the dog and are shed in the feces. When such feces contaminate human food or through intimate contact with dogs, the eggs hatch in the human intestine, the larvae penetrate the mucosa and are carried by the portal blood to the liver, lung, brain etc. where hydatid cysts may develop. Involvement of the liver occurs in 60% and of the lungs in 25% of cases.

The CNS is involved in only 1–2% of *E. granulosus* infections. The spinal cord may be involved causing cord compression. The larvae usually produce single, mass lesions within brain parenchyma that cause headache, convulsions, personality changes, memory loss, or focal neurological deficits. Hydatid disease usually affects young people, about 50–75% occurring in children as a space-occupying lesion of slow evolution. In the diagnosis serology is useful. CT would show a cystic lesion that is usually multiloculated with minute calcifications. Histology of excised lesions is diagnostic.

Carpio A; Caprio Arturo. Neurocysticercosis: an update. Lancet Infect Dis 2002;2(12):751–762

García HH, Evans CAW, Nash TE, et al. Current consensus guidelines for treatment of neurocysticercosis. Clin Microbiol Rev 2002;15(4):747–756

Nash TE, Garcia HH. Diagnosis and treatment of neurocysticercosis. Nat Rev Neurol 2011;7(10):584–594

Torgenson PR. The emergence of Echinococcus in central Asia. Parasitology 2013

Pedrosa I, Saiz A, Avvazola J, et al. Hydatid disease: radiology and pathology features and complications. Radiol Societ North America 2015;20(3)

13.5.3 Nematodes

1. Visceral larva migrans or toxocariasis
   a) *Toxocara canis*
      It is a canine parasite that causes accidental infection in man. It is distributed worldwide. Involvement of the CNS may be in the form of meningitis, encephalitis, or granuloma-like lesion. Rare but serious neurologic complications occur including headache, convulsions, or behavioral changes and hemiplegia.
   b) *T. cati*
   c) *Baylisascaris procyonis* (raccoon ascaridis)
2. Eosinophilic meningitis
   a) *Angiostrongylus cantonensis*
      It is found in Australia, Papua New Guinea, South East Asia, and Africa. *Angiostrongylus cantonensis* can infect man accidentally through the ingestion of snails, crabs, prawns, and vegetable if not properly cooked. Direct invasion of the CNS produces headache, vomiting, neck stiffness, fever, paraesthesias, convulsions, and cranial nerve palsies (CN VI or VII)

      The *differential diagnosis* of CSF eosinophilia includes:
      i. Foreign body

ii. CNS malignancy

iii. *Coccidioides immitis* meningitis

iv. Cysticercosis

v. Other parasitic infections (*Paragonimus westermani, Gnathostoma spinigerum,* or *Schistosoma* species)

3. Trichinosis

Infection is from eating meat of infected animals such as pigs, polar bear, and wild animals. Meningitis or cerebral hemorrhage may occur. Approximately 10% of patients with symptomatic trichinosis develop neurologic complications from the direct larval invasion of the brain (encephalitis) or CSF spaces (meningitis) producing personality changes, headache, meningismus, or lethargy. Later, focal signs such as motor or cranial nerve palsy predominate and correlate with larval encystment. Additionally, signs of cerebellar dysfunction, convulsions, or peripheral neuropathies may occur, indicating the broad spectrum of neurologic complications of symptomatic trichinosis. The disease causing organisms are species of genus *Trichinella*.

a) *Trichinella spiralis*—Temperate climates (Americas, Thailand)

b) *Trichinella nelsoni*—Africa

c) *Trichinella nativa*—Arctic

4. *Strongyloides stercoralis*

This nematode is endemic in tropical and subtropical regions and is excreted in the stools of 0.4–4% of the infected humans. The *Strongyloides stercoralis* larvae penetrate the skin and migrate to the intestines, lungs, or rarely the CNS; in the latter case producing meningitis, infarction, or brain abscess.

5. *Gnathostoma spinigerum*

It is found in tropical countries. Eating uncooked or undercooked food especially meat, fish, and chicken, as well as drinking contaminated water may cause infection. The infection may involve the brain and the spinal cord resulting in sensory and motor deficits. Massive cerebral hemorrhage has been reported.

6. Loa loa filariasis (*Loa loa*)

It is a microfilarial disease transmitted from man to man by flies of the genus *Chrysops* and it is endemic in West and Central Africa. Although it characteristically causes subcutaneous swelling known as "Calabar swelling," it may produce meningoencephalitis probably due to an allergic reaction to dead microfilaria causing occlusive thrombi.

Dupouy-Camet J, Kociecka W, Bruschi F, Bolas-Fernandez F, Pozio E. Opinion on the diagnosis and treatment of human trichinellosis. Expert Opin Pharmacother 2002;3(8):1117–1130

Pozio E. New patterns of Trichinella infection. Vet Parasitol 2001;98(1–3):133–148

Ramirez-Avila L, Slome S, Schuster FL, et al. Eosinophilic meningitis due to Angiostrongylus and Gnathostoma species. Clin Infect Dis 2009;48(3):322–327

13.5.4 Trematodes (Flukes)

1. Schistosomiasis (bilharziasis)

   Schistosomiasis is a neglected tropical disease or a man-made disease that is caused by species of blood flukes of the genus *Schistosoma,* which are endemic in tropical Africa, Middle East, Central and South America *(S. mansoni,* and *S. haematobium),* and in the Far East—Cambodia, Indonesia, Laos, Philippines, and China *(S. japonicum).* These *Schistosoma* species inhabit the human vascular system in the mesenteric veins *(S. mansoni* and *S japonicum)* or vesical plexus *(S. haematobium).*

   CNS involvement may cause scarring and epilepsy, cerebral hemorrhage, or transverse myelitis. Cerebral schistosomiasis is primarily caused by *S. japonicum,* whereas spinal cord lesions are due primarily to *S. mansoni* and *S. haematobium.* Neurologic complications are more frequent with *S. japonicum,* i.e., up to 3.5% of infections, including abrupt altered sensorium, extremity weakness, visual disturbances, incontinence, sensory disturbances, altered speech, ataxia, vertigo, neck stiffness and seizures. The diagnosis of neuroschistosomiasis is difficult because CNS symptoms are nonspecific and laboratory findings, such as eosinophilia and the presence of *Schistosoma* eggs in clinical samples may not be present.

   Neuroschistosomiasis should be included in the differential diagnosis in any patient who is from endemic area of schistosomiasis and who displays an acute encephalopathy of unknown origin. Biopsy of rectal wall, liver, or bladder wall may also reveal ova. The serologic test, ELISA is diagnostic.

2. Paragonimiasis

   a) *Paragonimus westermani*

      Endemic regions include West Africa, South and Central America, and South East Asia. Crabs and crayfish are intermediate hosts that harbor the encysted metacercariae and ingesting the infected crabs and crayfish infests man. *Paragonimus* immature or mature worms enter the cranium along perivascular tissues and reside in cerebral parenchyma, producing space-occupying lesions usually in the temporal, parietal, and occipital lobes or cause cord compression. Other presentations include meningitis, encephalopathy, cerebral infarct, focal or generalized convulsions, and transverse myelitis.

      Diagnosis depends on identifying the eggs in feces, sputum, and skin lesions. Serology may be of use and intracranial calcified lesions may be seen in radiographs or CT brain.

Sturrock RF. Schistosomiasis epidemiology and control: how did we get here and where should we go? Mem Inst Oswaldo Cruz 2001;96(Suppl):17–27

Barsoum RS, Esmat G, El-Baz T. Human schistosomiasis: clinical perspective: review. J Adv Res 2013;4(5):433–444

Fischer PV, Curtis KS, Folk SM, et al. Serologic Diagnosis of North American Paragonimiasis by Western Blot. Med Hyg (Geneve) 2013;88(6):1035–1040

13.5.5 Rocky mountain spotted fever (RMSF)

1. *Rickettsia rickettsii*

   It is transmitted via contact with the wood tick, the dog tick, or the lone star tick with an overall incidence of 0.2–0.5 cases per 100,000 population. The usual neurologic features consist of headache, neck stiffness, altered sensorium, and convulsions. Other neurologic abnormalities include ataxia, aphasia, neural hearing loss, and papilledema. The neuropathologic findings consist of cerebral edema, perivascular and meningeal lymphocytic infiltration, and an extensive necrotizing vasculitis. The presumptive diagnosis of RMSF should be entertained in a patient with a recent history of a tick bite or having crushed a tick. Especially in endemic areas, the absence of this history should not decrease the index of suspicion. Because of some areas more than 50% of the populace may have a history of tick bite, a positive history may not be particularly helpful either, especially if patients are misdiagnosed and are given antibiotic that is ineffective against rickettsiae. In this case the symptoms have progressed and a rush has developed, the diagnosis of drug eruption—rather than RMSF—is likely to be made. Within the first week of illness, finding a marked left shift in the differential count with a near normal number of leukocytes should suggest consideration of the diagnosis. Biopsy of a skin lesion (preferably petechial) for immunofluorescent staining could help in making a rapid diagnosis, if the results are positive, but is not helpful if negative. The rash may be helpful clinical sign, but it is not always classic or diagnostic in its presentation.

   Other illnesses that present with fever and petechial lesions that must be considered are: Meningococcemia, murine and epidemic typhus, typhoid fever, measles (especially atypical measles), dengue fever, emergent management of malaria, Group A streptococcal infection, Kawasaki disease, leptospirosis, paediatric rubella, paediatric syphilis, enteroviral infection with an exanthem, and vasculitis and thrombophlebitis.

Abramson JS, Givner LB. Rocky Mountain spotted fever. Pediatr Infect Dis J 1999;18(6):539–540

Edwards MS, Feigin RD. Rickettsial diseases. In: Feigin RD, Cherry JD, Demmler GJ, Kaplan SL, eds. Textbook of Pediatric Infectious Diseases. 5th ed. WD Saunders Co; 2004:2497–2515

Dumler JS, Walker DH. Rocky Mountain spotted fever--changing ecology and persisting virulence. N Engl J Med 2005;353(6):551–553

Azad AF. Pathogenic rickettsiae as bioterrorism agents. Clin Infect Dis 2007;45(Suppl 1):S52–S55

Walker DH. Rickettsiae and rickettsial infections. The current state of knowledge. Clin Infect Dis 2007;45(Suppl 1):S39–44

Walker DH. Rickettsiae and rickettsial infections: the current state of knowledge. Clin Infect Dis 2007;45(Suppl 1):S39–S44

Rovery C, Raoult D. Mediterranean spotted fever. Infect Dis Clin North Am 2008;22(3):515–530, ix

Biggs HM, Behravesh CB, Bradley KK, et al. Diagnosis and Management of Tickborne Rickettsial Diseases: Rocky Mountain Spotted Fever and Other Spotted Fever Group Rickettsioses, Ehrlichioses, and Anaplasmosis - United States. MMWR Recomm Rep 2016;65(2):1–44

13.6 Cat-Scratch Disease

Cat-scratch disease (CSD) is a common worldwide infection that usually presents as tender lymphadenopathy. It should be included in the differential diagnosis of fever of unknown origin and any lymphadenopathy syndrome. Asymptomatic, bacteremic cats with *Bartonella henselae* in their saliva serve as vectors by biting and clawing the skin, especially of children. Diagnosis is most often arrived at by obtaining a history of exposure to cats and a serologic test with high titers (> 1:256) of immunoglobulin G antibody to *B. henselae*. Most cases of CSD are self-limited and do not require antibiotic treatment. Infrequently, CSD may present in a more disseminated form with hepatosplenomegaly or meningoencephalitis, endocarditis, neuroretinitis or with biliary angiomatosis in patients with AIDS.

Encephalopathy is the most common neurologic manifestation, occurring in 2–3% of usually adult patients. The onset is usually abrupt and occurs 1–6 weeks after lymphadenopathy becomes apparent. Patients become confused and disoriented, and their condition can deteriorate to coma. About 50% of patients have a fever. Other neurologic complications consist of headache, convulsions (in 80%), altered level of consciousness, status epilepticus, spinal cord involvement with para- or tetraparesis and Brown–Sequard syndrome. CSF is usually normal, and so the CT scans. The EEG shows nonspecific slowing. Recovery is usually complete within 1 week or longer.

In the differential diagnosis other common diseases should be considered:
1. Infectious causes
   a) Infectious mononucleosis
   b) CMV lymphadenopathy
   c) Herpes zoster (shingles)
   d) Epstein–Barr virus lymphadenopathy
   e) Group A streptococcal adenitis
   f) HIV lymphadenopathy
   g) Nontuberculous mycobacterial lymphadenopathy
   h) *S. aureus* adenitis
   i) Toxoplasmosis lymphadenopathy
2. Noninfectious causes
   a) Malignancy (lymphoma, leukemia in children)
   b) Metastatic solid tumor

Klotz SA, Ianas V, Elliott SP. Cat-scratch Disease. Am Fam Physician 2011;83(2):152–155

Reynolds MG, Holman RC, Curns AT, O'Reilly M, McQuiston JH, Steiner CA. Epidemiology of cat-scratch disease hospitalizations among children in the United States. Pediatr Infect Dis J 2005;24(8):700–704

Sanguinetti-Morelli D, Angelakis E, Richet H, Davoust B, Rolain JM, Raoult D. Seasonality of cat-scratch disease, France, 1999–2009. Emerg Infect Dis 2011;17(4):705–707

13.7 Central Nervous System Infections in AIDS

1. Encephalitis: most common, approximately in 60% of HIV patients
2. Toxoplasmosis: most common opportunistic infection in 20–40% of AIDS sufferers
3. Cryptococcosis: in 5% of cases
4. PML: in 1–4% of cases
5. Miscellaneous
    a) CNS tuberculosis: incidence ranges from 2–18% in AIDS patients
    b) Neurosyphilis: present in 1–3% of HIV-infected patients
    c) CMV infection
    d) Herpes simplex (both HSV-1 and HSV-2)
    e) VZV: in less than < 1% of immunocompromised patients

Nissapatorn V, Sawangjaroen N. Parasitic infections in HIV infected individuals: diagnostic & therapeutic challenges. Indian J Med Res 2011;134(6):878–897

Smith AB, Smirniotopoulos JG, Rushing EJ. From the archives of the AFIP: central nervous system infections associated with human immunodeficiency virus infection: radiologic-pathologic correlation. Radiographics 2008;28(7):2033–2058

Cunha BA. Central nervous system infections in the compromised host: a diagnostic approach. Infect Dis Clin North Am 2001;15(2):567–590

Zunt JR. Central nervous system infection during immunosuppression. Neurol Clin 2002;20(1):1–22, v

13.8 Acute Bacterial Meningitis

Most common pathogens have been listed in the following tables by age group and by predisposing conditions.

Age group	Pathogenic organism
Birth to 6 weeks	*Escherichia coli,* other Gram-negative organisms
	Group B *Streptococcus*
	Klebsiella
	Listeria monocytogenes
	Salmonella
	Pseudomonas aeruginosa
	Staphylococcus aureus
	Haemophilus influenzae
	Citrobacter

(*Continued*)

Infections of the Central Nervous System

▶ (Continued)

Age group	Pathogenic organism
6 weeks to 3 months	E. coli
	Group B Streptococcus
	L. monocytogenes
	Streptococcus pneumoniae
	Salmonella species
	H. influenzae, type b
3 months to 6 years	H. influenzae, type b
	S. pneumoniae
	Neisseria meningitidis
	S. aureus
Adults and children (older than 6 years)	S. pneumoniae
	N. meningitidis
	L. monocytogenes
	E. coli, other Gram-negative organisms
Elderly adults	S. pneumoniae
	H. influenzae, type b
	L. monocytogenes

Chávez-Bueno S, McCracken GH, Jr. Bacterial meningitis in children. Pediatr Clin North Am 2005;52(3): 795–810, vii

Durand ML, Calderwood SB, Weber DJ, et al. Acute bacterial meningitis in adults. A review of 493 episodes. N Engl J Med 1993;328(1):21–28

Predisposing condition	Pathogenic organism
Intraventricular shunt infections	Coagulase-negative staphylococci (most commonly Staphylococcus epidermidis that accounts for more than 50% of all CSF-shunt infections)
	S. aureus (the second most common pathogen involved, up to 25% of CSF-shunt infections)
	Gram-negative organisms (are isolated in 5–20% of shunt infections, particularly in infants)
	Other pathogens Pseudomonas species Streptococcus species Propionibacterium acnes Diphtheroides Candidae

▶ (Continued)

Predisposing condition	Pathogenic organism	
Posttraumatic meningitis[a]		
Closed head injury	Streptococcus pneumoniae (Pneumococcus is the predominant organism, presumably due to its common presence in the upper airway)	(65%)
	Other streptococci	(10%)
	Haemophilus influenzae	(9%)
	Neisseria meningitides	(5%)
	S. aureus	(5%)
	Enteric Gram-negative bacilli	(4%)
	S. epidermidis	(2%)
	Listeria monocytogenes	
With CSF leak	Streptococcus pneumoniae	(56%)
	Aerobic Gram-negative bacilli	(26%)
	Enterobacter aerogenes	
	Serratia marcescens	
	Escherichia coli	
	Pseudomonas aeruginosa	
	Proteus mirabilis	
	Klebsiella species	
	H. influenzae	(8%)
	Streptococcus species	(6%)
	Neisseria meningitides	(2%)
	S. aureus	(2%)
Postoperative meningitis (Transsphenoidal hypophysectomy)	Aerobic Gram-negative bacilli	(46%)
	E. coli	
	P. mirabilis	
	P. vulgaris	
	P. aeruginosa	

(Continued)

▶ (*Continued*)

Predisposing condition	Pathogenic organism	
	Anaerobes Gram-positive (*Ppeptostreptococci, clostridia*, etc.)	(13%)
	Bacteroides fragilis	
	Anaerobes Gram-negative other than *B. fragilis*	
	Streptococcus species	(13%)
	S. epidermidis	(7%)
	S. aureus	(7%)
	H. parainfluenza	(7%)
	Diphtheroids	(5%)
Immunodeficiency states		
AIDS: opportunistic infections	*Toxoplasma gondii* (it causes the most common neurologic complications in patients with HIV infection. Cerebral toxoplasmosis was seen in 28–40% of AIDS patients)	
	Cryptococcus neoformans (cryptococcal meningitis is commonly associated with AIDS, with an estimated incidence varying from 2–11%)	
	Coccidioides immitis	
	Candida albicans (although 40–60% of AIDS patients develop oropharyngeal or esophageal candidiasis, it rarely affects the brains of patients with AIDS)	
	L. monocytogenes (a surprisingly low incidence of cerebral infection is seen compared to its very high frequency in patients with other causes of cell-mediated immunity)	
	Mycobacterium tuberculosis and *Mycobacterium avium-intracellulare* (involvement of the CNS is not as common as may be expected from the frequency of mycobacterial infection)	
	Treponema pallidum (syphilis takes a more aggressive course in HIV-seropositive persons and neurosyphilis is seen with increased frequency in the HIV-positive population)	
	Histoplasma capsulatum	
	Nocardia asteroides	
	S. pneumoniae	
	Gram-negative bacilli	

▶ (*Continued*)

Predisposing condition	Pathogenic organism
AIDS: type of cell deficiency	
• T-cell deficiency	*Salmonella*
	L. monocytogenes
	C. neoformans
	H. capsulatum
• B-cell deficiency	*S. pneumoniae*
	H. influenzae
• Neutropenia	*Pseudomonas aeruginosa*
	S. epidermis
	Streptococcus faecalis
Other causes of cell-mediated immunity deficiency	
• Bacteria	*L. monocytogenes* (Is the most common cause of bacterial meningitis in patients with cell-mediated deficiency, despite its rarity in AIDS patients. In renal transplant patients, meningitis appears in 75% of infected cases.
	N. asteroides (The CNS is involved in approximately one-third of all nocardial infections, being more common in immunocompromised patients)
	M. tuberculosis
• Fungi	*Cryptococcus neoformans*
	C. immitis
	H. capsulatum
• Parasites	*Toxoplasma gondii* (One of the most common CNS complications occurring in patients with immunodeficiency)
	Strongyloides stercoralis (CNS complications (meningitis, cerebritis, abscess, diffuse microinfarcts) are rare)
Defects of humoral immunity	Immunoglobulin deficiency or splenectomy
	S. pneumoniae
	H. influenzae
	N. meningitidis

(*Continued*)

▶ (*Continued*)

Predisposing condition	Pathogenic organism
Defects in neutrophils	Neutropenia or abnormalities in neutrophil function
• Bacteria	*P. aeruginosa*
	Other Gram-negative bacilli
	S. aureus
• Fungi	*Candida albicans*
	Aspergillus fumigatus
	Mucorales
Medical conditions	
• Diabetes mellitus	*S. pneumoniae*
	Gram-negative bacilli
	Staphylococci
	C. neoformans
	Mucorales
• Alcoholism	*S. pneumoniae*
	L. monocytogenes
• Pneumonia or upper respiratory infection	*S. pneumoniae*
	N. meningitidis
	H. influenzae
	Viruses
• Leukemia	Gram-negative bacilli
	S. aureus
• Lymphoma	*L. monocytogenes*

[a]From Hirschmann, J.V.: Bacterial meningitis following closed head injury. In Sande, MA: Smith AL, and Root RT, ed. Bacterial Meningitis. New York, Churchill Livingstone; 1985.

Leligdowicz A, Katwere M, Piloya T, Ronald A, Kambugu A, Katabira E. Challenges in diagnosis, treatment and follow-up of patients presenting with central nervous system infections in a resource-limited setting. McGill J Med 2006;9(1):39–48

Steinbrook R. The AIDS epidemic in 2004. N Engl J Med 2004;351(2):115–117

Cunha BA. Central nervous system infections in the compromised host: a diagnostic approach. Infect Dis Clin North Am 2001;15(2):567–590

Collazos J. Opportunistic infections of the CNS in patients with AIDS: diagnosis and management. CNS Drugs 2003;17(12):869–887

Thwaites G, Fisher M, Hemingway C, Scott G, Solomon T, Innes J; British Infection Society. British Infection Society guidelines for the diagnosis and treatment of tuberculosis of the central nervous system in adults and children. J Infect 2009;59(3):167–187

Renold C, Sugar A, Chave JP, et al. Toxoplasma encephalitis in patients with the acquired immunodeficiency syndrome. Medicine (Baltimore) 1992;71(4):224–239

Judah T. Uganda: The secret war. The New York Review 2004;51(14):62–64

Zahra LV, Azzopardi CM, Scott G. Cryptococcal meningitis in two apparently immunocompetent Maltese patients. Mycoses 2004;47(3–4):168–173

13.9 Chronic Meningitis

The term "chronic meningitis" was introduced to embrace a large number of illnesses causing meningoencephalitis (fever, headache, lethargy, confusion, nausea, vomiting, stiff neck) and CSF abnormalities (predominantly lymphocytic pleocytosis, elevated protein, and often low glucose) lasting at least 4 weeks. In previously healthy patients with chronic meningitis, the single most common cause was tuberculosis (40%) with cryptococcosis (7%), malignancy (8%) and other definable causes much less frequent. In one-third (30%) cases no cause was found. Chronic meningitides are very uncommon and account for less than 10% of all meningitis cases.

The key to diagnosis of chronic meningitis is early suspicion and lumbar puncture. CSF studies should include cryptococcus antigen, VDRL, PCR for *Mycobacterium tuberculosis*, AFB and fungal cultures, and cytospin cytology. All patients should also have a tuberculin skin test, chest X-ray, and imaging of the brain (CT or MRI with gadolinium enhancement to exclude abscesses, tumors, and nonmeningial infections). Additional studies should be targeted on the basis of thorough history and clinical examination and the results of initial laboratory tests. For example, tick exposure suggests Lyme disease, eosinophilia in the CSF suggests *Coccidioides*, parasites, lymphoma, or chemicals. (▶ Fig. 13.1 and ▶ Fig. 13.2)

The differential diagnosis of chronic meningitis is listed below:

13.9.1 Specific infectious causes

1. Bacterial meningitis
   a) *M. tuberculosis*
   b) *Treponema pallidum* (neurosyphilis)
   c) *Borrelia burgdorferi* (Lyme disease)
   d) *Brucella melitensis*
   e) *L. monocytogenes*
   f) *Nocardia asteroides*
2. Fungal meningitis
   a) *C. neoformans*
   b) *C. immitis*
   c) *Histoplasma capsulatum*

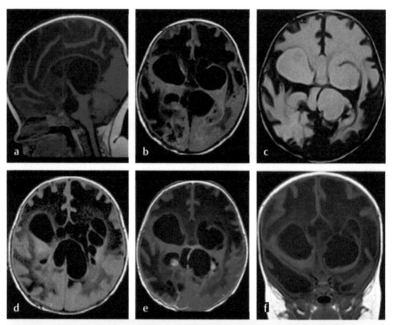

Fig. 13.1 (a–f) A 3-month-old female with multiloculated hydrocephalus secondary to bacterial meningitis and ventriculitis. The patient required multiple endoscopic procedures to connect the loculations and a ventriculoperitoneal shunt placement. (Reproduced from 11.4 Diagnosis and Imaging. In: Torres-Corzo J, Rangel-Castilla L, Nakaji P, ed. Neuroendoscopic Surgery. 1st edition. Thieme; 2016.)

- d) *Blastomyces dermatitidis*
- e) *Candida species*
- f) *Sporothrix schenckii*
- g) *A. fumigatus*
3. Parasitic meningitis
    - a) *Cysticercus cellulosae/racemosus*
    - b) *T. gondii*
    - c) *Angiostrongylus cantonensis/costaricensis*
    - d) Schistosomiasis
4. Viral meningitis
    - a) HIV
    - b) Echovirus

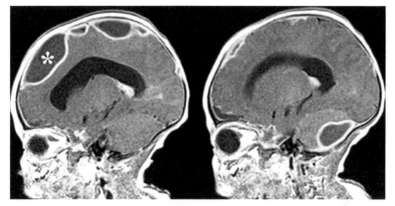

Fig. 13.2 This neonate developed subdural empyemas complicating *Escherichia coli* meningitis. The largest collection (*white asterisk*) was drained with a needle through the anterior fontanel. It was still culture-positive even though the cerebrospinal fluid (CSF) had been sterilized. Nevertheless, without any change in antibiotic therapy, after several weeks the other collections eventually resolved. The infant later required a CSF shunt for progressive hydrocephalus. (Reproduced from Meningitis. In: Albright A, Pollack I, Adelson P, ed. Principles and Practice of Pediatric Neurosurgery. 3rd edition. Thieme; 2014.)

13.9.2 Noninfectious causes

1. Sarcoidosis
2. Rheumatologic and vacsulitic diseases
   a) Granulomatous angiitis of the CNS
   b) Vasculitis associated with herpes zoster ophthalmicus
   c) Cogan's syndrome
3. Systemic vascilitides affecting the CNS
   a) Polyarteritis nodosa
   b) Systemic lupus erythematosus
   c) Sjogren's syndrome
   d) Behcet's syndrome
   e) Vogt–Koyanagi–Harada syndrome
   f) Wegener's granulomatosis
4. Chronic meningitis associated with malignancies
   a) Primary brain tumors (astrocytoma, glioblastoma, ependymoma, PNET tumors)
   b) Metastatic tumors (breast, lung, thyroid, renal, melanoma)

c) Meningeal carcinomatosis
d) Chronic benign lymphocytic meningitis
5. Chemical meningitis from the intrathecal injection of:
   a) Contrast agents for radiologic studies
   b) Chemotherapeutic agents
   c) Antibiotics (penicillin, trimethoprim, INH, ibuprofen)
   d) Local anesthetics

13.9.3 Immunocompromised patients

1. AIDS (HIV infection)
   The main infectious complications that present as chronic meningitis are:
   a) Toxoplasmosis
   b) Cryptococcosis
   c) Syphilis
   d) Aspergillosis
   e) Non-Hodgkin's systemic lymphoma
2. Hypoimmunoglobulinemia

Koski RR, Van Loo D. Etiology and management of chronic meningitis US Pharm 2010;35(1):HS-2–HS-8
Tan TQ. Chronic meningitis. Semin Pediatr Infect Dis 2003;14(2):131–139
Banarer M, Cost K, Rychwalski P, Bryant KA. Chronic lymphocytic meningitis in an adolescent. J Pediatr 2005;147(5):686–690
Cohen BA. Chronic meningitis. Curr Neurol Neurosci Rep 2005;5(6):429–439
Ginsberg L, Kidd D. Chronic and recurrent meningitis. Pract Neurol 2008;8(6):348–361

13.10 Recurrent Meningitis

Recurrent meningitis is defined as repetitive episodes of meningitis associated with an abnormal CSF followed by symptom-free periods during which the CSF is normal. An important differential diagnosis is *recurrent purulent meningitis* that is often attributable to a *congenital or traumatic defect* providing access to the subarachnoid space, such as congenital occult spina bifida or fracture of the base of the skull. A CSF leak may be apparent in about 50% of the cases with post-traumatic recurrent meningitis. The head trauma may have occurred many years earlier and a connection with the subarachnoid space may not be clinically apparent. Rarely, recurrent meningitis may arise from episodes of recurrent *sepsis of a parameningeal focus* (e.g., sinusitis, mastoiditis) or from a *complement deficiency.* Deficiency in a number of the components of the complement pathway has been detected in patients with recurrent meningitis. *Neisseria meningitidis* meningitis caused consecutively by different sero groups in the usual presentation in these cases. **Differential diagnosis** of recurrent meningitis is listed in the following section.

13.10.1 Specific infectious causes

1. Common bacterial meningitides
   a) Organisms
      i. *S. pneumoniae*
      ii. *H. influenzae*
      iii. *N. meningitidis*
   b) Pathophysiologic mechanisms
      i. Anatomical defects
         - Traumatic: basal skull fractures involving the paranasal sinuses, cribriform plate, petrous bone; postoperative
         - Congenital: myelomeningocele; dermoid sinus with midline cranial or spinal dermal sinus; petrous fistula; neurenteric cysts
      ii. Parameningeal infection
         - Paranasal sinusitis
         - Pyogenic otitis media with chronic mastoid osteomyelitis
         - Cranial or spinal epidural abscess
      iii. Idiopathic recurrent bacterial meningitis
      iv. Defective immune mechanisms
         - Hypoimmunoglobulinemia
         - Postsplenectomy susceptibility in children
2. Special bacterial meningitides
   a) *M. tuberculosis*
   b) *B. burgdorferi*
   c) *Brucella mellitensis*
   d) *Leptospira*
3. Fungal meningitides
   a) *C. neoformans*
   b) *C. immitis*
   c) *H. capsulatum*
   d) *B. dermatitidis*
   e) *Candida species*
   f) *S. schenckii*
4. Parasitic meningitides
   a) *Cysticercus cellulosae/racemosus*
   b) *T. gondii*
   c) *A. cantonensis/costaricensis*
   d) Schistosomiasis
5. Viral meningitides
   a) HIV
   b) Echovirus

13.10.2 Noninfectious causes

1. Sarcoidosis
2. Rheumatologic diseases and vasculitides affecting the CNS
   a) Systemic lupus erythematosus
   b) Polyarteritis nodosa
   c) Behcet's syndrome
   d) Sjogren's syndrome
   e) Vogt–Koyanagi–Harada syndrome
   f) Mollaret's meningitis (benign recurrent aseptic/lymphocytic meningitis)
3. Intracranial and intraspinal neoplasms
   a) Craniopharyngioma
   b) Ependymoma
   c) Cerebral hemangioma

Ginsberg L. Difficult and recurrent meningitis. J Neurol Neurosurg Psychiatry 2014;75(suppl I):i16–21

Wang H-S, Kuo MF, Huang SC. Diagnostic approach to recurrent bacterial meningitis in children. Chang Gung Med J 2005;28(7):441–452

Lieb G, Krauss J, Collmann H, Schrod L, Sörensen N. Recurrent bacterial meningitis. Eur J Pediatr 1996;155(1):26–30

13.11 Conditions Predisposing to Recurrent Bacterial Meningitis

Bacterial migration, along congenital or acquired pathways from skull or spinal dural defects, gains entrance into the CNS and should be taken into consideration when patients face recurrent bacterial meningitis. Without evidence of CSF leakage, a cranial symptom/sign or coccygeal cutaneous stigmata may suggest the approximate lesion site, diagnosis and detection remains difficult. To detect an occult dural lesion along the craniospinal axis, such as basal encephalocele, dermal sinus tract, or neurenteric cyst, a detailed clinical evaluation and the use of the modern diagnostic imaging methods is necessary. Because of the possibility of concomitant occurrence of more than one malformation, both of the frontal and the lateral skull base should be carefully evaluated. Precise localization of the dural lesion is a prerequisite for successful surgical repair. In addition, the bacteria specificity could leave significant clues; *Pneumococcus* or *Haemophilus* suggests cranial defects. *E. coli* or other Gram-negative bacilli suggests spinal dural defects, and meningococci suggest immunologic deficiency. Asplenia or immunodeficiency such as complement or immunoglobulin deficiency rarely causes recurrent meningitis without a history of frequent infection of non-CNS areas. *Salmonella* meningitis or brain abscess should not be treated incompletely or inadequately and could lead to recrudescence, relapse or recurrence of bacterial meningitis.

If no etiology is identified the following protocol is proposed:

1. An audiological evaluation—audiogram or brainstem auditory evoked potential.
2. A contrast enhanced CT scan of the head including coronal images of the sinuses and fine cuts through the temporal bone.
3. Spinal MRI if otherwise indicated
4. Immunological studies, including a complete blood count, total immunoglobulin levels, immunoglobulin G subclasses, and total hemolytic complement levels.

Anatomic communication with the nasopharynx, the middle ear, paranasal sinuses, the skin (e.g., congenital dermal sinus tracts), or prostheses (e.g., ventriculoperitoneal or lumboperitoneal shunts).

Parameningeal inflammatory foci which may drain to the meninges or cause repeated inflammatory meningeal reactions leading to clinical meningitis.

Immunodepression (e.g., hypogammaglobulinemia, splenectomy, leukemia, lymphoma, hemoglobinopathies such as in sickle cell anemia, or complement deficiencies).

13.12 Recurrent Nonpurulent (Aseptic) Meningitis

The differential diagnosis of recurrent episodes of nonpurulent meningitis is extremely broad. Diagnostic concerns may be divided into two broad groups:

1. Chronic meningitis with recurrent symptomatic episodes
   In these conditions CSF rarely, if ever, returns to normal between clinical attacks. Fungal meningitis, in particular due to *C. neoformans* or *C. immits*, comprises the major treatable group of infections. Chronic meningitis with sporadic exacerbations may also be caused by *Brucella*, syphilis, or Lyme disease. Noninfectious disorders include chronic inflammatory conditions such as sarcoidosis, Behcet's disease, vasculitis, drugs (nonsteroidal anti-inflammatory agents, metronidazole, amoxicillin), Sjogren–Larsson syndrome, and Vogt–Koyanagi–Harada syndrome. HIV infection is often accompanied by a persistent lymphocytic meningeal response. It is extremely important to remember, however, that recurrent meningitis in patients with AIDS may represent sequential infections by different organisms.

2. True episodic meningitis, Mollaret's meningitis
   In these conditions, episodes of nonpurulent meningitis are separated by periods in which CSF returns to normal. It is now recognized that the great majority of cases described as Mollaret's meningitis are due to reactivated herpes simplex virus type 2 or, rarely, herpes simplex virus type 1. Rare episodes of recurrent episodes of lymphocytic meningitis, with normalization of CSF between episodes, have also been reported in association with Epstein–Barr virus infection, with human herpes virus 6 and during chronic

infection with *T. gondii*. Noninfectious causes have included rupture of epidermoid cysts or teratomas, nonsteroidal anti-inflammatory drug use, and periodic disease.

3. Recurrent chemical meningitis
    Recurrent chemical meningitis (RCM) may be caused by leakage of intracranial or intraspinal epidermoid cysts causing erosion of the skull. RCM have also been reported with neuroepithelial cysts.

Bruyn GW, Straathof LJ, Raymakers GM. Mollaret's meningitis. Differential diagnosis and diagnostic pitfalls. Neurology 1962;12:745–753

Hermans P, Goldstein N, Wellman W. Mollaret's meningitis and differential diagnosis of recurrent meningitis Am J Med 1972;52:128–140

Mirakhur B, McKenna M. Recurrent herpes simplex type 2 virus (Mollaret) meningitis. J Am Board Fam Pract 2004;17(4):303–305

Forgacs P, Geyer CA, Freidberg SR. Characterization of chemical meningitis after neurological surgery. Clin Infect Dis 2001;32(2):179–185

Lancman ME, Mesropian H, Granillo RJ. Chronic aseptic meningitis in a patient with SLE Can J Neurol Sci 1989;16(3):354–356

Cascella C, Nausheen S, Cunha BA. A differential diagnosis of drug-induced aceptic meningitis Infect Med 2008;25:331–334

Fonseca Cardoso A, Rocha-Filho PA, Melo Correa-Lima AR. Neuro-Behçet: differential diagnosis of recurrent meningitis. Rev Med Chil 2013;141(1):114–118

13.13 Conditions Predisposing to Polymicrobial Meningitis

1. Fistulous communications
2. Tumors neighboring the CNS
3. Infections at contiguous foci
4. Disseminated strongyloidiasis.
    Following table lists the frequency of spinal epidural bacterial abscess.

Organism	Frequency (%)
Staphylococcus aureus	62
Gram-negative rods (aerobic) (*Escherichia coli, Klebsiella, Enterobacter, Serratia, Proteus, Providencia, Arizona* etc.)	18
Aerobic streptococci	8
Staphylococcus epidermidis	2
Anaerobes	2
• Gram-positive (peptococci, peptostreptococci, clostridia), *Bacteroides fragilis*	
• Gram-negative other than *B. fragilis*	
Other organisms	2
Unknown	6

Baker AS, Ojemann RG, Swartz MN, Richardson EP, Jr. Spinal epidural abscess. N Engl J Med 1975;293(10): 463–468

Hlavin ML, Kaminski HJ, Ross JS, Ganz E. Spinal epidural abscess: a ten-year perspective. Neurosurgery 1990;27(2):177–184

13.13.1 Neurologic complications of meningitis

Acute complications

They occur within the first one or two days of admission and result from the intense disruption of normal brain function. This is produced most likely from synergistic effects among the infecting organism or bacterial products, the host inflammatory response, and alterations of normal brain physiology that result in brain injury. The pathophysiologic changes that accompany acute meningitis are:

1. Brain edema
2. Intracranial hypertension
3. Abnormalities of cerebral blood flow, loss of cerebrovascular autoregulation and decreased CPP

Type of complication	Usually associated organisms	Usually associated conditions
Seizures		
Occur in 15–25% of patients. May be generalized (due to increased ICP or the irritative effects of the infection), or focal due to increased ICP, or venous or arterial infarcts	*S. pneumoniae* *H. influenzae* Group B streptococci Herpes simplex virus	Sarcoidosis Mass lesions Cortical vein thrombosis
Syndrome of inappropriate antidiuretic hormone release (SIADH)		
Occurs in 30% of children with purulent meningitis within the first 24 hours of admission to hospital	*N. meningitides* *S. pneumoniae*	
Ventriculitis		
Occurs in about 30% of patients and up to 50% of neonates with Gram-negative enteric organism infection		

Abbreviation: ICP, intracranial pressure.

Intermediate complications

These complications become manifest during hospitalization and may persist after discharge. Some of these problems either have been present earlier in the course of meningitis but not recognized until the patient has been in the hospital for a few days, or have not developed until the disease process has gone on for several days.

Type of complication	Associated organisms
Hydrocephalus	*H. influenzae*
a) Obstructive due to the obstruction of CSF resorption from postinflammatory adhesions of the arachnoid granulations	*Mycobacterium tuberculosis* Group B streptococci
b) Ex vacuo due to the diffuse brain injury and loss and resultant brain atrophy	
Subdural effusions	*H. influenzae*
Common in children; up 25%. Almost all sterile effusions resolve spontaneously, except for a small minority, which may cause pressure phenomena, require serial subdural taps	*Streptococcus pneumoniae*
Fever	
In cases with purulent meningitis, fever resolves within 3–4 days of drug therapy. About 10% of children with *H. influenzae* meningitis will have a delayed defervescence for 7–8 days. After a week of therapy, drug fever may occur, although this is most typical after 10–14 days	
Brain abscess	
Unusual complication to common bacterial meningitis, except with disease attributable to *Citrobacter* species, where abscesses develop in approximately 50% of cases, and, rarely, *Listeria*	Citrobacter species Listeria monocytogenes

Abbreviation: CSF, cerebrospinal fluid.

Long-term complications

Type of complication	Associated organism	Associated conditions
Cranial nerve abnormalities	*N. meningitidis* (CN VI, VII, VIII)	Sarcoidosis (nerve VII; also VIII, IX, X)
	M. tuberculosis (CN VI)	Meningeal carcinomatosis (variable)
	Borrelia burgdorferi	
	Lyme disease (CN VII)	
Motor handicaps	*S. pneumoniae*	
Range from isolated paresis to global injury leading to tetraplegia. Only 20% of these motor handicaps present at discharge persisted at 1-year follow-up		
Deafness, hearing loss		
It is the most common long-term injury in meningitis, with 5–25% of survivors suffering from some form of hearing impairment. It is age and pathogen specific, with neonates and children with *S. pneumoniae* meningitis having the highest incidence	*H. influenzae* *N. meningitidis* *M. tuberculosis* Mumps *S. pneumoniae*	
Impairment of cognitive function		
May range from milder forms "learning disabilities" in 25% approximately to more serious forms of injury in the range of 2% of the children with meningitis		

Namani S, Kuchar E, Koci R, et al. Acute Neurologic Complications on Long Term Sequelae of Bacterial Meningitis in Children. Internet J Infect Dis 2010;9(2)

Schuchat A, Robinson K, Wenger JD, et al; Active Surveillance Team. Bacterial meningitis in the United States in 1995. N Engl J Med 1997;337(14):970–976

Grimwood K, Anderson P, Anderson V, Tan L, Nolan T. Twelve year outcomes following bacterial meningitis: further evidence for persisting effects. Arch Dis Child 2000;83(2):111–116

Kaplan SL, Woods CR. Neurologic complications of bacterial meningitis in children. Curr Clin Top Infect Dis 1992;12:37–55

Tunkel AR. Bacterial meningitis. Philadelphia: Lippincott Williams& Wilkins; 2001

Bedford H, de Louvois J, Halket S, Peckham C, Hurley R, Harvey D. Meningitis in infancy in England and Wales: follow up at age 5 years. BMJ 2001;323(7312):533–536

Oostenbrink R, Maas M, Moons KG, Moll HA. Sequelae after bacterial meningitis in childhood. Scand J Infect Dis 2002;34(5):379–382

14 Pain

14.1 Myofascial Pain Syndrome

This condition is a regional musculoskeletal pain disorder which stems from the lack of obvious organic findings and characterized by tender trigger points in taut bands of muscle that produce pain in a characteristic reference zone.

14.1.1 Diagnostic clinical criteria[1]

1. Major criteria
   a) Regional pain complaint
   b) Pain complaint or altered sensation in the expected distribution of referred pain from a myofascial trigger point.
   c) Taut band palpable in an accessible muscle
   d) Exquisite spot tenderness at one point along the length of the taut band
   e) Some degree of restricted range of motion, when measurable
2. Minor criteria
   a) Reproduction of clinical pain complaint, or altered sensation, by pressure on the tender spot.
   b) Elicitation of a local twitch response by transverse snapping
   c) Palpation at the tender spot or by needle insertion into the tender spot in the taut band
   d) Pain alleviated by elongating (stretching) the muscle or by injecting the tender spot

14.1.2 Associated neurologic disorders

1. Neuropathies
   a) Radiculopathy
   b) Entrapment neuropathies
   c) Peripheral neuropathy
   d) Plexopathy
2. Multiple sclerosis (MS)
3. Rheumatologic disorders
   a) Osteoarthritis
   b) Rheumatoid arthritis
   c) Systemic lupus erythematosus

---

[1] Simons DG. Muscle pain syndromes. J Man Med 1991;6:3–23

4. Psychosocial factors
   a) Psychosomatic or somatoform disorders
   b) Secondary gain issues
   c) Adjustment disorders with depression and anxiety

14.1.3 Differential diagnosis

1. Mixed tension-vascular headaches: Associated with trigger points in the sternomastoid, suboccipital, temporalis, posterior cervical, and scalene muscles.
2. Thoracic outlet syndrome: Associated with trigger points in the scalene and pectoralis minor muscles.
3. Temporomandibular joint (TMJ) dysfunction: These conditions are often primarily myofascial in origin with particular trigger point involvement of the temporalis, masseter, and pterygoid muscles.
4. Piriformis muscle syndrome: Pseudosciatica with entrapment of the sciatic nerve by the involvement of the piriformis muscle and the trigger points identified within this muscle.

Gerwin RD. Differential diagnosis of myofascial pain syndrome and fibromyalgia. J Musculoskeletal Pain 1999;7:209–215 (The Haworth Medical Press)

Travell JG, Simons DG. Myofascial Pain and Dysfunction: The Trigger Point Manual. Vol. 1. 2nd ed. Baltimore: Williams and Wilins; 1998

Borg-Stein J, Simons DG. Focused review: myofascial pain. Arch Phys Med Rehabil 2002;83(3, Suppl 1):S40–S47, S48–S49

14.2 Fibromyalgia Syndrome

The American College of Rheumatology (ACR) set two criteria for the diagnosis of fibromyalgia syndrome (FMS). (1) chronic (i.e., persisting longer than 3 months) widespread pain, dull diffuse aching modulated by several factors, including weather changes, exercise, and stress. (2) Multiple localized areas of tenderness (trigger points), generally defined as 11 of 18 specific tender points of precisely determined location on examination. Patients with FMS report numerous additional—apart from pain—complaints: most common and more characteristic occur in over 75% of patients include fatigue, nonrestorative sleep pattern, and morning stiffness. Less common features (approximately 25% of cases) are irritable bowel syndrome, Raynaud's phenomenon, headache, subjective swelling, nondermatomal paresthesia. In addition, people with FMS often have neurotic, functional symptoms, including depression (20–80%), anxiety states (13–63%), emotional instability, and personality disorders.

The specific cause of FMS remains unknown; however, a number of events are known to be associated with this condition. These include trauma (particularly head and/or neck injury from motor vehicle accidents), recent infection, and stress. Sleep disturbances also play an important role in the pathology. FMS patients lack stage 4, non-REM (or slow-wave) sleep. Serotonin is considered the neurotransmitter that mediates slow-wave sleep. Inhibition of serotonin (or its precursor tryptophan) is associated with a decrease in slow-wave sleep and an increase in the somatic symptoms.

14.2.1 Diagnostic criteria of fibromyalgia syndrome

- Chronic widespread pain for more than 3 months (axial and 3 of 4 body quadrants)
- 11 out of 18 positive tender points

If both the criteria are fulfilled, FMS is confirmed. Other disease does not exclude FMS (sensitivity 95% and specificity 84%).

14.2.2 Differential diagnosis of fibromyalgia syndrome

1. Psychiatric disorders
   Common features: *depression* and *anxiety*
   But: In psychiatric disorders there are less somatic, functional symptoms and *no tender points* in clinical examination.
2. Sjogren's syndrome
   Common features: *Myalgia and arthralgia, dry mouth, dry eyes, Raynaud's phenomenon, paresthesia, mild psychological disturbances (e.g., mild depression).*
   But: In Sjogren syndrome positive Schirmer test, > antinuclear antibodies (ANA), and anti-La/Ro antibodies, abnormal salivary glands biopsies.
3. Systemic lupus erythematosus
   Predominate in both young and middle-aged female, widespread, nonspecific arthralgia and myalgia, Raynaud's-like peripheral acrocyanosis, debilitating fatigue, high sensitivity to light and noise, and menstrual irregularities.
   But: ANA not elevated > 1:640, no anti-dsDNS antibodies
4. Rheumatoid arthritis (RA)
   Common features: Arthralgia in hands and feet, prolonged morning stiffness, subjective puffiness of the hands and fingers, paresthesia in the fingers suggestive of carpal tunnel syndrome, Sicca syndrome (dry eyes, dry mouth).
   But: Elevated erythrocyte sedimentation rate (ESR), C-reactive proteins (CRP), anti-cyclic citrullinated peptide (CCP), and rheumatoid factor (RF).

5. Polymyalgia rheumatica (PMR)

   Out of FMS patients aged more than 60 years, 6% have previously been *misdiagnosed* as having PMR.

   But: Inflammatory markers (ESR and CRP) are frequently elevated. The ESR, however, can be normal in 6% to 20% of patients with PMR. Therefore, CRP may be more sensitive marker of inflammation in these patients. Rapid improvement after corticosteroid treatment is not seen in FMS. On the contrary, patients may even feel worse!

6. Polymyositis (PM)

   PM may have a very *indolent onset* with nonspecific fatigue, lethargy, weakness, an *acute-phase response* may be *absent, muscle enzymes* may be *normal* or only mildly increased, electromyography tests and biopsies may be necessary.

7. Hypothyroidism

   Symptoms include: Nonspecific aches and pain, chronic fatigue, intolerance of exercise and cold environments, may be associated with loss of concentration and menstrual upsets and constipation.

   But: Thyroxine levels are normal in FMS, myalgic symptoms respond to low dose thyroid replacement in hypothyroidism.

8. Hyperparathyroidism

   Common features: Insidious onset, reduced threshold for pain in the muscles, chronic fatigue, mild psychiatric disturbances (depression, attention)

   But: Calcium, alkaline phosphatase, and parathyroid hormone levels are normal in FMS.

9. Ehlers–Danlos benign hypermobility joint syndrome

   "Beighton score": Dorsiflexion of 2nd finger to 90°, apposition of thumb to volar aspect of forearm, hyperextension of elbow by 10°, hyperextension of knee by 10°, hands flat on floor with knees extended.

10. Musculoskeletal disorders (diffuse idiopathic skeletal hyperostosis (DISH), Paget's disease)

    Common features: muscle pain and exercise intolerance

    But: Physical examination may discriminate, good response to physiotherapy, in some cases of myopathy elevated creatine phosphokinase (CPK).

11. Statin myopathy

    Statins in general well tolerated: used > 100 million people worldwide.

    But: In 0.9% for all statins occurs clinically relevant myopathy (muscle pain with CPK > 10x of the norm and also more than 29 cases of statin-associated autoimmune disorders (e.g., PM, dermatomyositis).

    In daily practice: Stop statins if CPK > 5x norm and myalgia regresses after 2–3 months.

12. Cancer risk

No association between FMS and cancer found.

But: Increased risk of female breast cancer among unconfirmed cases who did not meet the ACR criteria for FMS.

13. Other diseases to differentiate FMS with, include: FMS-like syndromes (4–19%) in hepatitis C; inflammatory/autoimmune diseases; mitochondrial myopathies; FMG and aromatase inhibitor; generalized musculoskeletal pain is a feature of many malignant diseases, such as multiple myeloma, metastatic breast, lung, and prostatic cancers.

Chochowska M, Szostak L, Marcinkowski JT, et al. Differential diagnosis between fibromyalgia syndrome and myofascial pain syndrome (Review article). J PreClin Clin Res 2015;9(1):82–86

Wolfe F, Smythe HA, Yunus MB, et al. The American College of Rheumatology 1990 criteria for the classification of fibromyalgia. Report of the Multicenter Criteria Committee. Arthritis Rheum 1990;33(2):160–172

Bennett R. Fibromyalgia, chronic fatigue syndrome, and myofascial pain. Curr Opin Rheumatol 1998a;10(2):95–103

14.3 Postherpetic Neuralgia

It is one of the most common types of neuropathic pain. This syndrome is characterized by prolonged pain after an episode of herpes zoster (HZ), classically known as *shingles*. After the acute rash of HZ has resolved, pain can often persist at the site of the healed rash. This pain, termed *postherpetic neuralgia (PHN)*, is one of the most debilitating feature of HZ infection and can persist for months to years after initial HZ infection. The incidence of PHN varies between 9 and15% and increases with age, occurring in as many as 50% of the population older than 60 years. PHN is often defined as pain persisting for more than 3 months after the resolution of an HZ rash. (▶ Fig. 14.1)

PHN is caused by the varicella zoster virus (VZV), which causes two illnesses: the initial infection, known as *chickenpox*, and a reactivation illness known as *herpes zoster* or *shingles*. The virus gains access to and establishes latency within the dorsal root ganglia. Reactivation is associated with decline of cell-mediated immunity that may result from natural aging, AIDS, organ transplantation, or other causes of immunocompromised states.

The dermatomes from T3 to Le are most commonly involved in HZ (thoracic 55%, lumbar 10%, cervical 10%, and sacral 5%). However, in some cases, the virus may afflict the cranial nerves (trigeminal 20%) that leads to complications.

14.3.1 Diagnosis of PHN

Its diagnosis is based primarily on clinical features. Patients with PHN can exhibit a variety of pain and sensory patterns, including constant pain (burning or

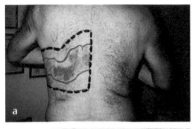
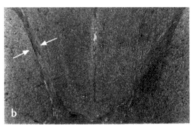
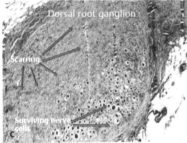

Fig. 14.1 **(a)** Postherpetic neuralgia 3 months after the rash. Skin lesions soon after rash healing surrounded by an area of anesthesia to punctate touch (*solid line*) and pinprick, with wider area of pain on moving touch of cotton or tissue (*interrupted line*). Moving the hair on this hirsute individual is exquisitely painful. Firm pressure is soothing. **(b)** Atrophy of the dorsal horn of the spinal cord in postherpetic neuralgia (*arrows*). **(c)** Scarring in the dorsal root ganglion with postherpetic neuralgia (*arrows*). (Reproduced from Practice. In: Burchiel K, ed. Surgical Management of Pain. 2nd edition. Thieme; 2014.)

throbbing), intermittent pain (shooting or stabbing), and allodynia (pain caused by a nonpainful stimulus). Areas of hypoesthesia and hyperesthesia can also be present in the affected area, sometimes in combination.

Although a clinical diagnosis is often sufficient to those patients presenting with the classic HZ rash, laboratory testing can be useful for atypical presentations. Both immunofluorescence VZV antigen detection and VZV detection by viral polymerase chain reaction are excellent tests with high specificity and sensitivity (90–100%). Serologic testing of acute and convalescent VZV immunoglobulin G (IgG) titers can also be used in establishing the diagnosis of HZ.

Johnson RW, Dworkin RH. Treatment of herpes zoster and postherpetic neuralgia. BMJ 2003;326(7392): 748–750

Gnann JW Jr, Whitley RJ. Clinical practice. Herpes zoster. N Engl J Med 2002;347(5):340–346

14.4 Atypical Facial Pain

The pain usually starts in the upper jaw. Initially pain spreads to the other side, and back to below and behind the ear. Later, pain may spread onto the neck and the entire half head.

1. PHN

   It occurs mainly with first-division herpes; although the whole zone hurts, the pain in the eyebrow and around the eye is especially severe. Pain is continual and burning, with severe pain added by touching the eyebrow or brushing the hair. The condition shows a tendency to spontaneous remission.

2. Temporal arteritis

   Swelling, redness, and tenderness of the temporal artery, and a headache in the distribution of the artery are the classic hallmarks of the disease. A diffuse headache can occur.

3. Cluster headache (migrainous neuralgia)

   Nocturnal attacks of pain in and around the eye, which may become bloodshot, and nose "stuffed up," with lacrimation and nasal watering. Bouts last 6–12 weeks and may recur at the same time each year.

4. TMJ dysfunction or Costen's syndrome

   Pain is mainly in the TMJ, spreading forward onto the face and up into the temporalis muscle. The joint is tender to touch and pain is provoked by chewing or just opening the mouth. The pain ceases almost entirely if the mouth is held shut and still.

5. Odontalgia

   A dull aching, throbbing, or burning pain that is more or less continuous and is triggered by mechanical stimulation of one of the teeth. It is relieved by sympathetic blockade.

6. Myofascial pain syndrome

   Aching pain lasting from days to months and elicited by palpation of trigger points in the affected muscle.

7. Atypical facial neuralgia

   Chronic aching pain involving the whole side of the face or even the head outside the distribution of the trigeminal nerve. This condition is much more common in women than in men and is often associated with significant depression.

Zakrzewska JM. Facial pain: neurological and non-neurological. J Neurol Neurosurg Psychiatry 2002; 72(Suppl 2):ii27–ii32

Nóbrega JCM, Siqueira SR, Siqueira JT, Teixeira MJ. Differential diagnosis in atypical facial pain: a clinical study. Arq Neuropsiquiatr 2007;65(2A):256–261

Agostoni E, Frigerio R, Santoro P. Atypical facial pain: clinical considerations and differential diagnosis. Neurol Sci 2005;26(Suppl 2):S65–S67

Quail G. Atypical facial pain—a diagnostic challenge. Aust Fam Physician 2005;34(8):641–645

14.5 Cephalic Pain

1. Migraine headache
   a) Classical migraine (hemicrania)
      A pulsatile headache which starts in the temple on one side and spreads to involve the whole side of the head. Usually self-limiting lasting from 30 minutes to several hours.
   b) Cluster headache (migrainous neuralgia)
      Nocturnal attacks of pain in and around the eye, which may become bloodshot and nose "stuffed up," with lacrimation and nasal watering. Bouts last 6–12 weeks and may recur at the same time each year.
   c) Chronic paroxysmal hemicrania
      Unilateral, shooting, boring headache, associated with lacrimation, facial flushing, and lid swelling that lasts 5–30 minutes day or night without remissions.
2. TMJ dysfunction or Costen's syndrome
   Pain is mainly in the TMJ, spreading forward onto the face and up into the temporalis muscle. The joint is tender to touch and pain is provoked by chewing or just opening the mouth. The pain ceases almost entirely if the mouth is held shut and still.
3. Odontalgia
   A dull aching, throbbing, or burning pain that is more or less continuous and is triggered by mechanical stimulation of one of the teeth. It is relieved by sympathetic blockade.
4. Tension headache
   Pain is believed to be due to spasm in the scalp and suboccipital muscles, which are tender and knotted. It is described as tightness like a "band" or "scalp too tight" is a frequent clue.
5. Temporal arteritis
   Swelling, redness, and tenderness of the temporal artery, and a headache in the distribution of the artery are the classic hallmarks of the disease. A diffuse headache can occur.
6. Psychotic headaches
   A specific spot on the head is isolated and bizarre complaints such as "bone is going bad," "worms crawling under the skin," quickly followed by an invitation to feel the increasingly large lump. Usually nothing other than normal bulge in the skull is palpable. This condition should always be suspected if the patient offers to locate the headache with one finger. A relentless pressure feeling over the vertex is typical of simple depression headache.
7. Pressure headache
   Occurs on waking and is aggravated by bending or coughing, produces a "bursting" sensation in the head and does not respond well to analgesics.

8. Posttraumatic headaches
   Pain occurs as a persistent and occasionally progressive and localized symptom following head trauma with an onset usually many months after the accident. It may relate to an entrapped cutaneous nerve neuroma, extensive base of skull fractures associated with injuries of the middle third of the face, stripping of the dura from the floor of the middle fossa, following diastatic linear fractures, etc.

9. Occipital neuralgia
   It is commonly a secondary manifestation of a benign process affecting the second cervical dorsal roots of the occipital nerves.

10. Carcinoma of the head and neck
    Often a deep, boring, headache, debilitating in its progressive persistence, regional or diffused and induced by carcinoma of the face, sinuses, nasopharynx, cervical lymph nodes, scalp, or cranium.

11. Headaches related to brain tumors or mass lesions
    A "cough" or "exertional" headache may be the sole sign of an intracranial mass lesion. Patients often wake up early in the morning with the headaches, which may be more frequent—daily versus episodically for migraine. Neurological examination may reveal focal abnormalities, as well as papilledema on fundoscopic examination.

12. Headaches related to ruptured aneurysms and arteriovenous anomalies
    The onset of pain is usually sudden and it is severe or disabling in intensity and located bi-occipital, frontal, and orbitofrontal.

13. Carotid artery dissection
    May present as an acute unilateral headache associated with facial or neck pain, Horner's syndrome, bruit, pulsatile tinnitus, and focal fluctuation neurologic deficits from transient ischemic attacks. Dissections occur in trauma, migraine, cystic medial necrosis, Marfan's syndrome, fibromuscular dysplasia, arteritis, atherosclerosis, or congenital anomalies of the arterial wall.

14. Spinal tap headaches
    Approximately in 20–25% of patients who undergo a lumbar puncture, irrespective of whether or not there was a traumatic tap and regardless of the amount of cerebrospinal fluid (CSF) removed. Characteristically, the headache is much worse when the patient is upright, often associated with disabling nausea and vomiting and improves dramatically when the patient lies flat in bed.

15. Postcoital headaches
    These occur before and after orgasm. The pain is usually sudden in onset, pulsatile, fairly intense, and involves the whole head. The International Headache Society classification defines three types:

a) Dull type: Thought to be due to muscle contraction and by far the most common type occurring prior to orgasm and located in the posterior cervical and occipital regions.

b) Explosive type: The pain is excruciating and throbbing and is thought to be of vascular origin occurring at the occipital region at or just after orgasm. There is a family history of migraine in 25% of cases.

c) Positional type: Secondary to low-CSF pressure presumed due to dural tear and CSF leak, becoming worst in the upright position.

16. Exertional headaches
These headaches tend to be throbbing, often unilateral, and of brief duration (1–2 hours). Generally, benign in nature and thought to be due to migraine, secondary to increased intracranial venous pressure, muscle spasm, sudden release of vasoactive substances, or very rarely due to structural intracranial abnormalities such as Chiari abnormalities, tumors, or aneurysms.

17. Headache related to analgesics and other drugs
    a) Analgesics, nonsteroidal anti-inflammatory
    b) Ergot derivatives
    c) Calcium antagonists
    d) Nitrates
    e) Hormones
        i. Progesterone
        ii. Estrogens
        iii. Thyroid preparations
        iv. Corticosteroids

14.6 Face and Head Neuralgias

1. Trigeminal neuralgia (TN)
The 2nd and 3rd divisions are most commonly involved and the attacks have trigger points. The symptoms may be due to tumors, inflammation, vascular anomalies or aberrations, and MS. TN is the most frequent of all neuralgias.

2. Glossopharyngeal neuralgia
Attacks of paroxysmal pains lasting for seconds or minutes, which are burning or stabbing in nature, and are localized to the region of the tonsils, posterior pharynx, back of the tongue, and middle ear. The causes may be idiopathic, vascular anatomic aberrations in the posterior fossa or regional tumors.

3. Occipital neuralgia
Attacks of paroxysmal pain along the distribution of the greater or lesser occipital nerve of unknown etiology.

4. Nasociliary neuralgia
   Paroxysmal attacks of orbital pain caused or exacerbated by touching the medial canthus and associated with edema and rhinorrhea. It is of unknown etiology.

5. Neuralgia of sphenopalatine ganglion (Sluder's neuralgia)
   Short-lived attacks of pain in orbit, base of nose. and maxilla associated with lacrimation, rhinorrhea, and facial flushing. It affects elderly females and the cause is idiopathic.

6. Geniculate ganglion neuralgia
   Paroxysmal attacks of pain are localized in the ear, caused by regional tumors or vascular malformations.

7. Greater superficial petrosal nerve neuralgia (Vidian's neuralgia)
   Attacks of pain in the medial canthus associated with tenderness and pain in the base of nose, and maxilla brought out or triggered by sneezing. The etiology is idiopathic or inflammatory.

8. Neuralgia of intermedius nerve
   Paroxysmal deep ear pain with trigger point in ear of unknown etiology. It may be related to varicella zoster virus infection.

9. Anesthesia dolorosa
   Continuous trigeminal pain in hypoalgesic or analgesic territory of nerve. It occurs following percutaneous radiofrequency lesions or ophthalmic HZ.

10. Tolosa–Hunt syndrome
    Episodes of retro-orbital pain lasting for weeks or months associated with paralysis of CNs III, IV, the 1st division of V, the VI, and rarely the VII. There is intact pupillary function. It is caused by a granulomatous inflammation in the vicinity of the cavernous sinus.

11. Raeder's syndrome
    Symptomatic neuralgia of the 1st division of CN V associated with Horner's syndrome, and possibly ophthalmoplegia from middle cranial fossa pathology.

12. Gradenigo's syndrome
    Continuous pain of the 1st and 2nd divisions of CN V with associated sensory loss, deafness, and CN VI palsy. It especially affects cases caused by inflammatory lesions in the region of the petrous apex after otitis media.

Zakrzewska JM. Differential diagnosis of facial pain and guidelines for management. Br J Anaesth 2013;111(1):95–104

Siccoli MM, Bassetti CL, Sándor PS. Facial pain: clinical differential diagnosis. Lancet Neurol 2006;5(3): 257–267

14.7 Trigeminal Neuralgia

It a neuropathic pain syndrome defined by the International Association for the Study of Pain (ISAP) as a "sudden and usually unilateral severe brief stabbing recurrent pain in the distribution of one or more branches of the fifth cranial nerve." It is an excruciating, short-lasting (< 2 minutes), unilateral facial pain that may be spontaneous or triggered by gentle, innocuous stimuli and separated by pain-free intervals of varying duration (▶ Fig. 14.2).

TN is classified as follows:

1. Primary or idiopathic (classic) that occurs in more than 85% of patients.
2. Secondary (symptomatic) that occur due to following reasons:
   a) *Compression*: Of all patients, 80–90% have a demonstrable focal compression of the trigeminal nerve root entry zone by a vascular loop (superior cerebellar artery and rarely by an aneurysm or an arteriovenous malformation, vertebrobasilar dolichoectasia). Post fossa tumors (brainstem neoplasm, trigeminal schwannoma, acoustic neuroma, cerebellopontine angle meningioma, metastatic infiltration of the skull base) and cavernous sinus lesions (cavernous carotid aneurysm, meningioma, pituitary adenoma, Tolosa–Hunt syndrome, metastasis) can also produce symptoms mimicking TN.

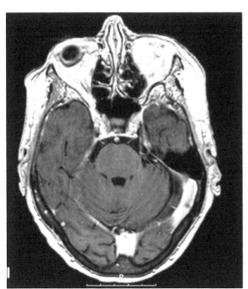

Fig. 14.2 MRI axial T1 image with contrast at the level of the midpons showing an aberrant loop of the superior cerebellar artery (*red arrow*) impinging on the root of the trigeminal nerve. The patient presented with clinical symptoms of trigeminal neuralgia. (Reproduced from 62.4 Trigeminal Neuralgia. In: Gasco J, Nader R, ed. The Essential Neurosurgery Companion. 1st edition. Thieme; 2012.)

b) *Demyelinating disease*: TN is 20 times more prevalent in MS sufferers compared with the general population. Demyelinating plaques are demonstrated in the pons, the root entry zone of trigeminal nerve by MRI of brain.

c) *Other brainstem lesions*: Rare cases of TN have been reported with brainstem infarcts and amyloid or calcium deposition along the trigeminal sensory pathway.

Diagnosis in typical cases of TN is straight forward; however, most patients suffer from misdiagnosis. Common conditions that mimic TN as well as their presenting features are listed in the following table.

Diagnosis	Important features
Dental infection or cracked tooth	Well localized to tooth, local swelling and erythema; appropriate findings on dental examination
Temporomandibular joint pain	Often bilateral and may radiate around ear and the neck and temples; jaw opening may be limited and can produce an audible click
Otitis media	Pain localized to ear, abnormalities on examination and tympanogram
Intracranial tumors	May have other neurologic symptoms or signs
Multiple sclerosis	Eye symptoms, other neurologic symptoms
Persistent idiopathic facial pain (atypical facial pain)	Often bilateral and may extend out of trigeminal territory (face, neck, ear); pain is often continuous, mild to moderate in severity, and aching or throbbing in character; provoking factors are stress and cold; sensory abnormalities may be present
Migraine	Often preceded by aura, severe unilateral headache often associated with nausea, photophobia, phonophobia, and neck stiffness
Paroxysmal hemicrania	Pain in forehead or eye, autonomic symptoms, responds to treatment with Indocid
Postherpetic neuralgia	History of herpes zoster or vesicular outbreak; continuous pain, tingling, often first division
Glossopharyngeal neuralgia	Pain is in the distribution of the glossopharyngeal nerve, classically oropharyngeal and otic

▶ *(Continued)*

Diagnosis	Important features
Temporal arteritis	Common in elderly people, temporal pain should be constant and often associated with jaw claudication, fever, and weight loss; temporal arteries may be firm, tender, and nonpulsatile on examination
Trigeminal autonomic cephalalgias (e.g., cluster headache, short-lasting unilateral neuralgiform headache with conjunctival injection and tearing (SUNCT) syndrome, chronic paroxysmal hemicrania)	Often have prominent autonomic features (e.g., conjunctival injection, lacrimation, nasal congestion, rhinorrhea, ptosis). Pain associated with cluster headaches typically retro-orbital

Bennetto L, Patel NKG, Fuller G. Trigeminal neuralgia and its management. BMJ 2007;334(7586):201–205

Casey KF. Role of patient history and physical examination in the diagnosis of trigeminal neuralgia. Neurosurg Focus 2005;18(5):E1

The International Classification of Headache Disorders. 2nd ed. Cephalalgia; 2004:24 (suppl)1:9–160

Gronseth G, Cruccu G, Alksne J, et al. Practice parameter: the diagnostic evaluation and treatment of trigeminal neuralgia (an evidence-based review): report of the Quality Standards Subcommittee of the American Academy of Neurology and the European Federation of Neurological Societies. Neurology 2008;71(15):1183–1190

Eller JL, Raslan AM, Burchiel KJ. Trigeminal neuralgia: definition and classification. Neurosurg Focus 2005;18(5):E3

14.8 Glossopharyngeal Neuralgia and Neuritis

A paroxysmal neuralgia with localized pain and trigger zones in the area of innervation of the glossopharyngeal nerve. The disease is quite rare and ranges from 0.75 to 1.1% of patients with TN.

Primary importance in the origin of the disease has a *compression factor* (hypertrophied styloid process of the temporal bone, ossified ligament, extended or elongated vessels, usually posterior inferior cerebellar and vertebral arteries).

Leading *clinical manifestation* are short-lived paroxysmal episodes of pain, the duration of which cannot exceed 1–2 minutes, but often they do not last more than 20 seconds. Patients describe the pain as burning, shooting, resembling an electric shock. Their intensity differs from mild to unbearable. Seizures are triggered by talking, eating, laughing, yawning, head movement, and change of position of the body. The number of attacks during the day range from a few to numerous (neuralgic status).

Initial localization of pain most often corresponds to the tongue, throat, tonsils, rarely is on the side of the neck, and behind the angle of the mandible. Trigger points are one of the most characteristic features of glossopharyngeal neuralgia. The most typical locations are in the tonsils, tongue, tragus in the ear. Pain often extend deep into the ear, throat, anterior to the tragus, and sides of the neck. Sensory disturbances in the form of hyper- or hypoesthesia detected in half of patients. Sensory disturbances are detected in most areas of pain, often at the root of the tongue, and in the back of the soft palate.

One of the most characteristic features of glossopharyngeal neuralgia is nerve tenderness around the corner point of the lower jaw.

Hiwatashi A, Matsushima T, Yoshiura T, et al. MRI of glossopharyngeal neuralgia caused by neurovascular compression. AJR Am J Roentgenol 2008;191(2):578–581

Teixeira MJ, de Siqueira SR, Bor-Seng-Shu E. Glossopharyngeal neuralgia: neurosurgical treatment and differential diagnosis. Acta Neurochir (Wien) 2008;150(5):471–475, discussion 475

Blumenfeld A, Nikolskaya G. Glossopharyngeal neuralgia. Curr Pain Headache Rep 2013;17(7):343

14.9 Painful Ophthalmoplegia

Pain localized in the eye, orbit, or forehead associated with ipsilateral ocular motor nerve palsies is the clinical hallmark of painful ophthalmoplegia, which is a group of disorders with various causes. Various pathologies localized in the orbit, the tip of the orbit, or cavernous sinus or the subarachnoid space can lead to this syndrome. Most commonly, painful disorders of the orbit are inflammatory in origin (45%), followed by vascular (24%), and neoplastic (20%). Infection (2%) and myopathy (1%) are rare.

14.9.1 Causes of painful ophthalmoplegia

1. Inflammatory (45%)
   a) Ocular myositis
   b) Idiopathic inflammatory pseudotumor of the orbit
   c) Tolosa–Hunt syndrome
   d) Sarcoidosis
   e) Wegener's granulomatosis
   f) Systemic lupus erythematosus
   g) Rheumatoid arthritis
2. Vascular (24%)
   a) Aneurysms of internal carotid artery
   b) Posterior communicating artery aneurysm

  c) Posterior cerebral artery aneurysm
  d) Arteriovenous malformations (orbit, cavernous sinus)
  e) Fistula (orbit, venous sinus)
  f) Carotid-cavernous thrombosis
  g) Pituitary apoplexy
  h) Ischemia (oculomotor nerve, brain stem)

3. Neoplastic (20%)
  a) Primary
    i. Meningioma
    ii. Pituitary adenoma/adenocarcinoma
    iii. Craniopharyngioma
    iv. Neurofibroma
    v. Sarcoma
    vi. Chordoma
    vii. Chondroma
  b) Metastases
    i. Melanoma
    ii. Lymphoma
    iii. Myeloma
    iv. Breast tumors
    v. Nasopharyngeal tumors

4. Infectious (2%)
  a) Mucormycosis
  b) Aspergillosis
  c) Pyogenic bacteria (e.g., complication of sinusitis)
  d) Syphilis
  e) Tuberculosis
  f) HZ
  g) HIV
  h) Cysticercosis

5. Traumatic
  a) Skull base fractures with lesion of the ocular motor nerves

Hunt WE. Tolosa-Hunt syndrome: one cause of painful ophthalmoplegia. J Neurosurg 1976;44(5):544–549

Smith JL, Taxdal DSR. Painful ophthalmoplegia. The Tolosa-Hunt syndrome. Am J Ophthalmol 1966;61(6):1466–1472

Gladstone JP. An approach to the patient with painful ophthalmoplegia, with a focus on Tolosa-Hunt syndrome. Curr Pain Headache Rep 2007;11(4):317–325

Schwarzman RJ. Differential Diagnosis in Neurology. Amsterdam-UK-USA: IOS Press Inc; 2006

14.10 Headache: World Health Organization Classification[2]

1. Migraine
   a) Migraine without aura
   b) Migraine with aura
      i. Migraine with typical aura
      ii. Migraine with prolonged aura
      iii. Familial hemiplegic migraine
      iv. Basilar migraine
      v. Migraine aura without headache
      vi. Migraine with acute onset aura
   c) Ophthalmoplegic migraine
   d) Retinal migraine
   e) Childhood periodic syndrome that may be precursors to or associated with migraine
      i. Benign paroxysmal vertigo of childhood
      ii. Alternating hemiplegia of childhood
   f) Complications of migraine
      i. Status migrainous
      ii. Migrainous infarction
   g) Migrainous disorder not fulfilling above criteria
2. Tension-type headaches
   a) Episodic tension-type headache
      i. Episodic tension-type headache associated with disorder of pericranial muscles
      ii. Episodic tension-type headache not associated with disorder of pericranial muscles
   b) Chronic tension-type headache
      i. Episodic tension-type headache associated with disorder of pericranial muscles
      ii. Episodic tension-type headache not associated with disorder of pericranial muscles
   c) Tension-type headache not fulfilling above criteria
3. Cluster headache and chronic paroxysmal hemicrania
   a) Cluster headache
      i. Cluster headache, periodicity undetermined
      ii. Episodic cluster headache
      iii. Chronic cluster headache

---

[2] International Headache Society of WHO (1988) Caphalgia, 8(Suppl. 7)

    b) Chronic paroxysmal hemicrania
    c) Cluster headache-like disorder not fulfilling above criteria
4. Miscellaneous headaches not associated with structural lesions
    a) Idiopathic stabbing headache
    b) External compression headache
    c) Cold stimulus headache
       i. External application of a cold stimulus
       ii. Ingestion of a cold stimulus (e.g., ice cream)
    d) Benign cough headache
    e) Benign exertional headache
    f) Headache associated with sexual activity
       i. Dull type
       ii. Explosive type
       iii. Postural type
5. Headache associated with head trauma
    a) Acute posttraumatic headache
       i. With significant head trauma and/or confirmatory signs
       ii. With minor head trauma and no confirmatory signs
    b) Chronic posttraumatic headache
       i. With significant head trauma and/or confirmatory signs
       ii. With minor head trauma and no confirmatory signs
6. Headache associated with vascular disorders
    a) Acute ischemic cerebrovascular disease
       i. Transient ischemic attack (TIA)
       ii. Thromboembolic stroke
    b) Intracranial hematoma
       i. Intracerebral hematoma
       ii. Subdural hematoma
       iii. Extradural hematoma
    c) Subarachnoid hemorrhage
    d) Unruptured vascular malformation
       i. Arteriovenous malformation
       ii. Saccular aneurysm
    e) Arteritis
       i. Giant cell arteritis
       ii. Other systemic arteritides
       iii. Primary intracranial arteritis
    f) Carotid or vertebral artery pain
       i. Carotid or vertebral dissection
       ii. Carotidynia (idiopathic)
       iii. Post endarterectomy headache

     g) Venous thrombosis
     h) Arterial hypertension
        i. Acute pressor response to exogenous agent
        ii. Pheochromocytoma
        iii. Malignant (accelerated) hypertension
        iv. Preeclampsia and eclampsia
7. Headache associated with nonvascular intracranial disorder
     a) High CSF pressure
        i. Benign intracranial hypertension
        ii. High-pressure hydrocephalus
     b) Low CSF pressure
        i. Postlumbar puncture headache
        ii. CSF fistula headache
     c) Intracranial infection
     d) Intracranial sarcoidosis and other noninfectious inflammatory diseases
     e) Headache related to intrathecal injections
        i. Direct effect
        ii. Due to chemical meningitis
     f) Intracranial neoplasm
     g) Headache associated with other intracranial disorders
8. Headache associated with substances or their withdrawal
     a) Headache induced by acute substance use or exposure
        i. Nitrate/nitrite-induced headache
        ii. Monosodium glutamate-induced headache
        iii. Carbon monoxide-induced headache
        iv. Alcohol-induced headache
        v. Other substances
     b) Headache induced by chronic substance use or exposure
        i. Ergotamine-induced headache
        ii. Analgesics abuse headache
        iii. Other substances
     c) Headache from substance withdrawal (acute use)
        i. Alcohol withdrawal headache (hangover)
        ii. Other substances
     d) Headache from substance withdrawal (chronic use)
        i. Ergotamine withdrawal headache
        ii. Caffeine withdrawal headache
        iii. Narcotics abstinence headache
        iv. Other substances
     e) Headache associated with substances but with uncertain mechanism
        i. Birth control pills or estrogens
        ii. Other substances

9. Headache associated with noncephalic infection
   a) Viral infection
      i. Focal noncephalic
      ii. Systemic
   b) Bacterial infection
      i. Focal noncephalic
      ii. Systemic (septicemia)
   c) Headache related to other infection
10. Headache associated with metabolic disorder
    a) Hypoxia
       i. High altitude headache
       ii. Hypoxic headache
       iii. Sleep apnea headache
    b) Hypercapnia
    c) Mixed hypoxia and hypercapnia
    d) Hypoglycemia
    e) Dialysis
    f) Headache related to other metabolic abnormality
11. Headache or facial pain associated with disorders of cranium, neck, eyes, nose, sinuses, teeth, mouth, or other facial or cranial structures
    a) Cranial bone
    b) Neck
       i. Cervical spine
       ii. Retropharyngeal tendinitis
    c) Eyes
       i. Acute glaucoma
       ii. Refractive errors
       iii. Heterophoria or heterotropia
    d) Ears
    e) Nose and sinuses
       i. Acute sinus headache
       ii. Other diseases of nose or sinuses
    f) Teeth, jaws, and related structures
    g) TMJ disease
12. Cranial neuralgia, nerve trunk pain, and deafferentation pain
    a) Persistent (in contact to tic-like) pain of cranial nerve origin
       i. Compression or distortion of cranial nerves and second or third cervical roots
       ii. Demyelination of cranial nerves
          – Optic neuritis (retrobulbar neuritis)
       iii. Infarction of cranial nerves
          – Diabetic neuritis

       iv. Inflammation of cranial nerves
- HZ
- Chronic postherpetic neuralgia

       v. Tolosa–Hunt syndrome
      vi. Neck–tongue syndrome
     vii. Other causes of persistent pain of cranial nerve origin

b) TN
       i. Idiopathic TN
      ii. Symptomatic TN
- Compression of trigeminal root or ganglion
- Central lesions

c) Glossopharyngeal neuralgia
       i. Idiopathic glossopharyngeal neuralgia
      ii. Symptomatic glossopharyngeal neuralgia

d) Nervus intermedius neuralgia
e) Superior laryngeal neuralgia
f) Occipital neuralgia
g) Central causes of head and facial pain other than tic douloureux
       i. Anesthesia dolorosa
      ii. Thalamic pain

h) Facial pain not fulfilling criteria in groups 11 or 12

13. Headaches not classifiable

International Headache Society of WHO.. Classification and diagnostic criteria for headache disorders, cranial neuralgias and facial pain. Cephalalgia 1988;8(Suppl. 7):1–96

14.11 Pseudospine Pain

The pain of back and/or leg pain as the presenting symptom of an underlying systemic (metabolic or rheumatological), visceral, vascular, or neurologic disease is known as pseudospine pain.

1. Vascular disorders
   a) Abdominal aortic aneurysm
      Patients are usually men over 50 years of age (1–4%) with abdominal and back pain (12%), pulsatile abdominal mass (50% sensitive; better in thin patients).
2. Visceral disorders
   a) Gynecologic disorders
      i. Endometriosis
         Patients are women of reproductive age (10%) with cyclic pelvic pain (25–67%), back pain (25–31%).

    ii. Pelvic inflammatory disease
       Predominate in young, sexually active women. Clinical features
       include:
- Ascending infection: endocervix to upper urogenital tract and symptoms of fever and chills, and leukocytosis
- Lower abdominal, back, and/or pelvic pain
- Vaginal discharge, leukorrhea
- Dysuria, urgency, frequency

    iii. Ectopic pregnancy
       Shows signs and symptoms of pregnancy, such as missed period (68%), breast tenderness, morning sickness. Other features include
- Abdominal pain (99.3%), unilateral in 33% (may mimic upper lumbar radiculopathy with radiation to thighs
- Adnexal tenderness (98%), unilateral adnexal mass (54%)
- Positive pregnancy test (83%)

b) Genitourinary disorders
    i. Prostatitis
      Occurs in men over 30 years of age; lifetime prevalence 50%. Acute febrile illness and leukocytosis, dysuria, lower back and/or perineal pain are its clinical features.
    ii. Nephrolithiasis
      Flank pain with radiation to groin, fever, chills, ileus, nausea, vomiting and microscopic hematuria.

c) Gastrointestinal disorders
    i. Pancreatitis
      Occurs in patients aged 35–45 years with alcohol abuse. Clinical features include:
- Midepigastric abdominal pain radiating through the back (90%)
- Systemic signs (fever, nausea, vomiting)
- Elevated serum amylase

    ii. Penetrating or perforated duodenal ulcer
      Abdominal pain radiating to the back and free air in abdominal radiography are the features.

3. Rheumatologic disorders
  a) Fibromyalgia
    The patients are mainly women (70–90%) aged 34–55 years. Clinical features include:
    i. Diffuse musculoskeletal pain typically including posterior neck, upper and lower back
    ii. Disturbed sleep, fatigue

      iii. Multiple (11 to 18) tender point sites on digital palpation (Important to demonstrate "negative" control points, i.e., midforehead or anterior thigh)

      iv. Normal radiographs and lab values

      Differential diagnosis: Polymyalgia rheumatica, hypothyroidism, Parkinson's disease, osteomalacia, chronic fatigue, and immunodeficiency syndrome.

b) Polymyalgia rheumatica

Occurs in elderly people aged 50–6 years (usually women). Clinical features include:

      i. Abrupt onset of shoulder, neck and upper back, hip, lower back, buttock, and thigh pain and morning stiffness

      ii. Elevated ESR (> 40 mmHg)

      iii. Dramatic response to low-dose prednisone

c) Seronegative spondyloarthropathies (ankylosing spondylitis; reactive arthritis or Reiter's syndrome; psoriatic spondyloarthropathy; enteropathic arthropathy

Males less than 40 years of age are more prone to these type of disorders with following clinical features:

      i. Dull, deep, aching back pain in the gluteal or parasacral area

      ii. Morning stiffness (gelling) in the back that improves with physical activity

      iii. Radiographic sacroiliitis

d) Diffuse idiopathic skeletal hyperostosis or Forrestier's disease (exuberant ossification of spinal ligaments)

Elderly people over the age of 50–60 years are prone to this disorder. Clinical features include:

      i. More of back stiffness (80%) than back pain (50–60%), pain is typically thoracolumbar

      ii. Flowing anterior calcification along contiguous vertebrae, preservation of disc height, and no sacroiliac involvement

      iii. Normal ESR or CRP

e) Piriformis syndrome

      i. Pseudosciatica—buttock and leg pain

      ii. Low back pain (50%)

      iii. Pain on resisted external rotation and abduction of hip

      iv. Piriformis muscle tenderness (transgluteal and transrectal)

f) Trochanteric bursitis, gluteal fasciitis

Predominant in females (75%) with features, such as gluteal and leg pain (64%), pain lying on affected side or with crossed legs (50%), and pain or tenderness over greater trochanter.

g) Scheuermann's disease (increased fixed thoracic kyphosis with anterior wedging of vertebrae and irregularity of vertebral endplates)
   Predominant in females (2:1) aged 12–15 years.
   i. Thoracic or thoracolumbar pain in 20–50% patients that is relieved by rest but increased with activity
   ii. Increasing fixed thoracic kyphosis
   iii. Anterior wedging of three or more contiguous thoracic vertebrae; irregular vertebral endplates

h) Adult scoliosis
   i. Back pain typically at apex of curve
   ii. Pseudoclaudication: spinal stenosis
   iii. Thoracic curve: uneven shoulders, scapular prominence, paravertebral hump with forward flexion
   iv. Lumbar curve: paravertebral muscle prominence

4. Metabolic disorders
   a) Osteoporosis
      i. Women over 60 years of age are more prone to this condition
      ii. Vertebral compression fractures, progressive loss of height, and increasing thoracic kyphosis
      iii. Pelvic stress fracture: weight-bearing parasacral or groin pain
      iv. Chronic mechanical spine pain: increased with prolonged standing, relieved rapidly in supine position

   b) Osteomalacia
      i. Diffuse skeletal pain: back pain (90%), ribs, long bones of the legs
      ii. Skeletal tenderness to palpation
      iii. Antalgic, waddling gait (47%)
      iv. Elevated alkaline phosphatase (94%)

   c) Paget's disease
      i. Bone pain: deep, aching, constant; back pain (10–40%)
      ii. Joint pain: accelerated degenerative disease
      iii. Nerve root entrapment: hearing loss, spinal stenosis
      iv. Deformities: enlarged skull, bowing of long bones, exaggerated spinal lordosis, kyphosis
      v. Increased alkaline phosphatase
      vi. Characteristic radiographic appearance

   d) Diabetic polyradiculopathy
      i. Older patients, over 50 years of age
      ii. Unilateral or bilateral leg pain, though diffuse, may resemble sciatica; typically worse at night
      iii. Proximal muscle weakness and muscle waste

e) Malignancy
    i. Patients usually over 50 years of age (75%)
    ii. Previous history of malignancy
    iii. Constant back pain unrelieved by positional change
    iv. Night pain
    v. Weight loss: 10 lb in 3 months
    vi. Elevated ESR (in 80% of patients), serum calcium, alkaline phosphatase (in 50% of patients)

Cole A, Herring S. Low Back Pain. Handbook end ed. Hanby & Bedfus; 2003

Speed C. Low back pain. BMJ 2004;328(7448):1119–1121

Deyo RA, Weinstein JN. Low back pain. N Engl J Med 2001;344(5):363–370

Pahl MA, Brislin B, Boden S, et al. The impact of four common lumbar spine diagnoses upon overall health status. Spine J 2006;6(2):125–130

Hazard RG. Failed back surgery syndrome: surgical and nonsurgical approaches. Clin Orthop Relat Res 2006;443:228–232

14.12 Back Pain in Children and Adolescents

Younger children (under the age of 10 years) develop back pain due to medical problems, such as infections, tumors, whereas older children and adolescents tend to have greater proportion of traumatic and mechanical disorders.

1. Developmental disorders
    a) Spondylolysis/spondylolisthesis
    b) Scoliosis
    c) Juvenile kyphosis (Scheuermann's disease)
2. Inflammatory disorders
    a) Discitis
    b) Vertebral osteomyelitis
    c) Sacroiliac joint infection
    d) Rheumatologic disorders
        i. Juvenile rheumatoid arthritis
        ii. Reiter's syndrome (reactive arthritis)
        iii. Psoriatic arthritis
        iv. Enteropathic arthritis
3. Tumors
    a) Intramedullary (31% of all paediatric spinal column tumors)
        i. Astrocytomas (60% of spinal cord tumors)
        ii. Ependymomas (30% of spinal cord tumors)
        iii. Drop metastases
        iv. Congenital tumors
        v. Hemangioblastomas

    b) Extramedullary tumors
       i. Eosinophilic granuloma
       ii. Osteoblastomas
       iii. Aneurysmal bone cysts
       iv. Hemangiomas
       v. Ewing's sarcoma
       vi. Chordoma
       vii. Neuroblastoma
       viii. Ganglioneuroma
       ix. Osteogenic sarcoma
    c) Intradural extramedullary tumors
       i. Nerve sheath tumors
       ii. Meningiomas
       iii. Mesenchymal chondrosarcomas
    d) Congenital tumors
       i. Teratomas
       ii. Dermoid and epidermoid cysts
       iii. Lipomas
4. Traumatic and mechanical disorders
    a) Soft-tissue injury
    b) Vertebral compression or endplate fracture
    c) Facet fracture and/ or dislocation
    d) Transverse process or spinous process fractures
    e) Chronic degenerative mechanical disorders
       i. Facet joint or pars interarticularis syndrome
       ii. Disc protrusion or herniation
       iii. Postural imbalances, asymmetries, and/or overload to functional spinal elements
       iv. Overuse syndrome
5. Nonspinal disorders
    a) Iliac fracture/apophyseal avulsion
    b) Renal disorder
    c) Pelvic/gynecologic disorder
    d) Retroperitoneal disorder
    e) Conversion reaction

Payne WK III, Ogilvie JW. Back pain in children and adolescents. Pediatr Clin North Am 1996;43(4):899–917

Taimela S, Kujala UM, Salminen JJ, Viljanen T. The prevalence of low back pain among children and adolescents. A nationwide, cohort-based questionnaire survey in Finland. Spine 1997;22(10):1132–1136

Balagué F, Troussier B, Salminen JJ. Non-specific low back pain in children and adolescents: risk factors. Eur Spine J 1999;8(6):429–438

14.13 Low Back Pain during Pregnancy

1. Herniated lumbar disc (HLD)
   The incidence of HDL is 1 in 10,000. The back pain may be worse when the woman is sitting and standing and relieved when she lies down.
2. Symphysiolysis pubis
   Pain in the groin, symphysis pubis, and thigh that may increase while rising from sitting to standing position and during ambulation.
3. Transient osteoporosis of the hip
   Pain in hip and groin areas that may increase on weight-bearing and a Trendelenburg gait, i.e., lateral limp during stance.
4. Osteonecrosis of the femoral head
   Groin or hip pain radiating to back, thigh, knee and aggravated by weight-bearing or passive hip rotation. May be related to excessive cortisol production in later stages of pregnancy.
5. Sacroiliac joint dysfunction, pelvic insufficiency, posterior pelvic pain
   It is the most common reason for low back pain and discomfort during pregnancy and may be related to excessive mobility of pelvic joints and altered stress distribution through pelvic ring.

Katonis P, Kampouroglou A, Aggelopoulos A, et al. Pregnancy-related low back pain. Hippokratia 2011;15(3):205–210

Wang SM, Dezinno P, Maranets I, Berman MR, Caldwell-Andrews AA, Kain ZN. Low back pain during pregnancy: prevalence, risk factors, and outcomes. Obstet Gynecol 2004;104(1):65–70

14.14 Back Pain in the Elderly Patients

1. Degenerative disorders of the spine
   The most common cause of back pain in the elderly is degenerative spondylosis of the spine.
   a) Disc herniations
   b) Spinal stenosis
   c) Degenerative spondylolisthesis
   d) Degenerative adult scoliosis
2. Neoplastic disorders of the spine
   a) Primary tumors
       i. Benign tumors
          – Hemangioma
          – Osteochondroma
          – Osteoblastoma
          – Giant cell tumor
          – Aneurysmal bone cyst

      ii. Malignant tumors
- Multiple myeloma
- Solitary plasmacytoma
- Chordoma
- Osteosarcoma
- Chondrosarcoma
- Ewing's sarcoma

  b) Metastatic tumors
- i. Lung
- ii. Colon/rectum
- iii. Breast
- iv. Prostate
- v. Urinary tract

3. Metabolic disorders of the spine

  a) Osteomalacia
Differential Diagnosis: Vitamin D deficiency, gastrointestinal malabsorption, liver disease, anticonvulsant drugs, renal osteodystrophy

  b) Paget's disease

  c) Osteoporosis

Kaye AD, Baluch A, Scott JT. Pain management in the elderly population: a review. Ochsner J 2010;10(3): 179–187

Rudy TE, Weiner DK. Lieber Sjet al: The impact of chronic low back pain in older adults Pain 2007;131(3): 293–301

Jarvik JG, Gold LS, Comstock BA, et al. Association of early imaging for back pain with clinical outcomes in older adults. JAMA 2015;313(11):1143–1153

15 Neurorehabilitation

Neurological rehabilitation programs are designed for people with injury or disorders of the nervous system and aim to improve function, reduce symptoms, and improve the well-being of the patient. It has been shown that brain is a dynamic organ capable of undergoing considerable modifications after suffering injuries or environmental changes—a property known as *neuroplasticity*. Due to this, great importance is currently being given to provide effective rehabilitation in cases of acquired brain injury and adequate stimulation to slow cognitive deterioration characteristic of pathologies.

Some of the conditions that may benefit from neurorehabilitation may include:

- Vascular disorders, such as ischemic and hemorrhagic strokes, and subdural hematomas
- Infections, such as meningitis, encephalitis, and brain abscesses
- Acquired trauma, such as brain and spinal cord injury
- Structural or neuromuscular disorders, such as brain or spinal cord tumors, peripheral neuropathy, muscular dystrophy, myasthenia gravis
- Neurodegenerative disorders, such as Parkinson's disease, multiple sclerosis, amyotrophic lateral sclerosis, Alzheimer's disease (AD), and Huntington's chorea
- Intellectual disability
- Mental illness
- Normal aging

15.1 Categories of Neurorehabilitation Scales

- Acute assessment (e.g., for admission/screening)
  - Consciousness/cognition (e.g., Glasgow Coma Scale, Mini-Mental State Examination (MMSE))
  - Stroke deficit (e.g., National Institute of Health Stroke Scale, Canadian Neurological Scale)
  - Global disability (e.g., Rankin Scale)
  - Activities of daily living (ADL)/outcomes (e.g., Barthel, Functional Independence measure (FIM), Supports Intensity Scale (SIS)- see below)
  - Health outcomes, physical and mental (e.g., Health Survey SF-36, on web)
  - Screening for rehab adherence (cognition, motivation, depression)
- Rehab admission/monitoring/outcomes
  - General scales such as ADLs (Barthel, FIM) or various quality of life (QOL) scales
  - Targeted functional assessment scales such as for balance, mobility, language/speech, dysphagia, hand function, cognition, depression, continence
- Stroke assessment scales overview

Type	Name and source	Approximate time to administer	Strengths	Weaknesses
Level-of-consciousness scale	Glasgow Coma Scale[1,2]	2 minutes	Simple, valid, and reliable	None observed
Stroke deficit scales	NIH Stroke Scale[3]	2 minutes	Brief, reliable, and can be administered by non-neurologists	Low sensitivity
	Canadian Neurological Scale[4]	5 minutes	Brief, valid, and reliable	Some useful measures omitted
Global disability scale	Rankin Scale[5,6,7]	5 minutes	Good for overall assessment of disability	Walking is the only explicit assessment criterion, low sensitivity
Measures of disability/activities of daily living (ADL)	Barthel Index[8,9]	5–10 minutes	Widely used for stroke, excellent validity and reliability	Low sensitivity for high-level functioning
	Functional Independence Measure (FIM)[10,11,12,13]	40 minutes	Widely used for stroke, measures mobility, ADL, cognition, functional communication	"Ceiling" and "floor" effects
Mental status screening	Folstein Mini-Mental State Examination[14]	10 minutes	Widely used for screening	Several functions with summed score. May misclassify patients with aphasia
	Neurobehavioral Cognition Status Exam (NCSE)[15]	10 minutes	Predicts gain in Barthel Index scores, unrelated to age	Does not distinguish right from left hemisphere, no reliability studies in stroke, no studies of factorial structure, correlates with education

(Continued)

▶ (Continued)

Type	Name and source	Approximate time to administer	Strengths	Weaknesses
Assessment of motor function	Fugl-Meyer[16]	30–40 minutes	Extensively evaluated measure, good validity and reliability for assessing sensorimotor function and balance	Considered too complex and time-consuming by many
	Motor Assessment Scale[17,18]	15 minutes	Good, brief assessment of movement and physical mobility	Reliability assessed only in stable patients. Sensitivity not tested
	Motricity Index[19,20]	5 minutes	Brief assessment of motor function of arm, leg, and trunk	Sensitivity not tested
Balance assessment	Berg Balance Assessment[21,22]	10 minutes	Simple, well established with stroke patients, sensitive to change	None observed
Mobility assessment	Rivermead Mobility Index[23,24]	5 minutes	Valid, brief, reliable test of physical mobility	Sensitivity not tested
Assessment of speech and language functions	Boston Diagnostic Aphasia Examination[25]	1–4 hours	Widely used, comprehensive, good standardization data, sound theoretical rationale	Time to administer long; half of patients cannot be classified
	Porch Index of Communicative Ability (PICA)[26]	1/2–2 hours	Widely used, comprehensive, careful test development and standardization	Time to administer long, special training required to administer, inadequate sampling of language other than one word and single sentences
	Western Aphasia Battery[27]	1–4 hours	Widely used, comprehensive	Time to administer long, "aphasia quotients" and "taxonomy" of aphasia not well validated

Depression scales	Beck Depression Inventory (BDI)[28,29]	10 minutes	Widely used, easily administered, norms available, good with somatic symptoms	Less useful in elderly and in patients with aphasia or neglect, high rate of false positives, somatic items may not be due to depression
	Center for Epidemiologic Studies Depression (CES-D)[30]	< 15 minutes	Brief, easily administered, useful in elderly, effective for screening in stroke population	Not appropriate for aphasic patients
	Geriatric Depression Scale (GDS)[31]	10 minutes	Brief, easy to use with elderly, cognitively impaired, and those with visual or physical problems or low motivation	High false negative rates in minor depression
	Hamilton Depression Scale[32,33]	< 30 minutes	Observer rated; frequently used in stroke patients	Multiple differing versions compromise interobserver reliability
	Quick Inventory of Depressive Symptomatology (QIDS)	5–10 minutes	Good internal consistency, correlates significantly with clinician ratings of depression severity, and is sensitive to change	
Measures of instrumental ADL	Philadelphia Geriatric Center Instrumental Activities of Daily Living[34]	5–10 minutes	Measures broad base of information necessary for independent living.	Has not been tested in stroke patients.
	Frenchay Activities Index[35]	10–15 minutes	Developed specifically for stroke patients, assesses broad array of activities	Sensitivity and interobserver reliability not tested, sensitivity probably limited

(Continued)

▶ (Continued)

Type	Name and source	Approximate time to administer	Strengths	Weaknesses
Family assessment	Family Assessment Device (FAD)[36]	30 minutes	Widely used in stroke, computer scoring available, excellent validity and reliability, available in multiple languages	Assessment subjective, sensitivity not tested, "ceiling" and "floor" effects
Health status/quality of life measures	Medical Outcomes Study (MOS) 36-Item Short-Form Health Survey[37]	10–15 minutes	Generic health status scale SF36 is improved version of SF20. Brief, can be self-administered or administered by phone or interview. Widely used in the United States	Possible "floor" effect in seriously ill patients (especially for physical functioning), it is suggested that it should be supplemented by an ADL scale in stroke patients
	Sickness Impact Profile (SIP)[38]	20–30 minutes	Comprehensive and well-evaluated, broad range of items reduces "floor" or "ceiling" effects	Time to administer somewhat long, evaluates behavior rather than subjective health; needs questions on well-being, happiness, and satisfaction

Sources:

1 Teasdale G, Jennett B. Assessment of coma and impaired consciousness. A practical scale. Lancet 1974;2(7872):81–84

2 Teasdale G, Murray G, Parker L, Jennett B. Adding up the Glasgow Coma Score. Acta Neurochir (Wien) 1979(Suppl 28):13–16

3 Brott T, Adams HP Jr, Olinger CP, et al. Measurements of acute cerebral infarction: a clinical examination scale. Stroke 1989;20(7):864–870

4 Côté R, Hachinski VC, Shurvell BL, Norris JW, Wolfson C. The Canadian Neurological Scale: a preliminary study in acute stroke. Stroke 1986;17(4):731–737

5 Rankin J. Cerebral vascular accidents in patients over the age of 60. II. Prognosis. Scott Med J 1957;2(5):200–215

6 Bonita R, Beaglehole R. Modification of Rankin Scale. Recovery of motor function after stroke. Stroke 1988;19(12):1497–1500

7 van Swieten JC, Koudstaal PJ, Visser MC, Schouten HJ, van Gijn J. Interobserver agreement for the assessment of handicap in stroke patients. Stroke 1988;19(5):604–607

8 Mahoney FI, Barthel DW. Functional evaluation: the Barthel Index. Md State Med J 1965;14:61–65

9 Wade DT, Collin C. The Barthel ADL Index: a standard measure of physical disability? Int Disabil Stud 1988;10(2):64–67

10 Guide for the uniform data set for medical rehabilitation (Adult FIM), version 4.0 Buffalo, NY 14214: State University of New York at Buffalo; 1993

11 Granger CV, Hamilton BB, Keith RA, Zielezny M, Sherwin FS. Advances in functional assessment for medical rehabilitation. Top Geriatr Rehabil 1986;1(3):59–74

12 Granger CV, Hamilton BB, Sherwin FS. Guide for the use of the uniform data set for medical rehabilitation. Uniform Data System for Medical Rehabilitation Project Office, Buffalo General Hospital, NY; 1986

13 Keith RA, Granger CV, Hamilton BB, Sherwin FS. The functional independence measure: a new tool for rehabilitation. In: Eisenberg MG, Grzesiak RC, ed. Advances in clinical rehabilitation. Vol. 1. New York: Springer-Verlag; 1987:6–18

14 Folstein MF, Folstein SE, McHugh PR. "Mini-mental state". A practical method for grading the cognitive state of patients for the clinician. J Psychiatr Res 1975;12(3):189–198

15 Kiernan RJ, Mueller J, Langston JW, Van Dyke C. The Neurobehavioral Cognitive Status Examination: a brief but quantitative approach to cognitive assessment. Ann Intern Med 1987;107(4):481–485

16 Fugl-Meyer AR, Jääskö L, Leyman I, Olsson S, Steglind S. The post-stroke hemiplegic patient. 1. a method for evaluation of physical performance. Scand J Rehabil Med 1975;7(1):13–31

17 Carr JH, Shepherd RB, Nordholm L, Lynne D. Investigation of a new motor assessment scale for stroke patients. Phys Ther 1985;65(2):175–180

18 Poole JL, Whitney SL. Motor assessment scale for stroke patients: concurrent validity and interrater reliability. Arch Phys Med Rehabil 1988;69(3 Pt 1):195–197

19 Collin C, Wade D. Assessing motor impairment after stroke: a pilot reliability study. J Neurol Neurosurg Psychiatry 1990;53(7):576–579

20 Demeurisse G, Demol O, Robaye E. Motor evaluation in vascular hemiplegia. Eur Neurol 1980;19(6):382–389

21 Berg KO, Maki BE, Williams JI, Holliday PJ, Wood-Dauphinee SL. Clinical and laboratory measures of postural balance in an elderly population. Arch Phys Med Rehabil 1992;73(11):1073–1080

22 Berg K, Wood- Dauphinee S, Williams JI, Gayton D. Measuring balance in the elderly: preliminary development of an instrument. Physiother Can 1989;41(6):304–311

23 Collen FM, Wade DT, Robb GF, Bradshaw CM. The Rivermead Mobility Index: a further development of the Rivermead Motor Assessment. Int Disabil Stud 1991;13(2):50–54

24 Wade DT, Collen FM, Robb GF, Warlow CP. Physiotherapy intervention late after stroke and mobility. BMJ 1992;304(6827):609–613

25 Goodglass H, Kaplan E. The assessment of aphasia and related disorders. Philadelphia: Lea and Febiger; 1972. Chapter 4, Test procedures and rationale. Manual for the BDAE. Goodglass H, Kaplan E. Boston Diagnostic Aphasia Examination (BDAE). Philadelphia: Lea and Febiger; 1983

26 Porch B. Porch Index of Communicative Ability (PICA). Palo Alto: Consulting Psychologists Press; 1981

27 Kertesz A. Western Aphasia Battery. New York: Grune & Stratton; 1982

28 Beck AT, Ward CH, Mendelson M, Mock J, Erbaugh J. An inventory for measuring depression. Arch Gen Psychiatry 1961 June;4:561–571

29 Beck AT, Steer RA. Beck Depression Inventory: manual (revised edition). NY Psychological Corporation; 1987

30 Radloff LS. The CES-D scale: a self-report depression scale for research in the general population. J Appl Psychol Meas 1977;1:385–401

31 Yesavage JA, Brink TL, Rose TL, et al. Development and validation of a geriatric depression screening scale: a preliminary report. J Psychiatr Res 1982–1983;17(1):37–49

32 Hamilton M. A rating scale for depression. J Neurol Neurosurg Psychiatry 1960;23:56–62

33 Hamilton M. Development of a rating scale for primary depressive illness. Br J Soc Clin Psychol 1967;6(4):278–296

34 Lawton MP. Assessing the competence of older people. In: Kent D, Kastenbaum R, Sherwood S, eds. Research Planning and Action for the Elderly. New York: Behavioral Publications; 1972

35 Holbrook M, Skilbeck CE. An activities index for use with stroke patients. Age Ageing 1983;12(2):166–170

36 Epstein NB, Baldwin LM, Bishop DS. The McMaster Family Assessment Device. J Marital Fam Ther 1983;9(2):171–180

37 Ware JE Jr, Sherbourne CD. The MOS 36-item short-form health survey (SF-36). I. Conceptual framework and item selection. Med Care 1992;30(6):473–483

38 Bergner M, Bobbitt RA, Carter WB, Gilson BS. The Sickness Impact Profile: development and final revision of a health status measure. Med Care 1981;19(8):787–805

Note: Instrument is available from the Health Services Research and Development Center, The Johns Hopkins School of Hygiene and Public Health, 624 North Broadway, Baltimore, MD 21205.

Taken from "Post-Stroke Rehabilitation: Assessment, Referral, and Patient Management Quick Reference Guide Number 16" and published by the US Agency for Health Care Policy and Research.

- Other useful instruments for measuring disability/ADL include the following:
  - Katz Index of ADL
    Katz S, Ford AB, Moskowitz RW, Jackson BA, Jaffe MW. Studies of illness in the aged. The index of ADL: a standardized measure of biological and psychosocial function. JAMA 1963;185:914–919
  - Kenny Self-Care Evaluation
    Schoening HA, Iversen IA. Numerical scoring of self-care status: a study of the Kenny self-care evaluation. Arch Phys Med Rehabil 1968;49(4):221–229
  - LORS/LAD
    Carey RG, Posavac EJ. Program evaluation of a physical medicine and rehabilitation unit: a new approach. Arch Phys Med Rehabil 1978;59(7):330–337
  - Picture Exchange Communication System (PECS)
    Harvey RF, Jellinek HM. Functional performance assessment: a program approach. Arch Phys Med Rehabil 1981;62(9):456–460
- Another useful instrument for assessing mental status is motor impersistence.
  Ben-Yishay Y, Diller L, Gerstman L, Haas A. The relationship between impersistence, intellectual function and outcome of rehabilitation in patients with left hemiplegia. Neurology 1968;18(9):852–861
- Instrument for assessing depression is the Zung Scale.
  Zung WW. A self-rating depression scale. Arch Gen Psychiatry 1965;12:63–70
- Useful instruments for measuring IADL include:
  - OARS-Instrumental ADL
    Duke University Center for the Study of Aging and Human Development. Multidimensional Functional Assessment: The OARS Methodology. Durham, NC: Duke University; 1978
  - Functional Health Status
    Rosow I, Breslau N. A Guttman health scale for the aged. J Gerontol 1966;21(4):556–559

15.2 Measures (Scales) of Disability

15.2.1 Glasgow outcome scale

The Glasgow Outcome Scale (GOS) has provided a high inter-rater reliability and has proved its usefulness in multicenter clinical studies of head injury.

Score	Outcome
1	Death
2	Vegetative state: unresponsive and speechless
3	Severe disability: depends on others for all or part of care or supervision because of mental or physical disability
4	Moderate disability: disabled, but independent in ADLs and in the community
5	Good recovery: resumes normal life; may have minor neurologic or psychologic deficits

Source: Jennett B, Bond M. Assessment of outcome after severe brain damage. Lancet 1975;1(7905):480–484

15.2.2 Disability rating scale (DRS)

Developed as an alternative to GOS which was thought to be insensitive. It was tested with older juveniles and adults with moderate and severe brain injuries in an inpatient rehabilitation setting.

It is an 8-item outcome measure; scoring is reversed from many scales. The scale is intended to measure accurately general changes over the course of recovery. It is widely used in brain injury research.

Category	Item	Instructions	Score
Arousability	Eye opening	0 = spontaneous	
		1 = to speech	
		2 = to pain	
		3 = none	
Awareness and responsivity	Communication ability	0 = oriented	
		1 =confused	
		2 = inappropriate	
		3 = incomprehensible	
		4= none	
	Motor response	0 = obeying	
		1 = localizing	
		2 = withdrawing	
		3 = flexing	

(Continued)

▶ (*Continued*)

Category	Item	Instructions	Score
		4 = extending	
		5 = none	
Cognitive ability for sef-care activities	Feeding	0 = complete	
		1 = partial	
		2 = minimal	
		3 = none	
	Toileting	0 = complete	
		1 = partial	
		2 = minimal	
		3 = none	
	Grooming	0 = complete	
		1 = partial	
		2 = minimal	
		3 = none	
Dependence on others	Level of functioning	0 = completely independent	
		1 = independent in special environment	
		2 = mildly dependent	
		3 = moderately dependent	
		4 = markedly dependent	
		5 = totally dependent	
Psychosocial adaptability	Employability	0 = not restricted	
		1 = selected jobs	
		2 = sheltered workshop (noncompetitive)	
		3 = not employable	

Total DR score

Source: Rappaport et al. Disability rating scale for severe head trauma patients: coma to community. Arch Phys Med Rehabil 1982;63:118–123.

Total DR score level and disability	
0	None
1	Mild
2–3	Partial
4–6	Moderate
7–11	Moderately severe
12–16	Severe
17–21	Extremely severe
22–24	Vegetative state
25–29	Extreme vegetative state

Source: Bellon K, Jamison L, Wright J et al. J Head Trauma Rehabil 2012;27(6):449–451.
Note: The maximum score a patient can obtain on the DRS is 29 (extreme vegetative state). A person without disability would score zero. The DRS rating must be reliable, i.e., obtained while the individual is not under the influence of anesthesia, other mind-altering drugs, recent seizure, or recovering from surgical anesthesia. In comparison with the GOS, 71% of trauma brain injury individuals showed improvement on DRS whereas 33% show improvement on GOS.

Advantages of DRS
- Brevity (scoring time can range from 30 seconds if familiar with scale or client to 15 minutes)
- Reliability and validity tested
- Ability to track an individual from coma to community
- Can be self-administered or scored through interview over the phone
- Expertise in the field is not needed to complete it accurately

Disadvantages of DRS
- "Difficult" to rate
  - Expertise required 4/5
  - Content difficulty 4/5
- Relative insensitivity at the low end of the scale (mild trauma brain injuries)
- Not meant to measure change over short periods of time

15.2.3 Rankin disability scale

The Rankin Disability Scale has a special niche in clinical trials of stroke; however, its assessment of both, disability and impairment makes it a little inswensitive. Therefore, it is best used for large population studies that require a simple assessment.

Score	Outcome
1	No disability
2	Slight disability: unable to carry out some previous activities, but looks after own affairs without assistance
3	Moderate disability: requires some help, but walks without assistance
4	Moderately severe disability: unable to walk and do bodily care without help
5	Severe disability: bedridden, incontinent, needs constant nursing care

15.2.4 Modified Rankin scale (MRS)

Score	Description
0	No symptoms at all
1	No significant disability despite symptoms; able to carry out all usual duties and activities
2	Slight disability; unable
4	Moderately severe disability; unable to walk without assistance and unable to attend to own bodily needs without assistance
5	Severe disability; bedridden, incontinent and requiring constant nursing care and attention
6	Dead

TOTAL (0–6): _____

Source: Rankin J. Cerebral vascular accidents in patients over the age of 60. Scott Med J 1957;2:200–215

15.2.5 The Barthel index

The Barthel Index (BI) is a weighted scale of 10 activities, with maximum independence equal to a score of 100. Patients who score 100 on the BI can survive without attendant care. Scores below 61 on hospital discharge after a stroke predict a level of dependence that makes discharge to home less likely.

The BI is a well-known scale for the assessment and outcome of disability. It has been used in the epidemiologic studies of stroke, such as the Framingham study where patients were evaluated over time after stroke, and to complement impairment measures in multicenter trials of acute interventions for stroke, traumatic brain injury, and spinal cord trauma.

The BI has its limitations: (1) It has no language or cognitive measure and, (2) as is the case with most functional assessments, a change by a given number of points does not mean an equivalent change in disability across different activities. The BI, however, is the best-known scale to which other new measures will be compared.

Activity	Score
Feeding	
0 = unable	
5 = needs help cutting, spreading butter, etc., or requires modified diet	
10 = independent	_____
Bathing	
0 = dependent	
5 = independent (or in shower)	_____
Grooming	
0 = needs to help with personal care	
5 = independent face/hair/teeth/shaving (implements provided)	_____
Dressing	
0 = dependent	
5 = needs help but can do about half unaided	
10 = independent (including buttons, zips, laces, etc.)	_____
Bowels	
0 = incontinent (or needs to be given enemas)	
5 = occasional accident 10 = continent	_____
Bladder	
0 = incontinent, or catheterized and unable to manage alone	
5 = occasional accident 10 = continent	_____
Toilet use	
0 = dependent	
5 = needs some help, but can do something alone	
10 = independent (on and off, dressing, wiping)	_____
Transfers (bed to chair and back)	
0 = unable, no sitting balance	
5 = major help (one or two people, physical), can sit	
10 = minor help (verbal or physical)	
15 = independent	_____
Mobility (on level surfaces)	
0 = immobile or < 50 yards	

(Continued)

► (*Continued*)

Activity	Score
5 = wheelchair independent, including corners, > 50 yards	
10 = walks with help of one person (verbal or physical) > 50 yards	
15 = independent (but may use any aid; for example, stick) > 50 yards	_____
Stairs	
0 = unable	
5 = needs help (verbal, physical, carrying aid)	
10 = independent	_____

TOTAL (0–100): _____

15.2.6 The Barthel ADL index: guidelines

1. The index should be used as a record of what a patient does, not as a record of what a patient could do.
2. The main aim is to establish degree of independence from any help, physical or verbal, however minor and for whatever reason.
3. The need for supervision renders the patient not independent.
4. A patient's performance should be established using the best available evidence. Asking the patient, friends/relatives, and nurses are the usual sources, but direct observation and common sense are also important. However, direct testing is not needed.
5. Usually the patient's performance over the preceding 24–48 hours is important, but occasionally longer periods will be relevant.
6. Middle categories imply that the patient supplies over 50% of the effort.
7. Use of aids to be independent is allowed.

Mahoney FI, Barthel DW. Functional evaluation: the Barthel Index. Md State Med J. 1965; 14:61–65

15.2.7 Mini-mental state examination

The MMSE is the most frequently used cognitive screening test, but it has limited sensitivity in detecting language dysfunction and in determining the cognitive basis for disability in the neurorehabilitation population. Scoring must be considered within educational and age-adjusted norms.

Maximum score	Patient's score	
		Orientation
5	( )	What is the (year) (season) (date) (day) (month)
5	( )	Where are we: (state) (country) (town) (hospital) (floor)?
		Registration
3	( )	Name three objects, 1 second to say each, then ask the patient to repeat all three after you said them. Give 1 point for each correct answer. Continue repeating all three objects until the patient learns all three. Count trials and record.
		Attention and calculation
5	( )	Serial 7's. One point for each correct response. Stop after five answers. Alternatively, spell word backward.
		Recall
3	( )	Ask for the three objects named in Registration. Give one point for each correct answer.
		Language
2	( )	Name a pencil and watch.
1	( )	Repeat the following: "No ifs, ands, or buts."
3	( )	Follow a three-stage command: "Take paper in your right hand, fold it in half, and put it on the floor."
1	( )	Read and obey the following: "Close your eyes."
1	( )	Write a sentence
1	( )	Copy a design
30	( )	

Assess level of consciousness along a continuum.

Alert	Drowsy	Stupor	Coma

Source: Folstein MF, Folstein SE, McHugh PR. "Mini-mental state". A practical method for grading the cognitive state of patients for the clinician. J Psychiatr Res 1975;12(3):189–198

15.2.8 The functional independence measure

The FIM was developed to resolve the long-standing problem of lack of uniform measurement and data on disability and rehabilitation outcomes (Granger 1998). The FIM emerged from a thorough developmental process, sponsored by the American Congress of Rehabilitation Medicine and the American Academy of Physical Medicine and Rehabilitation. A National Task force reviewed 36 published and unpublished functional assessment scales before agreeing on an instrument.

FIM(TM) scores range from 1 to 7: an FIM(TM) item score of 7 is categorized as "complete independence," while a score of 1 is "total assist" (performs less than 25% of task). Scores falling below 6 require another person for supervision or assistance.

The FIM(TM) measures independent performance in self-care, sphincter control, transfers, locomotion, communication, and social cognition. By adding the points for each item, the possible total score ranges from 18 (lowest) to 126 (highest) level of independence.

During rehabilitation, admission and discharge scores are rated by clinicians observing patient function. Functioning post discharge can be accurately assessed using a telephonic version of FIM(TM) when administered by qualified, trained interviewers.

Guide for the uniform data set for medical rehabilitation (Adult FIM), version 4.0 Buffalo, NY 14214: State University of New York at Buffalo; 1993

Granger CV, Hamilton BB, Keith RA, Zielezny M, Sherwin FS. Advances in functional assessment for medical rehabilitation. Top Geriatr Rehabil. 1986; 1(3):59–74

Granger CV, Hamilton BB, Sherwin FS. Guide for the use of the uniform data set for medical rehabilitation. Uniform Data System for Medical Rehabilitation Project Office, Buffalo General Hospital, NY; 1986

Keith RA, Granger CV, Hamilton BB, Sherwin FS. The functional independence measure: a new tool for rehabilitation. In: Eisenberg MG, Grzesiak RC, ed. Advances in clinical rehabilitation. Vol. 1. New York: Springer-Verlag; 1987:6–18

15.2.9 Hachinski ischemia score

The Hachinski Ischemic Score (HIS) is a simple 13-item clinical tool used for differentiating types of dementia (primary degenerative, vascular, or multi-infarct, mixed type). Patients with a score of 7 or higher are more likely to have a vascular dementia. A low HIS is less likely to indicate vascular dementia because ischemic lesions severe enough to produce a dementia would be expected to be severe enough to cause the accompanying neurologic changes and elevate the index.

Feature	Score
Abrupt onset	2
Stepwise deterioration	1
Fluctuating course	2
Nocturnal confusion	1
Relative preservation of personality	1
Depression	1
Somatic complaints	1
Emotional incontinence	1
History of hypertension	1
History of strokes	2
Evidence of associated atherosclerosis	1
Focal neurological symptoms	2
Focal neurological signs	2
TOTAL SCORE _____	

Source: Hachinski V, Oveisgharan S, Romney AK, Shankle WR. Optimizing the Hachinski Ischemic Scale. Arch Neurol 2012;69(2):169–175

Hachinski V, Oveisgharan S, Romney AK, Shankle WR. Optimizing the Hachinski Ischemic Scale Arch Neurol. 2012; 69(2):169–175

15.2.10 Stroke assessment scales

1. DSM-IV criteria for the diagnosis of vascular dementia
   a) The development of multiple cognitive deficits manifested by both:
      i. Memory impairment (impaired ability to learn new information or to recall previously learned information)
      ii. One or more of the following cognitive disturbances:
         – Aphasia (language disturbance)
         – Apraxia (impaired ability to carry out motor activities despite intact motor function)
         – Agnosia (failure to recognize or identify objects despite intact sensory function)
         – Disturbance in executive functioning (i.e., planning, organizing, sequencing, and abstracting)

b) The cognitive deficits in criteria A1 and A2 each cause significant impairment in social or occupational functioning and represent a significant decline from a previous level of functioning.

c) Focal neurological signs and symptoms (e.g., exaggeration of deep tendon reflexes, extensor plantar response, pseudobulbar palsy, gait abnormalities, weakness of an extremity) or laboratory evidence indicative of cerebrovascular disease (CVD) (e.g., multiple infarctions involving cortex and underlying white matter) that are judged to be etiologically related to the disturbance.

d) The deficits do not occur exclusively during the course of a delirium.

2. NINDS-AIREN criteria for the diagnosis of vascular dementia

   a) The criteria for the clinical diagnosis of *probable* vascular dementia include *all* of the following:

      i. **Dementia** defined by cognitive decline from a previously higher level of functioning and manifested by impairment of memory and of two or more cognitive domains (orientation, attention, language, visuospatial functions, executive functions, motor control, and praxis), preferably established by clinical examination and documented by neuropsychological testing; deficits should be severe enough to interfere with activities of daily living not due to physical effects of stroke alone. *Exclusion criteria*: Cases with disturbance of consciousness, delirium, psychosis, severe aphasia, or major sensorimotor impairment precluding neuropsychological testing. Also excluded are, systemic disorders or other brain diseases (such as AD) that in and of themselves could account for deficits in memory and cognition.

      ii. **Cerebrovascular disease**, defined by the presence of focal signs on neurologic examination, such as hemiparesis, lower facial weakness, Babinski sign, sensory deficit, hemianopia, and dysarthria consistent with stroke (with or without history of stroke), and evidence of not relevant CVD by brain imaging (CT or MRI) including *multiple large vessel infarcts* or a *single strategically placed infarct* (angular gyrus, thalamus, basal forebrain, or posterior cerebral artery or anterior cerebral artery territories), as well as *multiple basal ganglia* and *white matter lacunes*, or *extensive periventricular white matter lesions*, or combinations thereof.

      iii. **A relationship between the above two disorders**, manifested or inferred by the presence of one or more of the following: (a) onset of dementia within 3 months following a recognized stroke; (b) abrupt deterioration in cognitive functions; or fluctuating, stepwise progression of cognitive deficits.

b) Clinical features consistent with the diagnosis of probable vascular dementia include the following:
(a) Early presence of gait disturbance (small-step gait or marche a petits pas, or magnetic, apraxic-ataxic or Parkinsonian gait); (b) history of unsteadiness and frequent, unprovoked falls; (c) early urinary frequency, urgency, and other urinary symptoms not explained by urologic disease; (d) pseudobulbar palsy; and (e) personality and mood changes, abulia, depression, emotional incontinence, or other subcortical deficits including psychomotor retardation and abnormal executive function.

c) Features that make the diagnosis of vascular dementia uncertain or unlikely include: (a) early onset of memory deficit and progressive worsening of memory deficit and progressive worsening of memory and other cognitive functions such as language (transcortical sensory aphasia), motor skills (apraxia), and perception (agnosia), in the absence of corresponding focal lesions on brain imaging; (b) absence of focal neurological signs, other than cognitive disturbance; and (c) absence of cerebrovascular lesions on brain CT or MRI.

d) Clinical diagnosis of possible vascular dementia may be made in the presence of dementia ("DSM-IV Criteria for the Diagnosis of Vascular Dementia") with focal neurologic signs in patients in whom brain imaging studies to confirm definite CVD are missing; or in the absence of clear temporal relationship between dementia and stroke; or in patients with subtle onset and variable course (plateau or improvement) of cognitive deficits and evidence of relevant CVD.

e) Criteria for diagnosis of definite vascular dementia are: (a) clinical criteria for probable vascular dementia; (b) histopathologic evidence of CVD obtained from biopsy or autopsy; (c) absence of neurofibrillary tangles and neuritic plaques exceeding those expected for age; and (d) absence of other clinical or pathological disorder capable of producing dementia.

f) Classification of vascular dementia for research purposes may be made on the basis of clinical, radiologic, and neuropathologic features, for subcategories or defined conditions such as cortical vascular dementia, subcortical vascular dementia, Binswanger's disease, and thalamic dementia.

The term *AD with CVD* should be reserved to classify patients fulfilling the clinical criteria for possible AD and who also present clinical or brain imaging evidence of relevant CVD. Traditionally, these patients have been included with vascular dementia in epidemiologic studies. The term *mixed dementia*, used hitherto, should be avoided.

Román GC, Tatemichi TK, Erkinjuntti T, et al. Vascular dementia: diagnostic criteria for research studies. Report of the NINDS-AIREN International Workshop. Neurology. 1993; 43(2):250–260

15.3 Scales Used in Telerehabilitation and Human Performance Lab Related to Neurorehabilitation

For example, past MS research project of Adenine Stanislaus.

15.3.1 Functional impairment

Fugl-Meyer assessment

A systematic suite of tests using a 3-point ordinal scale that quantify motor recovery stages based on the scales of Brunnstrom and Twitchell (ontogenetic concept of motor recovery). In addition to motor recovery (100 points), balance (14 points), range of motion (44 points), sensation (24 points), and pain (44 points) are also assessed (total maximum score is 226). Movement is examined in and out of synergies. It is widely used for research studies. We tend to use the 66-point upper extremity portion of the assessment.

15.3.2 General ADL/independence

Functional independence measure

An 18-item test using a 7-level ordinal scale that targets functional assessment and independence. Roughly two-third of items target motor function and one-third target cognitive function. Documentation consists of observing and recording what a person actually does. It can be completed in approximately 15 minutes. Includes a very large national database, with strong federal buy-in (e.g., NIDRR funding, participation by VA hospitals).

Barthel index

A widely used 100-point assessment of independence in 10 daily activities (10 points for feeding, 5 for bathing, 5 for grooming, 10 for dressing, 10 for bowels, 10 for bladder, 10 for toilet use, 15 for transfers, 15 for mobility, 10 for stairs), originally designed for use with people with neuromuscular or musculoskeletal disorders. It is normally completed within 5–10 minutes.

15.3.3 Daily activity

Motor activity log (MAL)

This is a "real-world" measure of 30 different functional tasks, scored by self-report during a structured interview in terms of "how often" and "how well" they are performed (both on 0–5 scales in 0.5 increments), typically applied to the previous week. Developed by the group responsible for constraint-induced movement therapy. It can be completed in roughly 30 minutes.

15.3.4 Targeted functional performance

Nine-hole peg test

The nine-hole peg test is a simple timed test of fine motor coordination, involving placing dowels (9 mm in diameter and 32-mm long) in nine holes. Subjects are scored on the amount of time it takes to place and remove all nine pegs. Two scores are collected, one for each hand. It takes several minutes.

Jebsen-Taylor hand function test

Timed performance of seven test items designed to represent various aspects of hand function, using common activities such as writing, simulated feeding, holding objects, turning cards or pages as in reading, etc. The dimension used to measure each function is the length of time taken to complete each of the tasks. This test is performed in 10–15 minutes for both hands.

Wolf motor function test

This is a lab-based test focusing on arm function that involves 15 timed measures and 2 force-based measures which progress in complexity from engaging individual joints to use of the total arm. For the 15 timed tests, an ordinal score elated to the quality of movement is also scored. All are goal-directed, and several are functional (e.g., raising a can to the mouth). It can be completed in roughly 30 minutes.

15.4 Neuropsychological Evaluation and Differential Diagnosis of Mental Status Disturbances

Cognitive function	Amnesia (1)	Dementia (2)	Confusion (3)	Aphasia (4)	Aprosexia (5)
Attention	Normal	Normal	Impaired	Normal	Impaired
Memory	Impaired	Impaired	Impaired	Impaired verbal, normal nonverbal	Variably impaired
Intelligence	Normal	Impaired	Normal	Normal	Normal
Language	Normal	Normal early, impaired later	Normal	Impaired	Impaired
Visuospatial	Normal	Impaired	Impaired	Normal	Normal
"Executive"	Normal	Impaired	Impaired	Normal	Normal

Notes:

Attention: Tests of attentional capacity, such as digit span or mental arithmetic, will utilize subtests of the Wechsler Adult Intelligence Scale-Revised.

Memory: Short-term memory which has been viewed as "working memory," in which conscious mental processes are performed, and it is analogous to immediate or primary memory. "Memory tests" include verbal memory tasks, such as word list learning (Selective Reminding Test), digit supraspan (Serial Digit Learning), paragraph retention (Wechsler Memory Scale), and paired associate learning (Wechsler Memory Scale), and tests of nonverbal, visuospatial new learning, such as complex figure recall (Rey–Osterrieth Complex Figure), or learning simple geometric designs (Wechsler Memory Scale).

Intelligence: Testing is usually measured by the Wechsler Adult Intelligence Scale-Revised.

Language:	Core linguistic functions are measured by tests of visual naming, aural comprehension, sentence repetition, and verbal fluency from any common aphasia test battery.
Visuospatial:	Visuoperception, visuospatial reasoning, or judgment.
"Executive":	Functions such as abstraction, complex problem-solving, reasoning, concept formation, and the use of feedback to guide outgoing behavior. (Representing frontal lobe functions).

Differential diagnosis

1. Amnesia:	Dementia, acute confusional state, psychiatric disorders, psychogenic amnesia.
2. Dementia:	Mental retardation, acute confusional states, psychiatric disorders (depression)
3. Confusion:	Dementia
4. Aphasia:	Major aphasia syndromes

Aphasia subtype	Fluency	Comprehension	Repetition
Nominal	Normal	Normal	Normal
Conduction	Normal	Normal	Impaired
Broca's	Impaired	Normal	Impaired
Transcortical motor	Impaired	Normal	Normal
Wernicke's	Normal	Impaired	Impaired
Transcortical sensory	Normal	Impaired	Normal
Global	Impaired	Impaired	Impaired
Mixed transcortical	Impaired	Impaired	Normal

5. Aprosexia:	Amnesia and dementia in early stages, neurobehavioral disorders (attentional disability, insomnia, energy loss, and irritability)

15.5 Karnofsky Scale (Grading of Disability for Neoplastic Disease)

Functional status	Score (%)
Normal: no complaints and no evidence of disease	100
Able to carry on normal activity with only minor symptoms	90
Normal activity with effort; some moderate symptoms from disease	80
Cares for self but unable to carry on normal activities	70
Cares for most needs but requires occasional assistance	60
Requires considerable assistance to carry on activities of daily living; frequent medical care	50
Disabled: requires special assistance and care	40
Severely disabled: hospitalized, but death not imminent	30
Very sick: requires active supportive treatment	20
Moribund: death threatened or imminent	10

Source: Karnofsky DA, Abelmann WH, Craver LF, et al. The use of the nitrogen mustards in the palliative treatment of carcinoma: with particular reference to bronchogenic carcinoma. Cancer 1948;1:634–656

Index

Note: Page numbers set in **bold** or *italic* indicate headings or figures, respectively.

Index

Index

T

U